Textbook of Peripheral Vascular Interventions

Textbook of Peripheral Vascular Interventions

Richard R Heuser MD

Director of Research
St Lukes Medical Center
Phoenix AZ
USA

Michel Henry MD

Interventional Cardiologist
Cabinet de Cardiologie
Nancy, France
Chief Patron, Global Research Institute
Apollo Hospital
Hyderabad, India

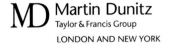
Martin Dunitz
Taylor & Francis Group
LONDON AND NEW YORK

© 2004 Martin Dunitz, an imprint of the Taylor & Francis Group

First published in the United Kingdom in 2004
by Martin Dunitz, an imprint of the Taylor & Francis Group,
11 New Fetter Lane, London EC4P 4EE

Tel: +44 (0) 20 7583 9855
Fax: +44 (0) 20 7842 2298
E-mail: info@dunitz.co.uk
Website: http://www.dunitz.co.uk

Although every effort has been made to ensure that all owners of copyright material have been acknowledged in
this publication, we would be glad to acknowledge in subsequent reprints or editions any omissions brought to
our attention.

A CIP record for this book is available from the British Library.

ISBN 1 85317 941 8

Distributed in the USA by
Fulfilment Center
Taylor & Francis
10650 Toebben Drive
Independence, KY 41051, USA
Toll Free Tel: +1 800 634 7064
E-mail: taylorandfrancis@thomsonlearning.com

Distributed in Canada by
Taylor & Francis
74 Rolark Drive
Scarborough, Ontario M1R 4G2, Canada
Toll Free Tel: +1 877 226 2237
E-mail: tal_fran@istar.ca

Distributed in the rest of the world by
Thomson Publishing Services
Cheriton House
North Way
Andover, Hampshire SP10 5BE, UK
Tel: +44 (0)1264 332424
E-mail: salesorder.tandf@thomsonpublishingservices.co.uk

Composition by Tek-Art
Printed and bound in Spain by Grafos SA Arte Sobre Papel

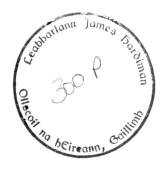

Contents

Contributors   ix

Preface   xvii

1 The natural history of peripheral arterial disease: indications for endovascular therapy   1
Michael R Jaff

2 Functional neuroradiologic and peripheral anatomy   5
Michael Wholey, Justin Zack

3 Peripheral arterial disease: clinical evaluation and non-interventional therapy   15
Michael R Jaff

4 Doppler scanning and imaging of the peripheral vasculature   19
Serge Kownator, François Luizy

5 The role of intravascular ultrasound in peripheral endovascular interventions   25
Khalid Irshad, Nawaf Rahman, Donald Bain, Peter Miller, Raj Velu, Donald B Reid

6 Endovascular equipment and interventional tools   35
Zvonimir Krajcer, Kathryn Dougherty

7 The endovascular interventional suite   51
Zvonimir Krajcer, Kathryn Dougherty

8 Certification and training in peripheral vascular intervention   57
Richard R Heuser

9 Surgical alternatives for peripheral vascular diseases   61
Evan C Lipsitz, William D Suggs, Frank J Veith

10 When to refer to surgery?   71
Osvaldo J Yano, Michael L Marin, Larry Hollier

11 Techniques of arterial access for endovascular intervention   79
Dwayne F Ledesma, Gregory S Domer, Frank J Criado

12 Transbrachial and transaxillary approach: indications, techniques, pitfalls and complications   87
Leon Gengler, Alain Rodde

13 Transradial approach   93
Isabelle Henry, Michel Henry

14 Popliteal access site   95
Michel Henry

15 Balloon angioplasty in peripheral arteries: techniques and results   101
Eberhard P Zeitler

16 Percutaneous peripheral atherectomy using the Rotablator   107
Isabelle Henry, Michel Henry

17 A new rotational thrombectomy and atherectomy catheter: the Rotarex system   119
Isabelle Henry, Michel Henry, Michèle Hugel

18 Open subintimal angioplasty of the superficial femoral and distal arteries   129
P Balas, Christos Klonaris

19 Percutaneous peripheral atherectomy   135
Manuel Maynar, Zhong Qian

20 Cutting balloon angioplasty in peripheral vascular diseases   149
Sanjay Tyagi

21 Chronic total occlusions: new therapeutic approaches   153
Philip A Morales, Richard R Heuser

22 Thrombolysis in peripheral vascular diseases   163
Krishna Kandarpa, Luis H Melendez Morales

23 Catheter-directed thrombolysis for lower extremity deep vein thrombosis   171
Mark W Mewissen

24 Drug-eluting stents for peripheral applications   177
Philip A Morales, Richard R Heuser

25 PTFE-covered stents   181
Richard R Heuser

26 Foreign body and stent retrieval   185
Dieter Liermann, Johannes Kirchner

27 Aortoiliac artery angioplasty and stenting   191
Christopher J White, Stephen R Ramee

28 Iliac occlusions   201
Isabelle Henry, Michel Henry

29 Interventional strategies for recanalization of chronic total iliac and   213
femoropopliteal artery occlusions
Sven Bräunlich, Dierk Scheinert, Giancarlo Biamino

30 Procedures for the hypogastric artery   231
Jacob Cynamon, Priya Prabhaker

31 Percutaneous endovascular treatment of femoropopliteal occlusive diseases   243
Michel Henry, Isabelle Henry, Christos Klonaris, Michèle Hugel

32 Infragenicular percutaneous transluminal angioplasty   263
Emilio Calabrese

33 Endovascular treatment for lower extremity bypass failure   269
Zvonimir Krajcer, Michael Levy

34 Renal artery stenosis: when and how to treat it   277
Christopher J White

35 Protected renal angioplasty and stenting with the PercuSurge Device   285
Michel Henry, Isabelle Henry, Christos Klonaris, Michèle Hugel

36 Renal angioplasty and stenting: techniques, indications and results   293
Emilio Calabrese, Luigi Inglese

37 Mesenteric and celiac angioplasty and stenting   305
Dieter Liermann, Johannes Kirchner

38 Percutaneous transluminal angioplasty of the subclavian arteries   309
Michel Henry, Isabelle Henry, Gérard Ethevenot, Michèle Hugel

39 Percutaneous transluminal angioplasty and stenting of extracranial vertebral artery stenosis   323
Michel Henry, Isabelle Henry, Christos Klonaris, Michèle Hugel

40 Carotid angioplasty and stenting   333
Debabrata Mukherjee, Jay S Yadav

41 Carotid angioplasty under cerebral protection with the PercuSurge device   341
Michel Henry, Isabelle Henry, Christos Klonaris, Michèle Hugel

42 Clinical trials in carotid angioplasty and stenting   355
Walter A Tan, Mark H Wholey

43 Endovascular surgery in multivascular atherosclerosis   363
LA Bockeria, BG Alekyan, AA Spiridonov, Yul Buziashvili, EB Kuperberg,
AV Ter-Akopyan, VF Kharpunov, MD Kirnus

44 Endovascular treatment of descending thoracic aortic aneurysms and dissections   371
Patrice Bergeron, Thierry De Chaumaray, Erica Taube, Nicola Mangialardi, Joël Gay

45 Abdominal aortic aneurysm: interventional treatment   385
Juan Carlos Parodi, Claudio J Schönholz

46 Complications of interventional treatment of aortic aneurysms   393
Luigi Inglese, Emilio Calabrese

47 Percutaneous endovascular treatment of peripheral aneurysms   401
Michel Henry, Isabelle Henry, Christos Klonaris, Michèle Hugel

48 Endovascular stent–grafts for the treatment of arterial disease   413
Nicholas J Morrissey, Michael L Marin

49 Interventions in aortoarteritis   425
KA Abraham, Sriram Rajagopal

50 Limb Salvage in critical limb ischemia   431
Emilio Calabrese

51 Embolization in peripheral territory   447
Claudio J Schönholz, Esteban Mendaro, Sergio Sierro, Denisse Hurvitz

52 Hemodialysis access intervention   457
Kamran Ahrar

53 Superior and inferior vena cava interventional management   469
João Martins Pisco

54 Restenosis in peripheal intervention   475
Luc Bilodeau, Jean-François Tanguay, Martin Sirois

55 Radioactive Therapy   485
Ron Waksman

56 Gene-based and angiogenesis therapy in cardiovascular diseases   493
Richard Baffour, Shmuel Fuchs, Ran Kornowski

57 Management of lipid disorders and other risk factors in patients with peripheral vascular disease   501
Deborah Levy, Thomas Pearson

58 Hemostasis and arterial 'closure' devices   513
     William G Kussmaul III, Marc Cohen

59 Our experience of endovascular treatment of some congenital heart defects   521
     BG Alekyan, VP Podzolkov, VA Garibyan, MG Pursanov, EY Danilov, KE Cardenas,
     VF Kharpunov, TN Sarkisova, AV Ter-Akopyan

60 Complications of peripheral interventions   533
     Philip A Morales, Richard R Heuser

61 Billing suggestions for peripheral vascular services   541
     Roseanne R Wholey

Index   547

Contributors

KA Abraham MD DM FACC FRCP
Senior Consultant and Interventional Cardiologist
Vijaya Heart Foundation
Chennai
India

Kamran Ahrar MD
MD Anderson Cancer Center
Department of Radiology
Houston TX
USA

BG Alekyan MD PhD
Professor, Head of Interventional Cardiology
and Angiology Department
President of Russian Scientific Society of
Interventional Radiology and Endovasular Surgery
Chief of Department of Endovascular Surgery
Bakoulev Scientific Center for Cardiovascular
Surgery
Moscow
Russia

Richard Baffour PhD
The Cardiovascular Research Institute
Washington Hospital Center
Washington DC
USA

P Balas MD
Vascular Surgeon
Henry Dunant Hospital
Athens
Greece

Donald Bain FRCS
Senior Registrar
Wishaw Hospital
Scotland
UK

Patrice Bergeron MD
Head, Department of Thoracic and
Cardiovascular Surgery
Saint Joseph Hospital
Marseille
France

Giancarlo Biamino MD
Clinical and Interventional Angiology
University of Leipzig, Heart Center
Leipzig
Germany

Luc Bilodeau MD
Division of Interventional Cardiology
Montreal Heart Institute
Montreal PQ
Canada

LA Bockeria MD PhD
Professor, Director of Bakoulev Scientific Center
for Cardiovascular Surgery
President of Russian Association of
Cardiovascular Surgeons
Moscow
Russia

Sven Bräunlich MD
Clinical and Interventional Angiology
University of Leipzig, Heart Center
Leipzig
Germany

Yul Buziashvili MD PhD
Head of Cardiology Department
Bakoulev Scientific Center
for Cardiovascular Surgery
Moscow
Russia

Emilio Calabrese MD
Director, National Center for Limb Salvage
Milan; Chief, Vascular and Endovascular Surgery
San Gaudenzio Clinic,
Novara
Italy

KE Cardenas MD PhD
Interventional Cardiologist, Senior Researcher
Bakoulev Scientific Center
for Cardiovascular Surgery
Moscow
Russia

Marc Cohen MD FACC
Director, Division of Cardiology
Newark Beth Israel Medical Center
Newark NJ
USA

Frank J Criado MD
Director, Center for Vascular Intervention
Chief, Division of Vascular Surgery
Union Memorial Hospital/MedStar Heath
Baltimore, Maryland
USA

Jacob Cynamon MD
Director, Division of Vascular Interventional
Radiology
Montefiore Medical Center
Bronx NY USA

EYu Danilov MD PhD
Interventional Cardiologist, Senior Researcher
Bakoulev Scientific Center
for Cardiovascular Surgery
Moscow
Russia

Thierry De Chaumaray MD
Department of Thoracic and Cardiovascular Surgery
Saint Joseph Hospital
Marseille
France

Gregory S Domer
Division of Vascular Surgery
Union Memorial Hospital/MedStar Heath
Baltimore, MD
USA

Kathryn Dougherty
Peripheral Vascular Interventional Research
St Luke's Episcopal Hospital
Texas Heart Institute
Houston, TX
USA

Gérard Ethevenot MD
Interventional Cardiologist
CHU de Brabois
Vandoeurvre-lès-Nancy
France

Shmuel Fuchs MD
The Cardiovascular Research Institute
Washington Hospital Center
Washington DC
USA

VA Garibyan MD PHD
Interventional Cardiologist
Bakoulev Scientific Center
for Cardiovascular Surgery
Moscow
Russia

Joël Gay MS
Scientific Coordinator
Department of Thoracic and Cardiovascular Surgery
Saint Joseph Hospital
Marseille
France

Leon Gengler MD
Radiologist
Department of Radiology
St Elisabeth Hospital
Luxembourg

Isabelle Henry MD
Interventional Cardiologist
Polyclinique de Bois Bernard
Rouvroy
France

Michel Henry MD
Interventional Cardiologist
Cabinet de Cardiologie
Nancy, France
Chief Patron
Global Research Institute
Apollo Hospital
Hyderabad
India

Richard R Heuser MD
Director of Research
Phoenix Heart Center
St Luke's Medical Center
Phoenix AZ
USA

Larry Hollier MD
Mount Sinai Medical Center
Department of Surgery
New York NY
USA

Michèle Hugel RN
Interventional Cardiologist
Cabinet de Cardiologie
Vandoeurve-lès-Nancy
France

Denisse Hurvitz MD
Department of Vascular and Interventional
Radiology
Abraxas Medica Clinica La Sagrada Familia and
Navy Hospital
Buenos Aires
Argentina

Luigi Inglese MD
Director, Cardiovascular Interventional Laboratory
Policlinic Institute
Professor, Dipartimento di Hemodinamica
Ospedale Clinicizzato San Donato
Milan
Italy

Khalid Irshad FRCS
Associate Surgical Specialist
Wishaw Hospital
Scotland

Michael R Jaff DO FACC
Medical Director
Vascular Ultrasound Core Laboratory
Morristown, NJ
USA

Krishna Kandarpa
Weill Medical College of Cornell University
Department of Radiology
New York NY
USA

VF Kharpunov MD PhD
Interventional Cardiologist
Bakoulev Scientific Center
for Cardiovascular Surgery
Moscow
Russia

Johannes Kirchner MD
Clinic of Radiology and Nuclaer Medicine
Marienhospital
University Hospital of the Ruhr-University
Bochum
Herne
Germany

MD Kirnus MD
Interventional Cardiologist
Bakoulev Scientific Center
for Cardiovascular Surgery
Moscow
Russia

Christos Klonaris MD
Vascular Surgeon
Henry Dunant Hospital
Athens
Greece

Ran Kornowski MD
Head, Cardiac Catheterization Unit
Department of Cardiology
Rabin Medical Center
Petach Tikva
Israel

Serge Kownator MD
Cabinet D'Explorations Cardio-vasculaires
Cardiologue
Thionville
France

Zvonimir Krajcer MD
Director, Peripheral Vascular Intervention
Texas Heart Institute
St Luke's Episcopal Hospital
Houston TX
USA

EB Kuperberg MD PhD
Vascular Surgeon
Bakoulev Scientific Center
for Cardiovascular Surgery
Moscow
Russia

William G Kussmaul III
Cardiac Catheterization Laboratory
Hahnemann University Hospital
Philadelphia PA
USA

Dwayne F Ledesma MD
Endovascular Fellow
Center for Vascular Intervention
And Division of Vascular Surgery
Union Memorial Hospital/Medstar Health
Baltimore MD
USA

Deborah Levy MD
Postdoctoral fellow in Preventive Cardiology
Department of Community and Preventive
Medicine
University of Rochester School of Medicine
and Dentistry
Rochester NY
USA

Michael Levy MS
Peripheral Vascular Intervention
Texas Heart Institute
St Luke's Episcopal Hospital
Houston TX
USA

Dieter Liermann MD
Chairman and Director
Radiology and Nuclear Medicine Clinic
Marienhospital
Herne
Germany

Evan C Lipsitz MD
Division of Vascular Surgery
Department of Surgery
Montefiore Medical Center
Albert Einstein College of Medicine
Bronx NY
USA

François Luizy MD
Centre D'Explorations Vasculaires
Paris
France

Nicola Mangialardi MD
Unita Operatia di Chirurgia Vascolare
ACO San Filippo Neri
Roma
Italy

Michael L Marin MD
Mount Sinai Medical Center
Department of Surgery
Vascular Division
New York NY
USA

João Martins Pisco MD
Professor of Faculty of Medical Sciences
Director of University Department of Radiology
Faculty of Medical Sciences
New University of Lisbon
Portugal

Manuel Maynar MD
Professor and Director
Diagnostic and Therapeutic Endoluminal Unit
Hospital Rambla Tenerife
Las Palmas de Gran Canaria University
Spain

Luis H Melendez Morales MD
Vascular and Interventional Radiology
Diplomate, American Board of Radiology
Santurce, San Juan
Spain

Esteban Mendaro MD
Department of Vascular and Interventional
Radiology
Abraxas Medica Clinica La Sagrada Familia and
Navy Hospital
Buenos Aires
Argentina

Mark W Mewissen MD
Wisconsin Heart and Vascular Clinics
Milwaukee WI
USA

Peter Miller RGN
Nurse in Charge of Endovascular Operating Room
Wishaw Hospital
Scotland
UK

Philip A Morales MD
Phoenix Heart Center
St Luke's Medical Center
Phoenix AZ
USA

Nicholas J Morrissey MD
Assistant Professor of Surgery
Division of Vascular Surgery
Mount Sinai School of Medicine
New York NY
USA

Debabrata Mukherjee
Director of Peripheral Interventions
Department of Cardiology
University of Michigan
Ann Arbor MI
USA

Juan Carlos Parodi MD
Director, Cardiovascular Institute of Buenos Aires
Chief, Vascular Surgery Department
Vice Director of the Postgraduate Training Program
in Cardiovascular Surgery
University of Buenos Aires
Clinical Professor, Department of Surgery
Wayne State University
Detroit MI
USA

Thomas Pearson MD PhD MPH
Professor and Chairman
Department of Community and Preventive
Medicine
University of Rochester School of Medicine
and Dentistry
Rochester NY
USA

VP Podzolkov MD PhD
Professor, Member of the Russian Academy of
Medical Sciences
Head of the Congenital Heart Disease Surgery
Department
Bakoulev Scientific Center for Cardiovascular
Surgery
Moscow
Russia

Priya Prabhaker
Division of Vascular Interventional Radiology
Montefiore Medical Center
Bronx NY
USA

MG Pursanov MD PhD
Interventional Cardiologist, Lead Researcher
Bakoulev Scientific Center
for Cardiovascular Surgery
Moscow
Russia

Zhong Qian MD
Associate Professor
Department of Radiology
School of Medicine
Louisiana State University Health Sciences Centre
New Orleans, LA
USA

Nawaf Rahman FRCS
Clinical Fellow and Honorary Consultant
Wishaw Hospital, Scotland
Consultant Vascular Surgeon
Irbid, Jordan

Sriram Rajagopal MD DM
Senior Cardiologist
Southern Railway Headquarters Hospital
Chennai
India

Stephen R Ramee MD
Director, Cardiac Catheter Laboratory
Ochsner Hospital
New Orleans LA
USA

Donald B Reid MD FRCS
Consultant Vascular and Endovascular Surgeon
Wishaw Hospital
Scotland
UK

Alain Rodde MD
Radiologist
Department of Radiology
St Elisabeth Hospital
Luxemburg

TN Sarkisova MD
Interventional Cardiologist
Bakoulev Scientific Center
for Cardiovascular Surgery
Moscow
Russia

Dierk Scheinert MD
Clinical and Interventional Angiology
University of Leipzig, Heart Center
Leipzig
Germany

Claudio J Schönholz MD
Director of Vascular Image-guided Interventions
Department of Radiology
LSU Health Sciences Center
Shreveport LA
Argentina

Sergio Sierro MD
Department of Vascular and Interventional
Radiology
Abraxas Medica Clinica La Sagrada Familia
and Navy Hospital
Buenos Aires
Argentina

Martin Sirois PhD
Departement de Chimie-Biologie
Universite du Quebec a Trois-Rivieres
Canada

AA Spiridonov MD PhD
Professor, Head of Vascular Surgery Department
Bakoulev Scientific Center
for Cardiovascular Surgery
Moscow
Russia

William D Suggs MD
Division of Vascular Surgery
Department of Surgery
Montefiore Medical Center
Albert Einstein College of Medicine
Bronx NY
USA

Walter A Tan MD MS
Director of Vascular Medicine Program
Assistant Professor of Medicine (Cardiology)
and of Radiology
University of North Carolina at Chapel Hill
USA

Jean-François Tanguay MD
Division of Interventional Cardiology
Montreal Heart Institute
Montreal PQ
Canada

Erica Taube MD
Department of Thoracic and Cardiovascular Surgery
Saint Joseph Hospital
Marseille
France

AV Ter-Akopyan MD PhD
Interventional Cardiologist
Bakoulev Scientific Center
for Cardiovascular Surgery
Moscow
Russia

Sanjay Tyagi MD
Department of Cardiology
GB Pant Hospital and Maulana Azad
Medical College
New Delhi
India

Frank Veith MD
Division of Vascular Surgery
Department of Surgery
Montefiore Medical Center
Albert Einstein College of Medicine
Bronx NY
USA

Raj Velu MB
Anaesthetist
Wishaw Hospital
Scotland
UK

Ron Waksman MD
Cardiovascular Brachytherapy Institute
Washington Hospital Center
Washington DC
USA

Christopher J White MD
Chairman, Department of Cardiology
Ochsner Clinic
New Orleans LA
USA

Mark H Wholey MD
Chairman
Pittsburgh Vascular Institute
Shadyside Hospital
Pittsburgh PA
USA

Michael Wholey, MD
University of Texas Health Science Center
San Antonio TX
USA

Roseanne R Wholey
President and Compliance Review Officer
Roseanne R Wholey and Associates
Oakmont PA
USA

Jay S Yadav MD
Director, Vascular Intervention
Department of Cardiology
Cleveland Clinic Foundation
Cleveland OH
USA

Osvaldo J Yano
Department of Surgery
Mount Sinai Medical Center
New York NY
USA

Justin Zack
University of Texas Health Science Center
San Antonio TX
USA

Eberhard P Zeitler MD
(Retired)
Institute of Diagnostic and Interventional Radiology
Nuremberg Hospital
Germany

Preface

This book grew from discussions of our earlier textbook entitled *Peripheral Vascular Stenting for Cardiologists*. The textbook was overwhelmingly well received; however, it had a limited focus. The earlier book was not intended as a comprehensive textbook nor did it address the fact that cardiologists are not the only physicians placing peripheral vascular stents. This textbook is a more comprehensive publication detailing endovascular treatment in all aspects of peripheral vascular disease. As the nature of medical care becomes more preventive rather than crisis-driven, the diagnosis and treatment of peripheral vascular disease becomes more relevant to everyday practice. Lifestyle changes for patients that are brought on by disease become more relevant as our population ages. As an example, consider that the incidence of peripheral vascular disease continues to increase. Approximately 1.5 to 2 million patients in Europe and the USA suffer from critical limb ischemia. Nearly half of these sufferers will require a major amputation within one year after the onset of limb ischemia. In addition, in the USA, prevalence of abdominal aortic aneurysm is quite significant. In 2002, 200 000 abdominal aortic aneurysms were diagnosed, adding to the estimated 1.5 million patients who currently experience this disease. In fact, 10% of men older than 80 years of age have a significant abdominal aortic aneurysm. Furthermore, 20% of patients who undergo coronary intervention have renal artery stenosis with as many as 50% of those patients having critical stenosis.

This publication, *Textbook of Peripheral Vascular Interventions*, will discuss therapies that can make a real difference in the lives of patients. Therapies for critical limb ischemia, chronic total occlusions, as well as therapies that in some subsets have been demonstrated more effective than the invasive surgical approaches will be discussed. New drug eluting stents for the coronary tree have revolutionized the care of patients with ischemic heart disease. These same drug eluting stents may have a wider range of application in the peripheral tree, particularly in the femoral arteries.

It is clear that patients need and are demanding less invasive procedures in the future. As our population ages, lifestyle limitations become more a question of 'quality of life'; as a result, increasing numbers of patients will come to our doors.

This textbook would not have been possible without our excellent authors as well as the people at Martin Dunitz who have smoothed our progress. Our sincere thanks to the many talented researchers and interventionists who have contributed to this textbook. Our thanks also to Alan Burgess, whose tireless efforts have helped to shape this text. This book stands as a tribute to the pioneering work of Charles Dotter and Andreas Grüntzig. Their initial vision and successful demonstration of early techniques for peripheral intervention have guided the developments of these endovascular interventions for the last 37 years.

We hope that *Textbook of Peripheral Vascular Interventions* serves as a practical source of information for students, physicians in training, radiologists, cardiologists, or vascular surgeons performing peripheral intervention, and that it provides a comprehensive introduction to endovascular techniques.

Richard R Heuser
Michel Henry

1

The natural history of peripheral arterial disease: indications for endovascular therapy

Michael R Jaff

Atherosclerosis is a widespread disorder, causing death and disability in many patients. Although most patients and physicians are familiar with the cardiac and cerebrovascular manifestations, peripheral arterial disease (PAD) escapes most healthcare professionals. In many cases, patients are instructed to use non-steroidal anti-inflammatory agents or enter physical therapy programs for their exertional limb pain. Physicians often ascribe exertional limb discomfort to 'old age'. In a recent series in which surveys were mailed to 843 internal medicine physicians in one segment of the USA, questions regarding the epidemiology and diagnosis of PAD were asked. Approximately 27% responded to the survey. Only 37% of the physicians obtained a history for intermittent claudication, and only 26% asked about a history of foot ulcerations. This is in contrast to obtaining a history of cardiac disease, which was performed in 92% of cases. During physical examination, the heart was examined in 95% of cases, but examination of peripheral pulses was actually performed in only 34–60% of cases.[1]

The most common clinical symptom of PAD is intermittent claudication, often interfering with the quality of life of patients. Although it is difficult to fully assess the prevalence of intermittent claudication in the general population, it is generally accepted that 1% of women and 2% of men aged 45–69 have clinical evidence of intermittent claudication.[2] As the population ages, however, the prevalence of intermittent claudication increases. Of 2415 initial cardiovascular events in the Framingham Study over 36 years of follow-up, 9.6% of the events in men were intermittent claudication; 9.7% occurred in women. However, in the subset of the population 65–74 years old, 11.6% of men and 9.4% of women had intermittent claudication.[3] If simple, non-invasive screening tests are utilized to diagnose PAD, the incidence clearly rises.

The United States National Institutes of Health suggests that PAD results in over 60 000 hospitalizations annually, each stay lasting an average of more than 11 days.[4] Other mani-festations of arteriosclerosis obliterans, namely diminished pedal pulses and carotid bruits, occur with increasing frequency as the population ages. While intermittent claudication occurs more often in men at any age, these physical examination findings occur with identical frequency in both men and women.[5] Approximately 50% of people with PAD have no symptoms, yet have abnormal peripheral pulses and/or the presence of arterial bruits. These patients do not require therapy for their PAD; however, an evaluation of their coronary and cerebrovascular status is critical, as patients with asymptomatic PAD are at markedly increased risk of early mortality and cardiovascular morbidity.

Classic factors that increase the risk for the development of PAD include hypertension, hypercholesterolemia, tobacco use, and diabetes mellitus, as well as non-modifiable risk factors including family history of atherosclerosis, male sex, and advancing age. Both the male and female hypertensive populations have an increased risk of developing intermittent claudication. The higher the systolic and diastolic blood pressures the greater the risk of claudication. In the Framingham study, for older men, the risk of intermittent claudication was 1.27 if the systolic blood pressure was 20 mmHg higher, and 1.62 if it was 40 mmHg higher. In older women, the effect of increasing systolic blood pressure and intermittent claudication was similar.[6]

Hypercholesterolemia doubles the incidence of intermittent claudication, and is found in as many as 50% of patients with PAD.[7] Aggressive lowering of elevated serum cholesterol levels has been shown to prevent progression of femoral and carotid atherosclerosis. Angiographic studies confirm that pharmacologic therapy, such as probucol, or combination treatment with colestipol and nicotinic acid, retards the progression of femoral atherosclerosis.[8,9] HMG-CoA reductase inhibitors such as lovastatin and pravastatin have been shown to reverse the progression of carotid intima–media thickness in comparison to placebo-treated patients.[10,11]

Tobacco use remains the most important modifiable risk factor for PAD. Hughson et al found that 56% of patients with intermittent claudication were active users of cigarettes, and 24% were former smokers.[1] In addition, active cigarette smoking causes more severe claudication pain and diminished peripheral circulation in comparison with patients who do not smoke, leading to a reduction in the exercise capacity of patients with claudication.[12] Finally, the risk of progression of PAD and atherosclerosis in other vascular beds is significantly greater in those patients who continue to smoke as compared to those who stop smoking. In 343 patients with intermittent claudication, only 11% stopped smoking 1 year after the diagnosis. Ischemic rest pain developed in 16% of continuing smokers after 7 years, while none of the former smokers suffered with rest pain. The incidence of myocardial infarction 10 years after the diagnosis of claudication was 11% in former smokers and 53% in active smokers. Ten-year overall survival rates were 82% in former smokers and 46% in active smokers.[13]

Diabetes mellitus and PAD is an ominous combination. Although the prevalence of PAD is higher in the diabetic than in the non-diabetic population, it is the relatively rapid progression to ischemic rest pain and ulceration that portends a poor prognosis for the patients with diabetes. There is a 2–3-fold increase in risk of intermittent claudication in diabetic patients when compared to the non-diabetic population.[14] This holds true for both men and women. The severity of PAD is also greater in the diabetic population. In a study of 47 patients with diabetes mellitus, all of whom had intermittent claudication at baseline, in comparison to 224 patients with intermittent claudication but no diabetes, the incidence of ischemic rest pain and/or gangrene after 6 years of follow-up was 40% and 18% respectively.[15] The duration of diabetes and the type of diabetes therapy (i.e. diet, oral hypoglycemic agent, and insulin) did not play a role in the incidence or severity of PAD.

Independent predictors of progression of PAD in diabetic patients include a decreased post-exercise ankle–brachial index, increased arm systolic blood pressure, and current smoking, demonstrating the additive effects of atherosclerotic risk factors on the natural history of PAD.[16] Interestingly, among the risk factors for amputation in patients with diabetes mellitus, neuropathic symptoms and lack of outpatient diabetes education are of importance, and must be viewed concomitantly with the location and severity of PAD.[17] Unfortunately, there remains no definitive evidence that strict glycemic control can prevent macrovascular complications from diabetes mellitus.[18]

As is the case with coronary artery atherosclerosis, the risk of PAD increases as the aggregate number of cardiovascular risk factors increases. However, in both female and male patients, tobacco use alone places patients at significant risk of PAD.[2]

There are several novel risk factors which have recently demonstrated potential impact in the presence of atherosclerosis. These include hyperhomocyteinemia, elevated fibrinogen levels, impaired fibrinolysis, platelet reactivity, hypercoagulability, lipoprotein(a), small dense low-density lipoprotein, infectious agents, and markers of inflammation (C-reactive protein, soluble intercellular adhesion molecule-1).[19] The clinical utility of these novel risk factors is evolving; however, at present, hyperhomocysteinemia should be identified in patients with early-onset atherosclerosis or atherosclerosis in the absence of 'classic' risk factors.

Non-invasive testing has been a helpful modality used to identify patients with PAD. The simplest method is the ankle–brachial index (ABI). The ABI is a measurement of the blood pressure in a pedal artery compared to the pressure in the brachial artery, as obtained with a hand-held continuous-wave Doppler. Although the ABI cannot localize areas of stenosis or occlusion, it is a very accurate measure of the overall severity of PAD, and can stratify patients' risk of wound healing and the development of ischemic rest pain.

The ABI has also been correlated as a marker of diffuse atherosclerosis, cardiovascular risk, and overall survival. In a study of 2023 middle-aged men screened with ABI, the relative risks of mortality from all causes, cardiovascular causes, and coronary causes was significantly higher in patients with an ABI ≤ 0.90 than in those patients with a normal ABI.[20] In a similar population of 1492 women over the age of 65, the relative risk of all-cause mortality, heart disease and cardiovascular disease was significantly greater when the baseline ABI was ≤ 0.90.[21] In a study of over 5000 men and women ≥ 65 years of age, the lower the ABI, the greater the incidence of cardiovascular risk factors, and clinical cardiovascular disease.[22]

Although the presence of intermittent claudication alone, without active tobacco use and/or diabetes, is generally believed to remain stable over subsequent years, severe PAD with claudication follows a more relentless course. If another non-invasive indicator of PAD severity, the toe pressure (TP), is used, the prognosis of patients with intermittent claudication and a low TP is poor. In a longitudinal study of patients with intermittent claudication and systolic TP $\leq 40\,mmHg$ followed for a mean of 31 months, 34% of patients progressed to ischemic ulceration, rest pain, or gangrene.[23] Of those patients who did progress, 26% required amputation. Comparing the two groups (stable versus progressive disease), only the presence of diabetes mellitus increased the probability of clinical deterioration.

Based on the presence of risk factors, a risk profile suggesting the likelihood of developing intermittent claudication over the subsequent 4 years has been proposed.[24] This risk factor profile underscores the impact of the presence of diabetes mellitus, coronary heart disease, high serum cholesterol and increasing amounts of tobacco consumption on the probability of developing intermittent claudication.

The decision to revascularize patients with iliac artery and/or superficial femoral artery (SFA) disease must be made based on the patients' clinical presentation and physical findings. Given the efficacy of endovascular therapy in stenotic common iliac arteries,[25,26] as well as long segment occlusive disease in the common and external iliac arteries,[27] patients with symptoms and physical findings consistent with iliac artery disease should undergo a thorough investigation. If symptoms are bothersome to the patient, the lesion appears amenable to endovascular therapy, and the operator has significant experience,[28] consideration should be given to stent-supported iliac angioplasty.

Intermittent claudication due to isolated SFA disease requires greater consideration, however, due to lack of durable benefit after endovascular therapy.[29,30] Consideration must be given to risk factor modification (specifically tobacco cessation and tight glycemic control in the face of diabetes mellitus) and supervised exercise as a viable alternative, unless critical limb ischemia ensues.

Endovascular revascularization for patients with femoropopliteal or infrapopliteal disease must be done based on the patients' clinical presentation and physical findings. Classically, patients with lifestyle-limiting intermittent claudication, ischemic rest pain, non-healing ischemic ulcerations or gangrene require some form of revascularization.

Results with PTA of the infrapopliteal vessels is variable. In a review of 14 reports of infrapopliteal PTA in patients with critical limb ischemia or disabling intermittent claudication, the limb salvage rate ranged from 56% to 95%.[31] In a surgical series of 25 patients who underwent infrapopliteal PTA, the 3-year success rate was only 20%, with 16 patients requiring subsequent revascularization procedures.[32]

There remain no prospective, controlled, randomized data demonstrating the long-term benefit of endovascular therapy on improving claudicating distance, and these data are crucial to our ability to provide firm recommendations concerning the timing of intervention in these patients.[33]

References

1 McLafferty RB, Dunnington GL, Mattos MA et al. Factors affecting the diagnosis of peripheral vascular disease before vascular surgery referral. *J Vasc Surg* 2000; **31**: 870–9.

2 Hughson WG, Mann JI, Garrod A. Intermittent claudication: prevalence and risk factors. *BMJ* 1978; **1**: 1379–81.

3 Kannel WB. The demographics of claudication and the aging of the American population. *Vasc Med* 1996; **1**: 60–4.

4 US Department of Health and Human Services. *Chartbook on cardiovascular, lung and blood diseases. Morbidity and Mortality.* Bethesda: NIH, NHLBI, 1994.

5 Abbott RD, Brand FN, Kannel WB. Epidemiology of some peripheral arterial findings in diabetic men and women: experiences from the Framingham Study. *Am J Med* 1990; **88**: 376–81.

6 Stamler J, Stemler R, Neaton JD. Blood pressure, systolic and diastolic, and cardiovascular risks. US population data. *Arch Intern Med* 1993; **153**: 598–615.

7 Kannel WB, Skinner JJ, Schwartz MJ, Shurtleff D. Intermittent claudication: incidence in the Framingham Study. *Circulation* 1970; **41**: 875–83.

8 Walldius G, Erikson U, Olsson AG et al. The effect of probucol on femoral atherosclerosis: the probucol quantitative regression Swedish trial (PQRST). *Am J Cardiol* 1994; **74**: 875–83.

9 Blankenhorn DH, Azen SP, Crawford DW et al. Effects of colestipol–niacin therapy on human femoral atherosclerosis. *Circulation* 1991; **83**: 438–47.

10 Furberg CD, Adams HP, Applegate WB et al. Effect of lovastatin on early carotid atherosclerosis and cardiovascular events. *Circulation* 1994; **90**: 1679–87.

11 Mercuri M, Bond MG, Sirtori CR et al. Pravastatin reduces carotid intima–media thickness progression in an asymptomatic hypercholesterolemic Mediterranean population: the carotid atherosclerosis Italian ultrasound study. *Am J Med* 1996; **101**: 627–34.

12 Gardner AW. The effect of cigarette smoking on exercise capacity in patients with intermittent claudication. *Vasc Med* 1996; **1**: 181–6.

13 Jonason T, Bergstrom R. Cessation of smoking in patients with intermittent claudication. Effects on the risk of peripheral vascular complications, myocardial infarction, and mortality. *Acta Med Scand* 1987; **221**: 253–60.

14 Brand FN, Abbott RD, Kannel WB. Diabetes, intermittent claudication, and risk of cardiovascular events. The Framingham study. *Diabetes* 1989; **38**: 504–9.

15 Jonason T, Ringqvist I. Diabetes mellitus and intermittent claudication. Relation between peripheral vascular complications and location of the occlusive atherosclerosis in the legs. *Acta Med Scand* 1985; **218**: 217–21.

16 Palumbo PJ, O'Fallon M, Osmundson PJ et al. Progression of peripheral occlusive arterial disease in diabetes mellitus. What factors are predictive? *Arch Intern Med* 1991; **151**: 717–21.

17 Reiber GE, Pecoraro RE, Koepsell TD. Risk factors for amputation in patients with diabetes mellitus. A case–control study. *Ann Intern Med* 1992; **117**: 97–105.

18 The Diabetes Control and Complications Trial (DCCT) Research Group. Effect of intensive diabetes management on macrovascular events and risk factors in the diabetes control and complications trial. *Am J Cardiol* 1995; **75**: 894–903.

19 Kullo IJ, Gau GT, Tajik AJ. Novel risk factors for atherosclerosis. *Mayo Clin Proc* 2000; **75**: 369–80.

20 Kornitzer M, Dramaix M, Sobolski J et al. Ankle/arm pressure index in asymptomatic middle-aged males: an independent predictor of ten-year coronary heart disease mortality. *Angiology* 1995; **46**: 211–19.

21 Vogt MT, Cauley JA, Newman AB et al. Decreased ankle/arm blood pressure index and mortality in elderly women. *JAMA* 1993; **270**: 465–9.

22 Newman AB, Siscovick DS, Manolio TA et al. Ankle–arm index as a marker of atherosclerosis in the cardiovascular health study. *Circulation* 1993; **88**: 837–45.

23 Bowers BL, Valentine RJ, Myers SI et al. The natural history of patients with claudication with toe pressures of 40 mmHg or less. *J Vasc Surg* 1993; **18**: 506–11.

24 Murabito JM, D'Agostino RB, Silbershatz H, Wilson PWF. Intermittent claudication: a risk profile from the Framingham heart study. *Circulation* 1997; **96**: 44–9.

25   Palmaz JC, Laborde JC, Rivera FJ et al. Stenting of the iliac arteries with the Palmaz stent: experience from a multicenter trial. *Cardiovasc Intervent Radiol* 1992; **15**: 291–7.

26   Sullivan TM, Childs MB, Bacharach JM et al. Percutaneous transluminal angioplasty and primary stenting of the iliac arteries in 288 patients. *J Vasc Surg* 1997; **25**: 829–39.

27   Henry M, Amor M, Ethevenot G et al. Percutaneous endoluminal treatment of iliac occlusions: long-term follow-up in 105 patients. *J Endovasc Surg* 1998; **5**: 228–35.

28   Ballard JL, Sparks SR, Taylor FC et al. Complications of iliac artery stent deployment. *J Vasc Surg* 1996; **24**: 545–55.

29   Stanley B, Teague B, Raptis S et al. Efficacy of balloon angioplasty of the superficial femoral artery and popliteal artery in the relief of leg ischemia. *J Vasc Surg* 1996; **23**: 679–85.

30   Gray BH, Sullivan TM, Childs MB et al. High incidence of restenosis/reocclusion of stents in the percutaneous treatment of long-segment superficial femoral artery disease after suboptimal angioplasty. *J Vasc Surg* 1997; **25**: 74–83.

31   Fraser SCA, Aghiad Al M. Percutaneous transluminal angioplasty of the infrapopliteal vessels: the evidence. *Radiology* 1996; **200**: 33–43.

32   Treiman GS, Treiman RL, Ichikawa L, Van Allan R. Should percutaneous transluminal angioplasty be recommended for treatment of infrageniculate popliteal artery or tibioperoneal trunk stenosis? *J Vasc Surg* 1995; **22**: 457–65.

33   Whyman MR, Fowkes FGR, Kerracher EMG et al. Is intermittent claudication improved by percutaneous transluminal angioplasty? *J Vasc Surg* 1997; **26**: 551–7.

2

Functional neuroradiologic and peripheral anatomy

Michael Wholey and Justin Zack

Introduction

Functional neuroanatomy is an important element in any diagnostic or interventional endeavor. It is crucial that interventionalists have a rudimentary knowledge of the carotids and vertebral arteries including the intracranial and extracranial anatomy. Should a complication develop it is essential that they know which vessel is involved and the extent of the damage. Similarly, should they uncover a pathologic abnormality such as an aneurysm or even a variant of the anatomy, the interventionalist must be able to describe its location and best oblique image to study the finding.

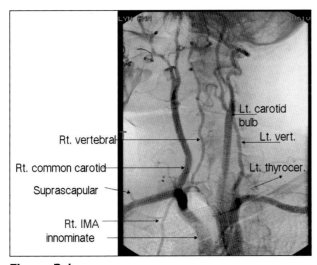

Figure 2.1
40 degree oblique view of aortic arch angiogram. Comments:
- We always begin the carotid angiograms with an aortic arch injection using a 5 or 6 French pigtail catheter for an injection of 25–30 cc/sec for 2 seconds.
- Objective: Beware of ostial stenoses; good view of both subclavians, vertebrals and other vessels.
Abbreviations:
Lt. thyrocer, left thyrocervical trunk;
Lt. vert, left vertebral artery;
Rt. IMA, right internal mammary artery.

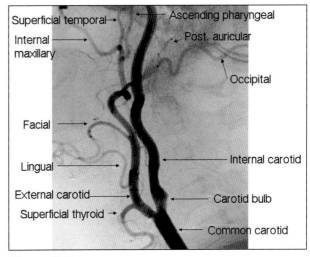

Figure 2.2
Lateral view of carotid bifurcation with catheter in the right common carotid. Comments:
- Usually hand injection of 6–8 cc.
- Lateral view usually opens up the bifurcation.

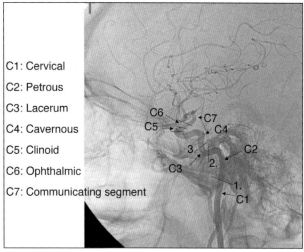

C1: Cervical

C2: Petrous

C3: Lacerum

C4: Cavernous

C5: Clinoid

C6: Ophthalmic

C7: Communicating segment

Figure 2.3
Right common carotid injection, lateral view, unsubtracted
Line demarcations:
1. Exocranial border of petrous carotid canal
2. Endocranial border of petrous carotid canal
3. Petrolingual ligament.

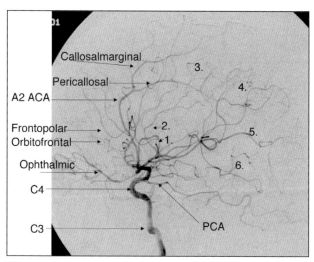

Figure 2.4
Right internal carotid injection, lateral view
Abbreviations:
ACA, Anterior cerebral artery;
PCA, Posterior cerebral artery;
Middle cerebral artery (MCA) branches,
1. Anterior temporal artery
2. Operculofrontal or 'Candelabra' artery
3. Central sulcus (Rolandic group) artery
4. Posterior parietal artery
5. Angular artery and branches
6. Posterior temporal artery.

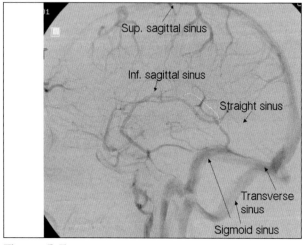

Figure 2.5
Right internal carotid injection, lateral view;
Venous phase.

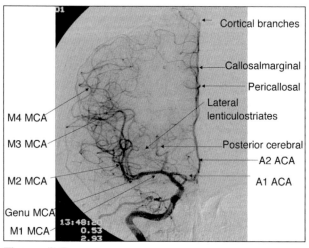

Figure 2.6
Right internal carotid injection; anteroposterior view. Comments:
- PCA (posterior cerebral artery) is easily detected in this image.
- Lateral lenticulostriate arteries arise from the M1 segment of the middle cerebral artery (MCA). These arteries supply the basal ganglia and other deep structures to the brain.

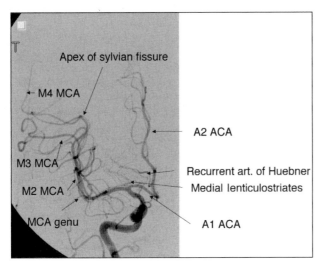

Figure 2.7

Right internal carotid injection; anteroposterior view (separate patient). Comments:
- Medial lenticulostriate arteries arise from A1 as well as close to the proximal medial cerebral artery (MCA).
- Recurrent artery of Huebner arises from A1 or A2 anterior cerebral artery (ACA).

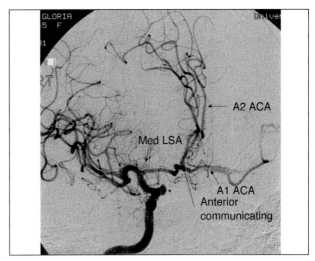

Figure 2.8

Right internal carotid injection, oblique anteroposterior view with cross compression of left common carotid artery (separate patient). Comments:
- This view through the orbits is a good way to visualize A1 segment of the anterior cerebral artery (ACA).

Abbreviations:

Med LSA, medial lenticulostriate arteries; *, small aneurysm off internal carotid artery.

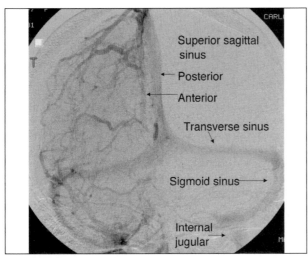

Figure 2.9

Right internal carotid injection; anteroposterior view; Venous phase.

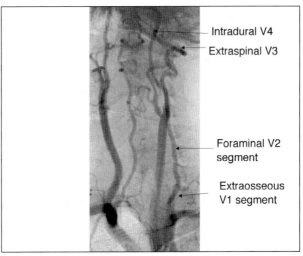

Figure 2.10

LAO projection from the initial aortic arch injection reveals the great vessels including both vertebral arteries. We will occasionally obtain an RAO view to visualize the vertebrals better, as well as to rule out stenoses at the origins of the great vessels. (In this figure the different segments of the vertebral artery are shown.)

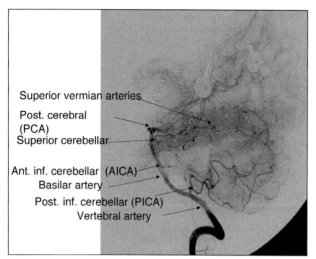

Figure 2.11

Left vertebral injection, lateral view (separate patient).
For standard four vessel angiograms, we will not usually engage
the vertebral artery; rather, we will place the diagnostic catheter
near the origin, inflate a blood pressure cuff on the arm and
obtain images with a rate of 8–12 cc/sec for 2 seconds.

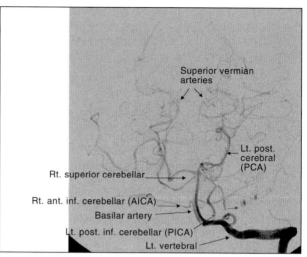

Figure 2.12

Left vertebral injection, anteroposterior view. Comments:
• There is cross filling of flow from the right vertebral artery.

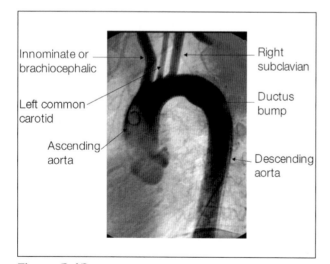

Figure 2.13

Normal thoracic aortogram.
Through a femoral approach, 5 or 6 French pigtail catheter placed
with tip in the ascending thoracic aorta. Injection rate was
25 cc/sec for total of 50 cc with an LAO 30-45 degree projection.

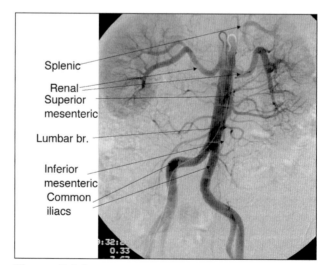

Figure 2.14

Abdominal angiogram.
A 5 French catheter was placed at approximately L1 vertebral
level with an injection rate of 15 cc/sec for total of 30 cc.

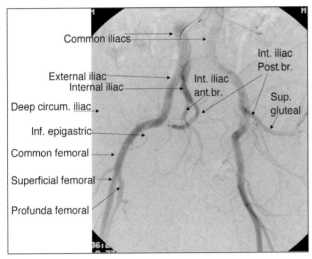

Figure 2.15
Pelvic angiogram.
A 5 French catheter was placed at approximately L3-4 vertebral level with an injection rate of 8 cc/sec for total of 15 cc with a 25 degree obliquity of the pelvis to open up the iliac arteries.

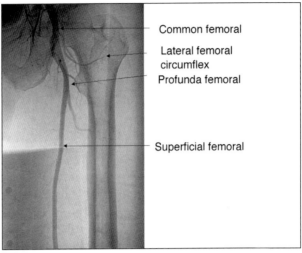

Figure 2.16
Left lower extremity angiogram (upper thigh).
A 5 French catheter was selected into the contralateral external iliac artery with an injection rate of 6 cc/sec for total of 12 cc. In this case, a straight AP projection was used, but a 15 degree RAO is often preferred to open up the PFA from the SFA.

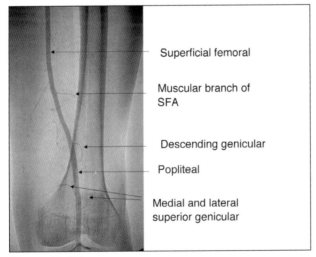

Figure 2.17
Lower extremity angiogram (lower thigh).
A 5 French catheter was selected into the contralateral external iliac artery with an injection rate of 8 cc/sec for total of 16 cc.

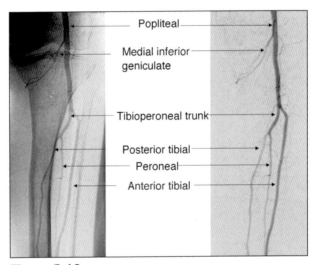

Figure 2.18
Lower extremity angiogram (knee joint).
A 5 French catheter was selected into the contralateral external iliac artery with an injection rate of 8 cc/sec for total of 20 cc. An approximate 15-20 degree LAO was used to open the trifurcation view.

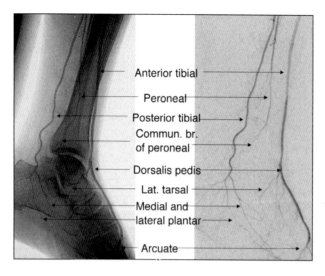

Figure 2.19
Lower extremity angiogram (lateral foot).
A 5 French catheter was selected into the contralateral external iliac artery with an injection rate of 8 cc/sec for total of 25 cc.

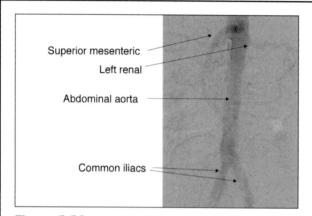

Figure 2.20
Abdominal aortogram with carbon dioxide injection.

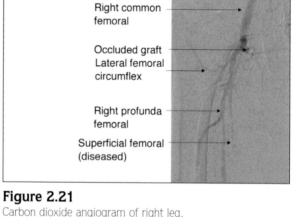

Figure 2.21
Carbon dioxide angiogram of right leg.

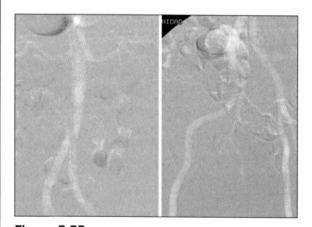

Figure 2.22
Carbon dioxide angiogram.

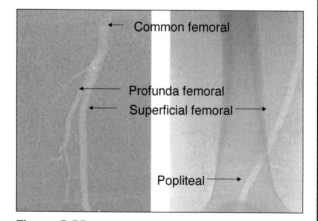

Figure 2.23
Carbon dioxide angiogram.

With the 5 French pigtail or omniflush catheter at approximately L1 vertebral body level, carbon dioxide was injected through the filtration and bag system (Mallinckrodt Medical, St. Louis, MO, USA). Carbon dioxide is used because of the elevated creatinine of this patient. Care must be given to make sure that the patient does not have an aneurysm. Also, some patients may complain of severe epigastric pain because of mild infarction caused by the gas bubbles in the SMA and IMA circulation. The catheter was then used to subselect the external iliac artery for the additional views. Note, the difficult interpretation as you go further down the leg.

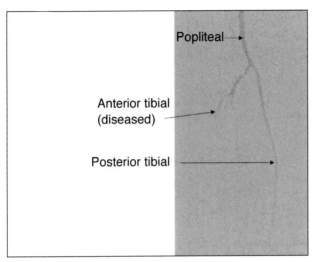

Figure 2.24
Gadolinium angiogram of popliteal artery and trifurcation.
We will frequently use another alternative: pure gadolinium
as in this image of the knee. Another alternative is a mixture of
1/3 saline, 1/3 contrast media and 1/3 gadolinium will be
injected into patients with renal impairment.

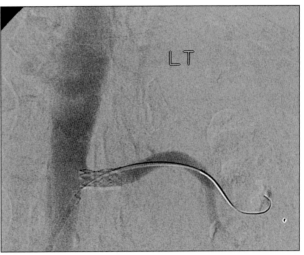

Figure 2.25
Gadolinium injection during and post renal stent placement.
Total dose of gadolineum should be kept under 60–80 cc to
avoid nausea. There have been a few cases of renal toxicity
regarding gadolinium injection.

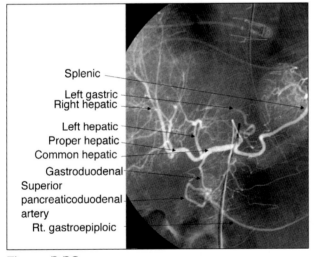

Figure 2.26
Celiac angiogram.
With an angled catheter, a 5 French Reuter catheter (Cook, Inc,
Bloomington, ID, USA), the celiac trunk was selected with
a rate of 8 cc/sec for 12 cc total in an AP projection.

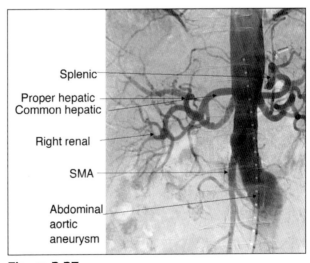

Figure 2.27
Abdominal aortic angiogram AP view.

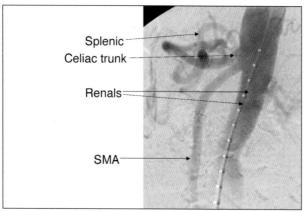

Figure 2.28
Abdominal aortic angiogram (lateral view).
Abdominal angiogram was obtained with a lateral view
to differentiate the origins of the SMA and celiac arteries.

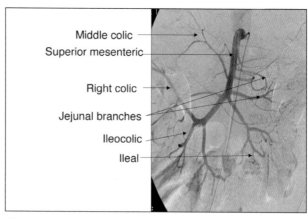

Figure 2.29
Superior mesenteric angiogram with the Reuter catheter placed
in the origin of the superior mesenteric artery. A delayed portal
vein phase was also shown.

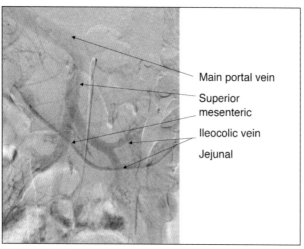

Figure 2.30
Portal phase of SMA injection.

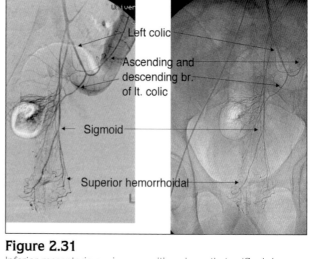

Figure 2.31
Inferior mesenteric angiogram with a rim catheter (Cook Inc,
Bloomington, IN, USA) at its origin in the arterial and venous phase.

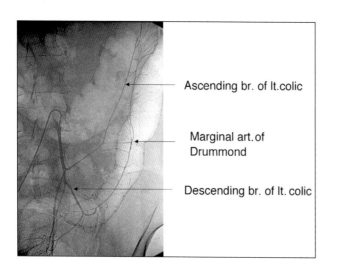

Figure 2.32
Inferior mesenteric angiogram.

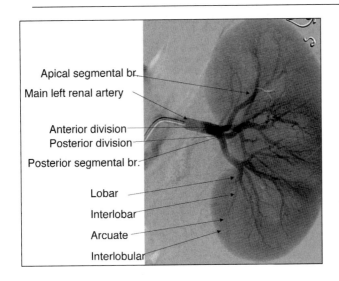

Figure 2.33
Selective renal angiogram with a 5 French cobra catheter.
Renal arterial anatomy: intrarenal branches
- Renal artery divides into anterior and posterior divisions prior to segmental branches.
- Kidney is divided into five vascular segments: apical, upper, middle, posterior and lower.
- Segmental artery divides into lobar, which subdivides into 2–3 interlobar (between the pyramids), then into arcuate at the corticomedullary junction, then into interlobular arteries.

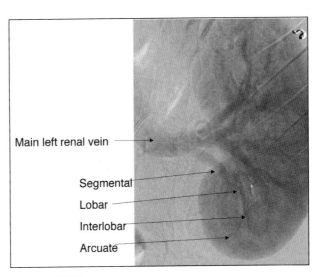

Figure 2.34
Venous phase of renal angiogram.

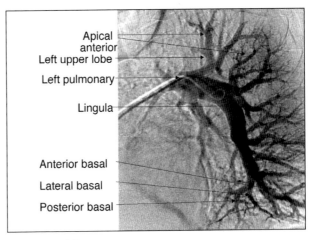

Figure 2.36
Left pulmonary angiogram.

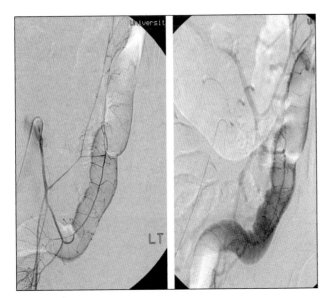

Figure 2.35
With the catheter placed at the origin of the inferior mesenteric artery, the inferior mesenteric artery is seen with the bifurcation into the left colic artery which then branches into the ascending and descending branches. The beginning of the sigmoid arteries with branches to the rectum are shown. The next image is the delayed run which shows the inferior mesenteric vein flowing to the portal vein.

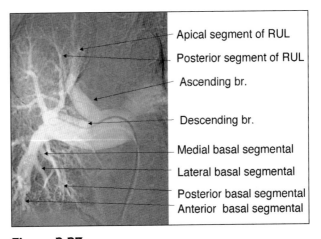

Figure 2.37
Right pulmonary angiogram.

3

Peripheral arterial disease: clinical evaluation and non-interventional therapy

Michael R Jaff

The evaluation of patients with peripheral arterial disease (PAD) begins with an understanding of the reason why the patient has sought evaluation. In patients with single-level disease (i.e. either iliac or superficial femoral artery (SFA) disease), the most likely presenting symptom will be intermittent claudication. Isolated iliac artery disease results in buttock or hip claudication, and is predominantly a lifestyle-limiting phenomenon. Patients with disease limited to the SFA generally present with calf claudication symptoms. However, if iliac artery, SFA and infrapopliteal disease occur in combination, critical limb ischemia (ischemic rest pain, non-healing ulcerations, gangrene) may occur in association with intermittent claudication.

The initial evaluation of patients with PAD must include a comprehensive history, eliciting exercise limitation, presence of ischemic rest pain, non-healing ischemic ulcers, and gangrene. In addition, a thorough review of other atherosclerotic risk factors and concomitant cardiovascular disease must be completed. On physical examination, a focused analysis of peripheral pulses, presence of audible bruits and evaluation of skin integrity of the feet and legs must occur. Cold feet, absent hair on the lower extremities and dystrophic toenails are not reliable physical findings for PAD. However, the presence of pallor on elevation of the feet, and dependent rubor, are accurate physical examination predictors of significant PAD. Physicians must be adept at detecting foot ulcerations that are due to limb ischemia. These ulcerations are commonly found over distal aspects of the feet and toes, and over bony prominences. They are dry, with a black/gray base, and no signs of viable granulation tissue, and are intensely painful.

Following this, an ankle–brachial index (ABI) should be performed in order to stratify the patient's level of ischemia. An abnormal ABI will also predict future risk of cardiovascular morbidity and mortality.[1] A full 'arterial profile' of the lower extremities includes the determination of segmental limb pressures and pulse volume recordings, both at rest and with exercise, using a standard treadmill protocol, and should be performed by an accredited vascular laboratory.[2] This series of tests provides physiologic and anatomic information about the patients' location and severity of peripheral arterial occlusive disease.

Arterial duplex ultrasonography is a useful test in patients with significant lower extremity arterial occlusive disease. Duplex ultrasonography can accurately predict the location and severity of arterial stenoses and occlusions in the peripheral arteries.[3] Direct interrogation of the iliac artery is preferable to analysis of the downstream common femoral artery doppler waveform.[4] There are specific duplex velocity characteristics which provide accurate categorization of degrees of stenosis.[5] Arterial duplex scanning, in certain scenarios, provides enough information to allow the interventionist to plan a revascularization strategy,[6] and can be reliably used as the sole imaging modality to plan infrainguinal revascularization, even in patients with critical limb ischemia.[7]

Alternative diagnostic options in patients with PAD disease include magnetic resonance arteriography[8] and contrast arteriography. Some have used carbon dioxide angiography in aortoiliac disease evaluation as well.

Non-interventional therapy for peripheral arterial occlusive disease is much more than unsupervised walking. Options for non-interventional therapy have now come to include supervised exercise therapy, new pharmacologic agents for intermittent claudication, novel angiogenic growth factors, and vascular brachytherapy to promote patency after intervention. Certainly, aggressive risk factor modification, such as tobacco cessation, normalization of hypercholesterolemia, control of hypertension, and aggressive glycemic control in diabetes mellitus, all are important primary maneuvers in the care of patients with vascular disease, and should represent the cornerstone of treatment, even if revascularization is required.[9]

Antiplatelet therapy has been used in patients with peripheral arterial occlusive disease, predominantly as a method of preventing coronary and cerebrovascular events and death.[10] Ticlopidine and clopidogrel are thienopyridine derivatives that inhibit platelet aggregation. Ticlopidine has been shown to decrease the incidence of myocardial infarction, stroke and transient ischemic attacks in patients with intermittent claudication.[11] In addition, as therapy for intermittent claudication, ticlopidine has demonstrated increases in the initial and absolute claudicating distances when compared to placebo.[12] Finally, in comparison to placebo, ticlopidine has been shown to improve the long-term patency of lower extremity saphenous vein bypass grafts. Patients assigned to placebo had a 2-year cumulative patency rate of 63%, compared to 82% in the ticlopidine-treated patients.[13]

The Clopidogrel versus Aspirin in Patients at Risk for Ischemic Events (CAPRIE) trial evaluated 19 000 patients with history of ischemic stroke, myocardial infarction, or symptomatic peripheral arterial occlusive disease, randomized to either clopidogrel or aspirin. Patients assigned to clopidogrel had a statistically significant reduction in the primary endpoint of stroke, myocardial infarction, or vascular death, compared to aspirin. The patients enrolled with symptomatic peripheral arterial occlusive disease gained the greatest benefit when using clopidogrel as compared with aspirin.[14] Clopidogrel appears to be an important adjunct in the management of patients with peripheral arterial occlusive disease to prevent cardiovascular events and vascular death.

A review of the published series of exercise therapy in PAD prior to 1993 demonstrated impressive improvement in pain-free walking distances (PFWD), despite the fact that two of these series reflected unsupervised exercise.[15] One early series of supervised exercise therapy for 4–6 months in 148 patients demonstrated a mean increase in walking ability of 234%, with 88% of patients demonstrating significant walking improvement.[16] Comparisons of supervised versus home exercise therapy among more current series have consistently revealed marked benefit in both the time to onset of intermittent claudication and maximum walking time among patients receiving supervised exercise therapy.[17,18] Supervised exercise therapy also offers improvement in functional status as measured by walking impairment questionnaires and physical activity recall surveys.[19] Addition of pentoxifylline[20] or strength training to exercise therapy[21] have not offered significant additive benefits in PFWD.

A meta-analysis of published studies of exercise rehabilitation programs for the treatment of intermittent claudication revealed increases in initial claudicating distance of 179% and absolute claudicating distance of 122%.[22] This analysis also suggests that an optimal exercise program should consist of three 30-min sessions per week for at least 6 months, supervised walking as the primary exercise modality, and near-maximal claudication pain as the pain endpoint.

Drug therapy for lower extremity arterial occlusive disease, and specifically intermittent claudication, has been viewed as ineffective. Between 1965 and 1985, 75 trials studied 33 pharmacologic agents to assess efficacy as primary therapy for intermittent claudication. Unfortunately, 75% of these trials were flawed by lack of a placebo-controlled arm, no double-blinding, inaccurate endpoints, or small sample sizes.[23]

Pentoxifylline has been the only medication approved by the United States Food and Drug Administration for treatment of stable intermittent claudication. Porter et al evaluated 128 patients in a randomized, double-blind, placebo-controlled fashion, and demonstrated a statistically significant increase in initial and absolute claudicating distances in patients assigned to pentoxifylline over placebo.[24] Given the large number of clinical trials of varying scientific merit, a meta-analysis was performed to determine the true benefit of pentoxifylline in patients with intermittent claudication.[25] In total, 12 studies met the criteria set forth by the authors. The analysis suggests that pentoxifylline is effective in improving walking capacity of patients with moderate intermittent claudication. However, when reviewing all trials, and all 'high-quality' trials, the results were not statistically significant.

The most exciting advance in the pharmacologic therapy for patients with intermittent claudication has been the advent of cilostazol. Cilostazol is a chemically unique compound with several mechanisms of action. The most important are inhibition of platelet aggregation and vasodilation. Clinical data have emerged demonstrating marked improvement in walking distances over both placebo and pentoxifylline.

In a multicenter, randomized, double-blind, placebo-controlled trial of 81 patients with chronic stable intermittent claudication, 54 were assigned to cilostazol, and 27 received matching placebo. All patients were evaluated with a constant-speed, constant-grade treadmill test, and were followed for 12 weeks. There was a 35% increase in initial claudicating distance (ICD), and a 41% increase in absolute claudicating distance (ACD), among patients who received cilostazol.[26]

A dose-ranging trial of cilostazol compared doses of 50 mg twice-daily versus 100 mg twice daily versus placebo in 394 patients with chronic stable intermittent claudication. After 24 weeks, both doses of cilostazol demonstrated superiority in ACD and ICD when compared with placebo, with the 100-mg twice-daily dose achieving optimal results.[27]

In another randomized, prospective, double-blind trial of 239 patients with intermittent claudication, 119 received cilostazol 100 mg orally twice-daily, and 120 received matching placebo. All patients were studied with constant-speed, variable-grade treadmill examinations, and were followed on their assigned medications for 16 weeks. In addition, standardized quality of life indicators were assessed. Patients receiving cilostazol demonstrated significant improvements in ACD. Those assigned to cilostazol had a 96.4 m increase in ACD, compared to only 31.4 m in the placebo group.[28]

Finally, a 24-week, multicenter, randomized, double-blind trial compared the effects of cilostazol 100 mg twice-daily, pentoxifylline 400 mg three times daily, and placebo in 698 patients with chronic stable claudication. Constant-speed, variable-grade treadmill testing was performed at 4–week intervals. Compared to placebo, cilostazol demonstrated a statistically significant increase in ICD (98.3% versus 55.1%) and ACD (53.9% versus 33.5%), whereas pentoxifylline did not (ICD, 68.4% versus 55.1%; ACD, 30.4% versus 33.5%). In addition, cilostazol was clearly and statistically significantly more effective in improving ICD and ACD than pentoxifylline.[29] As a result of these data, cilostazol has recently gained United States Food and Drug Administration approval for use in patients with chronic intermittent claudication to improve walking distances.

Surgical revascularization remains an important option in patients with infrainguinal arterial occlusive disease. This is classically limited to patients with critical limb ischemia, or in patients with severe, lifestyle-limiting intermittent claudication with limited alternatives. Interestingly, it has become the standard to search for pharmacologic and endovascular options prior to embarking on surgical revascularization.

Factors influencing the decision to undertake surgical revascularization include:

- The general health of the patient
- The anatomic distribution of peripheral arterial disease
- Suitable autogenous conduit
- Severity of the limb ischemia
- Expertise of the surgeon, and strength of the anesthesiologists/nurses
- Rehabilitation potential of the patient.

References

1. Vogt MT, McKenna M, Wolfson SK, Kuller LH. The relationship between ankle brachial index, other atherosclerotic disease, diabetes, smoking and mortality in older men and women. *Atherosclerosis* 1993; **101**: 191–202.

2. Jaff MR, Dorros G. The vascular laboratory: a critical component required for successful management of peripheral arterial occlusive disease. *J Endovasc Surg* 1998; **5**: 146–58.

3. Kohler TR, Nance DR, Cramer MM et al. Duplex scanning for diagnosis of aortoiliac and femoropopliteal disease: a prospective study. *Circulation* 1987; **76**: 1074–80.

4. Lewis WA, Bray AE, Harrison CL et al. A comparison of common femoral waveform analysis with aorto-iliac duplex scanning in assessment of aorto-illiac disease. *J Vasc Tech* 1994; **18**: 337–44.

5. de Smet AAEA, Ermers EJM, Kitslaar PJEHM. Duplex velocity characteristics of aortoiliac stenoses. *J Vasc Surg* 1996; **23**: 628–36.

6. Kohler TR, Andros G, Porter JM, et al. Can duplex scanning replace arteriography for lower extremity arterial disease? *Ann Vasc Surg* 1990; **4**: L280–7.

7. Ligush J, Reavis SW, Preisser JS, Hansen KJ. Duplex ultrasound scanning defines operative strategies for patients with limb-threatening ischemia. *J Vasc Surg* 1998; **28**: 482–91.

8. Cambria RP, Kaufman JA, L'Italien GJ, et al. Magnetic resonance angiography in the management of lower extremity arterial occlusive disease: a prospective study. *J Vasc Surg* 1997; **25**: 380–9.

9. Weitz JI, Byrne J, Clagett GP, et al. Diagnosis and treatment of chronic arterial insufficiency of the lower extremities: a critical review. *Circulation* 1996; **94**: 3026–49.

10. Antiplatelet trialists' collaboration. Collaborative overview of randomised trials of antiplatelet therapy – I: prevention of death, myocardial infarction, and stroke by prolonged antiplatelet therapy in various categories of patients. *BMJ* 1994; **308**: 81–106.

11. Janzon L, Bergqvist D, Boberg J et al. Prevention of myocardial infarction and stroke in patients with intermittent claudication; effects of ticlopidine. Results from STIMS, the Swedish Ticlopidine Multicentre Study. *J Intern Med* 1990; **227**: 301–8.

12. Balsano F, Coccheri S, Libretti A et al. Ticlopidine in the treatment of intermittent claudication: a 21-month double-blind trial. *J Lab Clin Med* 1989; **114**: 84–91.

13. Becquemin JP. Etude de la Ticlopidine après pontage fémoro-poplite and the Association Universitaire de recherche en Chirurgie. *N Engl J Med* 1997; **337**: 1726–31.

14. CAPRIE steering committee. A randomised, blinded, trial of clopidogrel versus aspirin in patients at risk of ischaemic events (CAPRIE). *Lancet* 1996; **348**: 1329–39.

15. Ernst E, Fialka V. A review of the clinical effectiveness of exercise therapy for intermittent claudication. *Arch Intern Med* 1993; **153**: 2357–60.

16. Ekroth R, Dahllof AG, Gundevall B, et al. Physical training of patients with intermittent claudication: indications, methods, and results. *Surgery* 1978; **84**: 640–3.

17. Williams LR, Ekers MA, Collins PS, Lee JF. Vascular rehabilitation: benefits of a structured exercise/risk modification program. *J Vasc Surg* 1991; **14**: 320–6.

18. Patterson RB, Pinto B, Marcus B, et al. Value of a supervised exercise program for the therapy of arterial claudication. *J Vasc Surg* 1997; **25**: 312–9.

19. Regensteiner JG, Steiner JF, Hiatt WR. Exercise training improves functional status in patients with peripheral arterial disease. *J Vasc Surg* 1996; **23**: 104–15.

20. Scheffler P, de la Hamette D, Gross J et al. Intensive vascular training in stage IIb of peripheral arterial occlusive disease. The additive effects of intravenous prostaglandin E_1 or intravenous pentoxifylline during training. *Circulation* 1994; **90**: 818–22.

21. Hiatt WR, Wolfel EE, Meier RH, Regensteiner JG. Superiority of treadmill walking exercise versus strength training for patients with peripheral arterial disease. Implications for the mechanism of the training response. *Circulation* 1994; **90**: 1866–74.

22. Gardner AW, Poehlman ET. Exercise rehabilitation programs for the treatment of claudication pain. *JAMA* 1995; **274**: 975–80.

23. Cameron HA, Waller PC, Ramsay LE. Drug treatment of intermittent claudication: a critical analysis of the methods and findings of published clinical trials, 1965–1985. *Br J Clin Pharmac* 1988; **26**: 569–76.

24. Porter JM, Baur GM. Pharmacologic treatment of intermittent claudication. *Surgery* 1982; **92**: 966–71.

25 Hood SC, Moher D, Barber GG. Management of intermittent claudication with pentoxifylline: meta-analysis of randomized controlled trials. *Can Med Assoc J* 1996; **155**: 1053–9.

26 Dawson DL, Cutler BS, Meissner MH, Strandness DE. Cilostazol has beneficial effects in treatment of intermittent claudication. *Circulation* 1998; **98**: 678–86.

27 Strandness DE, Dalman R, Panian S et al. Two doses of cilostazol versus placebo in the treatment of claudication: results of a randomized, multicenter trial. *Circulation* 1998 (suppl).

28 Money SR, Herd JA, Isaacsohn JL et al. Effect of cilostazol on walking distances in patients with intermittent claudication caused by peripheral vascular disease. *J Vasc Surg* 1998; **27**: 267–75.

29 Dawson DL, Cutler BS, Hiatt WR et al. A comparison of cilostazol and pentoxifylline for treating intermittent claudication? *Am J Med* 2000; **109**: 523–30.

4

Doppler scanning and imaging of the peripheral vasculature

Serge Kownator and François Luizy

Introduction

Ultrasound has been used in the evaluation of vascular diseases for more than 30 years. Continuous-wave Doppler was the original technique that facilitated the analysis of blood flow velocity. Initially, this technique was mainly used for the measurement of lower limbs blood pressures rather than for the diagnosis of stenosis along the arterial tree.

The incredible improvement in technology with the onset of real-time B-mode imaging, pulse Doppler, color Doppler and, more recently, power Doppler, allows an accurate evaluation of the arterial system, including the evaluation of the vessel wall and a hemodynamic quantification through the blood flow velocities.

Ultrasound imaging is now the most widely used imaging technique for vascular disease screening but is also seen more and more as the unique imaging method before surgery or angioplasty in some particular fields. In other fields the association with spiral computed tomography (CT) or magnetic resonance angiography (MRA) has replaced completion angiography. It is important to emphasize the critical need for all the ultrasound modalities – i.e., B-mode, color Doppler, pulse Doppler, and power Doppler. More recently, the advent of contrast agents has opened a new approach for ultrasound imaging.

Clinical applications

All the fields of vascular diseases are covered by color Doppler imaging. The most important applications are:

- carotid arteries, but also subclavian and vertebral arteries and the transcranial applications
- lower limb arteries, including the abdominal aorta
- visceral arteries and particularly renal arteries.

Carotid arteries (Figure 4.1)

Ultrasound imaging is recognized as being an accurate method for the diagnosis and the quantification of carotid artery stenosis, with a high rate of sensitivity and specificity. The prospective trials about internal carotid stenosis, NASCET and ECST for symptomatic patients,[1,2] ACAS and Veterans for asymptomatic patients,[3,4] focused their attention on diameter reduction, but there was no data regarding plaque composition.

Duplex scan and color flow Doppler are non-invasive techniques with the potential to assess both luminal features and arterial wall structure, before and after treatment.

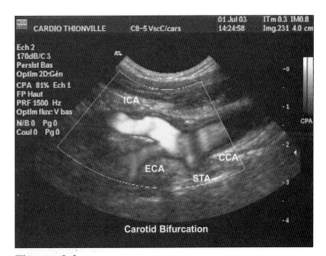

Figure 4.1
Carotid bifurcation: iso-echoic plaque from the anterior wall of the 2bifurcation and the internal carotid artery.
ICA, internal carotid artery; ECA, external carotid artery; CCA, common carotid artery; STA, superior thyroid artery.

Several studies comparing conventional angiography with Duplex scanning in the evaluation of carotid plaque morphology have confirmed the superiority of echography in this area.[5,6]

Doppler criteria for identifying carotid stenosis

Degree of stenosis

Hemodynamic quantification. Hemodynamic assessments commonly use peak systolic velocity (PSV) and end diastolic velocity (EDV) measurements to quantify the degree of stenosis:[7,8]

- For 70–99% carotid stenosis, PSV ≥ 240 cm/s and EDV > 100 cm/s provide a sensitivity of 91%, a specificity of 98%, a predictive positive value of 90%, a negative predictive value of 96%, and an overall accuracy of 95%.
- For 50–69% carotid stenosis, a PSV > 130cm/s and a EDV ≤ 100 cm/s proved to be the best combination, with a sensitivity of 92%, a specificity of 97%, a predictive positive value of 93%, a negative predictive value of 99%, and an accuracy of 97%.
- For 30–49% carotid stenosis, criteria are not as well defined, but a PSV range of 100 cm/s may be applicable.

Peak systolic velocity ratio: The ratio of the peak systolic velocity in the internal carotid artery to the peak systolic velocity in the ipsilateral common carotid artery can accurately identify patients with high-grade carotid stenosis.[9] An internal carotid artery/common carotid artery systolic velocity ratio (ICA/CCA ratio) of 3.5 or greater accurately predicts a greater than 70% internal carotid artery stenosis, with a sensitivity of 91%, a specificity of 90%, a predictive positive value of 87%, a negative predictive value of 94%, and an overall accuracy of 91%.

Anatomical quantification. The development of color Doppler and, in particular, power Doppler allows a good delineation between the surface of the plaque and the arterial lumen. This leads to an accurate measurement of diameters and surface.

Diameter reduction: The measurement of the diameter reduction is performed on a long-axis view at the tightest level of the stenosis, and compared with the diameter of the normal distal internal carotid (NASCET method), or with the diameter of the bulb (ECST method).[10]

Surface reduction: The surface reduction is measured on a short-axis view in order to compare the area of the residual lumen at the tightest level of the stenosis with the surface of the distal carotid (NASCET) or the surface of the bulb (ECST).

Brain hemodynamic incidence

The incidence of the stenosis depends not only on the degree of stenosis but also on the capacity of supply by the polygon of Willis. Transcranial color Doppler allows for a direct approach to hemodynamic repercussion of the cervical stenosis.[11] This technique facilitates the detection of intracranial stenosis.

Detection of high-intensity transient signals (HITS):

The presence of a cervical carotid stenosis is associated with a risk of cerebral events that depend on the degree of stenosis and the plaque morphology.

The benefit-risk ratio of treatment is often difficult to establish, and the detection of HITS might improve precision in predicting individual risk of cerebral vascular events, by determining the nature of the emboli and adapting the treatment to each patient.

Microemboli are most often detected beyond symptomatic carotid stenosis,[12] and the rate of microemboli is reduced by endarterectomy.

The relationship between HITS and structural modifications in the plaque has been often suggested, and there is a correlation between the hourly rate of HITS and the presence of an ulceration or an intraluminal thrombus.[13]

In the near future, patients with carotid stenosis should undoubtedly benefit from this technology, in order to predict the individual risk and determine the appropriate treatment.

Morphological approach

The importance of plaque morphology in the physiopathology of cerebral events is now well accepted: plaque structure has been implicated as an important factor in the development of embolic events.[14]

The characterization of the structure of the plaque has been made possible with the improvement of high-resolution B-mode ultrasound scanning, which is able to show the 'make-up' of the carotid plaque:

- fibrous or calcified material is more echogenic than lipid or intraplaque hemorrhage, which are more echolucent
- it has been estimated that intraplaque hemorrhage is 1.6–6.7 times more common in symptomatic patients
- lipid-laden or hemorrhagic plaques have the potential to ulcerate and to embolize
- plaque fracture over the site of a hemorrhage may lead to luminal thrombus formation.

The role of plaque morphology as an independent risk of cerebral events must then be evaluated and standardized. Various classifications have been proposed to characterize carotid plaques using ultrasonography, as, for example, homogenous and heterogenous plaques, or soft, dense, and calcified plaques.

The classification of Geroulakos et al.,[15] seems to be the most suitable to classify the echogenic structure, and differentiate between five types:

- Type I: uniformly echolucent plaques with or without a thin echogenic cap.
- Type II: predominantly echolucent plaques with less than 50% echogenic areas.
- Type III: predominantly echogenic plaques with less than 50% echolucent areas.
- Type IV: uniformly echogenic plaques.
- Type V: plaques that cannot be classified due to heavy calcifications producing acoustic shadows.

The use of color flow Doppler is an indispensable necessity to quantify the types I, II, and III.

Ulcerated plaque

The ulceration is characterized by an eccentric defect into the plaque, with smooth contours and abrupt limitations. The ulcer must be larger and deeper than 2 mm to be diagnosed by ultrasound, and color flow imaging is indispensable to have a better delineation of the plaque surface. In the future, 3D flow reconstruction should permit an easier interpretation of this kind of lesion.

To develop a clinical use of the plaque characterization, Nicolaides and his group have proposed a computerized method for the standardization of the gray scale. This method provides an objective measurement of echogenicity based on the grayscale median density value of the plaque. For the same degree of stenosis, patients with hypoechoic and/or ulcerated plaques are considered for a higher level of risk.[16,17]

Ultrasound and therapeutic strategy

Endarterectomy

The ACAS, NASCET, and ESCT studies have documented the benefit of carotid endarterectomy for treating asymptomatic or symptomatic patients with 70% or greater stenosis of the internal carotid artery.

The accuracy of ultrasound data has led more and more groups to perform carotid endarterectomy without angiography. This strategy provides a dramatic decrease in cost and avoids the risk directly dedicated to angiography (1.2% in ACAS).

Angioplasty and stenting[18,19]

Despite a growing number of cases performed all around the world (~6000) carotid angioplasty remains under evaluation and will remain until the results of randomized trials vs surgery.

Before the procedure, color Doppler is able to provide accurate measurements of the diameters of the internal and common carotid arteries required in the choice of the stent size. After the procedure, duplex (Figure 4.2) provides an immediate non-invasive status of the result, recording the PSV and measuring the diameters of proximal, median, and distal parts of the stent, and permeability of the external carotid artery through the stent network, if the stent covers its ostium.

These immediate results are important for the follow-up of the procedure and the evaluation of long-term results. Carotid ultrasound detects the different complications easily and accurately.

Follow-up. The long-term evaluation of carotid angioplasty requires a hemodynamic and a morphological follow-up and non-invasive methods using ultrasound are particularly suitable for this situation.

Measurements of the PSV and the stent diameters are compared with measurements of the immediate post-procedural status. The major complications are easily detected: unapply stent, restenosis, stent deformation, and external carotid artery thrombosis.

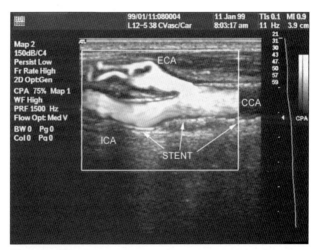

Figure 4.2
Control of a carotid stenting. The stent involves the common carotid artery and the internal carotid artery. The external carotid artery is patent through the network of the stent.

Lower limb arterial disease

The association between duplex and color Doppler now appears to be a tremendous progress in imaging lower limb arterial disease.[20] The purpose is no longer to evaluate the ankle–brachial index (ABI) but to provide an accurate mapping of the atheromatous lesions from the abdominal aorta to the distal arteries in order to determine the arterial status precisely and participate in the best choice of treatment.

Considering the evaluation of the degree of stenosis, the best specificity, sensitivity, and accuracy are provided by the velocity ratio between the PSV at the site of stenosis and the normal proximal site velocity. This ratio provides a pretty good performance, particularly for the discrimination of > 50% stenosis.[21] Even distal arteries are very well evaluated (Figure 4.3).

In a paper published in 1992 with duplex ultrasound, Moneta et al.[22] provided very interesting data on the feasibility and the accuracy of the technique (Table 4.1).

There is no doubt that the association of the color Doppler and the power Doppler increases the performance of the method. In the case of technical problems, the use of an intravenous contrast agent such as Levovist® (Schering AG) leads, in our experience, to a feasibility close to 100% in all the territories.

Considering the accuracy of Doppler ultrasound, we can propose in most cases the selection for surgery and the determination of the site of anastomosis based on ultrasound data.

Although contrast angiography remains necessary in a number of cases before surgery or angioplasty, duplex color ultrasound can replace it in some cases with very good efficiency: for example, in the case of a unique stenosis of an iliac artery, angioplasty can be performed, based on ultrasound data (Figure 4.4).

Table 4.1 Visualization of arterial segments by duplex scanning in 286 lower extremities studied by angiography

Artery	No. of segments satisfactorily visualized by angiography	Percent of angiographic visualized segments visualized by duplex scanning
Common iliac	269	95
External iliac	265	98
Common femoral	261	100
Deep femoral (origin)	246	99
Superficial femoral	616	100
Popliteal	380	99
Anterior tibial	539	94
Posterior tibial	525	96
Peroneal	506	83

In the case of a unique lesion of the superficial femoral artery, the punction can be oriented in the descending direction to perform angioplasty in one single stage. By avoiding routine arteriography, we are able to substantially reduce the risk and cost of a standard preoperative work-up for a lower extremity occlusive disease with ultrasound. If the duplex study reveals that the patient can be treated with a femoropopliteal bypass graft, then preoperative contrast angiography can be performed. After surgery or angioplasty, duplex color ultrasound is a useful technique for the follow-up.

In the case of angioplasty, restenosis is accurately detected with color Doppler. Quantification require pulse Doppler.

In the case of surgery, color duplex ultrasound can follow reliably the body of the bypass for the detection of

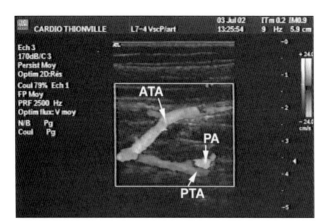

Figure 4.3
Infra popliteal arteries through an anterior access. ATA, anterior tibial artery; PTA, posterior tibial artery; PA, peroneal artery.

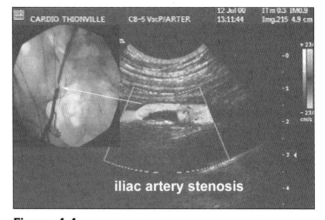

Figure 4.4
Tight stenosis of the right iliac artery due to a short iso-echoic plaque. Angiographic control before angioplasty.

thrombus. The velocities in the bypass predict the loss of patency when above 40 cm/s in the body of the venous bypass.

Doppler has been shown to be an accurate method for the diagnosis of restenosis at the site of anastomosis and for the detection of false aneurysm.

Duplex ultrasound is evolving into a useful tool for vascular imaging of lower limbs; in contrast to arteriography, it is inexpensive, risk-free, and well tolerated by patients.[23]

Renal arteries

The use of Doppler ultrasonography on patients with hypertension has led to an increase in the diagnosis of renal–artery stenosis (Figure 4.5).

Renal artery stenosis is often under-recognized.[24] Its frequency is linked to the underlying pathology. It is known that renal artery stenosis is more frequent in patients with diffuse atherosclerosis, particularly in patients with multivessel coronary artery disease. In addition, the incidence increases according to the pathology under consideration (Table 4.2).

The technique of renal artery duplex scanning has been validated for the detection of renal artery stenosis.[25–27] The feasibility is from 85% and rising to 95% when using a contrast agent. The diagnosis of renal artery stenosis is based on the maximum renal artery PSV and the renal-to-aortic ratio (RAR), which is defined as the ratio of the maximum PSV in the renal artery to the PSV in the adjacent abdominal aorta (Table 4.3).

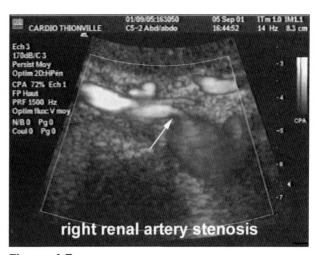

Figure 4.5
Power Doppler: right renal artery stenosis.

Using the criteria shown in Table 4.3, studies comparing the results of renal duplex scanning with the results of arteriography have shown that the overall accuracy for identifying renal artery disease is in the range of 80–96%.

We can now plan a renal artery stenosis for angioplasty on the basis of ultrasound examination. Completion angiography is performed at the first stage of the procedure to confirm the stenosis. Some renal artery stenosis are not suitable for angioplasty because of a poor expectancy for good results, particularly as regards blood pressure control and/or renal function. These patients can be identified by duplex scanning, as shown recently by Radermacher et al.[28] This identification is based on the evaluation of the resistance index at the level of intra-renal arteries.

Conclusion

With the dramatic improvement in technology, ultrasonography is now an accurate method for vascular imaging. It is widely used for the screening of vascular disease but also for the treatment strategy and the follow-up after endovascular procedure or surgery. Every vascular laboratory has to validate itself in order to optimize its performance; this procedure is one of the keys to accuracy.

Table 4.2 Incidence of stenosis	
Patient population	*Incidence %*
General population	0.1
Hypertensive population	4.0
Hypertensive and coronaropathy	23
Malignant hypertension	30
Malignant hypertension and renal insufficiency	40

Table 4.3 Diagnosis criteria for the quantification of renal artery stenosis by duplex scanning		
Renal artery diameter reduction	*Renal artery PSV*	*RAR*
Normal	< 190 cm/sec	< 3.5
< 60%	≥ 190 cm/sec	< 3.5
≥ 60%	< or ≥ 190 cm/sec	≥ 3.5
Occlusion	No signal	No signal

References

1 North American Symptomatic Carotid Endarterectomy Trial Collaborators. Beneficial effect of carotid endarterectomy in symptomatic patients with high grade stenosis. *N Engl J Med* 1991; **325**: 445–53.

2 European Carotid Surgery Trialists' Collaborative Group: MRC. European carotid surgery trial: interim results for symptomatic patients with severe (70–99%) or with mild (0–29%) carotid stenosis. *Lancet* 1991; **337**: 1235–43.

3 Asymptomatic Carotid Atherosclerosis Study Participants. Endarterectomy for asymptomatic carotid artery stenosis. *JAMA* 1995; **273**: 1421–8.

4 Hobson RW, Weiss DG et al. For the Veterans Affairs Cooperative Study Group. Efficacy of carotid endarterectomy for asymptomatic carotid stenosis. *N Engl J Med* 1993; **328**: 221–7.

5 Rubin JR, Bondi JA, Rhodes RS. Duplex scanning versus conventional arteriography for the evaluation of carotid artery plaque morphology. *Surgery* 1987; **102**: 749–55.

6 Srinivasan J, Mayberg MR, Weiss DG, Eskridge J. Duplex accuracy compared with angiography in the Veterans Affairs Cooperative Studies Trial for Symptomatic Carotid Stenosis. *Neurosurgery* 1995 **36**: 648–53; discussion 653–5.

7 Hood DB, Mattos MA, Mansour A et al. Prospective evaluation of new duplex criteria to identify 70% internal carotid artery stenosis. *J Vasc Surg* 1996; **23**: 254–61; discussion 261–2.

8 Carpenter JP, Lexa FJ, Davis JT. Determination of duplex Doppler ultrasound criteria appropriate to the North American Symptomatic Carotid Endarterectomy Trial. *Stroke* 1996; **27**: 695–9.

9 Moneta GL, Edwards JM, Papanicolaou G et al. Screening for asymptomatic internal carotid artery stenosis: duplex criteria for discriminating 60% to 99% stenosis. *J Vasc Surg* 1995; **21**: 989–94.

10 Steinke W. Classification of internal carotid artery stenosis by color Doppler flow imaging. *J d'Échographie et de Médecine par Ultrasons* 1995; **16**: 13–18.

11 Griewing B, Doherty C, Zeller JA, Kessler C. Power doppler. A new tool for transcranial duplex assessment of intracranial vasculature. *Imaging* 1996; **63**: 35–8.

12 Siebler M, Kleinschmidt A, Sitzer M, Steinmetz H, Freund HJ. Cerebral microembolism in symptomatic and asymptomatic high-grade internal carotid artery stenosis. *Neurology* 1994; **44**: 615–8.

13 Sitzer M, Muller W, Siebler M et al. Plaque ulceration and lumen thrombus are the main sources of cerebral microemboli in high-grade internal carotid artery stenosis. *Stroke* 1995; **26**: 1231–3.

14 Geroulakos G, Ramaswami G, Nicolaïdes A. Characterization of symptomatic and asymptomatic carotid plaques using high resolution real time ultrasonography. *Br J Surg* 1993; **80**: 1274–7.

15 Geroulakos G, Domjan J, Nicolaïdes A. Ultrasonic carotid artery plaque structure and risk of cerebral infarction on computed tomography. *J Vasc Surg* 1994; **20**: 263–6.

16 El-Barghouty N, Geroulakos G, Nicolaïdes A, Androulakis A, Bahal V. Computer-assisted carotid plaque characterisation. *Eur J Vasc Endovasc Surg* 1995; **9**: 389–93.

17 El-Barghouty N, Levine T, Ladva S, Flanagan A, Nicolaïdes A. Histological verification of computerised carotid plaque characterisation. *Eur J Vasc Endovasc Surg* 1996; **11**: 414–16.

18 Henry M, Amor M, Masson I et al. Angioplasty and stenting of the extracranial carotid arteries. *J Endovasc Surg* 1998 **5**: 293–304.

19 Henry M, Amor M, Henry I et al. Carotid stenting with cerebral protection: first clinical experience using the PercuSurge GuardWire system. *J Endovasc Surg* 1999 **6**: 321–31.

20 Hatsukami TS et al. Color Doppler imaging of infrainguinal arterial occlusive disease. *J Vasc Surg* 1992; **16**: 527–33.

21 Legemate DA, Teeuwen C, Hoeneveld H, Ackerstaff RGA, Eikelboom BC. Spectral analysis criteria in duplex scanning of aortoiliac and femoropopliteal arterial disease. *Ultrasound Med Biol* 1991; **17**: 769–76.

22 Moneta GL et al. Accuracy of lower extremity arterial duplex mapping. *J Vasc Surg* 1992; **15**: 275–84.

23 Wain RA et al. Can duplex scan arterial mapping replace contrast arteriography as the test of choice before infrainguinal revascularization? *J Vasc Surg* 1999; **29**: 100–9.

24 Olin JW, Melia M, Young JR, Graor RA, Risius B. Prevalence of atherosclerotic renal artery stenosis in patients with atherosclerosis elsewhere. *Am J Med* 1990; **88**: 46N–51N.

25 Kohler TR, Zierler RE, Martin RL et al. Noninvasive diagnosis of renal artery stenosis by ultrasonic duplex scanning. *J Vasc Surg* 1986; **4**: 450–6.

26 Taylor DC, Kettler MD, Moneta GL et al. Duplex ultrasound in the diagnosis of renal artery stenosis – a prospective evaluation. *J Vasc Surg* 1988; **7**: 363–9.

27 Radermacher J, Chavan C, Schäffer J et al. Detection of significant renal artery stenosis with color Doppler sonography: combining extrarenal, and intrarenal approaches to minimize technical failure. *Clin Nephrol* 2000; **53**: 333–43.

28 Radermacher J, Chavan A, Bleck J. et al. Use of doppler ultrasonography to predict the outcome of therapy for renal–artery stenosis. *N Engl J Med* 2001; **344**: 410–17.

5

The role of intravascular ultrasound in peripheral endovascular interventions

Khalid Irshad, Nawaf Rahman, Donald Bain, Peter Miller, Raj Velu and Donald B Reid

Introduction

Ultrasound was introduced into clinical medicine by Professor Ian Donald in the United Kingdom, an obstetrician who believed that the non-invasive imaging would provide safe and accurate diagnosis for mother and child.[1,2] Ultrasound is now universally adopted by all hospitals and many technological advances have helped its development. One specialized development is intravascular ultrasound (IVUS), a catheter-based technology where ultrasound is introduced into the vessel to provide imaging (Figure 5.1). Great detail is therefore possible because of the close proximity of the ultrasound catheter to the artery wall. This allows a significant magnification of the images compared to conventional extra corporeal ultrasound. Furthermore, intravascular ultrasound provides different information from angiography because it provides histological detail of the vessel wall[3,4] (see Figure 5.2).

Early IVUS probes mechanically rotated inside a catheter, sweeping an ultrasound signal around 360 degrees in the

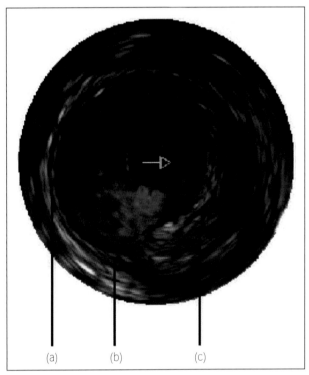

Figure 5.2
Two-dimensional cross-sectional image of an artery with histological detail of the vessel wall: a thin, white intima (a), a darker echolucent media (b), and homogeneous plaque (c).

same way as a radar sweeps around a ship at sea. The disadvantage of the early rotating catheters was that the probe did not configure co-axially with the guide wire and was in a 'side saddle' configuration. This meant that it did not track smoothly through the artery and could damage it. The more modern phased array probes are co-axial and do not require mechanical rotation.[5]

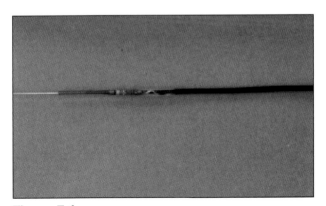

Figure 5.1
An intravascular ultrasound phased array catheter.

Interventional cardiologists pioneered the early use of IVUS, however its diagnostic accuracy was soon taken up and applied by peripheral endovascular specialists.[6,7] Its main use in peripheral interventions is to check the accuracy of stent deployment but it can also be used following percutaneous transluminal angioplasty (PTA), atherectomy, laser, thrombolysis, and endoluminal grafting.[8–11] As an institution we have also found that IVUS is particularly helpful diagnostically before the intervention by detecting disease and allowing accurate measurements of vessel diameters to assist the planning of treatment.[5] IVUS often detects significant disease that angiography has missed.[3] This chapter aims to explain the clinical role of IVUS in peripheral endovascular interventions and reports a study on its clinical value in patients with critical limb ischaemia that illustrates its benefit.

Technical aspects

There are two main systems that are commercially available. The Galaxy System (Boston Scientific, Natick, MA) utilizes mechanically rotating probes with two- and three-dimensional reconstructions. A newly developed mechanical catheter provides excellent 'black and white' IVUS imaging and luminal measurements of length with a mechanical pull back sled. The second system is the In-Vision system (Jomed, Beringen, Switzerland) which utilizes phased array imaging with probes that are co-axial (with fast exchange versions). Since this system was purpose made for the coronary market it uses 135-cm-long probes as small as 2.9 Fr (20 MHz) and 3.4 Fr (20 MHz) that go over 0.014- and 0.018-inch guide wires. A larger 8-Fr probe goes co-axially over a 0.035-inch wire. The smaller probes have a maximum range of 24 mm in diameter yet we use them for vessels as large as the iliac arteries. Indeed, we routinely stent on an 0.016-inch wire in most peripheral situations when we use these probes since this avoids time-consuming wire exchanges. The 8-Fr probe has a maximum diameter of 60 mm and is therefore useful for larger arteries such as in aortic aneurysms. The main advantage of the Jomed system is that it provides coloured blood flow imaging. This has significant diagnostic advantages over conventional 'black and white' IVUS.

Colour IVUS

ChromaFlo® is a computer software that detects blood flow and colours it red, which was developed by EndoSonics (Rancho Cordova, CA) and purchased by Jomed. The software detects differences between adjacent IVUS frames taken at up to 30 frames per second. As the red blood cells move through the artery they move through the IVUS image frames. The software detects differences between adjacent frames and colours the image. ChromaFlo® can detect fast-flowing blood and colours it yellow. However, at present flow velocities cannot be measured using this technique. ChromaFlo® does not use the Doppler effect.[5]

Three-dimensional reconstruction

Three-dimensional reconstruction of the IVUS images created during a pull back through an artery provides the interventionalist with very helpful additional information[12] (see Figure 5.3). Serial image frames taken during a single pull back are stacked by the computer and reassembled into a three-dimensional image. The three-dimensional images are presented either as 'longitudinal' or 'volume' views. The authors prefer the longitudinal images because they are immediately available in the operating room and enable the clinician to make rapid management decisions following a pull back. Longitudinal images are used in conjunction with the two-dimensional cross-sectional image and are similar in appearance to an angiogram, but also define the vessel wall anatomy and morphology. The images may be rotated around their longitudinal axis to provide lateral and oblique perspectives. The 'volume' images take 2–3 min to create but they provide a three-dimensional cylindrical picture of the vessel, which can be turned over or revolved around. The authors have found that the best computer software to create volume images is manufactured by Quinton Imaging (Sunnyvale, CA). This software allows hemisection of the cylinder along its length for inspection of the luminal aspect of the artery. In essence, three-dimensional reconstruction provides the IVUS operator with the maximum information in the operating room to assist him or her with clinical decisions and patient management.[13]

Operative and anatomical considerations

The IVUS catheter is chosen for the artery being treated based on the size of the artery and the range of ultrasound the catheter images. The selected probe is then flushed with heparinized saline before use. To obtain ChromaFlo® a 'reference' function should be performed on the IVUS

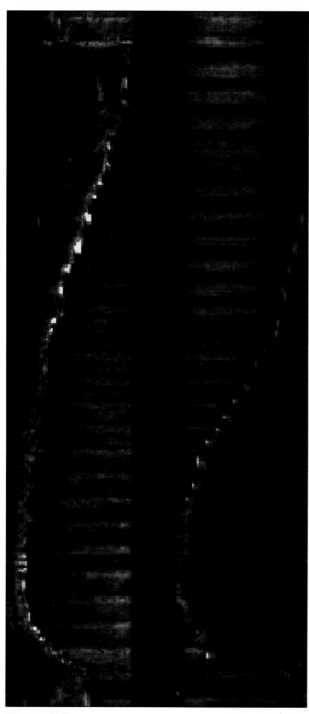

Figure 5.3

A longitudinal reconstruction of an iliac artery treated with an endoluminal graft to exclude a common iliac artery aneurysm. At the top of the picture the graft is tailored to the common iliac artery origin, while inferiorly it conforms with the narrower external iliac artery. Colour IVUS did not detect any endoleak outside the fabric of the graft, and the longitudinal reconstruction provides a more understandable picture than cross-sectional imaging alone.

machine when the probe is in the arterial lumen to remove near-field vision artefact – a characteristic of phased array IVUS. The catheter is passed into the artery under examination and (generally) pulled back through the area to interrogate the lesion. For many years we have always preferred a manual slow and steady pull back of the catheter to any commercially made mechanical device. Both the Boston Scientific and Jomed systems have user friendly software to measure diameters and cross-sectional areas. The Quinton equipment also calculates plaque volume.

Carotid arteries

IVUS has an important role in carotid artery stenting because it can detect inadequate stent deployment that may not be visible on the completion angiogram. In the carotid situation this is likely to be important by preventing acute occlusion and stroke.[14] We have also used it before angioplasty and stenting to measure the artery and therefore help achieve accurate stent placement (see Figure 5.4). However, in general, most endovascular specialists use IVUS very selectively in the carotid artery preferring to avoid over-instrumentation.[15]

Following stent placement the catheter is advanced into the distal internal carotid artery. Here the artery wall is usually free of disease and luminal diameters are measured. The catheter is pulled back through the stent so that deployment can be assessed and the minimum stent diameter measured. The deployed stent should be uniformly expanded along its entire length and there should be no space between the stent and the artery wall. The IVUS operator needs to confirm that the stent covers the lesion and no proximal or distal disease is left untreated. Careful examination for intimal dissection should also be made. In general a minimum internal carotid artery stent diameter of greater than 4 mm is required to avoid a haemodynamically significant stenosis remaining.[3]

Carotid stenting is difficult in cases with heavy calcification of the plaque or fibrotic tissue which resist complete stent expansion and this is often seen on IVUS as a mid-stent 'waisting'. A clinical decision then needs to be made whether to re-balloon or to leave be since repeated re-ballooning increases the risk of embolization to the brain.

Another way in which we have found IVUS to be helpful is when stenting the origin of the common carotid arteries. The curvature of the aortic arch makes accurate location of their origins difficult with angiography alone. The IVUS probe is used in combination with fluoroscopy and angiography to road map the exact location for stenting (see Figure 5.5).

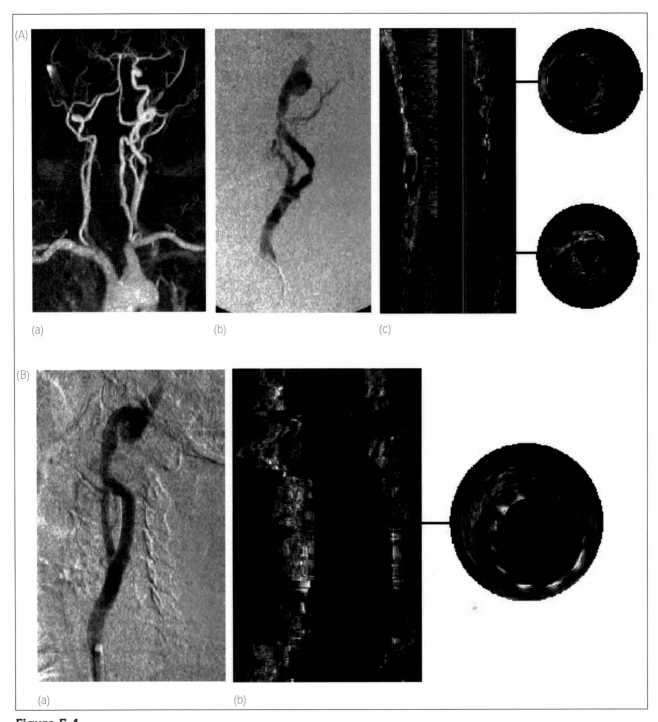

Figure 5.4
(A) Magnetic resonance angiogram (a) of the supra-aortic vessels showing a left internal carotid artery (ICA) stenosis before intervention. Operative digital subtraction provides a selective angiogram of the left ICA stenosis (b). Evaluation of the lesion with IVUS (c) shows a healthy ICA cephalad to a critically tight stenosis. In this situation IVUS dictated that primary stent deployment was not possible. (B) Following pre-dilatation the lesion was stented. The completion angiogram (a) and IVUS (b) both confirm satisfactory stent deployment.

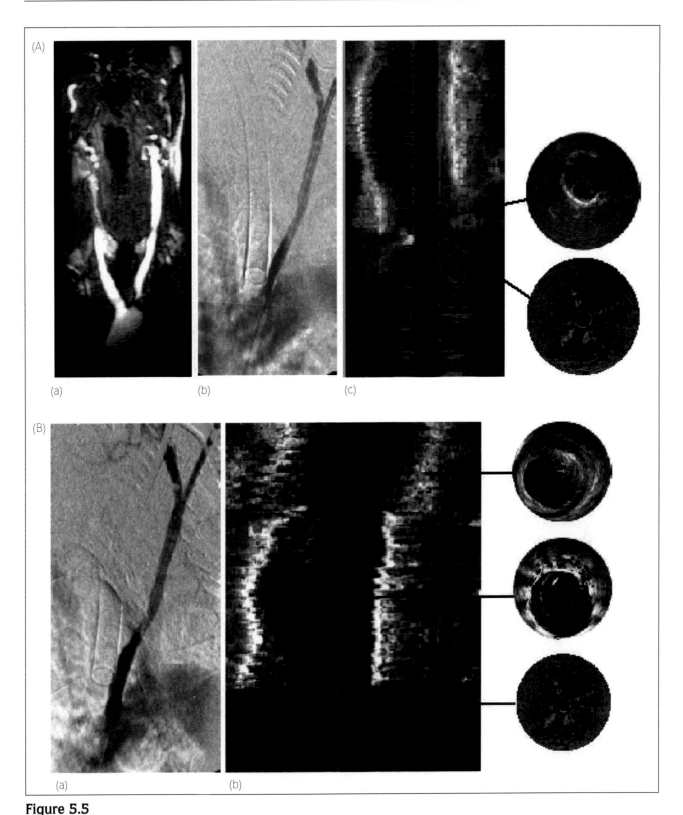

Figure 5.5

(A) Magnetic resonance angiography (a) and operative angiography (b) show a tight stenosis at the origin of the left common carotid artery – close to the tip of the endotracheal tube. At surgery an operative exposure of the carotid bifurcation allowed retrograde carotid access for an IVUS probe to be passed down assisted by road mapping: two- and three-dimensional colour IVUS (c) precisely locates the origin of the common carotid artery. (B) Following stenting the operative completion angiogram (a) and the colour two- and three-dimensional IVUS (b) show accurate deployment of the stent at the origin of the common carotid. (With permission from Irshad K, Bain D, Miller PH et al. Role of intravascular ultrasound in cartoid angioplasty and stenting. In: Henry M, Ohki T, Mathias K (eds). *Angioplasty and Stenting of the Carotid and Supra-aortic Trunks*, London: Martin Dunitz, in press.)

Subclavian and brachial arteries

A similar situation exists when stenting at the origin of the subclavian and innominate arteries. IVUS here can help locate the vertebral artery and the internal mammary artery as well as the origin. The pull back can estimate the length of the artery to be treated to protect the vertebral and mammary arteries.

Familiarization of the use of the brachial approach to the subclavian artery can have some advantages. In Figure 5.6, IVUS was used in an emergency procedure to accurately deploy an endoluminal graft in a torn and bleeding brachial artery. The probe provided measurements to size the endoluminal graft and check that it was well deployed. This case illustrates that it is worthwhile using IVUS routinely in the endovascular suite: it can then be utilized without delay in an emergency situation.

Aorta

In occlusive disease of the aorta IVUS is used to determine the correct balloon and device size to place. This is important because ballooning with too large a balloon, even at only a few atmospheres, can cause rupture of the aorta. IVUS is

diagnostic in aortic dissection where subtle tears may not be apparent on computed tomography (CT) or conventional angiography: colour IVUS can be used to find the correct lumen for endovascular repair.

In aortic aneurysm endoluminal grafting, accurate measurements, and evaluation of the proximal neck and distal arteries greatly assist the procedure and provide the operator with a much better understanding of the case than with CT alone. Once an endoluminal graft has been deployed it can be difficult to obtain good IVUS imaging in the aorta when tiny pockets of trapped air in the endoluminal prosthetic material and metal reflect the ultrasound signal. Further technological advances with IVUS are therefore necessary here since colour IVUS could potentially detect endoleaks[5,13] (see also Figure 5.3).

Renal artery

In a study of 131 patients undergoing IVUS-guided renal artery stenting, IVUS assessment determined the need for additional balloon dilation despite an adequate angiogram result in 36 (23.5%) cases: IVUS findings included 22 (14.4%) instances of incomplete stent apposition/expansion, 8 (5.2%) dissections, and 6 (3.9%) incomplete covered ostia (more than one condition was detected in some cases).[16]

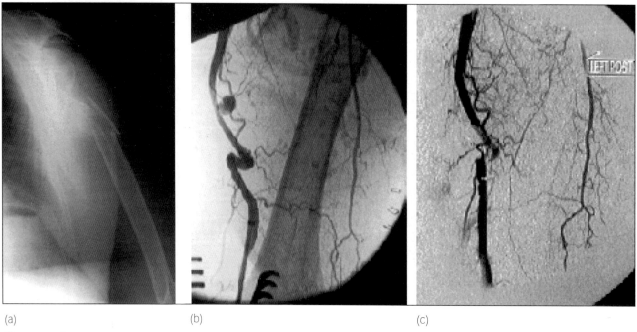

(a)   (b)   (c)

Figure 5.6
An 86-year-old man presented with a badly comminuted fracture of his left humerus (a) and a rapidly expanding false aneurysm of the brachial artery which was caused by puncture of the vessel by a bone fragment (b). IVUS rapidly provided accurate sizing of the vessel for endoluminal grafting and also confirmed satisfactory deployment. Completion digital subtraction angiogram confirmed seal (c).

Iliac arteries

The main use of IVUS in the iliac artery is to check the completeness of stent deployment (Figure 5.7). IVUS can also detect disease not apparent on angiography and we have found this particularly to be the case where there is a discrepancy between the clinical picture and the preoperative angiogram. We have found that IVUS often detects clinically

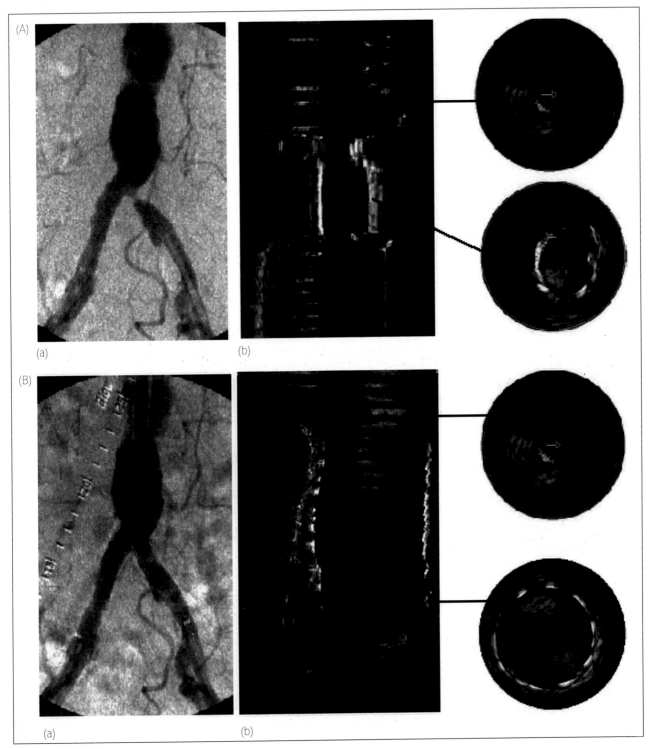

Figure 5.7

(A) A patient presenting with intermittent claudication and a tight stenosis of the left common iliac artery (a) had evaluation with colour IVUS (b). (B) Choosing the correct balloon size, a balloon expandable stent was deployed (a). IVUS confirmed excellent deployment which did not compromise the origin of the right iliac artery (b).

significant lesions where there was no significant arterial pressure gradient. The operator needs to use sound clinical judgement to decide how he or she treats the patient. This generally is best done based on the clinical picture in conjunction with 'triple assessment': IVUS, angiography, and pressure gradient measurements.

Superficial femoral and popliteal arteries

The coronary based colour IVUS probes produce elegant imaging in these smaller peripheral vessels. We have found

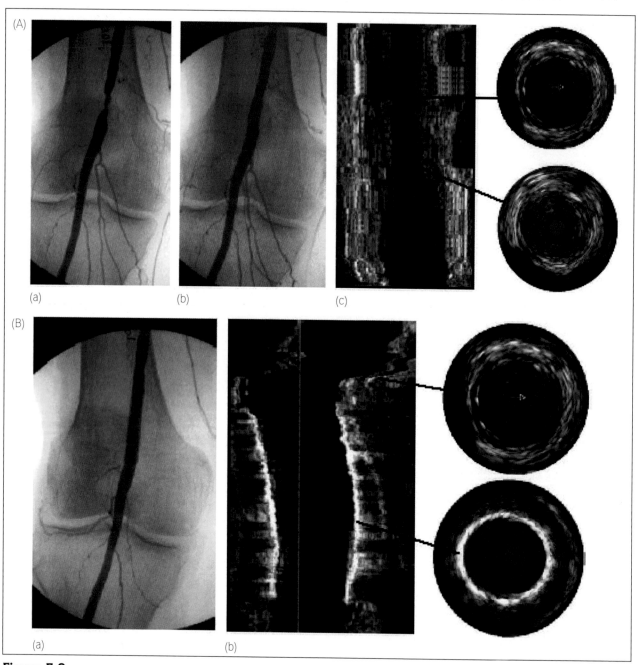

Figure 5.8

(A) An elderly women who presented with critical ischaemia had a tight stenosis of the popliteal artery (a). Percutaneous balloon angioplasty was performed with an apparently satisfactory completion angiogram (b). However, IVUS showed that there was still a large plaque volume remaining and obstructing the lumen (c). (B) An endoluminal graft was therefore deployed. Completion angiography was similar to the angiogram following PTA. IVUS showed perfect deployment of the endoluminal graft and a much better channel for blood to flow to the ischaemic limb.

that IVUS is helpful in detecting disease that the preoperative angiogram missed in the superficial and popliteal arteries, and have used IVUS routinely to accurately deploy endoluminal grafts (Figure 5.8).

Tibial arteries

Combination balloon/IVUS catheters originally designed for coronary angioplasty are large enough for tibial vessels. The IVUS transducer, which is just proximal to the balloon, immediately evaluates treatment, which is done without exchanging catheters or wires. We have found this particularly beneficial in patients with tibial artery disease seen in diabetic gangrene (see Figure 5.9), but in the future such combination probes are likely to be manufactured in larger sizes for use in all peripheral situations.

Clinical study

Our experience with colour flow three-dimensional intravascular ultrasound has shown that it detects arterial disease and maldeployment of stents, which are frequently not apparent on arteriography. Given that IVUS has this ability to provide maximum information about the disease process and its treatment at the time of the intervention, we felt it was appropriate to evaluate the role of IVUS in patients with the most severe arterial disease: critical limb ischaemia.

Fifty consecutive patients having IVUS guided endoluminal repair for critical limb ischaemia were prospectively studied for limb salvage over a 3-year period on an intention to treat basis. The patients (30 males, 20 females) were aged between 33 and 87 (mean 67) years and presented with ischaemic rest pain ($n=20$), ischaemic ulceration ($n=14$), and gangrene ($n=16$). One patient had bilateral leg ischaemia and one patient had critical ischaemia of her arm.

Colour flow IVUS was performed in all patients using balloon/IVUS combination catheters and standard IVUS

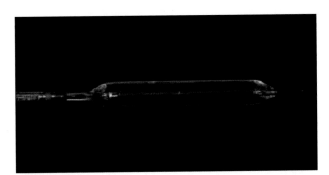

Figure 5.9
A combination balloon/IVUS probe catheter.

probes (Jomed) in order to evaluate the arterial disease and to assist endoluminal repair. In two patients IVUS showed that the arterial disease was too extensive for endoluminal repair and these patients were treated with open surgery. The remaining 48 patients were treated with 10 endoluminal grafts and 53 stents as well as simple balloon angioplasty.

IVUS was crucial in 16 patients (32%), being responsible for discovery of unsuspected disease ($n=11$) and inaccurately deployed stents ($n=5$). Thirty-day perioperative mortality was 2% ($n=1$). Twelve additional patients died during follow-up of natural causes (ischaemic heart disease, stroke, cancer, and fractured neck of femur). Only 11 patients underwent major amputation during the 3 years of follow-up (3 below knee and 8 above knee amputations). Kaplan–Mier survival graphs for limb salvage and mortality are shown in Figure 5.10A and B, respectively.

Summary

Our experience with IVUS over many years has led us to believe that IVUS is of benefit in many peripheral interventions. This is particularly so because it detects disease that other modalities cannot detect. It confirms satisfactory device

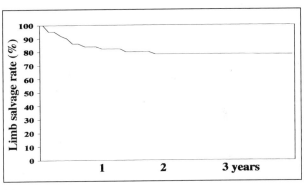

(a)

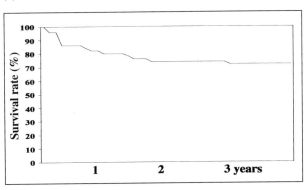

(b)

Figure 5.10
(a) Kaplan–Mier survival curve for limb salvage. (b) Kaplan–Mier survival curve for mortality.

deployment or the need for further treatment. It provides very accurate measurements of artery size and width. The addition of colour and three-dimensional reconstruction has enhanced its diagnostic ability and provides images similar to an angiogram which are easily understood by the operator. Our study of 50 patients with critical limb ischaemia had favourable limb salvage results. While we attribute much of this to intravascular ultrasound, it will be necessary to perform a clinical randomized trial in order to prove clinical outcome benefit from IVUS in peripheral interventions.

We have become sufficiently familiar with IVUS in that we use it in many patients who have renal failure or contrast allergy to treat them without angiography. With fluoroscopy alone the IVUS catheter can be used to road map intervention safely and accurately.[5]

Further technological advances are currently underway. One example is the introduction of combination balloon/IVUS probes with pre-mounted stents. A technology involving placement of the probe distal to the balloon is also being developed, reducing the number of times the lesion is crossed. Such advances are likely to encourage the more widespread use of IVUS in peripheral interventions, particularly if its cost effectiveness can be proved.

References

1   Donald I. How and why medical sonar developed. *Ann R Coll Surg Engl* 1974; **54**: 132–40.

2   Willocks J. Ian Donald and the birth of obstetric ultrasound. In: Neilson JB, Chambers SE (eds), *Obstetrics ultrasound 1*. Oxford: Oxford University Press, 1993: 1–18.

3   Reid DB, Diethrich EB, Marx P, Wrasper R. Clinical application of intravascular ultrasound in peripheral vascular disease. In: Seigel RJ (ed.), *Intravascular ultrasound imaging in coronary artery disease*. New York: Marcel Dekker, 1998: 309–41.

4   Nissan SE, Grines CL, Gurley JC et al. Application of a new phased array ultrasound imaging catheter in the assessment of vascular dimensions. *Circulation* 1990; **81**: 660–6.

5   Irshad K, Reid DB, Miller PH et al. Early clinical experience with color three-dimensional ultrasound in peripheral interventions. *J Endovasc Ther* 2001; **8**: 329–38.

6   Rosenfield K, Losordo DW, Ramaswamy K et al. Three-dimensional reconstruction of human coronary and peripheral arteries from images recorded during two-dimensional intravascular ultrasound examinations. *Circulation* 1991; **84**: 1938–56.

7   Heuser RR, Laas T, Prebble B et al. Computerised three-dimensional intravascular ultrasound reconstruction. In: Klein L (ed.) *Coronary stenosis morphology: analysis and clinical implications*. Norwell: Kluwer Academic Publishers, 1996.

8   Cavaye DM, Diethrich EB, Santiago OJ et al. Intravascular ultrasound imaging: an essential component of angioplasty assessment and vascular deployment. *Int Antgiol* 1993; **12**: 212–20.

9   Katzen BT, Benenati JF, Becker GJ et al. Role of intravascular ultrasound in peripheral atherectomy and stent deployment. *Circulation* 1991; **84**: 2152 (abstract).

10   Gussenhoven EJ, van der Lugt A, Pasterkamp G et al. Intravascular ultrasound predictors of outcome after peripheral balloon angioplasty. *Eur J Vasc Endovasc Surg* 1995; **10**: 279–88.

11   Laskey WK, Brady ST, Kussmaul WG et al. Intravascular ultrasonograhic assessment of the results of coronary artery stenting. *Am Heart J* 1993; **125**: 1576–83.

12   Reid DB, Douglas M, Diethrich EB. The clinical value of three-dimensional intravascular ultrasound imaging. *J Endovasc Surg* 1995; **2**: 356–64.

13   White RA, Scoccianti M, Back M et al. Innovations in vascular imaging; arteriography, three-dimensional CT scans and two- and three-dimensional intravascular ultrasound evaluation of an abdominal aortic aneurysm. *Ann Vasc Surg* 1994; **8**: 285–9.

14   Reid DB, Diethrich EB, Marx P et al. Intravascular ultrasound assessment in carotid interventions. *J Endovasc Surg* 1996; **3**: 203–10.

15   Diethrich EB, Marx P, Wrasper R, Reid DB. Percutaneous techniques for endoluminal carotid interventions. *J Endovasc Surg* 1996; **3**: 182–202.

16   Dangas G, Laird JR, Mehran R et al. Intravascular ultrasound-guided renal artery stenting. *J Endovasc Ther* 2001; **8**: 238–47.

6

Endovascular equipment and interventional tools

Zvonimir Krajcer and Kathryn Dougherty

Introduction

Since being first described in 1964 by Charles Dotter,[1] angioplasty and the management of peripheral vascular disease has undergone tremendous changes. It has not only proven effective and durable, but has also paved the way for a technological revolution that has applied percutaneous catheter techniques to progressively more complex clinical situations. This chapter reviews the basic equipment and current adjunctive endovascular therapies used to manage peripheral vascular disease.

Although coronary angioplasty and peripheral angioplasty procedures are similar, there are significant differences in interventional tools and treatment of the two disease states. The success of the intervention is determined by the physician's experience, level of training, type of lesion, and technique.

Overview of basic endovascular equipment

The disposable products required for peripheral vascular interventions, while similar to those used for coronary interventions, incorporate technological design features adapted to the anatomical variances of the arterial site being treated. Low-profile balloons and small-diameter shaft catheters allow access to the majority of lesions, even small-caliber arteries such as those below the knee.

Introducer sheath

Hemostatic introducer sheaths are generally used for all endovascular procedures. They establish a secure path from the skin to the vascular lumen. In addition to providing a safe port of access to the vascular system, they allow catheter instrumentation without ongoing blood loss or damage to the vessel. Sheath size is dependent upon the type of procedure, the outer diameter of the catheters, or equipment used during the intervention. Sheaths are generally 10–11 cm in length, although shorter and longer (7.5–100 cm) sheaths are used for a variety of purposes, such as straightening out the tortuous iliofemoral vessels, improving torque control, and facilitating the guide catheter, stent, and stent graft advancement. The Super Arrow-Flex® introducer sheath (Arrow International, Inc., Reading, PA) is popular for peripheral intervention because of its flexibility, numerous sizes, and lengths. It can provide all of the features of a guide catheter, with the added advantages of a built-in hemostatic valve and side-port. It incorporates a highly radiopaque coil-wire design that allows it to flex at any point, in any direction, without kinking. A hydrophilic coating added to the tip allows successful negotiation through the tortuous peripheral anatomy.

Many introducer sheaths can be used in place of guiding catheters for selective catheterization and visceral/branch artery intervention. Cook® Incorporated has a variety of peripheral introducer sheath sizes, lengths and configurations to accommodate radial, brachial, axillary, or femoral access. The Cook Flexor® (Cook, Inc., Bloomington, IN) introducer systems are thin walled, with large lumens. The Flexor® is equipped with a Tuohy-borst side-arm that allows contrast injections, prevents blood reflux, and permits unimpeded catheter and guidewire introduction. It is kink-resistant, with a hydrophilic coating, and easily accommodates contralateral access. The Balkin Contralateral® sheath is frequently used for contralateral iliofemoral approach. The Shuttle® has a radiopaque marker band in the distal tip that allows accurate positioning and facilitates endoluminal maneuvers in the supra-aortic vessels. Cook also makes the Extra Large (14F–24F) introducer. The 24F (French) Keller–Timmerman

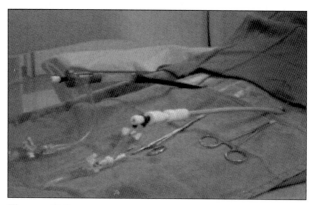

Figure 6.1
A 22F Keller–Timmerman sheath with the CheckFlow® valve is in the right femoral artery and a 16F Extra Large introducer is in the left femoral artery.

sheath is used to introduce large devices like endovascular stent – grafts for abdominal aortic aneurysm (AAA) exclusion. These sheaths range from 25 to 50 cm in length. They are equipped with a special hemostasis valve or Check Flow® valve that prevents blood reflux and allows flushing around the larger devices while they are positioned inside the sheath (Figure 6.1).

Guide wires

Guide wires permit safe transluminal navigation of catheters and devices. Guide wire design variables include tip configuration, length, diameter, stiffness, antifriction coatings, and radiopaque markers. The fundamental attributes of a guide wire include the ability to transmit torque, minimize friction, tip flexibility, and steerability. All guide wires should only be advanced under fluoroscopic guidance and never advanced against resistance. This will eliminate the risk of subintimal wire passage, vessel dissection, and perforation.

Guide-wire diameters are measured in inches. The standard range is 0.014–0.038 inches. The diameter of the guide wire should match the required diameter of the catheter: this provides better support of the catheter during manipulation and decreases the amount of leakage around the wire.

Guide wires are either straight, angled, or have a 'J'-shaped tip and have varying lengths of flexibility at the tip, ranging from 3 to 20 cm. The J-tipped wire is the most commonly used guide wire for initial passage into the vessel because of its low-risk of subintimal dissection. The main components of the traditional guide wire are the central core, which provides body, steerability, and torque control, and a tightly wound outer spring coil, which contains a forming ribbon for tip shaping and a Teflon outer coating to decrease friction. More

recently, a hydrophilic wire has been developed. Terumo Glidewire™ (Somerset, NJ) is using a unique design of a nitinol inner core, that is only minimally elastic, a markedly tapered distal tip that has a polyurethane outer surface instead of a spring coil, and a hydrophilic polymer coating.

The length of the wire is determined by its intended use. Most guide wires are 145–175 cm long. Exchange length guide wires, are 260–450 cm long and allow catheters, balloon, and other device exchanges while the guide wire is maintained in the distal position. The length of the guide wire will generally depend on the distance of the lesion from the access site and on the length of the catheter or the device that is being used.

For diagnostic procedures it is not necessary to use guide wires that are longer than 180 cm; however, during the interventional procedure it is generally recommended that exchange length (260 cm) guide wires are used. This length is necessary to have adequate length of the guide wire to be able to remove the device without losing the wire position across the lesion. It is occasionally necessary to use a 450-cm-long wire when brachial access is used for an intervention of femoral, popliteal, and tibioperoneal arteries. In this circumstance a 450-cm-long Geenan™ (Meditech, Boston Scientific Corp., Boston, MA) guide wire is very useful.

When attempting to traverse severely stenotic lesions or occlusions of vessels it is essential to select a guide wire that is flexible and can be easily steered, yet has sufficient body stiffness. There are several products that are commonly used for this purpose. A 0.035-inch Super stiff angled Glidewire™, because of good steerability and sufficient support is the wire of choice when crossing occluded vessels. The 0.018-inch angled Goldwire™ (Terumo, Glidewire™, Somerset, NJ) is another guide wire that has a hydrophilic coating and can be of a great advantage for crossing severely stenotic or occluded tibioperoneal arteries. One of the disadvantages of wires with a hydrophilic coating is their propensity to cause perforations of the vessels when not used with caution. For this particular reason it is not advisable to use these wires for renal or visceral interventions. Shorter guide wires are suitable for the renal and visceral interventions, such as the 0.014-inch Steel Core or the HI-TORQUE SPARTACORE™ 14 (Guidant Corp., Santa Clara, CA) with a 3- and 5-cm floppy tip for support.

Several guidewires offer even more support and stiffness of the body than the Super stiff Glidewire™. For endoluminal repair of AAA it is essential to have a sufficient support to advance a large profile stent–graft device across the iliac arteries. In this type of procedure a 0.035-inch Super Stiff Amplatz™ (Meditech, Boston Scientific Corp., Boston, MA) guide wire or, even stiffer, a 0.035-inch Lunderquist™ (Cook, Inc., Bloomington, IN) guide wire should be used.

The Bentsen™ (Cook, Inc., Bloomington, IN) wire is a 0.035-inch guide wire with a very soft body that allows easy tracking in a tortuous vessel. This wire is frequently used for advancing the catheter in the renal and other visceral vessels when other wires are not able to achieve this goal. It is also routinely used for advancing the vascular coils through the catheter for coil embolization.

The guide wires are available with different lengths of the flexible segments at their distal ends. Some of the products are available with 1 cm, 3 cm, 6 cm, and 10 cm flexible tip segments. The flexible segment of the wire enables the wire to conform itself to the vessel anatomy and avoid vessel trauma and spasm. The choice of length of the flexible segment will depend on the location of the vessel and the amount of support that will be needed to advance the device. For carotid and renal intervention, a 3 cm flexible segment length is commonly used. For endovascular AAA repair, a 10 cm flexible tip length should be used.

Other specialty guide wires include infusion wires such as the ProStream™ (Micro Therapeutics, Inc., San Clemente, CA), the Katzen™, and the Cragg™ (Meditech, Boston Scientific Corp., Natick, MA) (Figure 6.2), which have an outside diameter of either 0.035 or 0.038 inch and range from 145 cm to 180 cm in length. Multiple side-holes with various infusion port lengths from 3 cm to 15 cm and/or an open end-hole allow pharmacological agents to be delivered to distal vessels. This configuration also permits coaxial use through 5F infusion catheters (Meiwissen™, Meditech, Boston Scientific Corp., Natick, MA). A smaller 2.9F MicroMewi™ (Micro Therapeutics, Inc., San Clemente, CA) infusion catheter is inserted over a 0.018 inch guide wire and permits coaxial infusion. The Meiwissen™ catheter is a 5F infusion catheter, 150 cm long, that has an infusion length of either 5 or 30 cm.

For totally obstructed vessels, the Safe-Steer™ (IntraLuminal Therapeutics, Carlsbad, CA) guide-wire system incorporates guidance technology (optical coherence reflectometry) to help safely negotiate and prevent vessel perforation. The Safe-Steer™ is available in several diameters, ranging from 0.014–0.035 inches and straight or angled tip configurations. It has been used in conjunction with the excimer laser to safely redirect the laser catheter using real-time feedback and recanalize a totally occluded superficial femoral artery.[2]

The Flo Wire® Doppler wire and the Pressure Wire™ XT (RADI Medical Systems, Inc., Reading, MA) have become extremely useful tools when assessing flow disturbances and pressure gradients pre and post intervention.[3] Although both are 0.014-inch compatible wire systems, they were designed for use in the coronary vasculature, but may be beneficial when assessing limb ischemia in small distal branches below the bifurcation.

Finally, there are several guide-wire systems being tested that are designed to provide distal protection from embolization during coronary, supra-aortic, and peripheral interventions. Protective wire systems were developed in an effort to reduce the incidence of cerebral embolization during carotid artery stenting and distal embolization during coronary and saphenous vein bypass graft intervention. Wires currently under investigation include the NeuroShield™ (MedNova, USA, Topsfield, MA), the GuardWire (PercuSurge®, Sunnyvale, CA) (Figure 6.3), Angioguard™ (Cordis, Inc., Johnson & Johnson, Warren, NJ) (Figure 6.4), and the EPI™ filter wire (Embolic Protection, Inc., San Carlos, CA). Protective wires basically consist of a 0.014- or 0.018-inch wire with a filter basket or occluding balloon incorporated into the distal wire segment that captures any thromboembolic debris. Although still under FDA (Food and Drug Administration) investigation, these protective wires appear to be beneficial in reducing ischemic complications associated with the interventions.[4–6]

Diagnostic catheters

Diagnostic angiography is always performed prior to endovascular therapy, since it determines the complexity of the procedure, the access site, and the equipment that may be needed to successfully complete the intervention.

Diagnostic catheters, like guide wires, are available in multiple shapes, sizes, and materials and serve many purposes. Diagnostic catheters are usually introduced into the vasculature over a 'J' wire that has a soft distal tip. Diagnostic

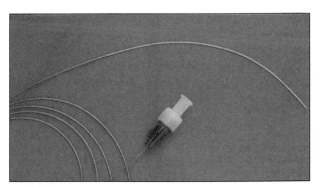

Figure 6.2
The Cragg Convertible™ (Meditech, Boston, Scientific Corp., Natick, MA) wire has an outer diameter of 0.038 inches and an inside diameter of 0.027 inches.

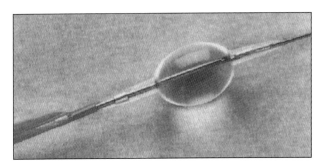

Figure 6.3
The GuardWire (PercuSurge®, Sunnyvale, CA) distal protection wire.

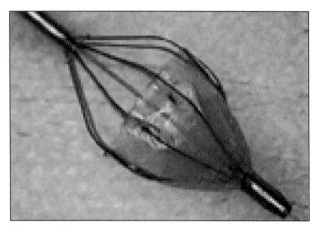

Figure 6.4
The AngioGuard™ (Cordis, Inc., Johnson & Johnson, Warren, NJ) cerebral protection wire.

Table 6.1   Pre-shaped catheter configurations

Area for visualization	Size	Suggested diagnostic catheter
Aortic arch and branches (vertebral, subclavian, carotid)	4–6F	H1, H2, SIM1, SIM2, SIM3, JB1, JB2, JB3, MANI, VITEK, HINCK, MPA, angled, vertebral (100–125 cm length)
Visceral (renal, celiac, superior mesenteric)	4–6F	C1, C2, RDC, RDC2, HS, MPA, SIM1, SIM2 (65 cm length)
Abdominal aorta and iliac run-off	5–6F	PT, Tennis Racket
Contralateral iliac	5–6F	MPA, hook, RIM, IM, SIM1, SIM2, (50 cm length)

catheters can be divided into two basic categories: selective and non-selective. Non-selective catheters are usually designed with multiple side holes, like the 'pigtail', 'Omniflush™' (AngioDynamics, Inc, Queensbury, NY), or 'Tennis Racket™' (Meditech, Boston Scientific Corp., Watertown, MA) and are placed within large vessels, such as the aorta or vena cava. These non-selective shapes provide high flow and dispersion of a contrast agent. Angiography of high-flow vessels requires contrast injection by a power injector to obtain adequate opacification. The 'pigtail' catheter is designed to protect the vessel walls from the whipping effect during power-injected boluses of contrast. Calibrated marker 'pigtail' catheters are used to determine accurate sizing of vessel lumen prior to endoluminal AAA repair. This is particularly important during endoluminal intervention. Radiopaque marker bands delineate a 20 cm segment, at 1 cm intervals, for precise measuring accuracy.

Catheter types and shapes are infinitely variable and choice is based on type and location of the lesion being treated. Selective catheters are pre-shaped to allow direct branch vessel engagement, pressure measurements, and contrast angiography. Specific catheters are recommended for specific anatomical locations and are designed to facilitate selective manipulation into branch vessels. Favorite pre-shaped catheter configurations are listed in Table 6.1. It is best to have a variety of catheter shapes available for challenging anatomical situations. Precise knowledge of the type of catheter is very important for angiography, so that appropriate and accurate information can be obtained prior to the intervention (Figure 6.5). Each company provides detailed product information on the catheters and their use. Hydrophilic catheters are useful for a selective approach of the carotid arteries, and to study the intracranial branches. Shorter-length catheters (50 cm) are used for visceral, renal, or contralateral iliac artery injections.

Catheters with side holes should be avoided. Selective catheters generally have a single hole, located at the tip, through which all injected contrast exits. Because of the single end hole, flow rates are much lower than non-selective catheters and, therefore, power injectors should not be used. Furthermore, high-flow power injection through an end-hole catheter carries a considerable risk of vessel injury due to the end-hole jet effect.

Catheter size or outer diameter is measured in 'French' units (1 mm = 3 F), whereas catheter inner lumen diameter is measured in inches. Common sizes range from 0.018 to 0.038 inch. This inner diameter measurement denotes the acceptable guide-wire size for the catheter. A mismatch in sizes can cause problems, such as either the guide wire not fitting inside the catheter or blood leakage around the guide wire. Diagnostic catheter size and length range from 4 to 6F, and from 50 to 125 cm, respectively. Most of these catheters are braided, with a soft tip, without braiding. Different catheter materials have specific functional characteristics such as stiffness or rigidity and kink-free torque control. Some catheters have inner and outer hydrophilic coatings to reduce friction for ease of passage and manipulation.

Guide catheters

Like diagnostic catheters, guide catheters come in a variety of lengths and shapes designed to facilitate their manipulation into branch vessels. However, they differ from diagnostic catheters by having a substantially larger luminal diameter.

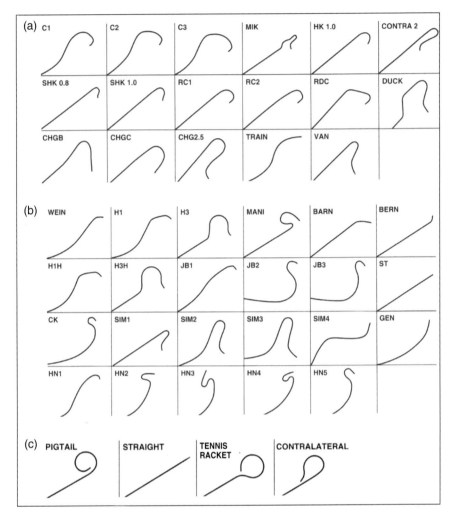

Figure 6.5
(a) Visceral and (b) cerebral pre-formed diagnostic shapes and (c) angiography catheters shapes.

Guide catheters are sized like diagnostic catheters with the outer diameter in French and the inner diameter in inches. But, to allow passage of the endovascular instruments, guide catheters must have a lumen diameter at least twice that of a typical diagnostic catheter. Guide catheters are similar to sheaths in that they provide protection to the vasculature when passing multiple devices into the same vessel. Important guide catheter characteristics include the ability to provide stable coaxial alignment between catheter tip and ostium of the vessel and kink-free torque control.

A properly selected guide should also provide back-up support for balloon catheter advancement, reliable pressure monitoring, and adequate contrast delivery during injections. In comparison to diagnostic catheters, guide catheters have reinforced construction and a much stiffer shaft to provide back-up support for the advancement of guide wires, balloons, and stents. Peripheral guide catheters are generally 6, 7, or 8F and range from 65 to 100 cm in length, with internal diameters ranging between 0.064 and 0.088 inches.

Balloon dilatation catheters

Balloon catheters are available in a wide variety of sizes, shapes, lengths, and compositions and are designed for different functions. They are the universal tool of endovascular intervention. The most important characteristic of a balloon dilatation catheter is its ability to inflate to a precisely defined diameter at a known pressure. Factors that determine balloon characteristics are dependent on balloon composition. All of the PTA (percutaneous transluminal angioplasty) balloons are made of plastic polymers, which are then altered to enhance the physical properties of the balloon. The balloon's composition dictates its performance and is the primary determinant of compliance, burst pressure, and scratch or puncture resistance. A balloon's compliance is a measure of how much it continues to grow beyond its predetermined size when pressure is applied. Compliant balloons will stretch and expand in the direction of least resistance. The more it expands beyond its predetermined size, the greater the reduction of dilating force on the stenosis and the greater the chance of transmitting that force and causing trauma to the healthy, non-diseased vessel.

Non-compliant balloons like those made of polyethylene terephthalate (PET) or nylon-reinforced polyurethane have minimal expansion and have a high rated burst pressure. Manufacturers use proprietary additives to strengthen the balloon material and improve puncture resistance. Non-compliant balloons are more desirable because they provide a high dilating force up to the stated diameter and length, which may be necessary for highly calcified lesions.

Balloon dilatation catheters are available in two basic designs: over-the-wire and on-the-wire systems. The balloon over-the wire system is when the wire and balloon move independently of each other. Fixed, or on-the-wire systems consist of a balloon mounted directly on a steerable wire core. Because of advances in balloon and catheter technology, over-the-wire systems are as low a profile and perform competitively with on-the-wire systems, thereby largely eliminating their use. Unfortunately, lower profile and smaller diameter shafts may allow access to smaller vessels but they may not be stiff enough to push through tight, heavily calcified lesions. Therefore, stiffer catheter shafts and lubricious coatings like silicone have been applied to the outside of balloon catheters to help prevent kinking and ease the passage through tortuous and tight lesions. The best results achieved with a balloon catheter are on short, concentric, and non-calcified lesions.

Balloons are available in several shapes, which vary by manufacturer and balloon type. Other important considerations when selecting a balloon is how long or short is the catheter tip, the length of taper to the shoulders of the balloon, and the length of the balloon. The use of short-tip, short-taper balloons minimizes the trauma to the adjacent non-diseased vessel wall and is especially useful at vessel branch points or at sites of acute angulation, which is commonly seen in the extracranial vasculature. Balloon lengths range from 2 to 10 cm and the shortest balloon that completely straddles the lesion should be used. Longer balloons may be necessary in the iliac, femoral, or popliteal area. The carotid, renal, celiac, and mesenteric vessels generally require shorter balloons; the kissing balloons are advisable when treating bifurcation vessels, such as in the aortoiliac region.

The balloon size is selected after measuring the diameter of the reference artery distal to the target lesion using digital subtraction angiography. Depending on the anatomy, balloon sizes can vary (Table 6.2) from 2 to 25 mm in diameter. The smaller balloons are generally used for dilating vessels below the knee. In many instances, e.g. in carotid intervention, a smaller coronary balloon (3–4 mm) is used to pre-dilate the stenosis prior to stent implantation and a larger balloon (5–6 mm) is used to post-dilate the stent. For post-dilating after endoluminal exclusion of AAA, larger balloons like the XXL™ (12–18 mm) (Meditech, Boston Scientific Corp.) and

the 'Impact' (20–25 mm) (Braun Medical, Inc., Bethlehem, PA) are used. Finally, placement or positioning of balloons should be accomplished under fluoroscopic guidance using road-mapping and anatomical landmarks.

Table 6.2   Balloon dilatation catheter sizes

Target vessel	Balloon diameter (mm)	Balloon length (cm)
Internal carotid	4–6	2
Common carotid	5–7	2–4
Subclavian	5–8	2–4
Vertebral	3–5	2
Abdominal aorta	10–26	2–4
Renal	4–8	2
Celiac and mesenteric	4–6	2
Common and external iliac	6–10	2–4
Common or superficial femoral	4–6	2–10
Popliteal	3–5	2–4
Tibial or peroneal	<4	2–4

Adjunctive endovascular tools

Stents

In spite of the significant improvements in technology, balloon angioplasty remains plagued with unacceptable restenosis rates for complex lesions, requiring re-intervention. Vascular stents were developed to deal with the major limitations of balloon angioplasty: unsuitability of some lesions, residual stenosis and failure due to dissection or recoil; and late failure due to restenosis. None of these problems, though, have been completely solved by using stents. Yet, increasing experience and clinical studies continue to shape our understanding of the role of stents. The concept of vascular stenting originated with Charles Dotter in 1969, but it did not become a clinical reality until the 1980s. Endovascular coils were first described in 1983 using a nitinol coil to support the arteries in an animal model.[7,8] These initial experiments were the catalyst for further development in stent to non-surgically treat vascular disease. Since that time, many stents have been designed and evaluated in both the animal laboratory and clinically. Stents have become the most important mechanical technique for percutaneous revascularization.

In 1985, Palmaz and colleagues[9] described preliminary results of balloon expandable stainless-steel stents in canine arteries. Of the 18 arteries stented, 22% developed thrombotic occlusion. It was in this small series that the need for adequate antithrombotic and antiplatelet therapy at the time of stent deployment was well recognized.[10]

Subsequently, an enhanced antiplatelet regimen is standard clinical practice for all stent procedures today and has had a pivotal effect in reducing the incidence of stent thrombosis. Although the rates today are low compared to early results, stent thrombosis is a disastrous complication with a high risk of ischemic sequelae and those who receive stents for high-risk indications should be considered for an even more intense antithrombotic regimen.

All stents share a common function of enlarging and supporting the vascular lumen and decreasing the incidence of complications and restenosis; however, they differ in their fundamental designs. There are two basic types of stents that differ considerably – balloon expandable and self-expanding. Balloon expandable are generally pre-mounted on a balloon and can be placed accurately, using less metal and greater radial strength. Balloon expandable stents, however, initially resist deformation, but can eventually yield under stress (compression) and become irreversibly deformed. Because of a risk of deformation or 'crush', balloon expandable stents are not recommended for use in extracranial carotid and femoropopliteal locations. Balloon expandable stents are best suited for accurate placement at the site of ostial lesions, such as in the renal, celiac, and mesenteric arteries and are ideal for ostial aortic arch lesions. Conversely, self-expanding stents, behave elastically and do not become deformed, however, they have less radial strength than balloon expandable stents to resist elastic recoil. In addition, they are less accurate than balloon expandable stents and have sharp strut ends.

Other stent characteristics include biocompatibility, which refers to the stents ability to resist thrombosis. The stent surface is an important determinant of its thrombogenic potential. All currently available stents are made of metal. The composition and characteristics of the stent itself have been shown to initiate a complex interaction between the blood components and the metallic surface of the stent. The nature of the flow in the vessel also determines the degree to which

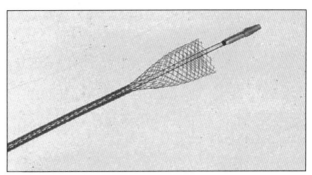

Figure 6.7
The self-expanding Wallstent (Boston Scientific, Watertown, MA).

blood elements interact with the structures on the vessel wall.[11] Special coatings have been added to metallic stents to provide a biologically inert barrier between the stent surface and the circulating blood to improve the hemodynamic compatibility as well as the biocompatibility of the stent.[12–15]

Flexibility is another very important stent characteristic because of tortuosity and angulation that is encountered in the periphery. The flexibility of a stent is the amount of force required to flex it a given amount, or the force with which it resists bending. A flexible stent can be deployed in a tortuous artery without altering its normal course, whereas an inflexible stent when deployed can straighten the vessel, forcing it to conform to its shape rather than vice versa. Most balloon expandable stents are less flexible than self-expanding stents. The least flexible stent is the non-articulated stent, such as the Palmaz® (Cordis, Inc., Johnson & Johnson, Warren, NJ) (Figure 6.6), and therefore the majority of the newer stent designs have articulations. Different types of stents are used for specific anatomical applications. The newer pre-mounted, low profile, balloon expandable stents such as the Megalink (Guidant Corp., Santa Clara, CA), and the Bridge (Medtronic AVE, Santa Rosa, CA) are well suited for iliac, renal, celiac and mesenteric arteries. The lower profile self-expanding nitinol stents such as the Wallstent (Figure 6.7), Memotherm Flexx™ stent (CR Bard, Covington, GA), Symphony (Meditech, Boston Scientific, Watertown, MA) or the 0.018 inch SMART™ (Cordis, Inc., Johnson & Johnson, Warren, NJ) are useful in extracranial carotid, subclavian, and iliac intervention. As far as femoral and popliteal stenting is concerned, the IntraCoil™ (IntraTherapeutics, Inc., St. Paul, MN) (Figure 6.8) has shown encouraging results.

Renal artery stenting has shown superior results to balloon angioplasty by avoiding recoil and dissection. In the early stages of renal artery stenting, the Palmaz® 15 mm, 20 mm, or 29 mm stent was mounted on a peripheral balloon that was from 5–8 mm in diameter and 20 mm in length. The current generation of stents are pre-mounted on a balloon that is lower in profile and specifically designed for renal artery stenting. They are available in over-the-wire or monorail

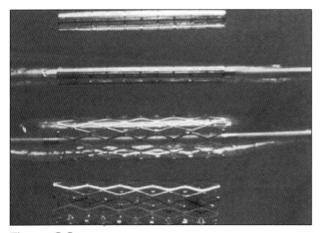

Figure 6.6
The non-articulated Palmaz® (Cordis, Inc., Johnson & Johnson, Warren, NJ) stent.

design. The Megalink stent (Guidant Corp., Santa Clara, CA) comes either mounted or unmounted. Pre-mounted stents come on a ViaTrax balloon that is 0.018 inch wire compatible and is available in the monorail design. The Bridge stent (Medtronic AVE, Santa Rosa, CA) and the Palmaz Corinthian IQ stent (Cordis, Inc., Johnson & Johnson, Warren, NJ) are pre-mounted over-the-wire systems.

Stent coatings are also being investigated as a way of decreasing neointimal hyperplasia. For reasons that remain unclear, some patients develop an aggressive neointimal hyperplasia, leaving restenosis as the main clinical obstacle of stent technology. In an attempt to deal with the shortcomings of stents, future strategies include:

- stents made of biological materials and stent grafts
- polymer-coated stents that are thrombo-resistant
- biodegradable stents that absorb, avoiding a permanent prosthetic implant
- drug-eluting stents
- radioactive stents or using adjunctive radiotherapy.

Endografts

The rapid evolution of transcatheter devices for the delivery of vascular prostheses has gotten non-surgical interventional radiologists and cardiologists involved in the vascular surgical arena. Endoluminal stent grafts and covered stents are now being used to treat aneurysmal and occlusive peripheral vascular disease.[16–21] Endoluminal grafts represent a joining of stent and surgical bypass technology. The bypass graft material is used to line or cover the stent. Although it is yet to be proven, it is believed that the covered stent may limit the ingrowth of intimal hyperplasia and improve long-term patency compared with balloon angioplasty and stenting.

Indications for using a covered stents include:

- arterial rupture
- arteriovenous fistulas
- arterial trauma
- aneurysms.

Possible indications for using covered stents:

- long occlusions or stenosis
- long dissections.

There are several covered stents in clinical investigation:

- the Cragg Endopro System or Passenger (Boston Scientific Corp., Natick, MA)
- the Hemobahn (WL Gore, Flagstaff, AZ)
- the Wallgraft™ (Boston Scientific Corp., Natick, MA)
- the JOSTENT® (JOMED International AB, Helsingberg, Sweden).

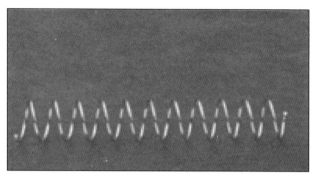

Figure 6.8
The IntraCoil™ (IntraTherapeutics, Inc., St. Paul, MN) stent.

For aneurysmal disease, stent grafts are used to exclude the aneurysm from the native circulation. All but one of the currently available endoluminal grafts used in the periphery are made of self-expanding nitinol. The JOSTENT® stent graft is a balloon expandable system (Figure 6.9). This system uses double-thin stainless steel with an expandable polytetrafluorethylene (PTFE) coating between the two layers. It ranges from 5 to 10 mm in diameter and from 28 to 58 cm long. It has been implanted successfully in iliac and femoral arteries.

The Wallgraft™, which is still in clinical trials in the United States, has been used to successfully treat iliac, femoral, and popliteal aneurysms and iliac artery occlusive disease.[22,23] It is composed of PET graft material covering a Wallstent (Figure 6.10). The UNISTEP™PLUS delivery system has a working length of 90 cm and is supplied with the Wallgraft™. The Wallgraft™ is available in diameters from 6 to 12 mm and lengths of 20, 30, 50, and 70 mm and the system accommodates a 0.035-inch guide wire.

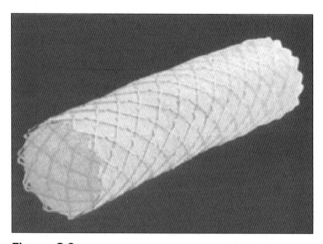

Figure 6.9
The JOSTENT™ (JOMED International AB, Helsingberg, Sweden) peripheral stent graft is stainless steel, balloon expandable and covered with an expandable PTFE coating.

The Viabahn (WL Gore, Flagstaff, Az) endoprosthesis showed, in an international trial, promising patency rates at 1 year when it was used to treat iliac and femoral occlusive disease.[24] This device is composed of a self-expanding nitinol stent, which is incorporated in an ultrathin polyester cover (Figure 6.11).

Endoluminal grafts for treating abdominal aortic aneurysms

Endoluminal grafts have also been gaining acceptance in the treatment of thoracic and abdominal aortic aneurysms. Initial experience with endovascular AAA exclusion was performed with straight, non-bifurcated devices.[25,26] The early prostheses were relatively inflexible and required a 24F internal diameter introducer sheath. However, few patients could be treated with the tube devices. Now, tube as well as bifurcated grafts are available; they are more flexible than the first-generation devices and are smaller in diameter. The stent grafts are either supported completely by a self-expanding stent or are unsupported, only stented at the attachment sites.

There are several systems being used around the world, but only four systems have been FDA approved for use in infrarenal AAAs in the United States: the Ancure™ Endograft System (Guidant EVT, Menlo Park, CA), the AneuRx™ device (Medtronic AVE, Santa Rosa, CA), the Excluder (WL Gore, Flagstaff, Az) and the Zenith (Cook Inc, Bloomington, IN). All of these systems are over-the-wire systems that require bilateral femoral artery access.

The Ancure™ is an unsupported single piece of woven Dacron (PET) fabric (Figure 6.12). The graft is bifurcated with no intragraft junctions. The device is delivered through a 24F introducer sheath; a 12F sheath is required to facilitate the deployment of the contralateral limb. The graft is attached by a series of hooks that are located at the proximal aortic end and at both the distal iliac limbs. The hooks are seated transmurally in the aorta and the iliac arteries and affixed by low-pressure balloon dilatation. Radiopaque markers are located on the body of the graft positioning and alignment.

The AneuRx™ device is a modular two-piece system (Figure 6.13) composed of a main bifurcation segment and a contralateral iliac limb. The graft is made of thin-walled woven polyester that is fully supported by a self-expanding nitinol exoskeleton. The main bifurcated body is delivered through a 21F or 22F sheath, and the contralateral limb requires a 16F sheath. The body of the graft has radiopaque markers for alignment, and positioning the attachment is accomplished by radial force.

Other stent graft systems being investigated include Vanguard (Boston Scientific Corp., Watertown, MA) and the

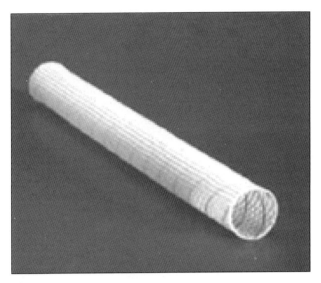

(a)

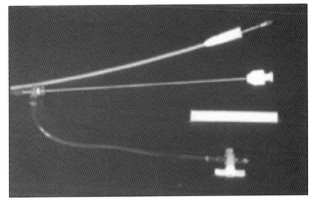

(b)

Figure 6.10
(a) The Wallgraft™ and (b) the UNISTEP™ PLUS system (Boston Scientific Corp., Watertown, MA).

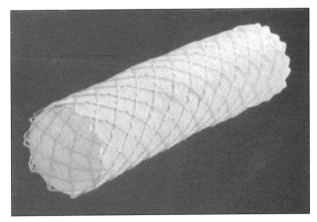

Figure 6.11
The Viabahn endoprosthesis.

Figure 6.12
The Ancure™ (Guidant EVT, Menlo Park, CA) bifurcated and tube graft systems.

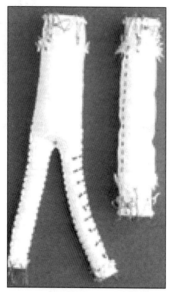

Figure 6.13
The AneuRx™ (Medtronic AVE, Santa Rosa, CA) modular stent graft system.

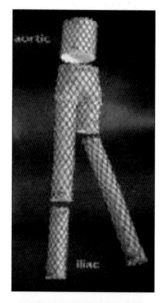

Figure 6.14
20F Bifurcated EXCLUDER Endoprosthesis (WL Gore, Inc., Sunnyvale, CA).

Figure 6.15
The Talent™ (Medtronic AVE) Bifurcated stent graft allows suprarenal fixation.

Figure 6.16
The Zennith™ (Cook, Inc., Bloomington, IN) AAA endovascular graft bifurcated three-component system.

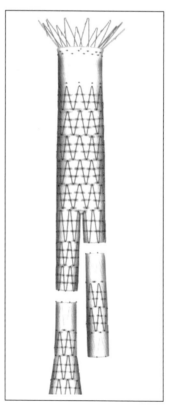
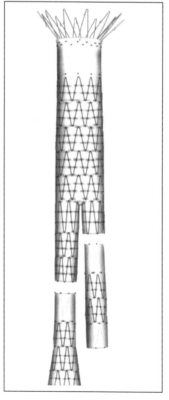
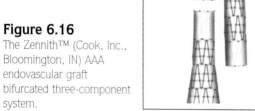

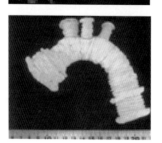

Figure 6.17
Inoue stent graft.

EXCLUDER Endoprosthesis (WL Gore, Inc., Sunnyvale, CA) (Figure 6.14). Two other systems, the Talent® (Medtronic, AVE, Santa Rosa, CA) (Figure 6.15) and the Zenith™ (Cook, Inc., Bloomington, IN) (Figure 6.16), incorporate a design feature that affixes the graft in a healthy segment in the suprarenal aorta with the proximal end of the graft left uncovered[27,28] are also being investigated.

Endovascular treatment of descending thoracic aortic aneurysms is limited.[29–31] Clinical trials are currently underway in the United States using the Thoracic EXCLUDER Endoprosthesis, (WL Gore, Inc., Sunnyvale, CA). The EXCLUDER stent graft is composed of a self-expanding nitinol stent exoskelton lined with an ultrathin-walled PTFE. Graft diameter ranges from 26 to 40 mm and is 7.5 to 20 cm in length. The grafts can be implanted singly or in multiples, according to the length of the diseased segment. In the initial feasibility trial,[30] there were no instances of deployment failure, conversion to open surgery, graft occlusion or paralysis. The Inoue stent graft (Figure 6.17) has been attempted in 52 patients, with a clinical success of 87.5% and a complications rate of 28%.

Mechanical thrombectomy devices

Mechanical thrombectomy has been developed to address a number of significant problems associated with chemical thrombolysis. These problems include bleeding complications, prolonged procedure times, the cost and the risk of the thrombolytic agent, and residual clot. A number of mechanical devices have been developed to disrupt and remove freshly formed thrombus from the circulation. There are three hydrodynamic devices that are currently in use. The AngioJet® Rheolytic™ Thrombectomy System (Possis Medical, Inc., Minneapolis, MN) is approved for use in the arterial circulation and is an over-the-wire system that uses high-velocity saline jets (Figure 6.18). Pulverized clot is then aspirated by the Bernoulli-effect induced vacuum at the tip of the catheter. Micro-fragments are discharged through the outflow lumen into the collecting bag.[32] Wagner et al., reported the success rate of 90% and low incidence of amputation and mortality with using rheolytic thrombectomy for treatment of limb ischemia.[33] Angiojet® catheters were first designed for coronary vessels 5F in size, requiring a 0.018-inch guide wire. The second-generation Angiojet Device (Xpeedior™) is 6F in size and 0.035-inch wire compatible; it offers greater effectiveness in thrombus removal and is better suited for treating larger peripheral vessels. There is now a 4F thrombectomy device (XPI™) that is available from the same manufacturer (Possis Medical, Inc., Minneapolis, MN).

The Hydrolyser™ Thrombectomy Catheter (Cordis Europa NV, Roden, the Netherlands) is another over-the-

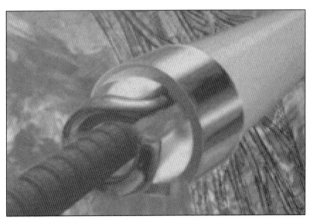

Figure 6.18
The AngioJet® Rheolytic™ thrombectomy catheter (Possis Medical, Inc., Minneapolis, MN).

wire hydrodynamic thrombectomy system. This system uses the Venturi principle for aspiration and removal of intravascular thrombus. Negative pressure pulls the thrombus into the heparinized saline stream, resulting in micro-fragments that are discharged through the outflow lumen into the collection bag. In reports from the European trials[34,35] this device may be of benefit in thrombus-containing lesions and in degenerated vein grafts.

The Oasis™ Thrombectomy System (Meditech, Boston Scientific Corp., Watertown, MA) is the third hydrodynamic system that has been used in the United States for obstructed renal dialysis grafts. It is also an over-the-wire system that works on the same Venturi principle as the Hydrolyser™.

There are several other systems that do not work on the hydrodynamic principle (Table 6.3). They include impeller devices, therapeutic ultrasound, clot-macerating, and suction devices, all of which all are designed to remove thrombus.

Debulking devices

There are a variety of debulking devices – including directional atherectomy, laser angioplasty, and rotational atherectomy – that have been investigated as a potential means of improving long-term patency and reducing restenosis. None, thus far, have clearly demonstrated an advantage for peripheral revascularization.[36–40] The technique of debulking (EVI™ Remote Endarterectomy Catheter, EndoVascular Instruments, Inc., Vancouver, WA) prior to endoluminal femoropopliteal bypass is now being tested as a means of increasing long-term patency rates after lower extremity bypass. In addition, atherectomy devices like the REDHA-CUT® (SherineMed, Irvine, CA), designed specifically to treat in-stent restenosis, are under investigation.

Table 6.3 Commercially available thrombectomy devices

Hydrodynamic devices
Thrombus is broken up by a high-velocity saline stream:
- Oasis™ Amplatz Thrombectomy System (Boston Scientific Corp., Natick, MA)
- AngioJet® Rheolytic™ Thrombectomy (Possis Medical Inc., Minneapolis, MN)
- Hydrolyser™ (Cordis Corp., Johnson & Johnson, Miami, FL)

Impeller devices
Thrombus is cleared by a rotating internal impeller:
- Clotbuster® Amplatz Thrombectomy (Microvena, White Bear Lake, MN)
- Straub Rotarex® (Straub Medical AG, Straubstrasse, CH-7323 Wangs)

Ultrasonic devices
Thrombus is dissolved with therapeutic ultrasound:
- Sonicath (Guidant Corp, St. Paul, MN)
- Acolysis System™ (Angiosonics, Morrisville, NC)

Suction devices
Thrombus is extracted by manual aspiration:
- Guardwire™ (PercuSurge, Sunnyvale, CA)

Clot-macerating devices
Thrombus is macerated:
- Arrow-Trotola® Thrombectomy Device (Arrow International, Inc., Reading, PA)
- Cragg Thrombolytic Brush™ (Micro Therapeutics, Inc., Irvine, CA)
- Gelbfish EndoVac (NeoVascular Technologies, New York, NY)
- PMT (Baxter, Irvine, CA)

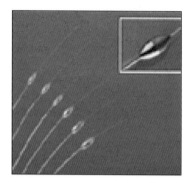

Figure 6.19
The Rotablator is an olive-shaped, nickel plated, brass burr. The leading edge of the burr is coated with 20–30 μm diamond chips.

Directional atherectomy

Directional atherectomy has the unique capability of resecting and retrieving intact atherosclerotic plaque. The atherectomy catheter (Atherotrack™, Mallinckrodt Inc., St. Louis, MO) is a coaxial multi-lumen catheter designed for percutaneous resection of atheromatous material. It consists of a catheter shaft, equipped distally with a balloon mounted opposite a housing unit and proximally with a central adapter and a battery-operated motor drive unit. The distal housing contains a rigid cutter within an open window. The balloon is used to support the rigid cutter housing and push the plaque into the housing window. A lever on the motor drive unit allows the operator to activate and slowly advance the cutter through the lesion as it rotates at 2000 rpm. Excised atheroma is stored in a distal nose cone collection chamber. Peripheral catheters are 7–11F, with working diameters of 5.3–9.7 mm. Directional atherectomy may be useful to debulk focal or eccentric stenosis, but there is no clear-cut long-term improvement over balloon angioplasty alone.

Rotational atherectomy

The Rotablator system (Boston Scientific, Northwest, Redmond, WA) consists of a reusable console that controls the rotational speed of an olive-shaped, nickel-plated, brass burr, which is coated on its leading edge with 20–30 μm diamond chips and is bonded to a flexible drive shaft (Figure 6.19). The rotating burr is regulated by a compressed air or nitrogen driven turbine. The rotating burr (160 000–170 000 rpm) is cooled by a saline flush as it is slowly advanced through a stenosis. Rotational atherectomy can achieve a lumen that is 90% of the selected burr size. It has not, however, been demonstrated to have an advantage for iliac and superficial femoral artery lesions but may be useful to debulk calcified lesions and branch stenosis in the smaller popliteal and tibioperoneal arteries.

Excimer laser ablation

The Excimer laser energy (Spectranetics Corp., Colorado Springs, CO) emits a pulsed, ultraviolet light at 308 nm. Ablation of inorganic material is achieved by photochemical mechanisms that involve the breakdown of molecular bonds without generating heat.[41] The role of laser angioplasty in peripheral revascularization is still investigational in the United States. Preliminary results of a phase I clinical trial (Laser Angioplasty for Critical Ischemia) indicate that excimer laser angioplasty was safe and feasible in popliteal occlusive disease with a 3-month patency rate of 88%.[42] Laser angioplasty may also be useful in total occlusions that are refractory to other techniques.

Radiation therapy

Low-dose radiation has been suggested to inhibit intimal hyperplasia. Recent clinical data indicate that peripheral vascular brachytherapy may be effective in the prevention of restenosis.[43]

The double-lumen PARIS Centering catheter (Guidant Corp., Santa Clara, CA) with multiple segmented centering balloons is used to deliver gamma radiation (^{192}Ir) to the target site. Radioactive stents with low-activity beta-emitters, e.g. phosphorus (^{32}P), have been suggested as a method of treatment for the larger peripheral vessels. Also, balloons filled with different isotopes, such as rhenium (^{188}Re or ^{186}Re), have been suggested as a way of delivering radiation to the vessel. All of these methods, however, are still under investigation. Future studies will focus on isotope selection, dosing strategies, and optimal stent designs for delivery of radiation.

Percutaneous closure devices

A variety of devices are available for arterial hemostasis after sheath removal. They include mechanical clamp (Compressar, Instrumedix, Hillsboro, OR), inflatable pressure device, the FemoStop™ (USCI, Billerica, MA), extravascular collagen plug (VasoSeal™ Datascope® Corporation, Montvale, NJ), intravascular anchor and collagen plug (St Jude Medical, Daig Division, Minnetonka, MN), bio-absorbable pledgets (Duet™ Thrombin, Vascular Solutions, Minneapolis, MN), and vessel suturing device (Perclose®, Abbott Corp., Redwood City, CA) deployed through specifically designed catheters.

The device of choice is the Prostar XL® Percutaneous Vascular Surgery (PVS) device (Perclose®, Inc., Menlo Park, CA). It is available in 6F, 8F, or 10F catheter systems and designed for percutaneous deployment of surgical sutures to common femoral artery puncture site. The 10F Perclose® has been used to repair large-bore sheath sites (16F) after endoluminal repair of AAAs.[44-46] The 10F device is advanced into the femoral artery over a 0.035-inch guide wire until adequate blood marking is achieved through the dedicated marker lumen, indicating the sutures and needles are within the vessel lumen (Figure 6.20a). Four needles are then deployed and sutures are removed from the hub (Figure 6.20b). The upper and lower sets of sutures are identified and remain untied. The device is then partially backed out of the femoral artery and a 0.035-inch guide wire is reinserted through the guide-wire port. The device is then removed and an 11F sheath is reintroduced over the guide wire. The sheath is then upsized to 16F. After completion of the procedure, the sutures are tied with a sliding knot and the knot pusher is used to assure approximation of the knot to the vessel wall for adequate hemostasis (Figure 6.20c). The subcutaneous tissues are then infiltrated with 1% lidocaine with epinephrine and the incision edges are approximated with adhesive steri-strips. An arterial tamper device may or may not be required.

Vascular occlusion devices

There are several types of vascular occlusion coils (Toronado™ Embolization Coils and Microcoils™, Gianturco-Grifka Vascular Occlusion Device, Cook, Inc., Bloomington, IN) that are used to occlude selective vessel supply to arteriovenous malformations, intrasaccular pseudo-aneurysms,[47] or collateral vessel branch flow feeding an aneurysmal sac. Coil embolization has successfully treated pulmonary artery branch rupture after Swan–Ganz catheterization.[48] Coil embolization has become a common procedure performed as an adjunct prior to endoluminal AAA repair, or after, to remedy collateral branch flow.[49] Coils (Figure 6.21) or embolization particles are deployed percutaneously through diagnostic catheters that are coated to prevent friction. Coils range from 2 to 14 cm in length with diameters from 0.018 to 0.038 inch. Platinum coils with synthetic fibers incorporated help to maximize thrombogenicity. The microcoil design permits delivery into the target vessel by saline flush or by push technique.

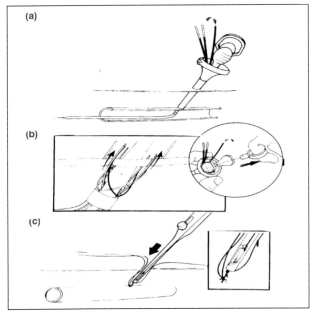

Figure 6.20
Perclose®, Inc., Abbott Corp., Redwood City, CA is a surgical suture method of arteriotomy closure. For explanation of the procedure (a–c), see text.

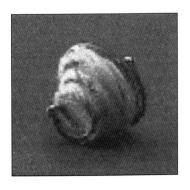

Figure 6.21
Fibered platinum embolization coil.

Vascular snares

Vascular snares are used to retrieve foreign objects from the vasculature. These include fractured catheters, guide wires, balloons, embolic coils, undeployed stents, or other foreign bodies. They are also used to manipulate or reposition catheters or to facilitate contralateral guide-wire pull-through during endoluminal AAA repair with the Ancure stent graft. Snare loops come in various sizes (2–35 mm), and loop size (Figure 6.22), depends on the size and the obstacle being snared.

Future developments remain focused on the issue of restenosis and neo-intimal hyperplasia. The field of 'smart' stents, which refers to drug-eluting and thrombo-resistent stents and stent grafts will have an important role in defining the future course of endovascular therapy. New opportunities being explored are those that would influence local vascular biology, such as cell-seeding, genes, and non-reactive polymer carriers that elicit optimal biological effects.

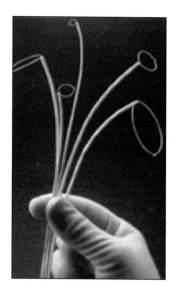

Figure 6.22
Loop snares come in various loop sizes for retrieval of foreign bodies from the circulation.

References

1 Dotter CT, Judkins MP. Transluminal treatment of arteriosclerotic obstruction: description of a new technique and preliminary results of its application. *Circulation* 1964; **30**: 654–70.

2 Biamino G, Schofer J, Tübler T, Schulter M. A new vascular approach to chronic total occlusions of the superficial femoral artery [abstract]. International Congress on Endovascular Interventions, 2000.

3 Beyer-Enke SA, Zeitler E. When to stop angioplasty in the peripheral vessels (arteries). *J Invas Cardiol* 1998; **10**(7): 425–31.

4 Roubin GS, Mehran R, Diethrich EB et al. Carotid stent-supported angioplasty with distal neuroprotection using the Guardwire™: 30-day results from the carotid angioplasty free emboli (CAFÉ-USA) trial. *J Am Coll Cardiol* 2001; **37** (suppl A): 829.

5 Diethrich EB, Rodriguez-Lopez J, Ramaiah V, Olsen D. Comparison of carotid stenting with and without cerebral protection versus carotid endarterectomy in a single center experience. *J Am Coll Cardiol* 2001; **37**(suppl A): 829.

6 Henry M, Klonaris C, Amor M et al. Stent supported carotid angioplasty. The beneficial effect of cerebral protection. *J Am Coll Cardiol* 2001; **37** (suppl A): 829.

7 Dotter CT, Buschmann PAC, Mckinney MK, Rösch J. Transluminal expandable nitinol coils stent grafting: preliminary report. *Radiology* 1983; **147**: 259–60.

8 Cragg A, Lund G, Rysavy J et al. Non-surgical placement of arterial endoprosthesis: a new technique using nitinol wire. *Radiology* 1983; **147**: 261–3.

9 Palmaz JC, Sibbit RR, Reuter SR et al. Expandable intraluminal graft: a preliminary study. *Radiology* 1985; **156**: 73–7.

10 Palmaz JC, Sibbit RR, Tio FO et al. Expandable intraluminal graft: a feasibility study. *Surgery* 1986; **99**: 199–205.

11 Williams DF, Surface interactions. In: Sigwart U (ed.), *Endoluminal stenting*. London: WB Saunders, 1996: 45–51.

12 Lu L, Jones MW. Diamond-like carbon as biological compatible material for cell culture and medical applications. *Bio Med Mat Engin* 1993; **3**: 223–8.

13 Amon M, Bolz A, Schaldach M. Improvement in stenting therapy with a silicon carbide coated tantalum stent. *J Mater Sci Mater Med* 1996; **7**: 273–8.

14 Beythien C, Gutensohn K, Kühnl P et al. Influence of 'diamond-like' and gold coating on platelet activation: a flow cytometry analysis in a pulsed floating model [abstract]. *J Am Coll Cardiol* 1998; **31** (suppl): 413A.

15 Aggarwal RK, Ireland DC, Ragheb A et al. Reduction in thrombogenicity of polymer-coated stents by immobilization of platelet targeted urokinase [abstract]. *Eur J Cardiol* 1996; **17** (suppl): 177.

16 Cragg AH, Dake MD. Percutaneous femoropopliteal graft placement. *J Vasc Interv Radiol* 1993; **4**: 445–63.

17 Parodi JC. Endovascular repair of abdominal aortic aneurysms and other arterial lesions. *J Vasc Surg* 1995; **21**: 549–57.

18 Diethrich EB, Papazoglou CO. Endoluminal grafting for aneurysmal and occlusive disease in the superficial femoral artery: early experience. *J Endovasc Surg* 1995; **2**: 225–39.

19 Marin ML, Veith FJ, Cynamon J et al. Transfemoral endovascular stent graft treatment of aortoiliac and femoropopliteal occlusive disease for limb salvage. *Am J Surg* 1994; **168**: 156–62.

20 Bergeron P. Stenting and endoluminal grafting of femoral and popliteal arteries. *J Endovasc Surg* 1995; **2**: 197–8.

21 Henry M, Amor M, Cragg A et al. Occlusive and aneurysmal peripheral arterial disease: assessment of a stent graft system. *Radiology* 1996; **201**: 717–24.

22 Howell MH, Krajcer ZK, Diethrich E et al. Percutaneous treatment of traumatic arterial injuries with the Wallgraft endoprosthesis. *J Am Coll Cardiol* 2001; **37** (suppl A): 1257.

23   Krajcer Z, Sioco G, Reynolds T. Comparison of Wallgraft™ and Wallstent for treatment of complex iliac artery stenosis and occlusion. *Tex Heart Inst J* 1997; **24**: 193–9.

24   Lammer J, Becker GJ, Cejna M et al. A prospective study of a transluminally placed self-expanding endoprosthesis (Hemobahn Endoprosthesis) for the treatment of peripheral arterial obstructions. *Cardio Vasc Interv Radiol* 1999; **22**(suppl 2): S134.

25   Parodi JC, Palmaz JC, Barone HD. Transfemoral intraluminal graft implantation for abdominal aortic aneurysms. *Ann Vasc Surg* 1991; **5**(6):491–9.

26   Lazarus HM. Endovascular grafting technique in the treatment of infrarenal abdominal aortic aneurysm. *Surg Clin North Am* 1992; **72**(4): 959–68.

27   Beebe HG, Blum U. Experience with the Meadox Vanguard Endovascular Graft. In: Yao JST, Pierce WH (eds), *Techniques in vascular and endovascular surgery*. New York: McGraw-Hill/Appleton and Lange, 1998: 421–32.

28   Taheri SA, Leonhardt HJ, Greenan T. The Talent™ Endoluminal Graft Placement System. In: Yao JST, Pierce WH (eds), *Techniques in vascular and endovascular surgery*. New York: McGraw-Hill/Appleton and Lange, 1998: 433–45.

29   Dake M, Semba C, Kee S et al. Endografts for the treatment of descending thoracic aortic aneurysm: results of the first 150 procedures. *J Endovasc Surg* 1999; **6**: 189.

30   Shim WH, Lee B-K, Yoon Y-S et al. Endovascular stent graft implantation for descending thoracic aortic dissection and aneurysm. *J Am Coll Cardiol* 2001; **37** (suppl):1230.

31   Dake MD. Thoracic Excluder: initial results of a feasibility study for stent-graft treatment of descending thoracic aortic aneurysms. 1999 Current Issues and New Techniques in Interventional Radiology.

32   Silva TA, Ramee SR, Collins TJ et al. Rheolytic thrombectomy in the treatment of acute limb-threatening ischemia: immediate results and six-month follow-up of the multi-center AngioJet registry. Possis peripheral Angiojet study investigators. *Cathet Cardiovasc Diag* 1998; **45**: 386–92.

33   Wagner HY, Muller-Hulsbeck S et al. Rapid thrombectomy with hydrodynamic catheter: results from a prospective multi-center trial. *Radiology* 1997; **205**: 675–81.

34   Henry M, Amor M, Henry I et al. The Hydrolyser thrombectomy catheter: a single-center experience. *J Endovasc Surg* 1998; **5**: 24–31.

35   van Ommen VG, van den Bos AA, Pieper M et al. Removal of thrombus from aortocoronary bypass grafts and coronary arteries using the 6F Hydrolyser. *Am J Cardiol* 1997; **79**: 1012–16.

36   Simpson JB, Selmon MR, Robertson GC et al. Transluminal atherectomy for occlusive peripheral vascular disease. *Am J Cardiol* 1988; **61**: 96G–101G.

37   Graor RA, Whitlow PL. Transluminal atherectomy for occlusive peripheral vascular disease. *J Am Coll Cardiol* 1990; 15: 1551–8.

38   Zacca NM, Raizner AE, Noon GP. Treatment of symptomatic peripheral atherosclerotic disease with a rotational atherectomy device. *Am J Cardiol* 1989; **63**: 77–80.

39   Isner JM, Rosenfield K. Redefining the treatment of peripheral artery disease. *Circulation* 1993; **88**: 1534–57.

40   Isner JM, Pieczek A, Rosenfield K. Untreated gangrene in patients with peripheral artery disease. *Circulation* 1994; **89**: 482–3.

41   Grundfest WS, Segalowitz J, Laudenslager J et al. The physical and biological basis for laser angioplasty: In: Litvack F (ed.), *Coronary laser angioplasty*. Oxford: Blackwell Scientific Publications, 1992.

42   Biamino G. Laser recanalization and debulking technique in popliteal and tibial occlusive disease [abstract]. International Congress on Endovascular Interventions, 1999.

43   Waksman R, Crocker IA, Kikeri D et al. Long-term results of endovascular radiation therapy for prevention of restenosis in the peripheral vascular system. *Circulation* 1996; **94**: 8, I-300: 1745.

44   Haas P, Krajcer Z, Diethrich E. Closure of large percutaneous access sites using the Prostar XL percutaneous vascular surgery device. *J Endovasc Surg* 1999; **6**: 168–70.

45   Krajcer Z, Howell M. A novel technique using the percutaneous vascular surgery device to close the 22 French femoral artery entry site used for percutaneous abdominal aortic aneurysm exclusion. *Catheter Cardiovasc Intervent* 2000; **50**: 356–60.

46   Krajcer Z, Howell M, Villareal R. Percutaneous access and closure of femoral artery access sites associated with endoluminal repair of abdominal aortic aneurysms. *J Endovasc Ther* 2001; **8**: 68–74.

47   Gottwalles Y, Wunschel-Joseph, Janssen M. Coil embolization treatment in pulmonary artery branch rupture during Swan Ganz catheterization. *Cardiovasc Intervent Radiol* 2000; **23**(6): 477–9.

48   Bush RL, Lin PH, Dodson TF et al. Endoluminal stent placement and coil embolization for the management of carotid artery pseudoaneurysms. *J Endovasc Ther* 2001; **8**: 53–61.

49   Halloul Z, Büger T, Grote R et al. Sequential coil embolization of bilateral internal iliac aneurysms prior to endovascular abdominal aortic aneurysm repair. *J Endovasc Ther* 2001; **8**: 87–92.

7

The endovascular interventional suite

Zvonimir Krajcer and Kathryn Dougherty

Introduction

Endovascular interventions have enjoyed an explosive growth in popularity since they were first introduced by Andreas Gruentzig in 1977.[1] The current state of endoluminal technology continues to alter therapeutic algorithms in favor of endovascular techniques, and they have already replaced 10–15% of vascular operations.[2,3] It is likely that the impact of reimbursement for medical care will stimulate even more interest, adding new endovascular procedures that involve

stents and stent grafts and will supplant an additional 40–70% of traditional vascular operations.[2,3] All these treatments involve the use of catheters, balloons, wires and imaging modalities, including digital subtraction angiography, road mapping and three-dimensional reconstruction. Therefore, a variety of factors must be considered when designing an endovascular surgical suite that can extend the limits of performance and clinical utility and accommodate today's managed-care environment.

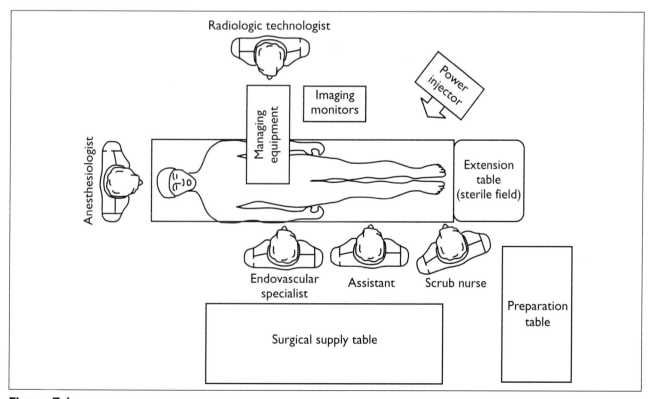

Figure 7.1
The endovascular suite set-up.

An endovascular suite must support full operative sterile conditions, particularly for procedures like endoluminal grafting that incorporate prosthetic materials. Procedures involving stents or stent–grafts can potentially result in catastrophic infections.[4–6] Additionally, if an endovascular intervention should require conversion to a surgical intervention, complete sterility is imperative to ensure patient safety and avoid unacceptable contamination. Furthermore, the interventional suite must be large enough to accommodate the equipment and staff needed if it were necessary to convert from an endovascular to a surgical procedure (Figure 7.1).[7–9]

Design of the procedure room

A number of essential design elements need to be considered that are beyond those of a traditional operating room or angiographic suite. First, in order to comfortably accommodate the core equipment, the suite should be at least 1000 square feet,[10] with 650 square feet devoted to procedure area (Figure 7.2) and 350 to the control/observation area (Figure 7.3). The ceiling height should be at least 10 feet[8] and the walls should be shielded with 1 mm of lead to provide radiation protection for personnel in surrounding work areas. Observation windows and doors should also be lead-treated.

Electrical supply and regulatory requirements are also a primary consideration. The suite should be equipped with emergency power outlets located on the operating table and all four walls of the suite. The endovascular suite should have compressed air, oxygen and suction outlets at both ends of the operating table. The operating table should be radiolucent, minimize radiation exposure and provide exceptional visualization. Communications capabilities should include in-room intercoms, video input and output links to a high-bandwidth image routing network, and video/audio recording.

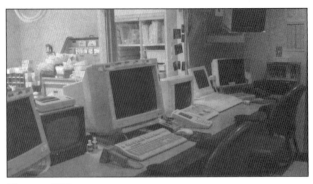

Figure 7.3
A separate control room/observation area protected with lead shielding allows staff members to process and record procedural data with out interrupting the intervention.

Since typical angiography suites and cardiac catheterization suites are primarily designed for catheter-based procedures, they do not meet operating room requirements. Until recently, there was no need to change the semi-sterile environment; however, because of potential need for surgical intervention when endovascular intervention has failed, the endovascular suite should be designed to accommodate strict sterile conditions. These should include laminar or negative airflow, seamless floors, and ceilings and walls that can be washed. It should also have multiple in-wall X-ray view boxes (Figure 7.4). The suite should be equipped with limited in-room storage, comprising stainless steel cabinets with glass doors. In addition, the suite should have operating room-certified, shatterproof lighting that allows low, medium and ultra-bright capabilities. Individual xenon head-lamps are also necessary for surgical procedures. Vascular instrumentation should be readily available in the room, as well as adequate space for the anesthesiologists, anesthesia equipment, circulators and instrument tables (Figure 7.1). The room should have controlled access and outside indicators to specify acti-

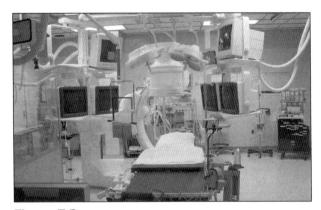

Figure 7.2
The endovascular suite must be large enough to accommodate all of the equipment needed to perform complex interventions.

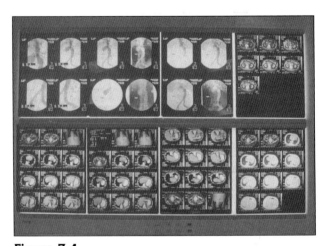

Figure 7.4
Multiple in-wall view box displays necessary diagnostic films readily available for review during the procedures.

vation of the fluoroscopic equipment, so that inadvertent radiation exposure is prevented.

Fluoroscopy equipment

The success of endovascular procedures is dependent on high-quality imaging equipment with high-resolution and high-frequency monitors that are designed to provide easy access to the patients.[7,8] Additional high-resolution monitors posi-

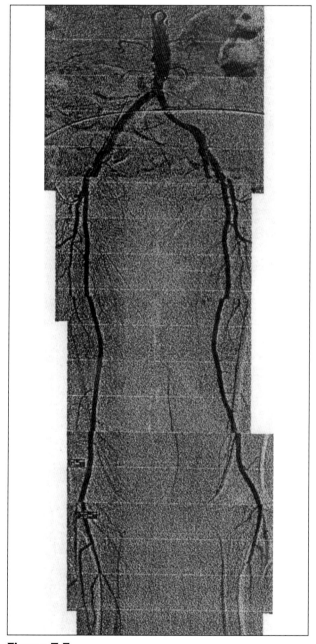

Figure 7.5
Abdominal angiography and ilio-femoral run-off using the bolus chase technique.

tioned for viewing on both sides of the operating table are essential (Figure 7.2). This allows visualization from multiple angles and/or access sites, either by surgical cut-down or percutaneously in the right or left femoral or right or left brachial vessels.

The operating table should be able to rotate on its center axis by 180° to allow antegrade, as well as retrograde, panning. In addition, the table should be motor-driven to allow remote high-speed bolus-chase digital peripheral studies, as well as digital stepping angiography (Figure 7.5). This allows the use of automated head-to-toe angiographic coverage with minimal contrast usage and optimal vessel opacification. The bolus-chase technique prevents dense contrast visualization in the proximal vessels with poor contrast visualization in the distal vessels. Digital unsubtracted and subtracted angiography is a very useful modality when evaluating intracranial vascular problems (Figure 7.6). In addition, this digital feature is extremely valuable when using other contrast agents such as CO_2 or gadolinium in patients who might be at increased risk for 'traditional' iodinated contrast angiography. CO_2 and gadolinium provide less contrast than iodinated (nephrotoxic) agents, but are indicated for patients with chronic renal insufficiency or congestive heart failure.

The fluoroscopy system can be single or bi-plane. Most currently used systems for peripheral vascular interventions are single-plane. They are either fixed or mobile. Unless a large number of pediatric procedures are to be performed, single-plane systems are adequate and are considerably less expensive. Fixed systems also use less radiation and less contrast than mobile systems. They provide automatic functions that include collimator adjustments, extended dynamic range filtering and injection triggering. Other advantages include excellent image quality (even during rapid panning), an adjustable source-to-intensifier distance and processing that results in immediate image availability. Fixed systems also allow image-review functions to be directly accessible from hand-held, in-room remote controls. This option can streamline procedures and minimize delays while archiving angiographic information. Post-processing, laser filming and digital image archiving is usually performed at the system console in the control/observation bay area.

Imaging techniques

Proper positioning of the equipment and good radiographic imaging technique are crucial to the safety and success of endovascular procedures. Calibrated marker catheters and a graduated marker tape are useful safety measures when deploying stents and stent–grafts. The imaging system used for endovascular procedures should also have a 12-inch or 16-inch image intensifier. Standard 7- or 9-inch image intensifiers that are used in the cardiac catheterization laboratories are inadequate for most endovascular procedures. During

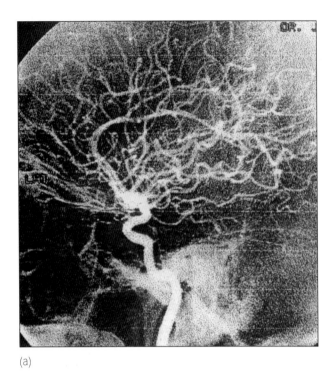

(a)

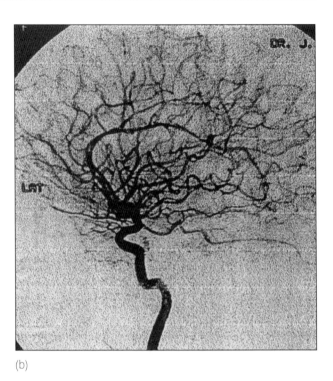

(b)

Figure 7.6
Digital unsubtracted (a) and subtracted (b) angiography of the intracranial anatomy from the left common carotid artery in the lateral projection.

endovascular abdominal aortic aneurysm repair, it is important that the entire field of endograft deployment can be seen on a single view, so the entire endograft can be seen as it is deployed (Figure 7.7).

'Road mapping' is an imaging technique that allows superimposition of a real-life fluoroscopy image on a previously recorded angiographic image. These images are retained as a road map and used to facilitate the positioning of interventional devices. They are also helpful to compare anatomy before and after intervention, and to perform on-line measurement of severity of stenosis. This technique is extremely beneficial when negotiating wires and catheters through tortuous vessels and when there is concern about contrast-induced renal dysfunction.

High-speed rotation is another useful imaging technique. This is especially helpful when evaluating the degree of stenosis and eccentricity of the vasculature, as in the extracranial carotid arteries. It can also be used effectively to evaluate the thoracic and abdominal aorta, and the iliac and femoral arteries. Like all digital images, however, the drawback of road mapping and high-speed rotation is that any motion of the vascular structures detracts from the quality of the image. Primary sources of movement include cardiac, diaphragmatic, ureteric, and interstitial. Pain is also a primary cause of movement of the patients and is commonly seen with high-osmolality contrast agents. Adequate sedation of patients and the use of lower-osmolality radiographic dyes can help reduce the motion artifact.

Another type of artifact is parallax, which is also exaggerated by movement. Because the X-ray beam is shaped like a cone, radial elongation or distortion of the structures occurs at the edges of the field, and this is called parallax. There is no distortion in the center of the field, but if the position changes from the road map, relative distances change dramatically, increasing parallax artifact. To avoid image artifact caused by parallax, it is important for the patient and the table to remain stationary during the crucial part of the intervention. Therefore, for precise placement of stents or stent–grafts, no movement should occur once the road map has been obtained and no measurements attempted in the outer 20% of the field of view.[10]

A variety of post-processing features are employed to clean images that have been degraded by patient movement, and these include pixel shifting, landmarking, on-screen measurements, annotation and image zooming. The advent of digital subtraction techniques has greatly enhanced visualization (Figure 7.6). Digital subtraction is a feature that eliminates static elements (bones and other structures) from the initial image contrast injection, allowing a clear image of the vessels.

Finally, angiography performed in multiple orthogonal views is paramount to the procedures, particularly in regions of vascular bifurcations or when bone edges overlie the area of interest. A thorough understanding of the principles of parallax, positioning and projections are instrumental when determining the precise placement of endovascular devices.

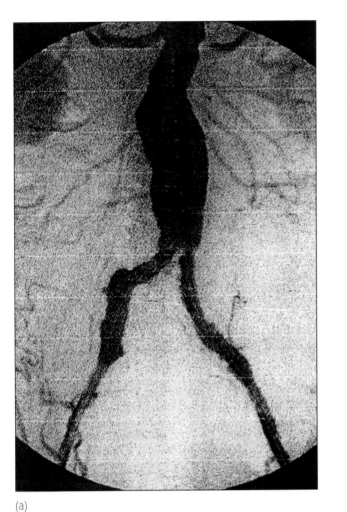

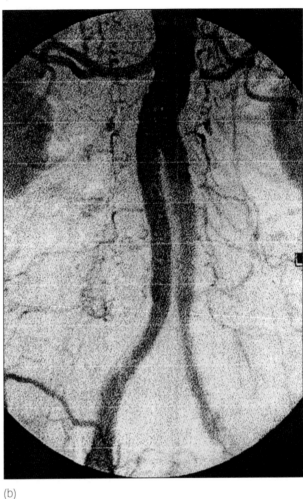

(a)   (b)

Figure 7.7
Using a 16-inch image intensifier, abdominal aortogram in the AP projection before and after aneurysm exclusion.

Record management and archiving

There continues to be a proliferation of digital technologies within the cardiovascular field. Despite continued efforts to move from cine film to all-digital approaches, there has to date not been adequate means for exchanging images between institutions in digital formats.

The American College of Cardiology, the American College of Radiology and the National Electrical Manufacturers' Association have combined efforts to implement standards for storing and retrieving digital images on recordable compact disks, as the replacement for cine-angiographic film as the dominant archival medium.[11,12] A refined standard, 'Digital Imaging and Communications in Medicine' (DICOM), was developed, and uses industry standard networking protocols, specifying mechanisms for image storage on removable media and added additional imaging modalities. DICOM is the key component addressed within the broader concept of comput-

erized patient records. Industries must develop software based on user-friendly operating systems (MacOS, Windows 95, and Windows NT) that are compatible with all major vendors so that images can be stored, manipulated and shared.

Digital images require a large hard disk for storage, while post-processing information is outputted to a compact disk and/or laser printer. This technology eliminates the need for wet processing. In fact, digital systems have largely replaced the need for videotape recorders and 'frame grabbers' (single-frame images).

Radiation safety and training

With the advent of stents and endoluminal grafts and other endovascular procedures, the time needed for fluoroscopy has significantly increased. High-quality, fixed imaging systems need high-heat-capacity tubes to minimize the need for heat-cooling delays that often occur with long imaging times.

Furthermore, there is an even greater need for significant lead shielding to ensure the safety of patients and healthcare personnel. Mechanisms to reduce radiation exposure can be divided into those directed at reducing the output of the X-ray unit and those designed to limit the amount of radiation contacting the interventionalist and the staff. Staff members should be properly trained in radiation safety principles, equipment, potential complications and trouble-shooting. Staff members should be able to demonstrate their understanding of the basic concepts of medical imaging and the use of newer imaging systems.

The most important method to reduce scatter radiation is to minimize patient dose and the ultimate source of scatter to the operator.[13–15] Staff members should monitor the judicious use of fluoroscopy and terminate imaging runs as soon as relevant information has been obtained. Other key elements to reduce radiation exposure include collimation, pulsed fluoroscopy, imaging acquisition, frame rates and last image hold. During long procedures the operator and staff members should stand as far back from the unit as possible to take advantage of the fact that radiation exposure decreases exponentially with increased distance from the source.

Lead shielding requirements are dictated by stringent radiation safety regulations. Protective lead aprons, thyroid shields, leaded glass screens and leaded eye glasses with side shields are the most effective way to reduce radiation exposure. The suite itself must be lead-lined, including the doors, glass and walls,[13–15] and all personnel in the room should wear film badges that detect radiation exposure.

Conclusion

Endovascular procedures have already changed the way arterial and venous diseases are managed. It is likely that these techniques will have an even greater influence in the future. Transluminal angioplasty has already proven to be a helpful adjunct to arterial reconstructive surgery rather than a competitive modality. It can be used to treat lesions that produce symptoms insufficient to justify open surgery and to simplify or help manage complicated or difficult cases.[16,17]

Endovascular intervention is the fastest growing area of vascular medicine and requires dedication on the part of practitioners. Endovascular techniques require specialized skills and training in peripheral vascular diseases, diagnostic angiography, interventional techniques and therapeutic alternatives. The challenge to the practitioner is intensified by the continual introduction of new products and methods. The establishment of a modern endovascular suite arranged in an ergonomically devised fashion is crucial to remaining in the forefront of developments in the treatment of patients with arterial and venous disorders.

References

1   Gruentzig AR. Transluminal dilatation of coronary artery stenosis. *Lancet* 1978; **1**: 263.

2   Veith FJ. Presidential address: Charles Darwin and vascular surgery. *J Vasc Surg* 1997; **25**: 12–18.

3   Veith FJ, Ohki T. Endovascular intervention and its impact on vascular practice: current and future perspective. In: Criado FJ, ed. *Endovascular Intervention: Basic Concepts and Techniques.* Armonk, NY: Futura Publishing Co., 1999: 181–6.

4   Heikkinen L, Valtonen M, Lepantalo M et al. Infrarenal endoluminal bifurcated stent graft infected with Listeria monocytogenes. *J Vasc Surg* 1999; **29**: 554–6.

5   Deitch JS, Hansen KJ, Regan JD et al. Infected renal artery pseudoaneurysm and mycotic aortic aneurysm after percutaneous transluminal renal angioplasty and stent placement in a patient with a solitary kidney. *J Vasc Surg* 1998; **28**: 340–344.

6   Weinberg DJ, Cronin DW, Baker AG Jr. Infected iliac pseudoaneurysms after uncomplicated percutaneous balloon angioplasty and (Palmaz) stent insertion: a case report and literature review *J Vasc Surg* 1996; **23**: 162–6.

7   Hodgson KJ, Mattos MA, Summer DS. Angiography in the operating room: equipment, catheter skills, and safety issues. In: Yao JS, Pearce WH, eds. *Techniques in Vascular and Endovascular Surgery.* East Norwalk, CT: Appleton and Lange, 1998: 25–45.

8   Queral LA. Operating room design for the future. In: Yao JS, Pearce WH, eds. T*echniques in Vascular and Endovascular Surgery.* East Norwalk, CT: Appleton and Lange; 1998: 1–5.

9   Diethrich EB. Endovascular suite design: an integrated approach for optimal interventional performance. In: Criado FJ, ed. E*ndovascular Intervention: Basic Concepts and Techniques.* Armonk, NY: Futura Publishing Co. 1999: 5–16.

10   Fillinger MF, Weaver JB. Imaging equipment and techniques for optimal intraoperative imaging during endovascular interventions. *Semin Vasc Surg* 1999; **12**: 315–26.

11   ACC/ACR/NEMA Ad Hoc Group. American College of Cardiology, American College of Radiology, and industry develop standards for digital transfer of angiographic images. *J Am Coll Cardiol* 1995; **25**: 800.

12   Elion J, Petrocelli R. DICOM Structured reporting: the future is now. *Cath Lab Digest* 2001; **9**: 66–8.

13   *Implementation of the principle of as low as reasonable achievable (ALARA) for medical and dental personnel.* NCRP Report No. 107. Bethesda, MD: National Council on Radiation Protection and Measurements, 1990.

14   Lowe FC, Auster M, Beck TJ et al. Monitoring radiation exposure to medical personnel during percutaneous nephrolithotomy. *Urology* 1986; **28**: 221–6.

15   Bush WH, Jones D, Brannen GE. Radiation dose to personnel during percutaneous renal calculus removal. *Am J Radiol* 1985; **145**: 1261–4.

16   Veith FJ, Gupta SK, Samson RH et al. Progress in limb salvage by reconstructive arterial surgery combined with new or improved adjunctive procedure. *Ann Surg* 1981; **212**: 386.

17   Brewster DC, Cambria RP, Darling RC et al. Long-term results after combined iliac balloon angioplasty and distal surgical revascularization. *Ann Surg* 1989; **210**: 324.

8

Certification and training in peripheral vascular intervention

Richard R Heuser

Introduction

The use of endovascular techniques for peripheral vascular intervention has evolved over a period of nearly 30 years. As new devices and techniques are developed, however, considerable controversy remains about who is best qualified to use them. A variety of specialists are now in the business of advancing guidewires and placing stents or endoluminal grafts. Cardiologists, vascular surgeons and radiologists all possess specialized training that makes them experts in one or more aspects of endovascular therapy. The cardiologist is skilled in working with catheters, sheaths, balloons, wires, and stents, while the vascular surgeon has considerable experience in the iliac and aorta, performing vascular cutdowns and managing complications in these arteries. The radiologist brings another kind of experience – that with imaging procedures such as angiography, and duplex and intravascular ultrasound.

While it is certainly clear that each of these clinicians brings important knowledge and capabilities to the operating table, the endovascular interventionist needs to combine experience from each discipline to provide optimal care in treating peripheral vascular disease. A handful of organizations, including the American College of Cardiology (ACC), American Heart Association (AHA), Society for Cardiac Angiography and Interventions (SCAI), Society of Cardiovascular and Interventional Radiology (SCVIR), and Society for Vascular Surgery/International Society for Cardiovascular Surgery (SVS/ISCVS), have explored the standardization of training and have made recommendations. There are now a number of fellowship programs that offer new trainees experience in all aspects of endovascular techniques. Continuing education workshops have provided learning opportunities for established clinicians for a number of years. While the latter are certainly valuable, endovascular expertise is acquired over the 'long haul' and requires considerable training and practice. In this chapter, a review of training and certification options is provided, and the minimum standards for endovascular facilities are reviewed.

Qualifications

The majority of the governing organizations in endovascular interventions have outlined educational requirements for certification in endovascular therapies. The 1989 SCVIR guidelines[1] were some of the first to formally address physician requirements, and state as follows: 'Physicians who perform angioplasty of the peripheral and renal vessels should have a thorough understanding of the clinical manifestations and natural history of peripheral and renovascular disease … They should be competent to interpret diagnostic peripheral and renal angiographic examinations and to perform arteriographic procedures via femoral (retrograde and antegrade), auxiliary, and translumbar approaches …' To this end, the SCVIR guidelines[1] recommend that the physician meet the following minimal criteria: (1) completion of an approved residency program; and (2) additional experience in a 1- or 2-year post-residency program in percutaneous interventions. The ACC Peripheral Vascular Disease Committee Recommendations[2] are somewhat more specific, stating that, 'Training in vascular medicine should be offered to physicians with training in internal medicine. The physician should have taken or be eligible to take the internal medicine examination of the American Board of Internal Medicine or its equivalent.' Clearly, the general idea is to ensure that the physician has adequate background and training to embrace the subtleties of additional education in endovascular treatment.

Training

In some cases, recommendations recognize the importance of instruction from more than one clinician or expert in the field. There is no doubt that the trainee benefits from a variety of experiences. In addition to related training as described above, the ACC suggests a trainee receive a minimum of 12 months of training in vascular medicine in a program that includes two different faculty members.[2] 'This 12 months of training could be incorporated into a cardiology fellowship program,' the guidelines state; however, each governing body (ACC, AHA, SCAI, SCVIR, SVS/ISCVS) has made recommendations regarding the number of angiograms, angioplasties and other procedures required to demonstrate competence in endovascular procedures (Table 8.1).

The ACC guidelines[2] suggest cognitive training and clinical exposure that includes patient care management, and experience in invasive and non-invasive imaging techniques. Didactic lectures are to include information on etiology, pathophysiology, signs and symptoms, diagnostic techniques, and treatment. Clinical rotations should allow trainees to spend a minimum of 3 months on a hospital service, where they are directly involved in patient care. In addition, 3 months should be spent in an outpatient facility. Imaging rotations should allow 3 months in the non-invasive vascular laboratory and at least 1 month in an area where angiography and catheter revascularization techniques are performed. While 1 month does not provide sufficient experience for ACC certification, it is intended to provide a basic background in arteriography, angioplasty, atherectomy, stenting, and other percutaneous procedures.[2]

Credentialing guidelines for vascular surgeons, as outlined by White et al,[3] describe the need for competence in lesion access techniques, image acquisition and interpretation, guidewire use, and experience with specific devices, such as balloons, atherectomy equipment, stents, and other devices being evaluated for endovascular application. There is no doubt that skill with various percutaneous access techniques is important to the endovascular surgeon, because nearly 100% of transluminal peripheral vascular interventions are performed percutaneously. Lesion access is determined by patient characteristics, the location of the target lesion, and the intended procedure. Establishing skill and dexterity with the equipment requires considerable practice; coordinating fluoroscopic imaging and guidance is extremely important in ensuring the success of balloon angioplasty and stenting, which are the primary techniques used to treat vascular lesions. The SCVIR guidelines[1] also stress the importance of formal instruction in radiation physics, radiation effects, and protection, which are clearly a vital part of understanding imaging principles and safety.

Obtaining privileges

The Joint Commission on Accreditation of Health Care Organizations mandates that specific privileges be outlined for all hospital staff. Staff qualifications are based on training in residency or fellowship, and other specialized training.[3]

According to ACC guidelines,[4] physicians who have completed a formal fellowship program should provide the hospital with a list of patients that includes the total number of cases performed, the sites treated, and the complications encountered. If the physician has not completed at least 100 diagnostic peripheral angiograms, 50 peripheral angioplasty procedures, and 10 cases of peripheral thrombolytic therapy (50% of these as the primary operator), he or she should complete the requirements for postgraduate physicians.

Recommendations for postgraduate physicians state that the physician should attend at least two peripheral angioplasty seminars and learn the nature and anatomy of peripheral vascular disease, as well as the indications for and risks of alternative therapies. The physician should perform non-invasive evaluation, visit a laboratory in which peripheral

Table 8.1 Guidelines for training in peripheral endovascular intervention

Organization	Angiograms	Angioplasties	Live Demo	Thrombolysis
ACC	100	50/25[a]	Yes	Yes
AHA	100	50/25[a]	Yes	Yes
SCAI	100/50[a]	50/25[a]	Yes	No
SCVIR	200	25	Yes	No
SVS/ISCVS	50[a]	10–15[a]	Yes	Yes

[a]As primary interventionist.

angioplasty is being performed by experienced personnel, and observe at least 10 peripheral procedures. Postgraduate physicians are then required to demonstrate they have completed at least 100 diagnostic peripheral angiograms, 50 peripheral angioplasty procedures, and 10 cases of peripheral thrombolytic therapy (50% of these as the primary operator) under supervision of an experienced interventionist.[4]

The maintenance of peripheral angioplasty privileges should be dependent on the physician's active participation in a Joint Commission on Accreditation of Health Care Organizations mandated quality assurance program.[4] This includes the establishment of a registry that enrolls all patients who undergo peripheral interventions and the compilation of data on clinical characteristics, pertinent medical and surgical history, and examination findings. Angioplasty data are to be recorded and coded with information on the site, acute success, procedural complications and clinical follow-up in a manner that allows only the director of the registry to know the identity of the physician being reviewed. 'Blinded' review is then performed on an annual or biannual basis by a peer-review panel, and observations are forwarded to the hospital committee. When the results are deemed acceptable, privileges may be renewed for 1- or 2-year periods.

Permission to study new devices in the hospital setting is dependent upon review of protocols by Institutional Review Boards and the Food and Drug Administration.[3]

Facilities

Design of the facility that houses the endovascular laboratory must provide for adequate space, electrical capacity, and lead shielding. Minimal requirements for angiographic facilities were outlined by the SCVIR in 1989.[1] According to these early guidelines, the angiographic facility should have the following: (1) a film changer capable of obtaining rapid serial film at least 14 inches in diameter with digital subtraction angiography capability, (2) a high-resolution image intensifier and television chain; (3) physiologic monitoring devices; (4) facilities to manage and resuscitate unstable patients; and (5) personnel trained to provide proper patient care and operate the equipment. More recently, the ACC guidelines have made additional recommendations regarding peripheral angioplasty laboratories.[4] These state that the laboratory should be equipped with the following:

- Ample balloon dilation catheters, calibrated balloon inflation devices, and a complete range of current guidewires allowing for differences in flexibility and steerability.
- A high-resolution fluoroscopic system and an optimal television chain that allows ready visualization of a 0.014-inch guide wire and in which still frames (road map images) can be displayed simultaneously with the real-time fluoroscopic image.

- An angulating X-ray tube image intensifier arm that allows ready determination of the anatomic position of a guidewire or balloon catheter.
- A physiologic recording system, high-resolution fluoroscope, cineangiographic and/or digital subtraction or acquisition angiographic and/or cut film angiographic equipment, a complete set of emergency resuscitation instruments, and a full complement of drugs.
- Radiation exposure control systems, including such items as an X-ray beam with automatic collimation, a carbon fiber scattered radiation grid, a carbon fiber tabletop, and a correct tube filter. Further reduction of radiation exposure can be achieved by gap filling and using a reference monitor. Lead aprons, eyeglasses, thyroid protection and additional shielding of the X-ray tube are also recommended.
- Peripheral angiography should include contrast material and should image the entire vascular distribution. The use of video fluoroscopy alone is not sufficient.
- The surgical operating suite should be equipped to provide general anesthesia, a full complement of instruments, as well as drugs for the management of the cardiovascular patient.

Although there are no published position statements on the use of intravascular ultrasound (IVUS), its value in the endovascular procedures should not be underestimated. IVUS allows both pre-procedural evaluation and post-interventional assessment, providing baseline luminal dimensions and accurate determination of arterial architecture and lesion pathology. In most cases, the IVUS data help determine the need for stenting and then evaluate the adequacy of device deployment. Proper training in IVUS techniques should be a requisite part of any training program for endovascular interventionists.

Conclusion

There are now a variety of recommendations aimed at standardizing training in peripheral vascular intervention. While each governing body has produced different guidelines, it is clear that all favor supervised training and subsequent demonstration of skills in imaging, angioplasty, and management of complications. There are minimum standards governing the choice of equipment in endovascular facilities, and adequate attention to radiation safety is clearly a priority. As new devices and techniques become available, additional training is always required. Physicians must provide evidence of competence to maintain hospital privileges and uphold the highest standards of patient care in the emerging discipline of endovascular intervention.

References

1 Society of Cardiovascular and Interventional Radiology (SCVIR). *Credentialing criteria number 1: peripheral, renal, and visceral percutaneous transluminal angioplasty*. SCVIR Criteria, 1989.

2 Spitell JA, Creager MA, Dorros G et al. Recommendations for training in vascular medicine. *JACC* 1993; **22**: 626–8.

3 White RA, Fogarty TJ, Baker WH et al. Endovascular surgery credentialing and training for vascular surgeons. *J Vasc Surg* 1993; **17**: 1095–102.

4 Spitell JA, Creager MA, Dorros G et al. Recommendations for peripheral transluminal angioplasty: training and facilities. *JACC* 1993; **21**: 546–8.

9

Surgical alternatives for peripheral vascular diseases

Evan C Lipsitz, William D Suggs and Frank J Veith

Introduction

Endovascular interventions for the treatment of both aneurysmal and occlusive disease represent an increasing proportion of vascular surgery practice. Although it has been estimated that in the near future the majority of vascular interventions may be performed by an endovascular method,[1,2] standard surgical procedures, especially those in the periphery, represent the benchmark against which these techniques must be measured. Despite the increase in endovascular interventions, the ultimate durability of these treatments is unknown. While there have been tremendous advances in some areas, in others the use of endovascular therapies may have outpaced the development and evaluation of the currently available devices and techniques.

Infrainguinal occlusive disease

Several endovascular techniques have been used in the treatment of chronic infrainguinal occlusive disease, including standard balloon angioplasty with or without stent placement, subintimal angioplasty, and atherectomy. These treatments have variable success rates and tend to become less efficacious as the lesions extend to the periphery.

Surgical techniques for the treatment of infrainguinal occlusive disease include standard bypass, endarterectomy, and patch angioplasty. Prior to intervening in any patient, a careful history and lower extremity physical examination must be performed. An accurate pulse examination can both predict the pattern of infrainguinal disease as well as the treatment required to relieve the symptoms. Non-invasive laboratory tests can also help to estimate the location of occlusive lesions as well as assess the degree of ischemia within the lower extremity. Such lesions can be well localized and defined using duplex scanning.[3,4] Recently, there has been a great deal of interest in planning infrainguinal revascularizations on the basis of arterial duplex mapping alone.[5,6]

Prior to performing any endovascular or standard surgical intervention, the patient's clinical presentation and staging must be considered. It is unjustified to intervene in patients without clinical symptoms (stage 0) and usually unjustified to intervene in patients with mild claudication and no physical changes (stage 1). The conservative approach to patients with stage 1 disease is supported by numerous reports that highlight the benign nature and slow progression of this process to more advanced stages. Without any treatment 10–15% of patients will improve over a 5-year period and 60–70% will show no progression of their disease over the same interval.[7,8] The remaining 10–15%, who do worsen, can best be treated with a primary operation or therapeutic intervention after the disease has progressed. Patients with disabling claudication and physical findings such as dependent rubor or temperature differential (stage 2) are a heterogeneous group and it is sometimes justified to intervene in these patients depending on the symptomatology and activity level of the patient. However, many patients respond to conservative therapy and may remain stable or even improve over a period of several years.

Patients with rest pain (stage 3) or non-healing ischemic ulcers or gangrene (stage 4) have threatened limbs, although occasionally mild ischemic rest pain can remain stable over a several-year period. In addition, patients with small gangrenous patches can occasionally go on to heal without any further intervention. Patients with stage 3 and 4 disease are likely to have occlusions at multiple levels and, as such, tend to be less amenable to endovascular methods. These patients generally require a bypass for treatment.

Recent improvements in imaging techniques and equipment coupled with the relative ease of percutaneous balloon angioplasty and other endovascular treatments have prompted some physicians to recommend lowering the therapeutic threshold for the treatment of infrainguinal disease. This includes treatments for stage 1 and even stage 0 disease for lesions which are detected incidentally during other physical examination or arteriography. Presently, this practice should be condemned because not only are mid- and long-term results of these newer treatments totally unknown but also the treatment itself may initiate a healing process within the artery that can cause either late failure or worse, acceleration of the ongoing occlusive process, and ultimately net harm to the patient. Studies from both the cardiology and peripheral vascular literature have often demonstrated that the tightest stenosis seen at the time of angiography is not necessarily the lesion which goes on to occlude.[9–12]

Endovascular and standard surgical techniques should be viewed as complementary. In fact, maximal benefit can often be gained by combining these modalities. For example, the use of intraoperative arteriography with angioplasty and stenting to eliminate gradient-producing inflow lesions in conjunction with lower extremity bypass is quite effective and allows the entire therapy to be performed in a single sitting. An additional advantage of this combined approach is that gradients can be more accurately assessed once proper outflow has been established.

The choice and configuration of various materials for the bypass has been a subject of much debate and is too lengthy to discuss in detail here. In general, conduits for bypass consist either of autogenous vein, prosthetic material, or cryopreserved vein. Autogenous vein is the preferred conduit for bypass. This is based on improved patency compared with other conduits. However, in the above knee popliteal position, there is not a significant difference in the patency of autogenous vein vs polytetrafluorethylene (PTFE).[13,14] Prosthetic grafts include tubular expanded PTFE grafts as well as polyester fabric grafts. The use of umbilical vein has been preferred by some in terms of handling; however, grafts of this material have had a tendency towards aneurysmal degeneration.[15]

Autogenous vein grafts can be placed in several different configurations without significant differences and primary patency, secondary patency, and limb salvage rates.[16] The saphenous vein may be harvested and used in a reversed position. Alternatively, veins can be left *in situ* with the branches clipped and valves lysed by various techniques. Composite grafts, either a vein–vein or vein with prosthetic material, can be utilized. When the greater saphenous vein is diseased of unavailable, lesser saphenous or arm veins may be used if of suitable quality.

Femoropopliteal bypass

Patients whose limbs are threatened should undergo femoropopliteal bypass when the superficial femoral or popliteal artery is occluded and the patent popliteal artery segment distal to the occlusion has luminal continuity with any of its three terminal branches. (Figure 9.1). This is true even if one or more of these branches ends in an occlusion anywhere in the leg. Even if the popliteal artery segment into which the graft is to be inserted is occluded distally, femoropopliteal bypass to this isolated segment can be considered when the segment is > 7 cm in length.[17,18] If the isolated popliteal segment is less than 7 cm in length or there is extensive gangrene or infection in the foot, a femoral-to-distal artery bypass or sequential bypass is sometimes performed in one or two stages.[19]

Femoropopliteal bypass performed with greater saphenous vein have 4-year primary patency rates that range from 68% to 80% and limb salvage rates ranging from 75 to 90%.[20] Femoropopliteal bypasses done with PTFE have patency rates that are similar to that with vein if the bypass is to the above-knee popliteal artery, but bypasses constructed with PTFE to the below-knee popliteal artery do not perform as well.[13]

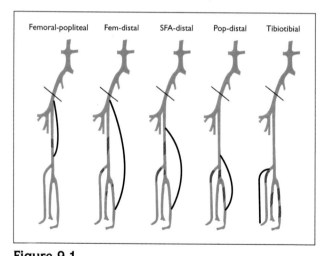

Figure 9.1
Various lower extremity bypasses as determined by the location and distribution of occlusions.

Infrapopliteal bypass

Bypasses to arteries beyond the popliteal (small vessel bypasses) are generally performed only when femoropopliteal bypass is not deemed possible, according to the foregoing criteria. Infrapopliteal bypasses may be performed to any of the three lower leg runoff vessels and can originate from either the common femoral, superficial femoral, or popliteal arteries, depending on the distribution of disease (Figure 9.1) A tibial artery is generally used for outflow only if its lumen runs without obstruction into the foot, although vein bypasses to isolated tibial artery segments and other disadvantaged outflow tracts have been performed and have remained patent over 4 years.[21,22] The peroneal artery is usually used only if it is continuous with one or two of its terminal branches which communicate with major arteries within the foot. Absence of a plantar arch and vascular calcification are not considered contraindications to a reconstruction. Some patients require a bypass to an artery or arterial branch in the foot.[23]

For both femoropopliteal and small vessel bypasses, stenosis of less than 50% of the diameter of the vessel may be acceptable distal to the site chosen for the distal anastomosis when the length of suitable autologous vein is a concern. Although an effort is made to find the most disease-free segment of artery to use for the distal anastomosis, this may be tempered by the advisability of using the most proximal patent segment possible to shorten the length of the bypass. Bypasses to tibial arteries should be performed with autogenous vein either by the reversed or in-situ technique. These bypasses should have 5-year primary patency rates that range from 60 to 70%, with limb salvage rates of 70–80%.[24,25] The secondary patencies of all of these grafts are improved with close patient follow-up and graft surveillance.[26]

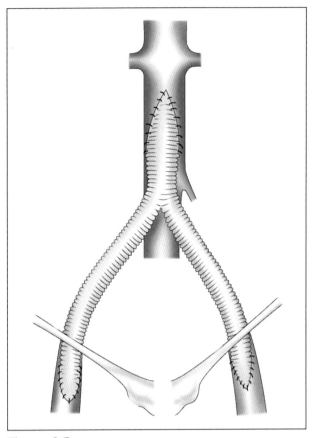

Figure 9.2
Aortobifemoral bypass with end-to-side proximal anastomosis.

Aortoiliac occlusive disease

The emergence of balloon angioplasty and stenting has greatly altered the face of treatment of aortoiliac occlusive disease. These are significant advantages to this less-invasive approach in the iliac system where the surgical approach, especially in an obese patient, can be quite challenging. The endovascular treatment of complex or long-segment aortoiliac occlusions or stenoses with a stent–graft has also been advocated. However, this approach has the major disadvantage of collateral sacrifice in an already compromised situation which is likely to leave the patient significantly worse in the event of graft failure.

Aortobifemoral bypass is the gold standard treatment for aortoiliac occlusive disease with cumulative 5-year patency rates in the 75–90% range.[27–32] Aortobifemoral bypass is generally performed through a limited midline abdominal incision and two small groin incisions. Depending on the disease pattern the proximal anastomosis is performed in either an end-to-end or end-to-side fashion to the aorta just inferior to the renal arteries. The end-to-end anastomosis has the theoretical advantage of a hemodynamically superior conformation, whereas the end-to-side anastomosis (Figure 9.2) has the advantage of preservation of flow to collateral vessels within the bypassed segment, including the lumbar arteries, the inferior mesenteric artery, and the internal iliac arteries when there is external iliac artery occlusion.[27,33] The distal anastomoses are generally performed to the common femoral arteries over the superficial femoral to deep femoral artery bifurcation for reasons of improved outflow. When there is a diseased or scarred common femoral artery and superficial femoral artery occlusion the distal anastomosis may be performed directly to the deep femoral artery. Other surgical options include axillofemoral or axillobifemoral bypasses and a femorofemoral bypass when the patient has anatomical contraindications or comorbid conditions which preclude the more stressful aortobifemoral bypass.

Femoral-to-femoral bypass

Crossover bypasses for unilateral iliac artery occlusion have been traditionally reserved for high-risk patients, but have been used more recently in good-risk patients (Figure 9.3). This procedure can easily be performed through two small groin incisions under regional or local anesthetic if required. Patency rates range from 60% to 90% at 5 years.[34–36] When

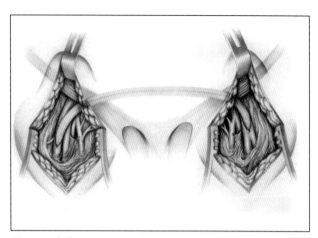

Figure 9.3
Femorofemoral bypass.

prostheses, patency rates of axillofemoral grafts improved.[39] Recent papers have demonstrated patency rates for axillary grafts that approach those from historic series for aortobifemoral grafts.[40,41] Passman et al.[35] also found that axillofemoral grafts compared favorably to aortic grafts in terms of limb salvage. In their comparative series of concurrently performed procedures, the aortic grafts had better long-term patency but equivalent results in terms or limb salvage. In this report the group of patients undergoing axillary to femoral artery bypasses were an older group of patients with a greater number of medical comorbidities and a significantly decreased life expectancy when compared to the patients undergoing aortic procedures. Therefore, one may anticipate that patients with limited life expectancy can achieve results from axillofemoral bypasses which should be equivalent to those of aortic reconstruction. However, younger, better-risk patients should undergo direct aortic reconstruction.[42]

concurrently performed femorofemoral bypasses were compared to aortobifemoral bypasses in low-risk patients, femorofemoral bypasses were inferior in terms of patency and hemodynamic performance to aortobifemoral bypasses (primary patency 61% vs 87% at 3 years). However, in this series, limb salvage rates were similar for both procedures in patients initially admitted with limb-threatening ischemia.[34] Femorofemoral bypass grafting may also be employed to treat a unilateral limb occlusion of a bifurcated standard or endovascular aortic graft.[37]

Direct iliofemoral bypass is another option for unilateral iliac artery occlusion. In a randomized study, aortofemoral and iliofemoral bypass were compared with femorofemoral or crossover iliofemoral bypass. Primary patency rates for direct reconstruction were better at 4 years (89%) than for crossover grafts (52%) with no difference in morbidity.[36] Five-year secondary patency rates for iliofemoral vs femorofemoral bypass were 69% vs 65%, respectively, in a report by Harrington et al.[38]

Axillofemoral bypass

Traditionally, high-risk patients with aortoiliac occlusive disease have been treated with axillofemoral bypasses (Figure 9.4). This 'extraanatomic' procedure uses the axillary artery as an inflow source, thus avoiding the need to expose and cross-clamp the aorta. The axillary artery should be evaluated preoperatively by either duplex or contrast arteriography. The artery is exposed in the infraclavicular area and the graft tunneled subcutaneously to the groin. The distal anastamoses are performed as for aortobifemoral bypasses. Axillofemoral grafts were considered inferior to aortobifemoral grafts in terms of long-term patency. However, after the introduction of externally supported

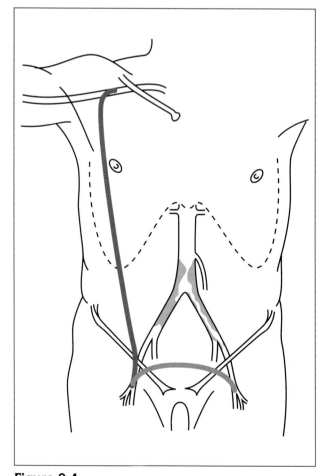

Figure 9.4
Right axillobifemoral bypass.

Abdominal aortic aneurysm

There has been an explosion over the past several years in the number of endografts placed for abdominal aortic aneurysm (AAA). This trend has been sparked by improvements in the industry-made grafts, as well as by the recent FDA (Food and Drug Administration) approval of two grafts for use in the United States. However, not all patients are suitable candidates for endovascular treatment. Patient selection, including graft configuration and artery size and tourtuosity, are of critical importance in planning these procedures.

The criteria for endovascular aneurysm repair are evolving based on improvements in devices as well as the availability of follow-up reports of their efficacy. Currently, there are several anatomic factors which may make endovascular treatment of AAA unadvisable or unwise.[43–49] An adequate proximal neck should consist of a normal aortic segment at least 1.5–2 cm in length and generally not more than 28–30 mm in diameter. This area should be free of thrombus and not have a reverse taper, i.e. have no more than 3–4 mm widening from the proximal to distal ends of the neck. The angle between proximal neck and the aorta should be less than 60 degrees. If the site selected for distal implantation is the common or external iliac artery, its morphology must be adequate for seating a distal attachment system. Patients with tortuousity of > 90 degrees at any point, significant dilatation to 16–20 mm, and/or severe iliac artery calcification are generally not candidates for endovascular repair. The presence of a short (< 30 mm) common iliac or the use of the external iliac as the target vessel may require embolization of the internal iliac(s), if patent, with or without re-implantation, to prevent back filling of the aneurysm. Perhaps most importantly, the common and external iliac and femoral arteries must be of sufficient caliber to allow passage of the introducer sheath or must be amenable to balloon dilation to facilitate passage. Aberrant vessels, particularly an indispensable accessory renal artery, must not be present in the segment of aorta to be excluded from the circulation. The patient cannot be dependent on the inferior mesenteric artery for perfusion of the intestine, since that artery will be excluded from the circulation. Finally, the patient must have the ability to comply with a more rigorous follow-up regimen than after standard repair.

Surgical repair generally proceeds via one of two approaches: transabdominal or retroperitoneal. The transabdominal approach is performed through a midline laparotomy and facilitates bilateral exposure of the iliac arteries, but requires entering the peritoneum (Figures 9.5–9.8). The retroperitoneal approach is performed through a left flank incision and has theoretically less pulmonary and gastrointestinal disturbances postoperatively but may preclude adequate exposure of the right iliac arterial system (Figure 9.9). In patients with short aneurysm necks, the retroperitoneal approach facilitates clamping within or above the visceral segment. These two approaches have been compared in several studies.[50–56]

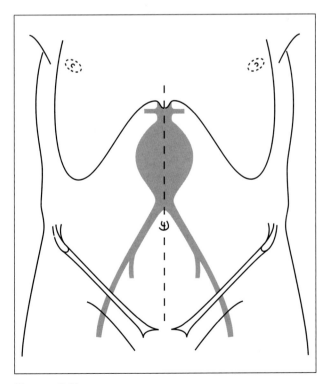

Figure 9.5
Midline transabdominal approach for abdominal aortic aneurysm repair.

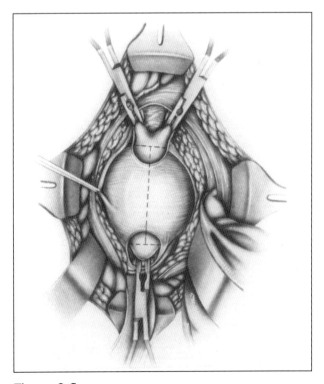

Figure 9.6
Exposure of the aneurysm and position of clamps for abdominal aortic aneurysm repair with tube graft.

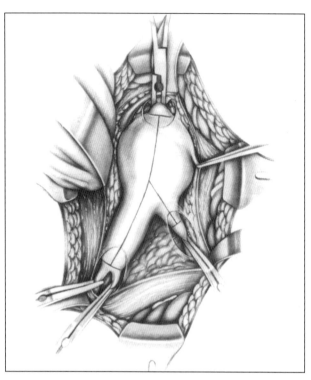

Figure 9.7
Exposure of the aneurysm and position of clamps for abdominal aortic aneurysm repair with bifurcated graft.

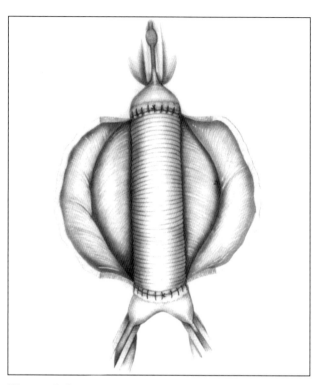

Figure 9.8
Completed abdominal aortic aneurysm repair with tube graft.

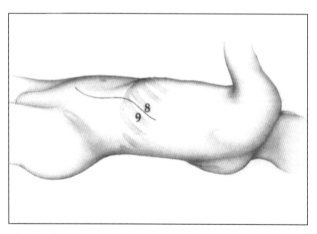

Figure 9.9
Retroperitoneal approach for abdominal aortic aneurysm repair. The position of the incision may be modified depending on the degree of para- or suprarenal involvement.

Carotid artery stenosis

The surgical treatment of carotid artery disease is based on extensive clinical observations and has been supported by a number of large studies. Patients with extracranial cerebral vascular disease may be either symptomatic or asymptomatic. Patients who have had a transient ischemic attack are at higher risk for developing a stroke in the future.[57] Since the mortality of such a stroke ranges from 15 to 33%, and since those who survive a stroke continue to remain at significant risk of subsequent stroke, treatment of this process is mandatory.[58–62] Also of note in patients who have suffered a stroke, the leading cause of death in these patients is recurrent stroke as opposed to myocardial infarction, which is the leading cause of mortality in all patients with extracranial occlusive disease.[62] The natural history of asymptomatic patients with carotid artery disease is more difficult to predict.

The pathophysiology of extracranial carotid disease and its symptomatology differs from that of arterial occlusive disease elsewhere in the body. The carotid artery bifurcation is one of many locations that are susceptible to the development of atherosclerotic plaque.[63] These plaques are susceptible to ulceration, intraplaque hemorrhage, and a variety of other processes which lead to local thrombosis and embolization. It is these emboli rather than the degree of stenosis and flow reduction which are responsible for the symptoms of carotid artery stenosis. Any treatment of carotid artery stenosis, therefore, must address these issues.

Prospective randomized trials can be divided into those evaluating asymptomatic patients and those evaluating symptomatic patients. The largest of the asymptomatic trials is the Asymptomatic Carotid Atherosclerosis Study (ACAS).[64] In this study over 1600 asymptomatic patients with greater than 60% carotid artery stenosis were randomized to endarterectomy plus best medical management vs medical management alone. After just over 2.5 years, a risk for ipsilateral perioperative stroke and death was 5.1% in surgical patients and 11% for medical patients, representing an absolute risk reduction of 53%, a difference which was highly significant. In this study the 30-day stroke and mortality rate in the surgical group was 1.52%.[65] One of the largest symptomatic trials is the North American Symptomatic Carotid Endarterectomy Trial (NASCET).[66,67] This study evaluated symptomatic patients who had had either a transient ischemic attack (TIA) or prior mild stroke and ipsilateral carotid stenosis, again randomized to surgery or medical management. The degree of stenosis was further subdivided into 30–69% and 70–99%. This trial was halted early by the Oversight Committee when in 18 months there was a 7% incidence of fatal and non-fatal strokes in the surgical group, but an incidence of 24% in the medical group. This difference again was significant ($p < 0.001$), representing an absolute risk reduction of 17%, and a relative risk reduction of 71%.

Based on the results from these prospective randomized trials as well as other retrospective reviews, a consensus conference from the Stroke Council of the American Heart Association has agreed on several indications for carotid endarterectomy.[68] For symptomatic good-risk patients, at a center with the surgical morbidity/mortality less than 6%, proven indications for endarterectomy include one or more TIAs within a 6-month period, and a carotid stenosis 70% or greater, or mild stroke with carotid stenosis 70% or greater. For asymptomatic good-risk patients treated at the center with surgical morbidity/mortality less than 3%, proven indications for endarterectomy include stenosis 60% or more. Other acceptable but non-proven as well as uncertain indications are also documented.

There are several variations in the operative technique for the treatment of carotid artery stenosis. These range in variations in the type of anesthesia used, the type of cerebral monitoring, whether or not a shunt is placed intraoperatively during carotid cross-clamping, and whether or not a primary or patch closure is performed, and within that group whether prosthetic or vein patches are used. Despite this variability, excellent surgical results with low morbidity and mortality, as outlined in the above studies, can be obtained with all of these methods at centers who use them.

In all cases a small incision is made along the anterior border of sternocleidomastoid and the dissection carried down to the common internal and external carotid arteries, which are dissected free. The artery is then opened and the plaque is removed using an endarterectomy spoon (Figure 9.10). Care is taken to avoid leaving any debris or distal intimal flaps; this may include the use of tacking sutures at the distal end point should these be required (Figure 9.11). The artery is then repaired with or without a patch and the incision closed in layers (Figure 9.12).

Recently, there has been significant enthusiasm generated for the treatment of carotid artery stenosis with angioplasty and stenting. This has developed because of the rare, but existing complication rate associated with carotid endarterectomy, including perioperative myocardial infarction, stroke, and cranial nerve injury. However, there is

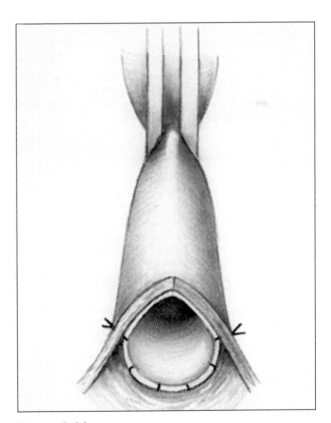

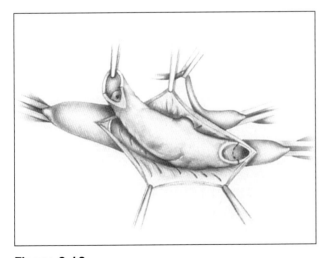

Figure 9.10
Removal of plaque from the carotid bifurcation. The dashed line indicates the end point of the endarterectomy.

Figure 9.11
Tacking sutures used to secure the distal end point and prevent the formation of flaps within the internal carotid artery.

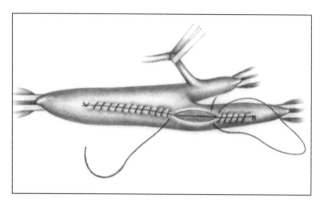

Figure 9.12
Closure of the carotid artery with primary anastomosis.

significant risk of embolization of plaque during carotid angioplasty and stenting, suggesting that at the present time this technique should only be used for high-risk cases.[69,70] There are a number of cerebral protection devices undergoing evaluation but these are also of unproven benefit.

References

1. Ohki T, Veith FJ, Sanchez LA et al. Can all abdominal aortic aneurysms be treated endovascularly: what is the role of a surgeon-made device? 23rd Annual Meeting of the Southern Association for Vascular Surgery, Naples, Florida, January 28–30, 1999.
2. Veith FJ. Presidential address: Charles Darwin and vascular surgery. J Vasc Surg 1997; **25**: 8–18.
3. Langsfeld M, Nepute J, Falls B et al. Duplex scanning to predict hemodynamically significant aortoiliac stenoses. J Vasc Surg 1988; 7: 395–9.
4. Moneta GL, Yeager RA, Antonovic R et al. Accuracy of lower extremity arterial duplex mapping. J Vasc Surg 1992; **15**: 275–84.
5. Ascher E, Mazzariol F, Hingorani A et al. The use of duplex ultrasound arterial mapping as an alternative to conventional arteriography for primary and secondary infrapopliteal bypasses. Am J Surg 1999; **178**(2): 162–5.
6. Wain RA, Berdejo GL, Delvalle WN et al. Can duplex scan arterial mapping replace contrast arteriography as the test of choice before infrainguinal revascularization? J Vasc Surg 1999; **29**(1): 100–7.
7. Coran AG, Warren R. Arteriographic changes in femoropopliteal arteriosclerosis obliterans: a five year follow-up study. N Engl J Med 1966; **274**: 643–5.
8. Imparato AM, Kim GE, Davidson T, Crowley JG. Intermittent claudication: its natural course. Surgery 1975; **78**: 795–7.
9. Walsh DB, Powell RJ, Stukel TA et al. Superficial femoral artery stenoses: characteristics of progessing lesions. J Vasc Surg 1997; **25**(3): 512–21.
10. Ambrose JA, Winters SL, Arora RR et al. Arteriographic evolution of coronary artery morphology in unstable angina. J Am Coll Cardiol 1986; 7: 472–8.
11. Haft JI, Al-Zarka AM. The origin and fate of complex coronary lesions. Am Heart J 1991; **121**: 1050–61.
12. Little WC, Constantinescu M, Applegate RJ et al. Can coronary arteriography predict the site of a subsequent myocardial infarction in patients with mild-to-moderate coronary artery disease? Circulation 1988; **78**: 1157–66.
13. Veith FJ, Gupta SK, Ascer E et al. Six year prospective multi center randomized comparison of autologous saphenous vein and expanded polytetrafluoroethylene grafts in infrainguinal arterial reconstructions. J Vasc Surg 1986; **3**: 104–14.
14. Bergan JJ, Veith FJ, Bernhard VM et al. Randomization of autologous vein and polytetrafluoroethylene in femoral distal reconstruction. Surgery 1982; **92**: 921–30.
15. Cranley JJ, Karkow WS, Hafner CD, Flanagan LD. Aneurysmal dilatation in umbilical vein grafts. In: Berrgan JJ, Yao JST (eds), Reoperative arterial surgery. Orlando, FL: Grune & Stratton, 1986, 343–58.
16. Wengerter KR, Veith FJ, Gupta SK et al. Prospective randomized multicenter comparison of in situ and reversed vein infrapopliteal bypasses. J Vasc Surg 1991; **12**: 189–99.
17. Veith FJ, Gupta SK, Daly V. Femoropopliteal bypass to the isolated popliteal segment: is polytetrafluoroethylene graft acceptable? Surgery 1981; **89**: 296–303.
18. Kram HB, Gupta SK, Veith FJ et al. Late results of 217 femoropopliteal bypasses to isolated popliteal segments. J Vasc Surg 1991; **14**: 386–90.
19. Flinn WR, Flanigan DP, Verta MJ et al. Sequential femoral-tibial bypass for severe limb ischemia. Surgery 1980; **88**: 357–00.
20. Taylor LM, Edwards JM, Porter JM. Present status of reversed vein bypass grafting: five-year results of a modern series. J Vasc Surg 1990; **11**: 193–206.
21. Lyon RT, Veith FJ, Marsan BU et al. Eleven-year experience with tibiotibial bypass: an unusual but effective solution to distal tibial artery occlusive disease and limited autologous vein. J Vasc Surg 1994; **20**: 61–8; discussion 68–9.
22. Ascher E, Veith FJ, Gupta SK. Bypasses to plantar arteries and other tibial branches: an extended approach to limb salvage. J Surg 1988; **8**: 434–41.
23. Andros G, Harris RW, Salles-Cuhna SX et al. Bypass grafts to the ankle and foot. J Vasc Surg 1988; 7: 785–94.
24. Rosenthal D, Arous EJ, Friedman SG et al. Endovascular-assisted versus conventional in situ saphenous vein bypass grafting; cumulative patency, limb salvage, and cost results in a 39-month multicenter study. J Vasc Surg 2000; **21**: 60–8.
25. Watelet J, Soury P, Menard JF et al. Femoropopliteal bypass: in situ or reversed vein grafts? Ten-year results of a randomized prospective study. Ann Vasc Surg 1997; **11**: 510–19.
26. Bandyk DF, Bergamini TM, Towne JB et al. Durability of vein graft revision: the outcome of secondary procedures. J Vasc Surg 1991; **13**: 200–10.
27. Brewster DC, Darling RC. Optimal methods of aortoiliac reconstruction. Surgery 1978; **84**: 739–48.
28. Crawford ES, Bomberger RA, Glaeser DH et al. Aortoiliac occlusive disease: factors influencing survival and function following reconstructive operation over a twenty-five year period. Surgery 1981; **90**: 1055–67.

29 Malone JM, Moore WS, Goldstone J. The natural history of bilateral aortofemoral bypass grafts for ischemia of the lower extremities. *Arch Surg* 1975; **110**: 1300–6.

30 Mozersky DJ, Summer DS, Strandness DE. Long-term results of reconstructive aortoiliac surgery. *Am J Surg* 1972; **123**: 503.

31 Piotrowski JJ, Pearce WH, Jones DN et al. Aortobifemoral bypass: the operation of choice for unilateral iliac occlusion? *J Vasc Surg* 1988; **8**: 211–18.

32 Szilagyi DE, Elliot JP, Smith RF et al. A thirty-year survey of the reconstructive surgical treatment of aortoiliac occlusive disease. *J Vasc Surg* 1986; **3**: 421–36.

33 Pierce GE, Turentine M, Stringfield S et al. Evaluation of end-to-side v end-to-end proximal anastomosis in aortobifemoral bypass. *Arch Surg* 1982; **117**: 1580.

34 Schneider JR, Besso SR, Walsh DB et al. Femorofemoral versus aortobifemoral bypass: outcome and hemodynamic results. *J Vasc Surg* 1994; **19**: 43–57.

35 Passman MA, Taylor LM Jr, Moneta GL et al. Comparison of axillofemoral and aortofemoral bypass for aortoiliac occlusive disease. *J Vasc Surg* 1996; **23**: 263–71.

36 Hanafy M, McLoughlin GA. Comparison of iliofemoral and femorofemoral crossover bypass in the treatment of unilateral iliac arterial occlusive disease. *Br J Surg* 1991; **78**: 1001–2.

37 Nolan KD, Benjamin ME, Murphy TJ et al. Femorofemoral bypass for aortofemoral graft limb occlusion: a ten-year experience. *J Vasc Surg* 1994; **19**: 851–7.

38 Harrington ME, Harrington EB, Haimov M et al. Iliofemoral versus femorofemoral bypass: the case for an individualized approach. *J Vasc Surg* 1992; **16**: 841–2.

39 Kenney DA, Sauvage LR, Wood SJ et al. Comparison of noncrimped, externally supported (EXS) and crimped, nonsupported Dacron prostheses for axillofemoral and above-knee femoropopliteal bypass. *Surgery* 1982; **92**: 931–46.

40 El-Massry S, Saad E, Sauvage LR et al. Axillofemoral bypass with externally supported, knitted Dacron grafts: a follow-up through twelve years. *J Vasc Surg* 1993; **17**: 107–15.

41 Taylor LM Jr, Moneta GL, McConnell DB et al. Axillofemoral grafting with externally supported polytetrafluoroethylene. *Arch Surg* 1994; **129**: 588–95.

42 Harrington ME, Harrington EB, Haimov M et al. Axillofemoral bypass: compromised bypass for compromised patients. *J Vasc Surg* 1994; **20**: 195–201.

43 Faries P. Clinical experience with endovascular grafts for aneurysmal arterial disease. In: Marin ML, Veith FJ, Levine BA (eds), *Endovascular stented grafts for the treatment of vascular diseases*. Austin RG Landes, 1995.

44 Chuter TAM, Nowygrod R. Bifurcated endovascular grafts for aortic aneurysm repair in: Parodi JC, Veith FJ, Marin ML (eds), *Endovascular grafting techniques*. St Louis: Quality Medical Publishing, 1996.

45 Moore WS. The EVT tube and bifurcated endograft systems: technical considerations and clinical summary. *J Endovasc Surg* 1997; **4**: 182–94.

46 Chuter TAM, Risberg BO, Hopkinson BR et al. Clinical experience with a bifurcated endovascular graft for abdominal aortic aneurysm repair. *J Vasc Surg* 1996; **24**: 655–66.

47 Schumacher H, Eckstein HH, Kallinowski F, Allenberg JR. Morphometry and classification in abdominal aortic aneurysms: patient selection for endovascular and open surgery. *J Endovasc Surg* 1997; **4**: 39–44.

48 Lipsitz EC, Ohki T, Veith FJ. What are the indications for endovascular stent-graft repair of abdominal aortic aneurysms: present status. In: Greenhalgh (ed.), *Indications in vascular and endovascular surgery*. London: WB Saunders, 1998.

49 Brewster DC. Clinical and anatomical considerations for surgery in aortoiliac disease and results of surgical treatment. *Circulation* 1991; **83**: I-42–I-52(suppl I).

50 Sicard GA, Reilly JM, Rubin BG et al. Transabdominal versus retroperitoneal incision for abdominal aortic surgery: report of a prospective randomized trial. *J Vasc Surg* 1995; **21**: 174–83.

51 Cambria RP, Brewster DC, Abbott WM et al. Transperitoneal versus retroperitoneal approach for aortic reconstruction: a randomized prospective study. *J Vasc Surg* 1990; **11**: 314–25.

52 Shepard AD, Scott GR, Mackey WC et al. Retroperitoneal approach to high-risk abdominal aortic aneurysms. *Arch Surg* 1986; **121**: 444–9.

53 Arko FR, Bohannon WT, Mettauer M et al. Retroperitoneal approach for aortic surgery: is it worth it? *Cardiovasc Surg* 2000; **9**(1): 20–6.

54 Leather RP, Shah DM, Kaufman JL et al. Comparative analysis of retroperitoneal and transperitoneal aortic replacement for aneurysm. *Surg Gynecol Obstet* 1989; **168**: 387–93.

55 Quinones-Baldrich WJ, Garner C, Caswell D et al. Endovascular, transperitoneal, and retroperitoneal abdominal aortic aneurysm repair: results and costs. *J Vasc Surg* 1999; **30**: 59–67.

56 Peck JJ, McReynolds DG, Baker DH, Eastman AB. Extraperitoneal approach for aortoiliac reconstruction of the abdominal aorta. *Am J Surg* 1986; **151**: 620–3.

57 Whisnant JP, Matsumoto M, Elveback LR. The effects of anticoagulant therapy on the prognosis of patients with transient cerebral ischemic attacks in community. Rochester, Minnesota, 1965–1969. *Mayo Clin Proc* 1973; **48**: 844.

58 Mohr JP, Caplan LR, Meski JW et al. The Harvard Cooperative Stroke Registry: a prospective registry. *Neurology* 1978; **28**: 754–62.

59 Sacco RL, Wolf PA, Kannel WB, McNamara PM. Survival and recurrence following stroke: the Framingham Study. *Stroke* 1982; **13**: 290–5.

60 Soltero I, Lin K, Cooper R et al. Trends in mortality from cerebrovascular diseases in the United States, 1960 to 1975. *Stroke* 1978; **9**: 549.

61 Enger E, Boysen S. Long term anticoagulant therapy in patients with cerebral infarction: a controlled clinical study: *Acta Med Scand* 1965; **178**(Suppl 438): 1–61.

62 Robinson RE et al. Natural history of cerebral thrombosis. 9–19 year follow-up. *J Chronic Dis* 1968; **21**: 221.

63 Schwartz CJ, Mitchell JRA. Observations on localization of arterial plaques. *Circ Res* 1962; **11**: 63.

64 The Executive Committee for the Asymptomatic Carotid Artherosclerosis Study. Endarterectomy for asymptomatic carotid artery stenosis. *JAMA* 1995; 273: 1421–8.

65 Moore WS, Young B, Baker WH et al. Surgical results: a justification of the surgeon selection process for the ACAS Trial. *J Vasc Surg* 1996; **23**: 323–8.

66   North American Symptomatic Carotid Endarterectomy Trial (NASCET) Steering Committee. North American Symptomatic Carotid Endarterectomy Trial: methods, patient characteristics, and progress. *Stroke* 1991; **22**: 711–20.

67   North American Symptomatic Carotid Endarterectomy Trial Collaborators. Beneficial effect of carotid endarterectomy in symptomatic patients with high-grade carotid stenosis. *N Engl J Med* 1991; **325**: 445–53.

68   Moore WS, Barnett HJ, Beebe ME et al. Guidelines for carotid endarterectomy: a multidisciplinary consensus statement from the ad hoc committee, American Heart Association. *Stroke* 1995; **26**: 188–201.

69   Ohki T, Marin M, Lyon RT. Ex vivo human carotid artery bifurcation stenting: correlation of lesion characteristics with embolic potential. *J Vasc Surg* 1998; **27**: 463–71.

70   Veith FJ, Amor M, Ohki T et al. Current status of carotid bifurcation angioplasty and stenting based on a consensus of opinion leaders. *J Vasc Surg* 2001; **33**: 111–16.

10

When to refer for surgery?

Osvaldo J Yano, Michael L Marin and Larry Hollier

Introduction

Endovascular techniques, once considered as only a diagnostic modality, have now been used to treat complex vascular pathologies, as a result of the recent advances in endovascular technology with the introduction of more sophisticated interventional equipment. Despite these advances, endovascular techniques are still in their embryonic phase of development. Thus, the clinical applications and limitations, as well as durability, of the various endovascular procedures are unknown issues that need to be studied on a long-term basis. This chapter focuses on the definition of difficult vascular anatomy, which initially may not be suitable for catheter-based therapy. One must be conscious of the fact that technology will rapidly overcome the various endovascular limitations that are currently present, thus allowing more patients to be treated by this minimally invasive technique. This chapter also describes various situations in which open surgical techniques are combined with endovascular techniques to create a hybrid type of intervention, both endovascular and surgical, with the intent of optimizing inadequate anatomy for endovascular repairs, and thus increasing the pool of patients that can be treated by this technology.

Aneurysms of the aorta

Following the introduction of stent–graft repair of abdominal aortic aneurysms (AAA) by Parodi in 1991,[1] this minimally invasive technique became an alternative modality of treatment for aortic aneurysms. The basic concepts of this technique are based on the ability to navigate the compartmentalized devices or delivery systems through remote access vessels and ultimately anchor them in a normal-caliber aortic

segment to achieve complete exclusion of the aneurysm from the arterial circulation.

In our experience with 421 patients treated by stent–graft exclusion of their AAA, 12% required some form of auxiliary maneuver to either allow navigation of the device or to achieve appropriate anchoring of the device to an adequate landing site to attain long-term durability.[2] The minimal invasiveness of this method provides advantages to patients, who are exposed to a less morbid procedure with shorter time of recovery. The eligibility of patients for endovascular stent–grafting, however, hinges upon the presence of favorable arterial anatomy of the aneurysm and its surrounding vessels. Conversely, in the case of open conventional repair of aortic aneurysms, the patient's physical fitness comes first as the determining factor as to whether or not one would be able to undergo a major operation. However, there are patients with difficult anatomy who might initially be deemed ineligible for endovascular techniques, yet who have such severe medical comorbidities that open repair seems inordinately risky. In the majority of these patients, instead of rejecting a patient as unsuitable for endovascular treatment, we often use a minor surgical procedure to improve anatomic conditions to make the patient eligible for endovascular stent–grafting. The various secondary procedures necessary to allow device navigation and proper device anchoring are listed below.

Device navigation issues

The iliofemoral route is the one most often used to introduce and navigate a stent–graft for the repair of aortic aneurysms. Unfortunately, this arterial segment is usually atherosclerotic, which could lead to serious obstacles in the implementation of endovascular repairs. Specific anatomic difficulties include the combination of tortuosity and occlusive disease, especially with calcification of varying degrees of severity. The various surgical maneuvers should be designed to address each of these problems according to their magnitude. For minor isolated segmental occlusion, a simple balloon angioplasty can be performed to dilate the access vessel to permit device insertion. When tortuosity prevents device navigation, a digital dissection of the external iliac artery can be done, with mobilization the redundant artery downwards and straightening of the tortuosity that was initially encountered (Figure 10.1).

In cases of severe occlusive disease in the iliofemoral region, a stent–graft could be deployed at the iliac bifurcation to allow subsequent balloon angioplasty of the long, nearly occlusive segment (Figure 10.2). In extreme conditions in which severe tortuosity is present in conjunction with occlusive disease, an arterial bypass conduit anastomosed from the common iliac artery can be used to insert the device and concomitantly augment bloodflow perfusion into the distal limb circulation (Figure 10.3). Thus, one must be sufficiently familiar with identifying the possible anatomic challenges as well as proficient enough to intervene according to the degree of anatomic difficulty prior to the development of iatrogenic complications during device insertion. Obviously, since stent–grafting technology is rapidly evolving to include smaller devices that can be carried in more flexible delivery systems, which are capable of negotiating sharp curves and tortuosities, one may speculate that the need for these auxiliary maneuvers will decrease in the future.

Attachment site issues

Endovascular repair of AAAs is a rapidly evolving technique that continues to undergo both procedural and device-related modifications. The feasibility of implanting stent–grafts by inserting them into the arterial tree via a remote site hinges upon the ability to choose the appropriate arterial location and then being able to fix the grafts there with appropriate

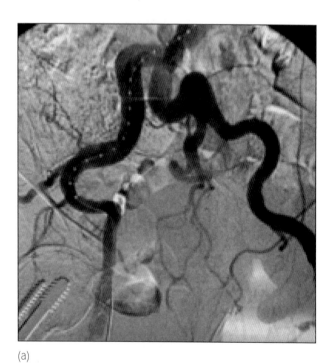

(a)

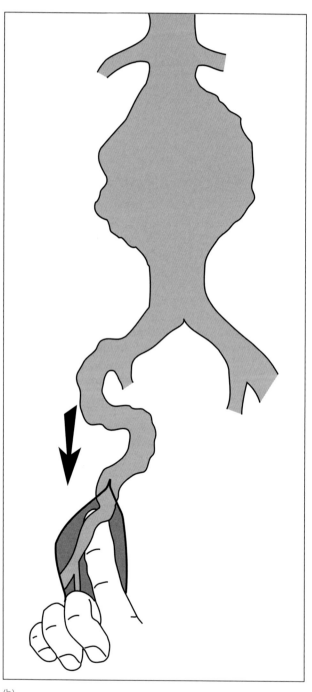

(b)

Figure 10.1
Angiogram of a tortuous external iliac artery (a), and schematic representation of a dissection to eliminate the redundancy of the artery (b).

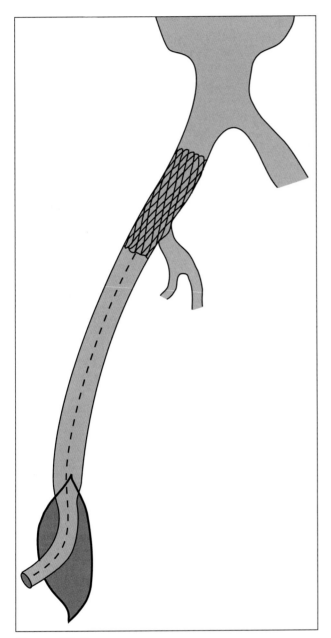

Figure 10.2
Schematic view of an iliac artery stent-graft to allow passage of the delivery system in a severely diseased iliac artery.

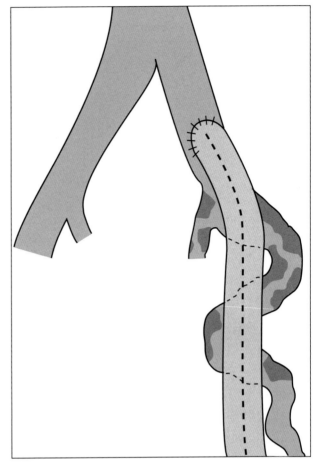

Figure 10.3
Schematic representation of an open iliofemoral bypass used to allow device navigation in an extremely diseased iliofemoral system.

attachment systems. These anchoring sites are defined as the aneurysm necks. Although approximately 85% of all aortic aneurysms are in the infrarenal position, on close inspection many of these lesions present with insufficient normal aorta immediately below the renal arteries, so that secure, long-term attachment of an aortic endograft is not possible.[3,4] To ensure long-term durability of stent–graft repair of aortic aneurysms, the attachment sites of the device must anchor on an aneurysm-free segment. Ideally, the necks should be long and not dilated in order to achieve complete exclusion of the aneurysm from the main arterial circulation. It is estimated that, as the population ages, the anatomy in these elderly patients also becomes more complex, usually with short, dilated and angulated aneurysm necks, which clearly impose difficulties for conventional stent–graft repair.

Aneurysm neck issues

In attempting to define what neck length is suitable for endovascular repair, the length of 15 mm or more was arbitrarily used as one of the inclusion criteria in various United States Food and Drug Administration investigational device trials (Vanguard, Boston Scientific Co., Natick, MA, USA). However, based on the versatility of the device employed to handle a short proximal neck, many surgeons as well as medical societies have accepted considerably shorter lengths. Despite enormous variations in anatomy and devices, the key components for successful deployment of an endograft include achieving total seal of the proximal and distal necks adjacent to the aneurysm. This simplistic approach takes into consideration many other factors that are necessary for achieving a successful endovascular procedure, such as correct morphometric measurements of the aneurysm and the choice of an appropriate device. Failure to obtain complete exclusion of the aneurysm will result in a type I endoleak (a leak from one end of the device) and may even lead to device migration.

We believe that transrenal deployment of a bare stent endograft allows us to increase the number of patients eligible for endovascular repair, and it has obliged surgeons to pay particular attention to precise device positioning. Furthermore, Sonesson et al.[4] reported infrarenal neck expansion rates in 44 patients who underwent endovascular exclusion of their AAAs. However, dilation in diameter was rarely seen in the suprarenal aortic segment (<5%). It is common knowledge that the suprarenal aorta is often spared in the majority of AAA repairs. Thus, one may rationalize that the attachment system for stent–grafts should be extended and anchored at the suprarenal portion of the aorta. In patients with extremely short necks who are at a prohibitively high risk for open conventional repair, a laparoscopic banding of the aortic neck can be performed to reinforce an otherwise suboptimal attachment site.

Iliac artery issues

Abdominal aortic aneurysms are frequently encountered with coexisting iliac artery aneurysms, which can further compli-

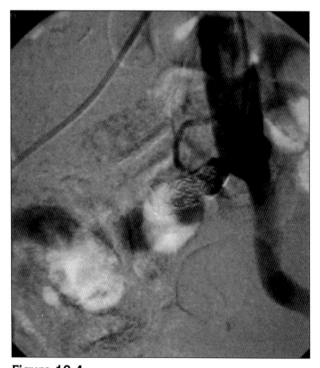

Figure 10.4
Coil embolization angiograms of an internal iliac artery with its orifice originating from the sac of a common iliac artery.

cate the choice of an adequate distal attachment site. In this situation, endovascular stent–grafting can still be employed by coil embolization of one internal iliac artery with preservation of the contralateral artery for continuous prograde pelvic blood perfusion (Figure 10.4). More complex reconstructions are reserved for cases in which bilateral common iliac arteries are dilated with aneurysm degeneration; in these situations, our preferred method of preserving pelvic perfusion is the construction of a bypass graft from the external iliac artery to the internal iliac artery with proximal hypogastric artery ligation, and extending the distal attachment site across the orifice of the native internal and into the external iliac artery, thus allowing concomitant preservation of pelvic circulation (Figure 10.5).

The second method used in these situations is a primary aneurysm repair with an aorto-uni-iliac device inserted across a previously embolized internal iliac artery with subsequent surgical disconnection of the iliac bifurcation contralateral to the side of the device followed by a construction of a femorofemoral bypass to restore circulation to the lower extremities (Figure 10.5).

Supra renal and thoracic aortic aneurysms

Currently, patients with thoracoabdominal or suprarenal aortic aneurysms are not usually candidates for endovascular repair, because of the involvement of essential branches of the aorta that cannot be covered by a stent–graft. Thus, open aneurysm repair has been the procedure of choice for patients who are adequately fit to undergo this approach. In general, however, patients with suprarenal or thoracoabdominal aortic aneurysms are elderly and often have multiple medical comorbidities which significantly increase the complications directly related to the procedure. To circumvent this obstacle, in selective patients a two-stage operation is performed, with initial remote revascularization of the essential vessels of the aorta such as the visceral and renal branches; these are directly bypassed and their aortic origin disconnected (Figure 10.6). This maneuver permits extension of the anchoring site to a segment of the aorta that is free of aneurysm involvement. Lawrence-Brown has also described the use of fenestrated stent–graft devices to allow perfusion of essential branches of the aorta when aneurysm involves the origin of essential aorti §c branches.[5] This technique, although successful in many patients who were initially deemed to be unsuitable for endovascular therapy, requires a great deal of technical expertise to access these side-branches. In addition, caution must be exercised in terms of patient selection and the proximity between the attachment site in question and the side-branch. When this distance is considerable and the aneurysmic process clearly involves the

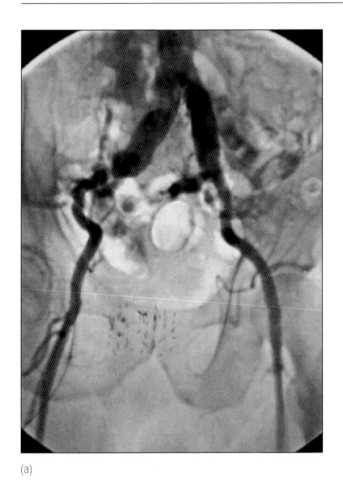

(a)

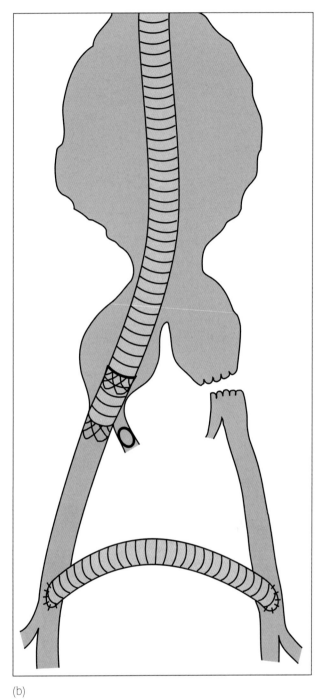

(b)

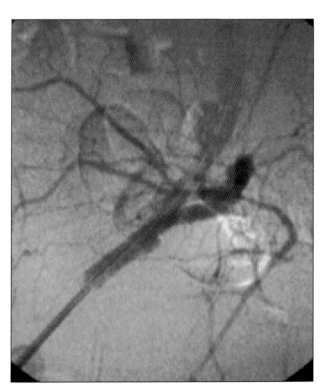

(c)

Figure 10.5

Different surgical strategies used in patients with bilateral iliac artery aneurysms. (b) Common iliac transection and plication to exclude the contiguous iliac aneurysm. (c) Angiogram following a relocation of the orifice of the internal to external iliac artery to allow full exclusion of the aorto-iliac aneurysm.

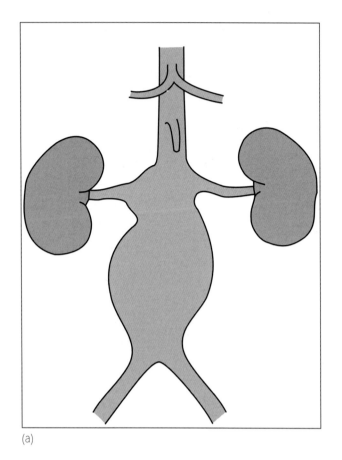

(a)

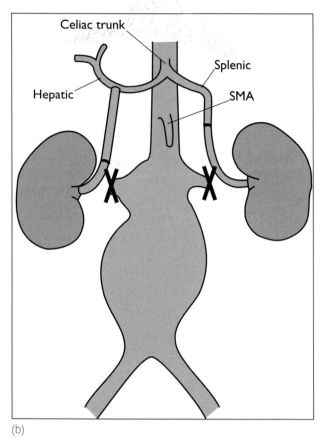

(b)

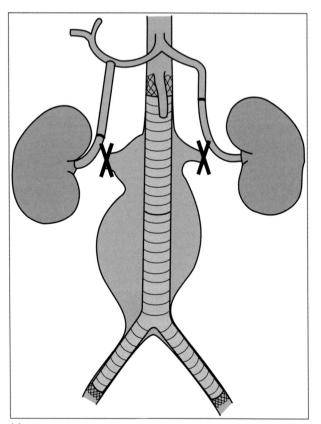

(c)

Figure 10.6

Schematic representation a suprarenal aortic aneurysm (a) treated by extra-anatomic bypass of renal arteries with disconnection of renal artery orifices from the aneurysm sac (b), to allow subsequent insertion of a stent–graft (c) SMA, superior mesenteric artery.

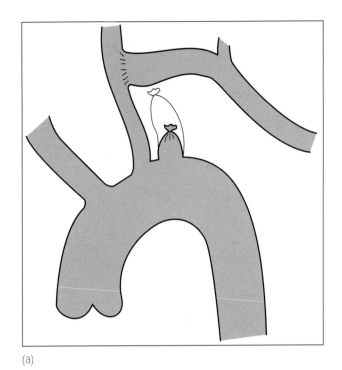

(a)

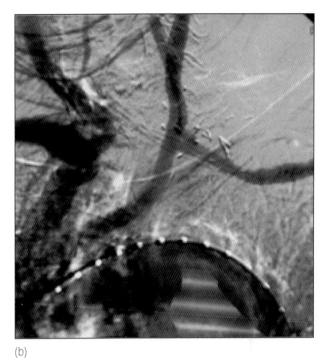

(b)

Figure 10.7
Schematic (a) and angiogram (b) of a subclavian-carotid transposition to expand the length of the anchoring segment for more secure stent–graft attachment.

orifice of the branch in question, the use of a branched stent–graft, such as the Inoue device for aneurysms involving the aortic arch,[6] would be more appropriate and probably more durable.

In patients with thoracic aortic aneurysm with insufficient proximal necks, a transposition of the left subclavian artery to the left carotid artery is frequently performed in patients with high descending aortic aneurysms (Figure 10.7). This adjunctive maneuver allows the device to cover the orifice of the left subclavian artery, which is usually free of aneurysmal disease. In our series, we performed subclavian artery transposition or bypass in more than five patients without major morbidities.

For patients with more proximal aneurysmal disease, bypasses via median sternotomy can be constructed from the ascending aorta to the aortic arch branches with subsequent disconnection of these vessels from the aneurysm sac. This maneuver also allows deployment of a stent–graft device at the aortic arch without ischemic consequences since the arch vessels have been transposed to a more proximal area at the ascending aorta.

Aortic dissection can be problematic in both the acute and chronic stages. Endovascular intervention appears attractive to avoid propagation of the dissection both proximally and distally in the acute stage. Some patients, acute or chronic, may need elephant trunk repair for extensive aneurysmal changes. We had the opportunity to treat three such patients. When the anatomy allows, a stent–graft can be employed to exclude the aneurysm by using the end of the elephant trunk

graft as the proximal neck site (Figure 10.8). The choice of a distal landing zone is usually more problematic, and hinges upon the site of the termination extension of the aortic dissection, or at least of the aneurysmal dilation; however, there is often an acceptable landing zone near the diaphragm. If the endpoint is far distal, perhaps into the iliac arteries, one can consider endovascular fenestration of the endpoint if false lumen bloodflow is significant.

Surgery still has its day

Although the endovascular options for patients with aortic aneurysms have been expanded by use of this hybrid approach, which combines open conventional surgery and endovascular technology, there are patients with such difficult anatomy that at the present time open aneurysm repair remains the only option.

Obviously, as device technology progresses along with improved operator skills, many patients who were initially labeled as non-candidates may be included in the pool of subjects amenable to treatment by future endovascular techniques.

In conclusion, based on our experience with more than 400 cases of aortic aneurysms repaired by endovascular means, we believe that is possible for a majority of patients with suboptimal anatomy to undergo secondary, less invasive interventions to manipulate the initial anatomic difficulty and to

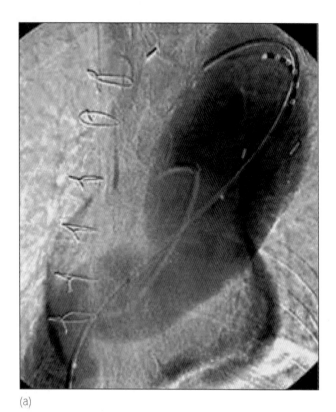
(a)

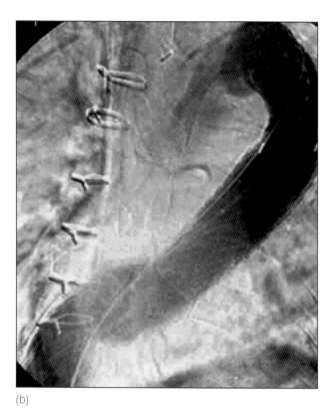
(b)

Figure 10.8
Angiograms of a patient with a previously performed elephant trunk repair and its descending thoracic aneurysm. (a) before and (b) following stent–graft repair.

allow subsequent endovascular treatment. This hybrid approach has permitted more patients to be treated by endovascular technology without exposing them to a high-morbidity procedure that would otherwise be the only option. We remain hopeful that rapid innovation and the natural evolution of second- and third-generation devices, which are more steerable and with available side-branches, will allow the treatment of patients with challenging anatomies whose only treatment option at this time is open surgery.

References

1   Parodi JC, Palmaz JC, Barone HD. Transfemoral intraluminal graft implantation for abdominal aortic aneurysms. *Ann Vasc Surg* 1991; **5**: 491–9.

2   Yano OJ, Morrisey N, Teodorescu V et al. Supplemental surgical techniques to facilitate endovascular repair of abdominal and thoracic aortic aneurysms. Presented at the 24th Annual Meeting of the Midwestern Vascular Surgical Society, Scottsdale, AZ, 2000.

3   White GH, Yu W, May J. Endoleak – a proposed new terminology to describe incomplete aneurysm exclusion by an endoluminal graft. *J Endovasc Surg* 1996; **3**: 124–5.

4   Sonesson B, Resch T, Lanne T et al. The fate of the infrarenal aortic neck after open aneurysm surgery. *J Vasc Surg* 1998; **28**: 889–94.

5   Browne TF, Hartley D, Purchas S et al. A fenestrated covered suprarenal aortic stent. *Eur J Vasc Endovasc Surg* 1999; **18**: 445–9.

6   Inoue K, Hosokawa H, Iwase T et al. Aortic arch reconstruction by transluminally placed endovascular branched stent graft. *Circulation* 1999; **100**: II–316–21.

11

Techniques of arterial access for endovascular intervention

Dwayne F Ledesma, Gregory S Domer and Frank J Criado

Introduction

Catheter-based endoluminal therapies have had an enormous impact on the practice of modern medicine and surgery. Ensuring appropriate intraluminal access is essential to achieve a safe and successful intervention. The fact that the majority of complications in endovascular intervention are access-related[1] further emphasizes the subject's importance. Proficiency with all available arterial puncture techniques is therefore a basic requirement for every vascular interventionalist. In this chapter, we intend to discuss the various puncture techniques and their associated complications.

Femoral access

The common femoral artery is the preferred access site for the majority of endoluminal interventions. Important reasons for this include the facts that the arterial pulse can be easily palpated for simple puncture, and that the artery can be effectively compressed after the introducer is withdrawn. Additionally, most arterial territories can be accessed via this approach. It is relatively simple, safe, and well tolerated.

Retrograde femoral catheterization

- The first consideration is the level of vessel entry, which must be at the infrainguinal position.
- The needle-to-vessel angle should be in the 30–45° range, in order to facilitate guidewire passage into the target vessel (Figure 11.1).

- Finding the femoral artery is usually straightforward, guided simply by the palpable femoral pulse. However, vessel puncture can be challenging in the setting of significant obesity or a diminished/absent pulse (see below).
- After obtaining pulsatile blood return, guidewire placement into the vascular lumen establishes access and permits over-the-wire insertion of the introducer sheath (Seldinger technique).
- In most cases, it is appropriate to use a J-tip steel wire and a 5F introducer sheath to begin the intervention. Use of a Glidewire (Terumo, Somerset, NJ, USA) after initial needle

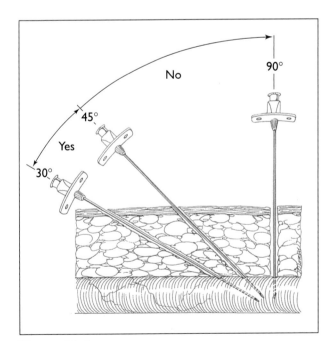

Figure 11.1
Proper arterial puncture angle is 30–45°.

introduction is fraught with complications, as its outer coating can be stripped or cut by the sharp end of the needle when trying to retract and reposition the wire.[2]

- The routine use of an introducer sheath is recommended for several reasons. First, it secures and maintains intraluminal access for safe and rapid catheter exchanges; second, it facilitates contrast injections, and the administration of heparin and other pharmacological agents.

Antegrade femoral catheterization

Antegrade femoral access is usually used in superficial femoral artery (SFA) or below-knee vessel interventions. The technique is challenging and involves certain limitations; as a result, it is only infrequently used. The major difficulty is with the angle of vessel entry. The ideal angle is between 30° and 45° (see below). The anterior abdominal wall and inguinal ligament may prevent vessel puncture at this angle. Once entry into the vessel lumen has been achieved, injection of contrast through the needle may help define the femoral bifurcation anatomy (Figure 11.2). Occasionally, direct puncture of the SFA is feasible, but it should be considered a less optimal site because of the reported greater potential for complications.[3]

Needle selection

There are two types of puncture needle available for percutaneous arterial access. The single-wall needle is usually preferred; the beveled needle tip is advanced towards the vessel, finding the lumen upon entry (Figure 11.3a). The potential disadvantage of this needle is that the bevel can be partially placed within the vessel wall (Figure 11.4); if not recognized, wire advancement (with the needle in this position) may result in subintimal dissection.

The double-wall puncture needle was designed to secure intraluminal position with little risk of subintimal dissection. The needle has a blunt tip and contains an inner beveled stylet that becomes the leading point. Transfixing puncture of the vessel is followed by removal of the stylet. The needle is gradually withdrawn until luminal entry is signaled by pulsatile blood return (Figure 11.3b). The principal drawback of the double-wall puncture needle is potential bleeding caused by the creation of a hole in the backwall of the artery. This can be troublesome when using thrombolytic agents, puncturing a synthetic graft (PTFE in particular), and when puncturing the vessel directly after surgical cutdown and circumferential exposure. Use of the single-wall technique is recommended in all such situations.

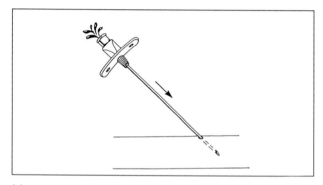

(a)

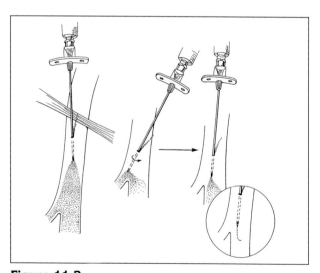

Figure 11.2
Antegrade puncture of the common femoral artery. Injection of radiocontrast through the needle defines the anatomy of the bifurcation, and may help to redirect the access pathway down the superficial femoral artery.

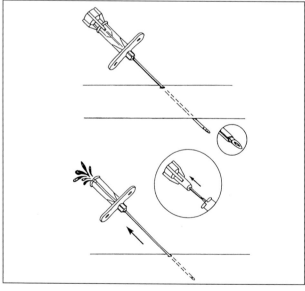

(b)

Figure 11.3
Single-wall puncture needle (a), and double-wall needle (b).

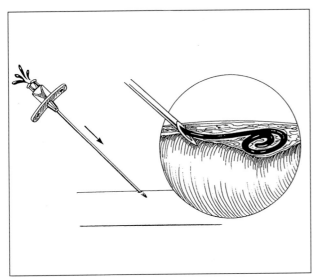

Figure 11.4
Subintimal dissection with the guidewire can occur when the long bevel of the single-wall needle ends up partially across the vessel wall, even when obtaining 'adequate' pulsatile arterial flow through the hub of the needle.

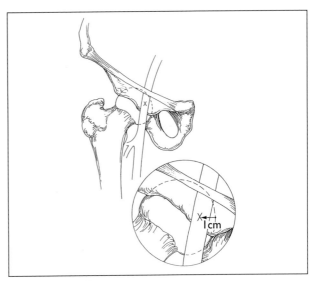

Figure 11.5
Rupp's method to target the infrainguinal common femoral artery for percutaneous puncture. Positioning the femoral head in the center of the fluoroscopic frame is essential.

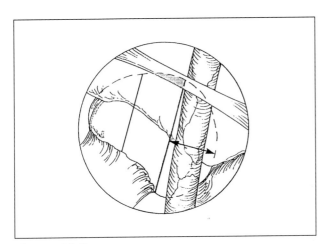

Figure 11.6
Alternative methodology to target the common femoral artery.

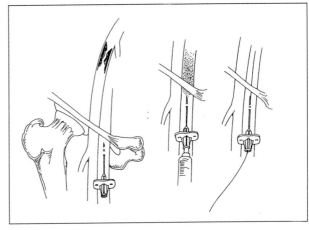

Figure 11.7
Use of the femoral vein as a reference for femoral arterial puncture when opacified with contrast or marked with an intraluminal guidewire.

Complications and troubleshooting

Failure to localize the femoral artery

The ability to localize the femoral artery may be difficult in the setting of obesity or diminished/absent pulses. There are several maneuvers that may be employed:

- A hand-held Doppler or ultrasound probe can be useful for vessel visualization.
- The anatomical relationship between the fluoroscopically visualized femoral head and the femoral artery has been described by Rupp et al:[4] the midpoint of the infrainguinal femoral artery puncture site is targeted 1 cm lateral to the most medial cortex of the femoral head (Figure 11.5). A similar approach relies on the medial third of the femoral head as a reference point (Figure 11.6).[5]
- Purposeful or inadvertent entry of the femoral vein can be used to help locate the femoral artery. Placement of a guidewire into the vein lumen or obtaining a 'radiographic mask' with contrast for road mapping can facilitate subsequent arterial puncture just lateral to the marked vein (Figure 11.7).

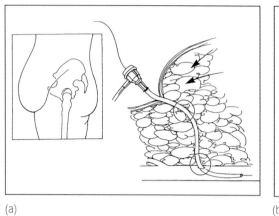
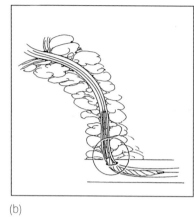
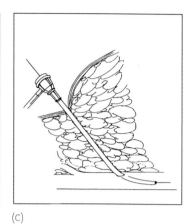

(a)   (b)   (c)

Figure 11.8
(a) S-shape deformity of the access pathway can occur in difficult groins and obesity. (b) The potential exists for mechanical complications and obstruction to the introduction of rigid devices. (c) Correction or prevention by use of a stiff guidewire.

The difficult groin

The 'difficult groin' is usually the result of significant obesity, or multiple surgical scars. In the obese patient, shifting of tissue layers between the skin and target artery may result in an S-shaped deformity of the access sheath. These angulations and kinks make the passage of a more rigid device difficult and may set the stage for serious technical complications (Figure 11.8a,b). The use of an extra-stiff guidewire will prevent or correct this angulation and create a smooth, gently curved access pathway (Figure 11.8c).

Failure to visualize

Fluoroscopic visualization and guidance are mandatory whenever wires, catheters and other devices are being introduced transluminally. Failure to visualize may result in loss of guidewire access, percutaneous puncture difficulties, and possible vessel dissection or perforation.

High (suprainguinal) puncture

Suprainguinal access should be avoided. It incurs unnecessary risks of retroperitoneal bleeding and pseudoaneurysm formation related to ineffective external compression of the puncture site due to mechanical interference from the inguinal ligament.

Low puncture

Although this contradicts the senior author's (FJC's) experience, gaining access through the proximal SFA has been reported to result in a higher than expected complication rate.[3] The groin crease is a poor marker of the position of the inguinal ligament. Guidelines described in Figures 11.5 and 11.6 should be of help to target the common femoral artery more precisely, especially when dealing with a diminished or absent pulse, and in obese patients. Femoral bifurcation anatomy can also be defined by injecting contrast through the needle prior to introducing the guidewire or catheters. This maneuver will immediately reveal whether the artery has been entered at the desired location, and may provide clues about corrective measures if necessary.

Angle of vessel entry

As described, the angle of vessel puncture should be between 30° and 45° (Figure 11.1). An angle >45° may lead to significant bending of the access pathway between the skin and vascular lumen, resulting in troublesome angulation of the introducer sheath (Figure 11.8a,b).

Subintimal dissection

Subintimal dissection should be suspected whenever smooth intraluminal passage of the wire is impaired, particularly when the guidewire curls a very short distance after emerging from the needle (Figure 11.4). This situation underscores the importance of fluoroscopically visualizing the access site whenever the introduction of a wire or catheter proves difficult. Removal of the wire is usually necessary, followed by injection of a small amount of contrast to confirm the location of the needle. A new puncture may be necessary.

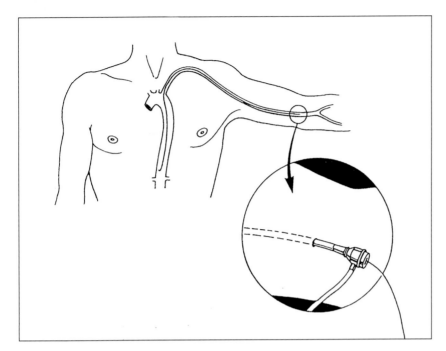

Figure 11.9
Antecubital site is preferred for brachial
artery puncture (using micropuncture set).

Brachial artery access

Puncture of the brachial artery is the second most frequently
used access site. It is a useful alternative for diagnostic angiography and interventional therapy in several vascular
territories. 5–7F systems are very well tolerated by the
brachial artery, with little risk of significant complications. The
left brachial artery is preferred whenever possible in order to
avoid crossing the flowpath to the cerebral circulation.

Technique

- Puncture of the distal brachial artery at or immediately
  above the antecubital fossa is our technique of choice
  (Figure 11.9). The artery is superficial and relatively fixed
  at this level, thus facilitating puncture. More importantly,
  it can be securely compressed against the humerus to
  obtain hemostasis upon removal of the sheath.
- A 21G needle/wire/catheter system (Micropuncture Kit,
  Cook, Bloomington, IN, USA) is used for initial entry.
  This is subsequently exchanged for a standard 0.035-inch
  guidewire and 5F introducer sheath. A Bentson, Storq or
  Wholey-type wire is preferred. Retrograde guidewire
  advancement is monitored and guided by fluoroscopy.
- Directing the guidewire down the descending thoracic
  aorta requires use of a pre-shaped selective (or pigtail)
  catheter (Figure 11.10). Otherwise, the wire is more
  likely to pass in the direction of the ascending aorta.
- A long 6F or 7F sheath is frequently used for brachiocephalic, visceral and renal procedures, and well
  tolerated in most instances.

- Hemostasis is achieved by simple manual compression of
  the puncture site for 15–20 min. Pseudoaneurysms and
  large hematomas occur only rarely, but ecchymoses are
  frequently observed.

The *axillary artery* is a very poor choice for percutaneous
arterial access, because of a definitely increased risk of inse-
cure hemostasis that can lead to intrasheath hematoma and
compressive neuropathy with (possibly) disastrous functional
sequelae. We see no reason to use this site – ever!

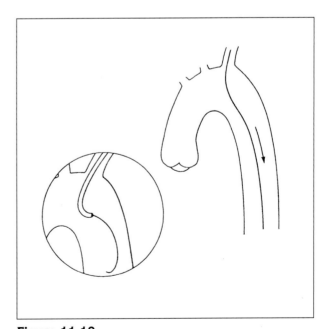

Figure 11.10
Steering of guidewire down the descending thoracic aorta is
facilitated by use of a selective 5F curved or pigtail catheter.

Retrograde popliteal artery puncture

Percutaneous retrograde puncture of the popliteal artery is an infrequently employed but useful alternative for endoluminal therapy of iliofemoral lesions that are in close proximity to the usual femoral puncture site. Requirements for safe popliteal artery puncture include absence of marked obesity or a very large extremity, and patency of a reasonably sized (>4 mm) popliteal artery that is relatively free of disease. Angiography and/or color-flow duplex scanning provide useful information to determine the appropriateness of using this puncture technique.

Technique (Figure 11.11)

- With the patient in the supine position, a 5F introducer sheath is placed (and secured) in the groin via retrograde femoral artery puncture. The patient is then turned to the prone position.
- The intended popliteal artery puncture target is placed in the center of the fluoroscopic field.
- Needle puncture is achieved under fluoroscopic guidance as the popliteal artery is visualized angiographically through a contrast injection in the (proximal) femoral sheath.

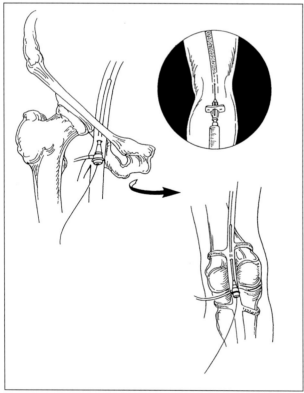

Figure 11.11

Technique of retrograde popliteal artery puncture, guided by angiographic visualization of the vessel following proximal injection of radiocontrast through the retrograde femoral sheath.

- Successful arterial puncture is followed by introduction of a guidewire, a 5–7F sheath, and transluminal intervention in standard fashion.
- Secure hemostasis is particularly important at this site. The following are helpful guidelines: use systemic heparin in small doses only (3000 U or less), reverse heparin with protamine sulfate if necessary prior to sheath removal, remove the sheath immediately at the end of the intervention, and follow by meticulous manual compression of the puncture site for 20–30 min.

Percutaneous closure devices[6,7]

Achieving puncture site hemostasis is an essential step, with potential for significant complications. The increasingly frequent use of larger-profile devices and aggressive anticoagulation, have brought puncture site management into focus.[6] There are several closure devices currently available: Perclose (Abbott), Duett (Vascular Solutions), VasoSeal (Datascope), Angio-Seal (Daig/St. Jude), and Matrix Vascular Sealing Gel (Access Closure). The Perclose device relies on transmural sutures, while the others use collagen to promote rapid formation of a thrombotic plug to seal the puncture hole.

Indications for use of a closure device[6]

Like other new technologies, closure devices offer attractive advantages but, at the same time, carry risks of complications and incur additional cost. The characteristics of each device need to be carefully considered as well. It would be safe to state that vascular closure is unnecessary and likely counter-productive when using an introducer sheath <6F. Puncture holes 7F and larger may be considered for closure, especially in the face of aggressive anticoagulation with heparin and/or IIb/IIIa glycoprotein inhibitors.

New developments

Biointerventional Corp. has developed the DISC-Close-Sure product with a catheter-based design that features an impermeable disk that is deployed intraluminally to locate the inner vessel wall and occlude the puncture hole temporarily while natural hemostasis occurs. The second-generation design (DISC-Close-Sure+) incorporates the capability of delivering a hemostatic agent to the puncture site.

The Scio Clo-Sur PAD (by Scion Cardio-Vascular) provides an alternative to the traditional closure devices. The product consists of naturally occurring biopolymer polyproleate acetate. This linear biopolymer is cationically charged in its dry state. It is the chain of positive charges along with the polymeric structure and molecular weight that endow polyprolate with its blood coagulating properties.

Another suture-based approach has been developed by Sutura, Inc. under the brand name SuperStitch. The device can be used to close puncture sites ranging from 6F to 24F. However, it is only approved for open or endoscopic procedures, and has not been approved for percutaneous vascular closure. Along the same lines is the Vascular Closure System (Angiolink Corporation). This device consists of three components: a titanium staple, a one-piece three-step introducer and a trigger-activated staple deployment mechanism. The result is an extraluminal purse-string staple closure. The device can be engineered for both small and large puncture sites, even those exceeding 20F. It is scheduled to enter phase I trials in the US in 2003.

Matrix VSG (vascular sealing gel; Access Closure Inc., Palo Alto, CA) is a tissue-adherent, flexible sealant consisting of two fully synthetic, nonthrombogenic liquids that – when mixed together – cause rapid cross-links to form a biocompatible absorbable gel that solidifies within seconds of injection and provides secure hemostasis within one minute.

Overview and conclusions

Endovascular access techniques and puncture site management are being recognized increasingly as critical components in angiographic and interventional procedures. Sound judgement in choosing a particular site, and skilled achievement of luminal access, rank among the most important steps, perhaps eclipsed only by the pivotal importance of securing prompt and reliable hemostasis after removal of the introducer sheath. New technologies and innovative techniques are now available to help us achieve these goals. However, in the end, it is the physician's interventional judgement and impeccable technical execution that carry the most weight at the time of preventing complications and produce a successful outcome.

References

1   Criado FJ, Abul-Khoudoud O, Wellons E. Complications and Troubleshooting. In: White RA, Fogarty TJ, eds. *Peripheral Vascular Intervention*, 2nd edn. New York: Springer-Verlag, 1999: 445–54.

2   Reagan K, Matsumoto AH, Teitelbaum GP. Comparison of the hydrophilic guidewire in double- and single-wall entry: potential hazards. *Cathet Cardiovasc Diagn* 1991; **24**: 205–8.

3   Altin RS, Flicker S, Naidech HJ. Pseudoaneurysm and artiovenous fistula after femoral artery catheterization: association with lower femoral punctures. *Am J Radiol* 1989; **152**: 629–31.

4   Rupp SB, Vogelzang RI, Nemcek AA et al. Relationship of the inguinal ligament to pelvic radiographic landmarks: anatomic correlation and its role in femoral arteriography. *J Vasc Intervent Radiol* 1993; **4**: 409–13.

5   Criado FJ. Percutaneous arterial puncture and endoluminal access techniques for peripheral intervention. *J Invas Cardiol* 1999; **11**: 450–6.

6   Criado FJ, Abul-Khoudoud O, Martin JA, Wilson EP. Current developments in percutaneous arterial closure devices. *Ann Vasc Surg* 2000; **14**: 683–7.

7   Achieving closure: a comprehensive overview of vascular closure technology (multiple articles). *Endovascular Today*, Wayne, PA: Bryn Mawr Communications, April 2003.

12

Transbrachial and transaxillary approach: indications, techniques, pitfalls and complications

Leon Gengler and Alain Rodde

Indications

Diagnostic and therapeutic procedures of the cervical arteries, of the arteries of the upper and lower extremities as well as of the abdominal aorta and branch vessels may be performed through the left brachial or axillary artery, but also through a right-sided approach.

The following indications are best suited for the left transbrachial approach, because of contraindications or failure of the femoral route or simply because of an easier approach from the upper extremity:

- Stenosis or occlusion of the left subclavian artery, in particular for ostial and paraostial lesions
- Renal artery stenosis in case of a sharp downward angle of the artery (2 out of 85 renal artery stents for Henry et al[1]). Some authors prefer the left brachial approach as a routine method for renal artery stenting[2]
- Stenosis of the celiac trunk and mesenteric arteries
- Occlusion of the abdominal aorta[3]
- Bilateral common iliac artery stenoses
- Stenosis or occlusion of the iliac arteries after failure of the femoral approach
- Postoperative scars of the groin
- Common femoral artery aneurysm
- Absent femoral artery pulses

The right brachial approach is best indicated for the treatment of stenoses of the right subclavian or the innominate artery as well as in cases of failure of the left brachial approach.

The axillary as well as the proximal brachial approach are possible options in case of small brachial arteries, or major atherosclerosis of the abdominal aorta,[4] or because of the use of a 7F or 8F arterial sheath.

Techniques

For diagnostic studies through the transbrachial approach mostly performed on outpatients, no anticoagulation is necessary.

For percutaneous angioplasty, anticoagulation with heparin (7500–10 000 U per 12 h) is started the previous evening, associated with antiplatelet therapy (aspirin 100–250 mg/day).

Spasmolytic therapy may be performed locally through the arterial sheath with 0.5 mg isosorbide dinitrate.

Transbrachial approach

At the antecubital fossa

No premedication is necessary. Slight sedation or neuroleptanalgesia may, however, be useful. The patient lies supine on the X-ray table, with the arm supinated and extended on an arm board in a 30–90° abduction. A superficial injection of 2% lidocaine is administered at the puncture site. The puncture is performed with a 19G Cordis one-piece needle, allowing the insertion of a 0.035-inch guidewire. This type of needle mostly avoids transfixion of the artery by immediate blood reflux. The puncture is performed superficially and obliquely in a proximal and internal direction along the axis of the brachial and radial artery. The entry site of the puncture needle is located 1–3 cm beneath the elbow bent in the antecubital fossa, where manual artery compression is easiest at the end of the procedure (Figure 12.1).

In case of a proximal bifurcation of the brachial artery, puncture may involve the proximal radial artery, which continues the axis of the brachial artery.

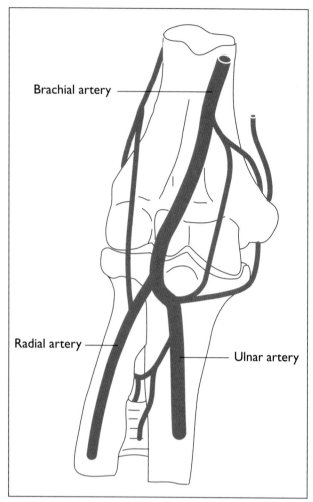

Figure 12.1
Elbow: normal arterial anatomy.

No arterial sheath is necessary for diagnostic studies with a 4F or 5F catheter. For angioplasty, it is advisable to stay with a 6F or possibly a 7F arterial sheath (Cordis 10 cm with a 0.038-inch guidewire) constantly perfused with heparin. After insertion of the sheath, a 1.5-mm J-shaped, 0.035-inch, 150-cm-long teflon-coated guidewire (Cordis) is routinely used.

In case of a tortuous brachial, axillary, subclavian or innominate artery, a hydrophilic guidewire is used (0.035-inch, 150-cm Terumo guidewire with a 3-cm flexible tip). Since significant arterial stenoses are infrequent, advancement of the guidewire and catheter to the thoracic aorta is mostly easy. Placement is fluoroscopically monitored as soon as the guidewire is advanced with difficulty.

On the left side, in most patients, the wire is advanced into the ascending arch of the aorta rather than into the descending aorta.

On the right side, mostly the wire passes into the ascending aorta, but in case of a large atheromatous aortic arch or left atheromatous displacement of the innominate artery, the guidewire may occasionally pass into the descending thoracic aorta. We find that manipulation of the guidewire into the descending aorta is made easier by using two types of catheters, whether the approach is through the right or the left brachial artery:

• Pigtail catheter (PIG Cordis Super Torque 5.2F or 4F 0.038 inch, 100 cm long). The curvature of the catheter allows the guidewire to slide along the upper wall of the aortic arch down to the descending aorta. Most standard guidewires are too stiff and have to be changed to a hydrophilic guidewire (0.035 inch, 150 cm Terumo with a 3-cm flexible tip).
• Simmons 2 catheter (Cordis Super-Torque 4F or 5F 100 cm long). The catheter is passed into the ascending aorta as far as the aortic valves and advanced so as to bend back on itself. Then the catheter is slowly withdrawn along the aortic arch, far enough to allow its tip to bend to the descending aorta. The guidewire is advanced along the upper wall of the aortic arch down to the descending aorta, the catheter then being advanced over the guidewire. In most cases, a hydrophilic guidewire is necessary (Figures 12.2 and 12.3).

Another technique may be useful, as follows. A 1.5-mm, J-shaped teflon-coated guidewire is pushed down to the aortic valves far enough to allow the wire to bend at the junction of the left subclavian artery with the aorta. A further push of the wire allows the proximal portion of the bend to advance down the descending aorta. The catheter is then advanced down the proximal bend of the guidewire.

After placement of the catheter into the inferior thoracic or upper abdominal aorta, the guidewire is changed to a 0.035-inch, 260-cm-long straight guidewire (Cordis exchange). Sometimes a stiff guidewire is necessary to prevent bending of the balloon catheter at the junction of the subclavian artery with the aorta (0.035-inch, 260-cm Amplatz Super Stiff with a 7-cm flexible tip). The 5F balloon catheter is inserted through the brachial sheath and advanced into the abdominal aorta, its branch vessels or the iliac arteries. Angiography to control the result of angioplasty may be done after retrieval of the balloon catheter by means of an angiography catheter advanced over a second guidewire. However, it is helpful to change the 10-cm arterial sheath to a 6F 90-cm-long sheath (Daig Corp, Minneapolis, MN, USA) which allows easy contrast injections. The long arterial sheath has to be used in case of stenting, in particular with Palmaz stents.

At the proximal brachial artery

The puncture site is at the upper third of the arm supinated and extended in a 60–90° abduction. This approach is an alternative to the axillary puncture and allows the insertion of a sheath superior to 6F. We do not use it.

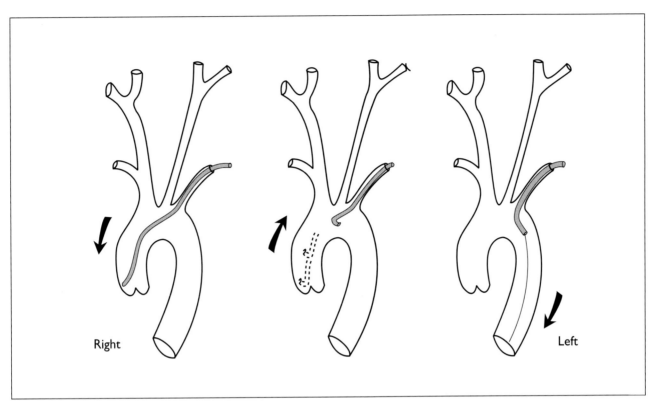

Figure 12.2
Left subclavian artery.

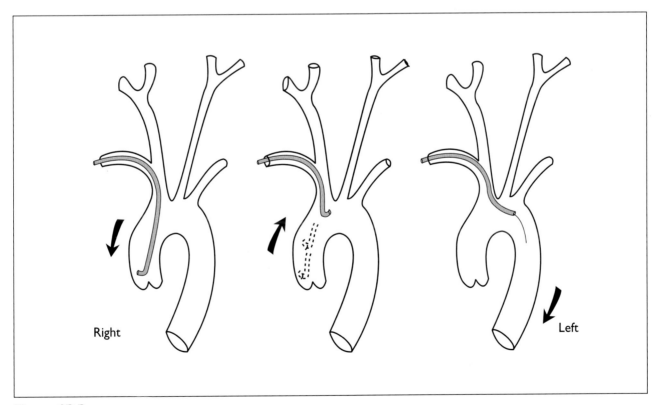

Figure 12.3
Right subclavian artery.

Transaxillary approach

The patient lies supine on the X-ray table with his hand underneath his head, with the arm supinated and extended from 90° to 180°, according to the physician's routine. The best positioning is the one which allows easy palpation of the arterial pulse, which is found in the axillary fossa along the anterior border of the pectoral muscle. After local anesthesia with 10 ml of lidocaine 2%, the axillary artery is punctured at the best arterial pulse at the level of or above the lesser pectoral muscle, proximal to the median nerve.

We do not use the axillary approach anymore for diagnostic studies, since the brachial route is most convenient.

For angioplasty, the axillary artery allows insertion of a 7F or 8F sheath.

Maneuvers to advance guidewire and catheter into the descending thoracic aorta are approximately the same as for the brachial approach.

Pitfalls

Technical difficulties seldom occur: brachial puncture is easy and applies mainly to patients with a palpable brachial pulse. In case of spasm of the left brachial puncture site, we recommend performing the procedure through the axillary or through the right brachial artery.

Unwanted catheterization of axillary side-branches, internal mammary artery or thyrocervical trunk may happen with a standard J-shaped guidewire. The use of a hydrophilic guidewire implies fluoroscopic monitoring to avoid possible injury of brachial or axillary side-branches. Tortuosity of the innominate artery may allow the catheter to advance to the right common carotid artery. Fluoroscopic monitoring is recommended for guidewire advancement in the subclavian and innominate artery.

Adequate advancement of the guidewire may be helped by the use of a Simmons catheter. Advancing the guidewire from the aortic arch to the descending thoracic aorta may be very difficult in case of a large atheromatous aorta. Only the use of a hydrophilic guidewire may allow advancement down the thoracic aorta. The guidewire has to be pushed down to the lower abdominal aorta to avoid recoil when the catheter is subsequently advanced over the guidewire.

Complications

Arterial spasm

Spasm may happen while puncturing the brachial artery. The failure rate due to arterial spasm is 4 out of 438 patients for Barnett et al.[5]

In case of spasm, the left brachial approach has to be given up in favor of the right brachial or the left axillary approach. Spasm is more frequent in smokers and women.[6]

The brachial approach has to be avoided in younger patients, especially women, because of a higher risk of spasm.

Temporary loss of radial pulse is found in 1.6% of cases, while a prolonged loss of radial pulse is found in 0.2% of diagnostic angiographies with 4F catheters.[5] Spasm might be more frequent with larger 6F or 7F arterial sheaths.

Arterial spasm may be treated medically by:

* Intra-arterial injection of nitroglycerin: isosorbide dinitrate 1 mg per injection up to 4 mg with continuous monitoring of blood pressure
* Sublingual or oral nifedipine (10 mg)

Diminution or loss of the radial pulse after removal of the catheter or during manual compression of the brachial artery is usually managed by us with immersion of the patient's hand and wrist in a moderately hot water bath.

While manual compression is continued, the radial pulse soon returns because of peripheral vasodilation.

Thrombosis

Spasm favors arterial thrombosis, in particular in a small brachial artery. To avoid spasm and thrombosis:

* Avoid double-wall puncture by using a one-piece needle
* Avoid forcing the guidewire in; advance it gently into the brachial and axillary artery by avoiding dissection of the arterial wall
* Use a sheath not larger than 6F in a brachial artery, and a 7F or 8F sheath in an axillary artery

In small numbers of patients, precise evaluation of the risk of thrombosis is not possible with a 6F or 7F sheath. With 4F catheters, no thrombosis was noted by Rodde et al[7] and Morin et al.[8] One case of thrombosis out of 660 patients was reported by Gritter et al.[9]

Hematoma at the puncture site

Manual brachial artery compression is easier than femoral artery compression because the pulse is easier to locate even in obese patients and because of a solid bone support underneath the artery.

Increased risk of hematoma is seen in cases of:

* Arterial wall damage while introducing the guidewire, the catheter or the sheath
* Larger arterial sheath (6F or 7F)
* Shorter compression or immobilization time
* Low platelet count ($<50\,000/mm^3$)

- High anticoagulation with heparin associated with aspirin
- High blood pressure

During diagnostic angiography with a 4F catheter, hematomas at the puncture site needing surgical drainage are infrequent: 0.15%[9] to 0.28%,[7] while spontaneously resorbing hematomas are more frequent 1.4%, 1.8%, 3.2% or 9.5%.[5,7,8,9]

Hematomas tend to be more frequent with larger sheaths, because the surface of the puncture hole is 64% higher with a 5F than with a 4F catheter, two times higher with a 6F catheter, and three times higher with a 7F catheter.

Some rare complications

- Arteriovenous fistula or traumatic aneurysm[10]
- Distal embolism: rare in the upper extremities
- Local infection[8] or phlebitis
- Arterial wall dissection: 0.2%[5] at the puncture site or during advancement of the catheter into a side-branch, in particular of the axillary artery. An axillary hematoma after a brachial approach may be a delayed complication as a result of damage to a side-branch
- Minor hazards, requiring no specific treatment, but generating some discomfort to the patient:[9] local arm pain (7.5%); transient paresthesia (7.3%); ecchymosis (50.4%)
- Neurologic complications: related to vertebrobasilar emboli with subsequent transient lateral hemianopsia and emboli to the right carotis with amaurosis fugax, sensory or motor symptoms, mostly transient
- Complications of the axillary approach are as follows: hematoma at the puncture site with possible nerve compression in the axilla or thrombosis (1.2%);[11] neurologic symptoms in the median and ulnar nerve territory are reported in 2.8% of the cases with axillary hematomas, and in 8% of the cases[12] where the procedure is performed with a 6.5 or 7.1F catheter; general hazards not related to the axillary route (1.2%)[11]

Conclusion

The left transbrachial artery approach is a valuable technique and has to be used instead of the transfemoral route in selected indications.

The right transbrachial, transaxillary and proximal transbrachial approach have few indications as an approach for the abdominal aorta and its branch vessels or for the iliac arteries.

References

1 Henry M, Amor M, Allaoui M et al. Renal arterial stent placement: single center experience, personal communication.

2 Dorros G, Prince C, Mathiak L. Stenting of a renal artery stenosis achieves better relief of the obstructive lesion, than balloon angioplasty. *Catheter Cardiovasc Diagn* 1993; **29**: 191–8.

3 Iyer S, Hall P, Dorros G. Brachial approach to management of an abdominal aortic occlusion with prolonged lysis and subsequent angioplasty. *Catheter Cardiovasc Diagn* 1991; **23**: 290–3.

4 Tegtmeyer CJ, Ayers CA, Wellons HA. The axillary approach to percutaneous renal artery dilatation. *Radiology* 1980; **135**: 775–6.

5 Barnett FJ, Lecky DM, Freiman DB, Montecalvo RM. Cerebrovascular disease: outpatient evaluation with selective carotid DSA performed via a transbrachial approach. *Radiology* 1989; **170**: 535–9.

6 Becker GJ, Hicks ME, Holden RW. Patient selection, catheters and contrast agents in intravenous and intraarterial DSA. II Appl. *Radiology* 1986; **15**: 69–73.

7 Rodde A, Bazin C, Blum A et al. Artériographie sélective des troncs supra-aortiques par voie humérale droite avec un catheter 4F. *J Radiol* 1993; **74**(12): 657–60.

8 Morin ME, Willens BA, Kuss PA. Carotid artery: percutaneous transbrachial selective arteriography with a 4-F catheter. *Radiology* 1989; **171**: 868–70.

9 Gritter KJ, Laidlaw WW, Peterson TN. Complications of outpatient transbrachial intraarterial digital subtraction angiography. *Radiology* 1987; **162**: 125–7.

10 Fodor G, Bonatti G, Psenner K, Ortore P. Un caso di fistola artero-venosa come complicanza tardiva di puntura percutanea dell'arteria omerale in angiografia vertebrale: diagnosi con color Doppler. *Radiol Med Torino* 1990; **80**(3): 367–9.

11 McIvor J, Rhymer JC. Transaxillary arteriograms in arteriopathic patients: success rate and complications. *Clin Radiol* 1992; **45**: 390–4.

12 Smith DC, Mitchell DA, Peterson GW et al. Medial brachial fascial compartment syndrome: anatomic basis of neuropathy after transaxillary arteriography. *Radiology* 1989; **173**: 149–54.

13

Transradial approach

Isabelle Henry and Michel Henry

Introduction

Femoral access is the most often used approach way for peripheral arterial procedures. However, the management of sheath removal and the prevention of vascular access complications still remain a practical day-to-day problem, including personnel involved to compress, cost of mechanical compression device or percutaneous closure device, and nursing time and in-hospital stay time, particularly after interventional procedures which require an aggressive anticoagulation therapy.

Furthermore the femoral approach is sometimes impossible for anatomical reasons: e.g. iliac stenosis or occlusion, tortuosities, aneurysm.

The transradial approach was first described for coronary procedures and is currently largely used with a very low rate of vascular complications, allowing an early discharge of the patient. The approach should be well known and should be used more frequently for some good indications.

Technique

Patients' selection

The major inclusion criteria are a good pulsating right or left radial artery, associated with a good cubital artery pulse and the absence of digital ischemia by Allen's test. This test is considered as normal if, after compression of both ulnar and radial arteries, hand color returned to normal within 10 s after releasing the ulnar artery.

Exclusion criteria are the following:

- absence of radial or ulnar pulse
- digital ischemia by Allen's test
- lesions which can necessitate techniques requiring large guiding catheters. A 7F (French) guiding catheter is possible in 70% of the patients, an 8F in 60%.

Which radial artery?

A right transradial approach is easier to perform for a right-handed operator. The left radial approach may be used with equal success.

Patient's position

The patient's arm may be extended a few inches from the body for the puncture, but the arm may rest along the body. The patient hand may be hyperextended in supine position, or in a relaxed supine position without hyperextension.

Artery puncture

A neuroleptanalgesia is performed in addition to local anesthesia with a superficial injection of 1–2 ml lidocaine followed by a light massage.

The puncture of the radial artery may be done with an 18–22 gauge bare needle (needle diameter selected in relation to the guide wire) at a 30–45° angle approximately 1 cm from the styloid process. Puncture with a venous catheter is possible and allows injections of antispastic medications before sheath insertion.

Several kits – (Arrow kit, Cordis kit) – are now on the market and can facilitate the technique.

Insertion of sheath

The operator may use a long (23 cm), standard (13 cm), or short (7 cm) sheath. A long sheath may serve to mechanically prevent spasm and facilitate movements of a guiding catheter, although it is harder to withdraw.

Following puncture using a bare needle, a straight Teflon 0.025 inch wire, 1.50 m in length, is used to catheterize the ascending aorta and permits identification of antebrachial or brachial loops. The extremity of the wire is slightly bent manually in order to facilitate insertion in the artery and crossing of tortuous segments.

The needle is then withdrawn and the introducer advanced into the artery over the wire (a cut in the skin may be made cautiously).

Following puncture with a venous catheter or a kit, the guide is inserted through the small catheter already in place. This wire may be short as it is only used to insert the introducer.

Medication cocktail

Medication is administered for prevention of spasm and radial thrombosis. We combine fast-acting nitrates (isosorbide dinitrate, molsidomine) and prolonged action verapamil (3–5 mg) injected simultaneously in the radial artery through the side lumen of the introducer. Subsequently, 5000 IU heparin are injected to prevent radial thrombosis.

Catheterization of the aorta and other arteries

This procedure is performed by the combined action of the guide wire and angiographic or angioplasty catheter. In the presence of severe loops (antibrachial, brachial) or tortuous subclavian arteries, hydrophilic wires may be used.

Any catheters, guiding catheters, or guide wires can be used in this approach, allowing the catheterization of not only coronary arteries but also renal, mesenteric, vertebral, carotid, and subclavian arteries.

Catheterization of the iliac and femoropopliteal arteries is limited by the length of the devices.

Introducer sheath removal and hemostasis

The arterial sheath is removed immediately after the withdrawal of the guiding catheter at the end of the procedure. The artery is manually compressed only for the time necessary to place a tourniquet set over the puncture site.

Local compression is held in place for 30–45 min and then pressure is gradually released until hemostasis is obtained. A compressive bandage is applied for 6 hours. The patient may be allowed to stand up for 1 hour after the end of the procedure and the radial pulse is checked by clinical examination.

Indications for radial approach

Femoral artery access may be difficult in obese patients, extensive postoperative scarring, and severe peripheral disease, is impossible in case of aortic or iliac occlusion, or relatively contraindicated (coagulopathy). For these patients the radial approach may be useful to catheterize supraortic, mesenteric, renal, or iliac arteries. Angiography and interventional procedures may be performed in this way and most of the stents can be implanted through 6–8F introducers.

This method should be more often used to treat supraortic and renal arteries.

Advantages

There are several advantages of the transradial approach. The sheaths are removed immediately after the procedure and no personnel are needed to compress the radial artery. The patient is able to ambulate 2 hours after the procedure and, if after an observation period of 6 hours no access site-related complications occur, an early discharge in carefully selected patients is possible. Peripheral procedures on an outpatient basis can now be performed, which reduces cost and patient discomfort.

Complications

Vascular access complications are reduced compared with femoral access and may occur in 1–2% of the cases, mainly forearm or arm hematomas. Asymptomatic radial artery occlusion has been reported in 6–10%, although 40% appear to spontaneously recanalize after 1 month.

Conclusion

Radial access is a new approach for peripheral procedures and indications should widen as a result of the new generation of miniaturized equipment, fewer access site complications, and the development of the procedures on an outpatient basis.

14

Popliteal access site

Michel Henry

Introduction

In endovascular treatment of peripheral arterial disease, the antegrade or retrograde femoral approach is the most often used access.

Lesions at the femoral bifurcation prevent guide wires and introducers from being placed. This leads to the use of other approaches such as the brachial, radial, controlateral or popliteal accesses. Described herein are the antegrade and retrograde popliteal approaches, as well as the present author's experience, so defining the current technique and its indications.[1–9]

Techniques

Retrograde percutaneous popliteal approach

The popliteal artery, together with the sciatic nerve and the popliteal vein, goes upward along the diagonal of the **popliteal triangle**. The superficial location of the popliteal artery allows retrograde puncture, which is usually performed just above the joint. The patient is preferably in the ventral decubitus position but may alternatively be in the lateral decubitus position. The procedure is usually performed under local anesthesia and complemented by intravenous sedation. General anesthesia, which may still be performed, is rarely required.

Before choosing the popliteal approach, one should check that the artery is free from any atheromatous lesion or significant stenosis. Angiography may be sufficient. However, echography provides more information regarding the state of the artery, particularly the presence of an aneurysm, which is a strict contraindication to puncture.

Due to overlying lesions, the artery may not be pulsatile. It should then first be located, for which several techniques may be used:

- **Angiography**: a 4 or 5F catheter is placed in the abdominal aorta, generally through contralateral access. Contrast media is injected to visualize the course of the popliteal runoff. 'Road mapping' renders the puncture more easily
- **Doppler** echocardiography (EchoDoppler): Angiography and/or EchoDoppler assists in locating the popliteal artery and the puncture site
- **'Smart Needle'**: A Doppler probe is connected to the needle. The sound of the Doppler helps in locating the popliteal artery.

Once the artery is punctured, an introducer, generally 6 or 7F, is placed in the artery. Larger introducers (8 or 9F) may be used in cases where larger devices are needed, such as burrs or covered endoprostheses, as long as the artery is at least 6 mm in diameter.

Although contrast media injections are performed through a contralateral access, the femoral bifurcation and the origin of the deep femoral artery are usually well opacified. The introducer is withdrawn at the end of the procedure. Hemostasis is obtained with manual compression of the puncture site for 10 to 20 min, and then a bandage is applied for 24 hours. Arterial puncture-site-closure devices may also be used at this level.[10]

Antegrade percutaneous popliteal approach

The popliteal artery may be accessed through an antegrade approach in the case of femoral artery obstruction, by using short introducers from 6 to 8 cm in length. This allows access to lesions in the leg, which may be helpful for limb salvage.

Applicable endovascular techniques

All angioplasty techniques may be performed through this approach, including balloon angioplasty atherectomy, such as rotational atherectomy (Rotablator),[11] or recanalization devices, such as the laser fiber. All stents that may be implanted in the femoral artery may be introduced through this access. This also allows placement of covered stents,[13] as compared to the contralateral access which is limited due to the rigidity of the introduction materials. Intravascular ultrasound examinations may also be performed through this access and all mechanical thrombectomy devices may be used e.g. Hydrolyser, AngioJet.[14]

In situ fibrinolysis may be attempted for limb salvage.[4–6]

However, it should be performed carefully due to risks of compression hematomas at this level. Small-diameter introducers should used with preference.

Drugs (pharmacological milieu)

The pharmacological environment for an angioplasty performed through the popliteal approach is the same as for any angioplasty performed from another approach. The day before the procedure, patients are given heparin IV (10 000 units/day), in addition to aspirin and calcium blockers, e.g. nifedipin (30 mg/day) or diltiazem (180 mg/day).

During the procedure a bolus injection of 5 000 units of heparin is given intravenously after the introducer is placed. Following the procedure, they are given aspirin indefinitely and ticlopidine or clopidogrel if stents are implanted.

Indications to popliteal approach

Retrograde femoral approach

There are two major classes of indications.

Popliteal approach as first choice

There are three types of indications.
(1) The femoral approach is contraindicated or may not be performed due to severe atheromatous lesions at the puncture site or due to heavy calcifications. An arterial EchoDoppler examination at the puncture site should be performed prior to the procedure to reveal lesions that were previously undetected, thus contraindicating the femoral approach.
(2) The other contralateral or brachial approach may not be used or are contraindicated. The contralateral approach may be difficult due to tortuous, stenosed, very atheromatous arteries, or an aortobifemoral bypass at a very acute aortic angle. They may also prevent the introduction of some devices. Certain atherectomy devices may not be used or long covered stents may not be placed through contralateral access due to the rigidity of the materials that may not cross the bifurcation.
As well, risks through the brachial access are even higher (thrombosis at the puncture site, cerebral embolization risks, etc.)
(3) The popliteal approach may be chosen as first choice due to the localization of the lesions.
   (a) Ostial lesions of the superficial femoral artery; (i) lesions in the proximal part of the artery; (ii) diffuse lesions (proximal and mid-third).
   (b) Lesions of the common femoral artery; (i) associated lesions (common femoral, proximal part of the superficial femoral artery); (ii) stenosis of a superior anastomosis of a bypass graft (Figure 14.1).

Arteries using an antegrade popliteal puncture. The present author has used this limb salvage procedure, but it requires skill and experience. The puncture site is localized through 'road mapping'. It may therefore be the only therapeutic access if surgery more proximally (e.g. femoropopliteal bypass graft) may not be performed and if the patient suffers from critical ischemia.

Author's personal experience

A total of 153 patients under this group's care have benefited from transluminal angioplasty using the percutaneous retrograde popliteal approach. During the same period, 5230 peripheral angioplasties were performed by the group, so transluminal angioplasties represent 2.8% of our procedures. These patients comprised 124 males and 29 females, with a mean age of 63 years (range 39–86 years). Risk factors were: diabetes ($n = 29$), hypertension ($n = 76$), smoking ($n = 120$), dyslipidemia ($n = 84$).

Of these patients, 117 were in stage II of Fontaine's classification, 24 in stage III, and 12 in stage IV. Lesion locations were as given in Table 14.1: 67% of the lesions were heavily calcified.

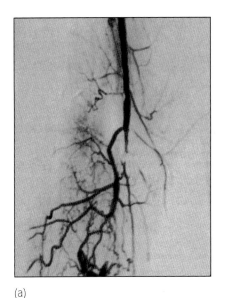 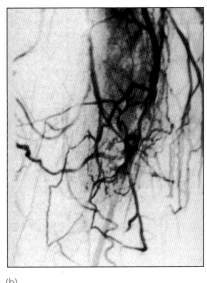 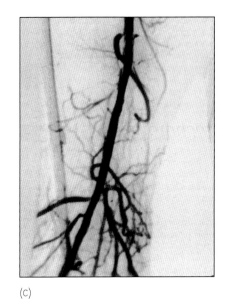

(a)   (b)   (c)

Figure 14.1

Table 14.1	Location of lesions	
Location		**Number**
Superficial femoral		133
Ostial lesions (2–4 cm)		7
Diffuse lesions > 15 cm		27
Thromboses		97
< 4 cm		5
4–8 cm		12
> 8 cm		80
aneurysm		1
post-surgery chronic dissection		1
Common femoral		17
Stenoses (2–4 cm)		10
Thromboses (4–6 cm)		7
Superior anastomosis stenosis of a bypass graft		3

Distal arterial runoff

Distal arterial runoff was as follows:

three patent vessels:	70 patients	(stage IIb)
two patent vessels:	46 patients	(stage IIc)
	13 patients	(stage III)
one patent vessel:	16 patients	(stage III)
	8 patients	(stage IV)

Seventy-five patients underwent angioplasty through the popliteal access as first choice and 78 as second choice after failure of recanalization, either antegrade through the ipsilateral femoral despite the use of hydrophilic guide wires, laser fibers or Kensey catheters, or through brachial or contralateral access sites.

Technical success

Success of the popliteal access was as follows:

No puncture failure	
Immediate success	138/153 (90%)
Success of first choice:	69/75 (92%)
Success of second choice:	69/78 (88%)

The ankle brachial index increased from 0.52 ± 0.15 before the procedure to 0.92 ± 0.13 after the procedure.

Failures occurred in 15/153 (10%) of cases and were mostly observed in long calcified lesions.

Techniques used

Laser recanalization	24 patients
Recanalization with Kensey catheter	four patients
Simpson atherectomy device	one patient
Rotablator	16 patients
Stent placement	87 patients

(Palmaz, $n = 36$; Strecker, $n = 2$; Nitinol stents, $n = 28$; covered stents, $n = 26$: several stents were implanted in the same patient.)

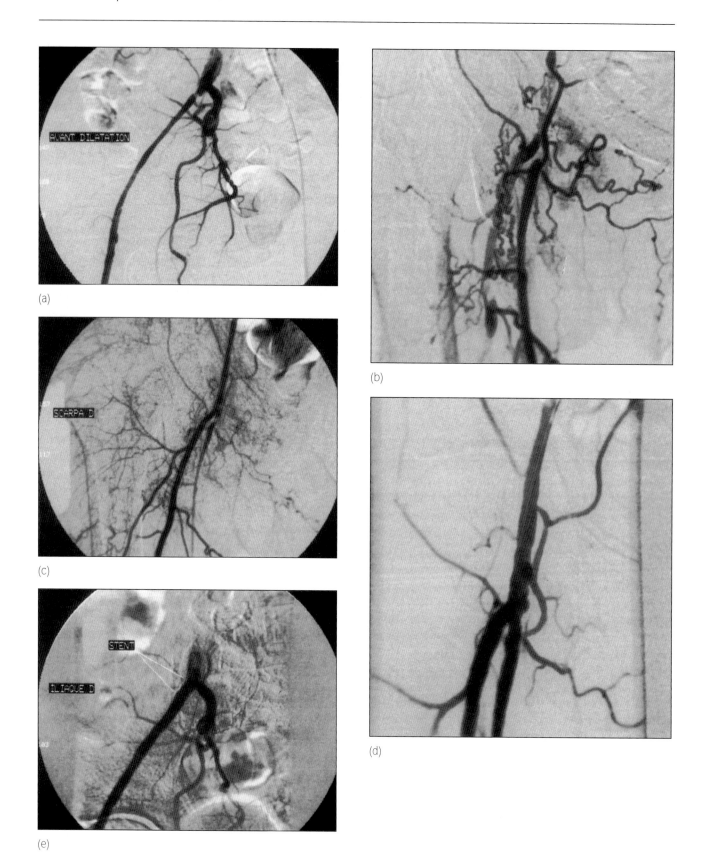

(a)

(b)

(c)

(d)

(e)

Figure 14.2

Complications

Two hematomas were reported at the puncture site; they did not lead to compression symptoms and did not require surgery. Nine acute thromboses in the superficial femoral artery appeared at the angioplasty site during the first day; five required a bypass, two were successfully treated with mechanical thrombectomy (hydrolyser) and/or thrombo-aspiration, and two patients who refused surgery were treated with drugs. Six thromboses appeared during the first month following the procedure; three were treated successfully with fibrinolysis and a new angioplasty, and three required a bypass graft.

Six arteriovenous fistulas without hemodynamic consequences were also reported.

Discussion

The popliteal access is still not often used, although it is reliable thanks to a good localization techniques (e.g. road mapping, EchoDoppler). Indeed, in a series of 50 angioplasties, Tonnesen et al.[1] reported results equivalent to ours, with an immediate success rate of 100%.

Some contraindications must be respected (e.g. respiratory insufficiency, obesity) which would prevent obtaining a satisfactory ventral decubitus position. Other cases were also encountered where this approach could not be used, such as an inability to hyperextend the knee. Anatomical characteristics may also prevent popliteal access such as a thin popliteal artery, femoral or femoropopliteal obstruction near the puncture site. However, even when these contraindications are taken into account, this still very often a usable approach.

As a first-choice treatment, this approach competes with the contralateral femoral and brachial accesses. However, those are not always usable for anatomic reasons and certain techniques may be difficult to use through these two access sites, whereas the popliteal access allows nearly all endovascular techniques. All endoprostheses currently available may be implanted through popliteal access, especially covered stents, which allow the creation of internal bypass through a percutaneous access. The stent may be implanted very precisely at the femoral ostium through the popliteal access, whereas this not always easy through contralateral access. The popliteal approach may be used to treat aneurysms in the leg arteries[2-3] or for in-situ fibrinolysis for limb salvage.[4-6]

This approach has high technical success rates and 88% of the antegrade femoral access failures could be recovered.

Complications of this access are rare as long as a pre-procedure EchoDoppler is performed to check the patency of the artery and that there is no aneurysm at this level. Risk of thrombosis at the puncture site is rare, never being

observed by this group. The hematomas observed were without any consequence and new arterial puncture site closure devices should decrease the risk. Tonnesen et al.[1] reports two popliteal hematomas in 50 cases, neither of which required surgery. Those hematomas caused edema and pain for 2–3 months. There remains an unsolved problem: the arteriovenous fistulas, which seem to be frequent. They are, however, without any obvious hemodynamic consequence.

Long-term results of the procedure do not depend on the approach but on the technique itself and on the lesions treated. The place of the popliteal access as compared to the contralateral and brachial approach ways is still debatable. The other two access sites allow manual compression remote from the treatment site, which is not associated with a decrease in flow related to the compression, which can result in the complication of thrombosis. Since the contralateral approach permits the use of large introducers, it thus also allows for procedures such as the 'kissing' technique in the femoral bifurcation, which is not usable through the popliteal access.

The brachial access, although useful, is limited by the diameter of the introducers. With preference, this group uses the popliteal access to treat superficial femoral lesions which may not be treated at first or second choice by an upper access. The antegrade popliteal approach enables treatment of popliteal lesions or threatening leg lesions.

Conclusions

The popliteal access seems reliable and efficient, enabling the operator to recover numerous failures of the antegrade femoral access. However, because of the lack of familiarity with this technique, it has not been widely used in the treatment of peripheral arterial diseases. Its complication rate is low, as long as one adheres to a strict technique and locates the artery precisely. Its indications should be compared with those of the other access sites, i.e. contralateral and brachial. The popliteal approach accommodates all of the endovascular techniques and, by broadening the indications for angioplasty, it improves the success rate of the procedures. This approach should be better known and more frequently used by interventionists.

References

1   Tonnesen KH, Sager P, Karle A et al. Percutaneous translumi-nal angioplasty of the superficial femoral artery by retrograde catheterization via the popliteal artery. *Cardiovasc Intervent Radiol* 1988; 11:127–31.

2   Edwards H, Martin E, Nowygrod R. Nonoperative manage-ment of a traumatic peroneal artery false aneurysm. *J Trauma* 1982; 22:323–6.

3   McIvor J, Treweeke PS. Case report: direct percutaneous embolisation of a false aneurysm with steel coils. *Clin Radiol* 1988; **39**:205–7.

4   Perler BA, Osterman FA. Immediate postoperative urokinase infusion: extending the limits of limb salvage surgery. *J Cardiovasc Surg* 1990; **31**:184–8.

5   Schroeder J. Catheter lysis and percutaneous transluminal angioplasty below the knee via the popliteal artery in a patient with femoral artery obstruction: technical note. *Cardiovasc Intervent Radiol* 1989; **12**:344-345

6   Weisman ID, Standchfield WR, Herzog CA Jr et al. Left ventricular thromboembolic occlusion of the popliteal artery treated nonoperatively with local urokinase infusion. A case report. *Angiology* 1988; **39**:179–86.

7   Zeitler E, Richter EJ, Roth FJ et al. Results of percutaneous angioplasty. *Radiology* 1983; **146**:57–60.

8   Henry M, Amicabile C, Amor M et al. Angioplastie artérielle périphérique. Intérêt de la voie poplitée. A propos de 30 cas. *Arch Mal Cœur* 1993; **88** :463–9 (abstract).

9   Henry M, Amor M, Henry I et al. Percutaneous transluminal angioplasty of peripheral arteries with retrograde catheterization through the popliteal artery: series of 63 cases. *Radiol* 1994; **193**:192 (abstract).

10 Henry M, Amor M, Allaoui M et al. A new access site management tool: the AngioSeal haemostatic puncture closure device. *J Endovasc Surg* 1995; **2**:289–96.

11 Henry M, Amor M, Ethevenot G et al. Percutaneous peripheral atherectomy using the Rotablator. *J Endovasc Surg* 1995; **2**:51–66.

12 Henry M, Amor M. Stenting of femoral and popliteal arteries. In: (Sigwart U, ed) *Endoluminal Stenting* WB Saunders: London, 1996; 476–86.

13 Henry M, Amor M, Cragg A et al. Clinical experience with a new stent-graft for treatment of occlusive and aneurysmal peripheral arterial disease. *Radiology* 1996; **201**:717–24.

14 Henry M, Amor M, Porte JM et al. La thrombectomie par le catheter Hydrolyser. A propos de 50 cas. *Arch Mal Cœur,* in press.

15

Balloon angioplasty in peripheral arteries: techniques and results

Eberhard P Zeitler

Percutaneous transluminal angioplasty (PTA) as a new type of treatment of peripheral occlusive vascular disease (POVD) with a limited trauma to the inner arterial wall was initiated by Charles Dotter and Melvin Judkins in 1964.[1] While dilatation with the bougienage technique and recanalization with guide wires and simple catheters are the basics of treatment, dilatation with balloon catheters according to Andreas Grüntzig[2] has improved the results and reduced the complications of PTA. Balloon angioplasty has provided the possibility of treating arteries with a diameter larger than the catheter itself, thus enabling the dilatation. The mechanism of dilatation is very complex[3,4] and the success depends on:

- rupture of the intimal and medial layers
- stretching of the arterial wall, including media fibers and adventitia
- compression and dilatation of parts of the media layers and the non-calcified organized thrombus.

Dilatation is also effected by several influences of the vasa vasorum in the adventitia and restoration by formation of a new intima, like a fibrotic scar.[5]

Depending on the vessel diameter, the scar caused by the smooth muscle cells that produce intimal hyperplasia is highly important. The clinical situation has shown that intimal hyperplasia in iliac arteries with a diameter of about 8 mm is less important than in small arteries.[6,7] Therefore, without additional types of treatment such as stent application or pharmacological local infusion of special drugs through infusion balloons, restenoses occur in a lower percentage in the aorta, iliac, and common femoral arteries than in the middle and distal third of the superficial femoral artery after balloon dilatation.

While restenosis or reocclusion within the first post-procedural days are mainly thrombi and the result of technical failure or intimal flaps and subintimal dissection, restenosis during the 3rd to the 9th month can mainly be identified histologically or by angioscopy as intimal hyperplasia.[8,9]

Stenoses or occlusions that occur later are mainly, again, arteriosclerotic lesions at the same site or in different areas.

Technique of balloon angioplasty in extremity arteries

After puncture of the common femoral artery in the retrograde or antegrade direction using the Seldinger technique,[10] nowadays mainly a 5F (French) or 6F sheath is introduced, followed by the intra-arterial injection of 5000 IU of heparin.

Under X-ray-TV control, angiography is necessary for localization of the significant obliterations, the definition of the grade of stenosis, and demonstration of the run-off arteries.

Following this, stenoses are bypassed by guide wires with a flexible or steerable guide wire,[11] or occlusions are recanalized with a catheter-controlled floppy guide wire (Terumo). The tip of the guide wire used in stenoses is sometimes curved, but in occlusions it is mostly straight. After successful guiding of all hemodynamic lesions, the pilot catheter is exchanged for a balloon catheter of the selected balloon diameter and length over a more rigid guide wire.

Balloon catheters

The first balloon catheter by Andreas Grüntzig was made out of polyvinyl chloride – shaft and balloon consisting of the same material – and the balloon looked sausage-like, without a shoulder. Later, the Grüntzig balloon catheters were made

Table 15.1   Catheter materials
Grüntzig balloon catheter: polyvinyl chloride // coaxial same material
Grüntzig balloon catheter: polyethylene shaft and balloon
High-pressure balloon catheters: two different materials – also polyolefin
Low-profile balloons: materials are thinner

out of polyethylene (Table 15.1). By contrast, high-pressure balloon catheters nowadays are made of two different materials, which can be polyethylene, polyolefin, or some other. The low-profile balloons consist of considerably thinner plastic materials, enabling the use of balloon catheters of a smaller diameter.

A different type of balloon catheter was introduced by Fritz Olbert in 1977.[12] This catheter consists of two different materials, and the inner catheter stretches the balloon, so that it clings close to the shaft, without producing sharp edges.

The use of a sheath is of great importance in all types of angioplasty, because with a sheath the trauma to the arterial wall can be reduced,[13] so that complications at the puncture site are less common. In addition, with the sheath, the exchange of balloon catheters of varying diameters or the application of stents, as well as the use of infusion balloon catheters for the delivery of special drugs and the aspiration embolectomy for peripheral emboli, can be managed easily and without additional risks.

In addition to the simple dilating balloon catheters, several modifications with two or three balloons on one shaft, balloons with a chamber in between two balloons for local chamber thrombolysis, and balloons providing the possibility of application of special drugs, with the intention to influence both the intima and the media to reduce acute thrombus formation and also intimal proliferation, are on the market.

Indications for balloon angioplasty in peripheral arteries

According to the recommendations by the SCVIR[14] and, in Germany, by the AGIR,[15] the obliterations of extremity arteries are classified in four categories in each anatomical area (Figures 15.1–15.4). According to these classifications, isolated or multiple local stenoses correspond to categories 1 and 2, which are angiographically defined as amenable to balloon angioplasty with a successful outcome.

Under category 2 also, short occlusions have been defined as indications amenable to recanalization and balloon angioplasty.

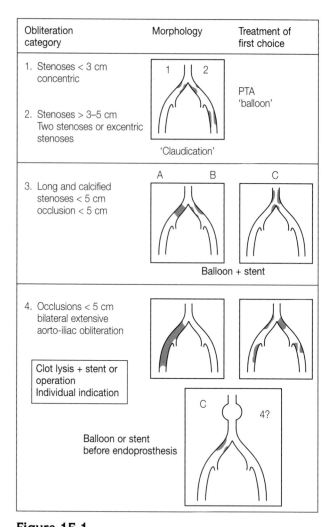

Figure 15.1
Categories of obliteration (SCVIR/AGIR Guidelines 1998) in iliac arteries. PTA, percutaneous transluminal angioplasty.

Category 3, with highly irregular and multiple stenoses in several areas of the arterial system or occlusions longer than 5 cm in the iliac arteries and longer than 10 cm in the superficial femoral artery, are regarded as less suitable for balloon angioplasty, since complications are more common and long-term results are less favorable.

For patients with claudication, physical training in addition to the treatment of the risk factors is therefore preferred. But in patients with rest pain or gangrene, or if the patient wishes it, after discussion with the vascular surgeon as a partner, a decision is necessary between primary vascular surgery with application of a bypass graft or angioplasty with special recanalization procedures, followed by balloon angioplasty. In several patients with occlusions in iliac arteries and in all patients after balloon PTA with residual stenosis, dissection, or intimal flap the application of a stent is necessary, because balloon angioplasty alone does not yield the best long-term results.

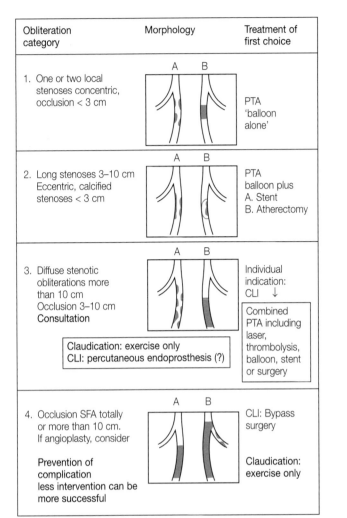

Figure 15.2
Categories of obliteration (SCVIR/AGIR Guidelines 1998) in femoral arteries. CLI, critical limb ischemia; PTA, percutaneous transluminal angioplasty; SFA, superficial femoral artery.

Obliteration category	Morphology	Treatment of first choice
1. Isolated stenoses Short occlusion < 3 cm After imaging in B: Atherectomy or balloon	A B	A. Angioplasty B. Imaging; US, MRI or CT individual
2. Long stenoses < 3 cm Occlusion < 3 cm Also obliterations below knee Critical limb ischemia: femorocrural bypass	A B	A. PTA B. Combined PTA including clot lysis and balloon and aspiration (RAT-PAT)
3. Diffuse stenotic obliterations One stenosis + short occlusion Critical limb ischemia: femorocrural bypass	A B	A. Conservative or laser-assisted PTA B. PTA + urokinase 100 000 IU(?)
4. Total occlusion Aneurysmatic stenoses Individual indication Age Symptoms Endoprosthesis Femorocrural bypass	A B	A. Surgery or conservative B. Surgery or conservative or endoprosthesis

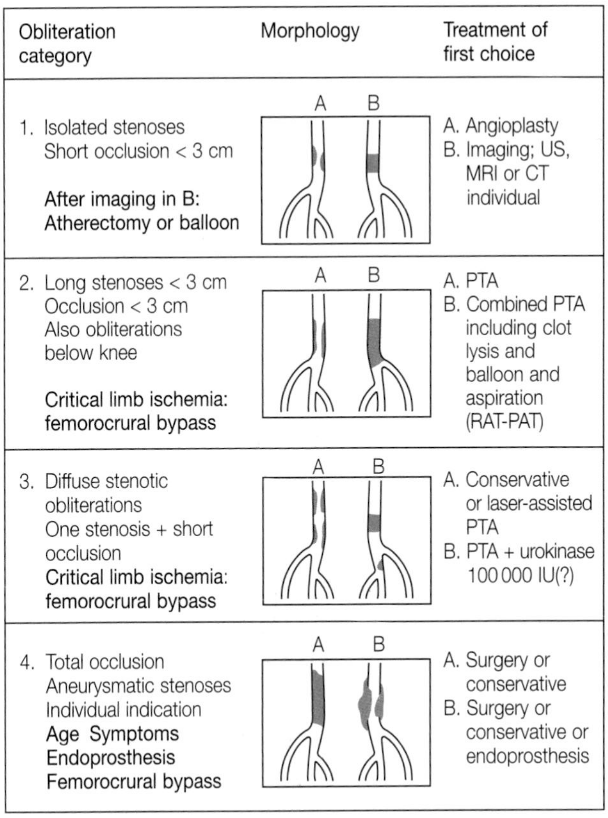

Figure 15.3
Categories of obliteration (SCVIR/AGIR Guidelines 1998) in the popliteal artery. US, ultrasonography; MRI, magnetic resonance imaging; CT, computed tomography; PTA, percutaneous transluminal angioplasty; RAT-PAT, rotational aspiration thromboembolectomy-percutaneous AT.

Since the indications for balloon angioplasty are mainly made in categories 1 and 2, whereas those for bypass surgery are mainly made for categories 3 and 4, real prospective studies enabling a comparison between surgery and balloon angioplasty cannot be carried out.

Results

The results of balloon angioplasty have been reported in numerous publications.

Primary success is mainly described as a reduction of the stenosis in the angiography below 25% and normalizing of the ankle blood pressure. The ankle blood pressure gradient is close to normal, or above 0.9. But the hemodynamics is also improved by a lowering of the ankle–arm pressure gradient (to more than 0.2 in single stenoses and 0.15 in combined obliterations in two anatomical areas). The clinical change is the reduction by one grade in the Fontaine or Rutherford classification. In many papers the long-term results are only defined on the basis of patients with primary success, not including all patients with intention to treat.

Table 15.2 demonstrates the results of 1771 balloon angioplasties[16] in different locations performed in Nuremberg. Primary success, including the angiographic, hemodynamic, and clinical change of the situation before the introduction of slippery guide wires, was between 85 and 95% in stenoses. The results were above 80% in occlusions of the superficial femoral artery (SFA), provided these were not longer than 12 cm. In the case of reocclusion, the primary success was only 60%, and 5-year patency only 18%. Short occlusions of the SFAs and single and multiple stenoses in contrast had similar 5-year patency rates, between 60 and 65%, but after balloon angioplasty of iliac artery stenoses without stent, the 5-year patency rate was 80%.

Obliteration category	Morphology	Treatment of first choice
1. Isolated stenoses Exercise	A B	Only in addition to femoropopliteal PTA and rest pain or CLI: balloon PTA small balloons
2. Two or more stenoses Treatment of risk factors	A B	A. As in Category 1 B. Conservative or femorocrural bypass
3. Occlusion < 3 cm Two or three stenoses in two tibiofibular arteries Individual indication Critical limb ischemia: femorocrural bypass	A B	A. As in Category 1 B. Small balloon PTA Small balloons or laser-assisted PTA
4. Multiple occlusions Diffuse arterioscleroses of two or three arteries If last alternative in patients interest after consultation: Rotablator	A B	A + B CLI: femoropedal bypass and/or sympathi-colysis or laser-assisted PTA

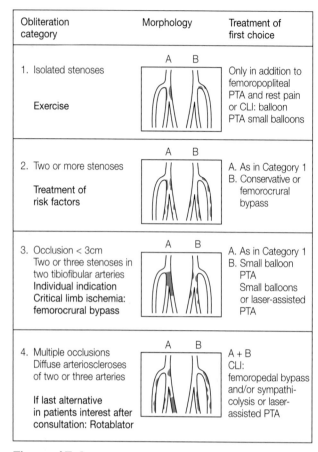

Figure 15.4
Categories of obliteration (SCVIR/AGIR Guidelines 1998) in infrapopliteal arteries. CLI, critical limb ischemia; PTA, percutaneous transluminal angioplasty.

Table 15.2   Results of balloon angioplasty (n = 1771). From Zeitler et al.[16]

Obliteration	Primary success (%)	Five-year patency (%)
Iliac artery stenoses	95	80
SFA stenoses	85	65
SFA occlusion, 1–5 cm	85	60
SFA occlusion, 6–12 cm	80	48
SFA occlusion, 12 cm and more	60	18

SFA, superficial femoral artery.

Table 15.3   Results of balloon angioplasty (n = 421). From Gallino et al.[17]

	Iliac artery stenoses		Femoropopliteal obliterations	
	1 year	5 years	1 year	5 years
Cure rate (%)	86	83	61	58
Patency (%)	91	87	70	67

In the specialized clinic for vascular diseases, Roth et al.[19] in Engelskirchen, Germany, were able to show, in 1996, that complications at and after balloon angioplasty occur in 8% in patients over 65 years of age, in contrast to younger patients with less than 2% of complications. (Table 15.4)

Table 15.4   Iliofemoral percutaneous transluminal angioplasty – complications and lethality (n = 2668). From Roth et al.[19]

	Complications		Lethality
Age	Without operation	With operation	
Below 65 years	38 (1.85%)	1 (0.05%)	1 (0.05%)
Above 65 years	49 (8%)	5 (0.8%)	5 (0.8%)

As a result of the enhanced quality of the equipment, with hydrophilic guide wires, long introducers, and high-pressure and low-profile balloons, the primary success rate for balloon-alone angioplasty has risen markedly over the last 10 years.

Henry et al.[20] have documented primary success and a 4-year patency in iliac and femoropopliteal stenoses in 95–100%, and in occlusions with stents in 82–92%, such as in the former years of angioplasty,[21] with the combination of balloon angioplasty and local thrombolysis in SFAs with occlusions up to 12 cm and in acute and subacute obliterations.

The primary and long-term results in aorto-iliac obliterations with the double-lumen balloon catheters inserted from both groins[22–26] have shown excellent primary success and long-term results with less than 10% residual stenoses. The aorto-iliac bifurcational stenoses are more common in younger patients between 45 and 65 years of age, but residual stenoses with intimal flap, dissection, or a pressure gradient above 10 mmHg and angiographically confirmed residual stenoses above 30% – more precisely defined by intravascular ultrasound (IVUS) – indicate a second balloon dilatation with a balloon of a bigger diameter, or primary stent application.

Table 15.3 demonstrates the patency and cure rates of the angiology department in Bern, by Gallino et al.,[17] with the most patients with stenoses or femoropopliteal occlusions smaller than 5 cm.

In 1989, Mahler[18] did not recommend outpatient angioplasty.

Outpatient balloon angioplasty

Between 1996 and 2001 (Table 15.5) we performed, in an outpatient clinic, 748 balloon angioplasties for single or multiple stenoses in 676 patients (545 in males and 203 in females) – more commonly in leg arteries (Table 15.6) than in iliac arteries (Table 15.5).

Applying clear exclusion and inclusion criteria, we treated patients in the iliac, femoral, and popliteal arteries in 92% with claudication and 8% with gangrene, mainly elderly patients with diabetes. The primary success rate of stenoses was above 95% and, in occlusions up to 10 cm in length, we were successful in 51 out of 54 extremities.

In femoropopliteal occlusions, however, we have experienced most of the complications with peripheral embolus. The additional treatment with percutaneous aspiration of peripheral embolisms (PAT) using the technique of Starck et al.[27] was necessary in 9 cases.

In most of these cases, additional local thrombolysis with 100 000 IU of urokinase was used, as in all patients with SFA occlusions longer than 5 cm.

Table 15.5 Angioplasty with balloon catheters in an outpatient clinic (January 23, 1996 to March 1, 2001)

748 PTAs in 676 patients: 545 males and 203 females (age between 40 and 91 years)
Iliac arteries: 102 patients   Leg arteries: 637 patients 139 PTAs: with stent 24 (17%) 695 PTAs: with stent 14 (2%)
PTA, percutaneous transluminal angioplasty.

Table 15.6 Percutaneous transluminal angioplasty (PTA) in leg arteries (1996–2001)

Single and two to three stenosis: 556 Bilateral SFA – stenosis: 46 Restenosis: 35 Femoral occlusions up to 10 cm length: 49 Short popliteal occlusions: 5 Deep femoral artery stenosis: 1 Additional lower leg arteries (stenosis): 23 Isolated lower leg arteries: 3 PAT: 9 patients to treat acute thromboembolism Local thrombolysis: with Urokinase in all PAT patients + SFA occlusions longer than 5 cm
PAT, percutaneous aspiration of peripheral embolisms.

The modern types of stents (see Chapters 24, 25) undoubtedly offer some advantages, as can be seen from the long-term patency rate in iliac arteries, which is about 10% better than after primary balloon-alone angioplasty.

Without question, stent application is necessary in iliac artery occlusions, in several types of bilateral iliac artery obliterations, as also, but very seldom, in cases of complications after balloon-alone angioplasty in femoropopliteal arteries.

In patients with category 3 and 4 of iliac and femoropopliteal arteries and with clinical contraindications or elevated risk for surgery, the recanalization of obliterations and balloon dilatation can also be used, but under these circumstances the need for stenting and in-clinic follow-up becomes more important.[28]

In our outpatient balloon angioplasty technique, out of 748 PTAs, stent application was only necessary in 31 patients (Table 15.7).

Table 15.7 Indications for stent application: 31 patients

Iliac arteries: unilateral 17 Bilateral + aortic bifurcation: 3 Common + external iliac artery: 1 Femoropopliteal arteries: 14 Dissection: 3 SFA occlusion: 10 Residual stenosis: 1
SFA, superficial femoral artery.

In the Nuremberg clinic (Ritter, pers. comm.), in patients who underwent angioplasty under clinical conditions for iliac artery obliterations, stents became necessary in 1999 in about 40%, by contrast, in superficial femoral and popliteal arteries, stents were necessary in only 12%.

Conclusion

Balloon angioplasty of arteries of the lower extremities in patients presenting the clinical symptoms of claudication, rest pain, or gangrene is indicated in angiographically confirmed single and multiple stenoses, but not in totally irregular arteries and long-distance occlusions.

As a result of modern equipment, the primary success rate is high; the long-term patency rate depends on the anatomical region and is excellent in the iliac arteries and good in the superficial femoral and popliteal arteries. The results in the tibioperoneal arteries are acceptable and the indication is mainly made to avoid amputation, and to shorten the healing time of ulcers.

Without question, the additional pharmacological treatment in the peripheral arteries lacks excellent randomized long-term studies which could provide clear recommendations.

Nevertheless, taking into account, that arteriosclerosis is a systemic disease, the long-term application of aspirin and other modern platelet-aggregation inhibitors and local low-molecular heparin for 3 to 5 days after angioplasty, is recommended.

The follow-up control is therefore mandatory both within the first week following angioplasty and, in the long run, at intervals of at least 6 months, to detect possible restenoses requiring a second intervention in time.

References

1   Dotter CT, Judkins MP. Transluminal treatment of arteriosclerotic obstructions: Description of a new technique and a preliminary report of its application. *Circulation* 1964; **30**: 654–70.

2   Grüntzig AR, Hopff H. Perkutane Rekanalisation chronischer arterieller Verschlüsse mit einem neuen Dilatationskatheter Modifikation der Dotter-Technik. *Dtsch med Wschr* 1974; **99**: 2502–5.

3   Leu HJ, Grüntzig A. Histopathologic aspects of transluminal recanalization. In: Zeitler E, Grüntzig AR, Schoop W (eds), *Percutaneous vascular recanalization*. Berlin: Springer, 1978: 39–50.

4   Castaneda-Zuniga WR, Formanek A, Tadavarthy M et al. The mechanisms of balloon angioplasty. *Radiology* 1980; **135**: 565–71.

5   Zollikofer Ch, Redha FH, Brühlmann WF et al. Acute and longterm effects of massive balloon dilation on the aortic wall and vasa vasorum. *Radiology* 1987; **164**: 145–9.

6   Roth F-J, Scheffler A, Krings W et al. Ballonangioplastie peripherer Gefäße. In: Günther RW, Thelen M (eds), *Interventionelle radiologie*. 2nd edn. 1996: 81–7.

7   Lafont A, Guzman A, Whitlow PL et al. Restenosis after experimental angioplasty. Intimal, medial and adventitial changes associated with constrictive remodeling. *Circ Res* 1995; **76**: 996–1002.

8   Beck A, Milic S, Spagnoli AM et al. The clinical value of percutaneous transluminal angioscopy. Angioscopical findings in primary vascular diagnosis and interventional radiology. *Clin Ter* 1989; **131**: 93–105.

9   Murray RR, Hewes RC, White J Jr et al. Long-segment femoropopliteal stenoses: is angioplasty a boon or a bust? *Radiology* 1987; **162**: 473–6.

10 Seldinger SJ. Catheter replacement of the needle in percutaneous arteriography. *Acta Radiol* 1953; **39**: 368–76.

11 Kadir S. *Teaching atlas of interventional radiology*. Stuttgart: Thieme, 1999.

12 Olbert F, Hanecka L. Transluminale Gefäßdilatation mit einem modefizierten Dilatationskatheter. *Wien Klein Wochenschr* 1977; **89**: 281–4.

13 Söldner HJ, Mittelmeier HD, Beyer-Enke S, Zeitler E. The reduction of the extent of vascular lesion during angioplasty by the use of a sheath. *Fortschr Röntgenstr* 1995; **163**: 341–4.

14 SCVIR. Guidelines for percutaneous transluminal angioplasty. Standards of the Practice Committee of the SCVIR. *Radiology*; **177**: 619–26.

15 AGIR. Leitlinien zur Gefäßrekanalisation der Arbeitsgemeinschaft für interventionelle Radiologie der Deutschen Röntgenstr 1997: L4–L13.

16 Zeitler E, Feng G, Oldendorf M et al. Ergebnisse der perkutanen transluminalen Angioplastie. *Herz* 1989: 22–8.

17 Gallino A, Mahler E, Probst E, Nachbur B. Percutaneous transluminal angioplasty of the arteries of the lower limbs: 5-year follow-up. *Circulation* 1984; **70**: 619–23.

18 Mahler F. *Katheterintervention in der Angiologie*. G. Thieme Verlag, Stuttgart: 1989.

19 Roth F-J, Scheffler A, Krings W et al. Ballonangioplastie peripherer Gefäße. In: *Interventionelle radiologie*. Günther RW, Thelen M (eds) 2nd edn: 81–7.

20 Henry M, Amor M, Henry I et al. Percutaneous endovascular treatment of aorto-iliac occlusive disease. In: *Tenth Interventional Course of Peripheral Vascular Intervention*. Paris Course Directors: Henry M, Amor M; Co-Directors: Biamino G, Ramee St, White C.

21 Hess H, Mietaschk A, Brückl R. Peripheral arterial occlusions: a 6-year experience with local low dose thrombolytic therapy. *Radiology* 1987; **163**: 753–8.

22 Grollmann JH, Del Vicario M, Mittal AK. Percutaneous transluminal abdominal aortic angioplasty. *Am J Roentgenol* 1980; **134**: 1053–4.

23 Tegtmeyer CJ, Wellons HA, Thompson RN. Balloon dilation of the abdominal aorta. *J Am Med Ass* 1980; **244** 2636–7.

24 Velasquez G, Castaneda-Zuniga WR, Formanek A et al. Nonsurgery angioplasty in Leriche syndrome *Radiology*; **134**: 359–60.

25 Zorn-Bopp E, Ingrisch H, Mietaschk A, Frey KW. Transluminale Gefäßdilatation der distalen Bauchaorta, der Arteriae iliaca communis und externa. *Forschr Röntgenstr* 1981; **134**: 471–5.

26 Ingrisch H, Seyferth W, Küffer G. Percutaneous transluminal angioplasty of the infrarenal abdominal aorta and aortoiliac bifurcation. In: Dotter CT, Grüntzig AR, Schoop W, Zeitler E (eds), *Percutaneous transluminal angioplasty*. Berlin: Springer, 1984: 127–30.

27 Starck EE, McDermott JC, Crummy A et al. Percutaneous aspiration thromboembolectomy. *Radiology* 1985; **156**: 61–6.

28 Günther RW. Ambulante periphere Angioplastie – Sicherheit und Grenzen. *Fortschr Röntgenstr* 1993; **158**: 391–2.

29 Zeitler E. Angioplasty: overview of techniques and results. In: Kadir S (ed.), *Teaching atlas of interventional radiology* Stuttgart: Thieme, 1999: 21–8.

16

Percutaneous peripheral atherectomy using the Rotablator

Isabelle Henry and Michel Henry

Introduction

Balloon angioplasty alone or completed with stent implantation is the most effective procedure to treat peripheral arterial diseases. However, this technique is still limited by the complexity of certain lesions (e.g. calcified, long, bifurcated, diffuse, and those in small vessels)

High-speed rotational ablation has been developed as a means of removing rather than simply displacing the occluding atherosclerotic material. It was postulated that this debulking process would improve results as compared to balloon dilatation.

The Rotablator was developed by David Auth and used for the first time in humans by Zacca.[1]

We report here our experiences and results of a 150 patient study using the Rotablator in the peripheral arteries for a variety of pathologies.

Methods

The Rotablator™ (Boston Scientific & Co, Boston, MA) is a flexible, nonradiopaque catheter fitted with a diamond-encrusted metal burr that selectively cuts away inelastic tissue during high-speed rotation. The catheter, which tracks coaxially over a 0.009-inch (0.23-mm) guide wire to prevent deflection, is encased in a 4.3F sheath that protects the vessel wall during drive shaft rotation. Saline is infused through this sheath to lubricate and cool the catheter, burr, and guide wire. The drive shaft is connected to a compressed air turbine that rotates the burr at speeds varying from 50 000 to 200 000 rpm. The diameters of available burrs range from 1.5 to 4.5 mm.

Atherectomy procedure[1]

Patient preparation

On the day prior to the procedure, patients receive 250 mg aspirin and 180 mg diltiazem and/or 60 mg nifedipine. They are also begun on intravenous heparin (15 000 units over 24 hours). In addition to the standard pre-angioplasty baseline testing, measurements of free hemoglobin (blood and urine), haptoglobin, and lactic dehydrogenase are made to monitor hemolysis that may be provoked by rotational ablation.

Approach techniques

All procedures are carried out under local anesthesia and neuroleptanalgesia. The most frequently used access technique to treat femoral, popliteal, or distal artery lesions is the ipsilateral antegrade femoral approach. An introducer is selected to accommodate the maximum size of the burr to be used (maximum size of the burr multiplied by 3 equals the French size of the introducer). For percutaneous access, a 9F is usually the largest sheath used in our facility (allows passage of a 3-mm burr).

Once the introducer is in place, baseline imaging is conducted, including control angiography as well as endovascular ultrasound and/or angioscopy. The 0.009-inch guide wire is carefully passed through the lesion site(s) as far as possible down the artery so that any complications (spasm, distal embolism) may be dealt with promptly. If the femoral artery is tortuous or if there is a stenosis at the origin of the anterior tibial artery, a straight or angled 4F catheter can be used to cross the proximal obstacles and/or to strengthen the guide wire.

When selecting the first burr, the diameter is usually 75–85% of the arterial diameter below the stenosis. With the guide wire positioned, this burr is slowly advanced along the wire to about 1 cm above the stenosis (because the burr advances spontaneously when rotation begins). The rotational speed should not be allowed to dip below 2000–5000 rpm, and ablation sequences must be short (15–30 s) to reduce heat accumulation and ensure appropriate downstream dispersion of the particles produced. The total rotation time depends on the lesion (15–450 s in our experience), but a note of caution is warranted. Inasmuch as the total ablation time has a major influence on hemolysis, spasm frequency, and distal embolism, rotation time must be strictly limited. Once the lesion has been cleared with the Rotablator, the burr is withdrawn, and angiography is used to evaluate the results. If the remaining stenosis is >50%, a larger burr is used. If <20% luminal narrowing remains, the procedure is stopped. Residual stenoses between 20 and 50% are always treated by adjunctive balloon dilatation. (As a rule the results of Rotablator therapy in the femoral segment are always insufficient, whereas in the distal arteries the outcome is almost always adequate.) If a complementary dilatation is necessary, the balloon chosen is equal in diameter to the size of the non-diseased artery, and the inflation pressure must remain below 4–5 atm. This low pressure is sufficient to remove the residual stenosis while avoiding a dissection. A completion angiogram documents the final results at the treatment site(s) as well as the distal runoff.

If no thrombogenic incident occurred during the procedure, the introducer is immediately withdrawn, and the postoperative care of the patient ensues as for other peripheral angioplasties. However, in addition to clinical and Doppler surveillance, the hematologic tests must be repeated to check for hemolysis. If this occurs, the patient is hydrated, and a bicarbonate solution is infused.

Other approach techniques may sometimes be used with the Rotablator. For example, the retrograde femoral procedure is required to treat iliac lesions. However, the size of this artery requires large burrs and introducers that increase procedural complications.

The retrograde popliteal approach, on the other hand, is excellent for treating common femoral artery lesions, stenoses at the origin of the superficial femoral artery (SFA), and after failure of a standard femoral approach. In this technique, a 7F or 8F introducer is inserted to accommodate up to a 2.5 mm burr if long, calcified femoral lesions are to be treated. The procedure is the same as the one described above.

Alternatively, the contralateral femoral approach can be used to treat lesions at the femoral bifurcation, in the common femoral artery, or at the origin of the SFA or profunda. An 8F or 9F guiding catheter may assist in crossing the aortic bifurcation. The guide wire is placed far into the contralateral SFA or profunda, and the burr is gently advanced along the guide wire. In particular, this approach allows access to sites (e.g., femoral bifurcation) that were herefore

unapproachable by other standard techniques except surgery.

The popularity of the radial or the brachial approach for balloon dilatation of axillary or subclavian artery lesions would appear feasible for rotational atherectomy treatment; however, we have never used it.

Special treatment scenarios

Multilevel disease (Figure 16.1) in the femoropopliteal and distal segments may be treated concurrently with endovascular techniques. The Rotablator guide wire is placed down the leg artery, and proximal lesions are treated first. Bilateral lesions, on the other hand, are always treated sequentially with a few days' interval between treatments to minimize the side effects.

In the case of an arterial occlusion, it is generally impossible to pass the Rotablator guide wire, and a channel must first be created through the obstruction. Currently, in 70–90% of cases, it is possible to recanalize with a hydrophilic guide wire, certain laser devices, or other recanalization devices. After creating a channel, the Rotablator guide wire can be inserted using a 4F or 5F catheter. Because even a recanalized calcified occlusion may not respond to balloon dilatation, the Rotablator can effectively debulk the lesion, reducing the delamination risk and possibly avoiding the need for a stent. It is preferable to use incrementally sized burrs to progressively pulverize the atheroma, and there should be no hesitation in using smaller burrs if resistance is encountered. Whereas recanalization of SFA occlusions remains controversial, the evolving Rotablator techniques for distal lesions require that the SFA remain open for access to these distal arteries. The immediate use of the Rotablator after angioplasty failure has not been investigated thoroughly. Poor radiological visibility may predispose to a high risk of complications, e.g., dissection extension, perforation, or plaque embolism.

Intraluminal imaging techniques, such as angioscopy or intravascular unltrasound, may assist in the decision to perform a simultaneous procedure ; however, when there is doubt, it is preferable to wait until the lesion has healed before using this technique.

Patient information

A total of 150 patients (94 males, 56 females; mean age 73 ± 1 years, range 42–90) were candidates for percutaneous rotational ablation in the lower limbs. Details of the patient population are shown in the Table 16.1. Thirty-two percent of the patients were diabetic; 85% had other atherosclerotic disease (cerebrovascular, coronary, renal). Twenty-one percent had undergone previous vascular surgery. Sixty-five percent had severe claudication, and one quarter of the patients had rest pain and/or ulceration. Adequate runoff (no stenosis >50% in three vessels) was present in only 28

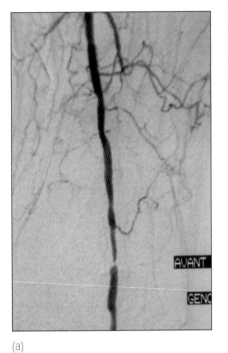 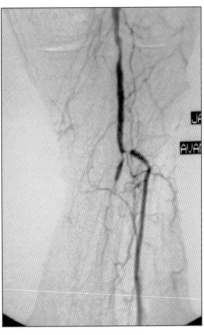 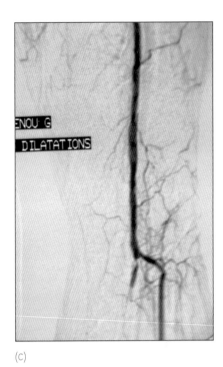

(a)   (b)   (c)

Figure 16.1
(a) Arteriogram showing a very tight popliteal stenosis. (b) Arteriogram at the origin of the anterior tibial artery. (c) After treatment with the Rotablator and balloon dilatation, both lesions show satisfactory flow.

patients (19%), and 51% of the patients had flow-limiting disease in all three distal arteries. Eighty-nine patients (59%) were being evaluated for failure to show improvement with other techniques (angioplasty, surgery, medical treatment), 39 patients (26%) for symptom progression or limb salvage, and the remainder for angioplasty restenosis or for the treatment of distal lesions in multilevel endovascular procedures.

Results

All 150 patients underwent rotational atherectomy using the Rotablator according to the methods described above. A total of 212 lesions were attempted in the iliac, femoral, popliteal, or distal arteries (Tables 16.2–16.4). There were 193 stenoses (91%) and 19 chronic occlusions; 93% were

Table 16.1   Patient characteristics

150 patients; mean age (years):	73 ± 1 (range 42–90)
94 male; mean age (years):	68 ± 1 (range 42–86)
56 female; mean age (years):	77 ± 1 (range 61–90)

Characteristic Parameters	No. of patients.
Risk factors:	
Diabetes	48 (32%)
Multivascular diseases (cerebral, coronary, renal, abdominal aorta)	128 (85%)
Previous vascular surgery	32 (21%)
Clinical stage:	
Moderate claudication	16 (11%)
Severe claudication	98 (65%)
Rest pain	28 (24%)
Minor tissue loss, nonhealing ulcer	8
Runoff status:	
Number of occluded arteries:	
3	21
2	40
1	40
0	49
Number of stenosed arteries (≥50%):	
3	76
2	28
1	18
0	28

Table 16.2   Lesion characteristics

	No.	Percent	Above knee (%)	Below knee (%)
Bifurcation or branches	134	63	62	64
Calcified	192	93	98	87
Occluded	19	9	14	4
Stenosed	193	91	86	96

Table 16.3 Lesion characteristics by location

Location	No.	Mean length (cm)	Range	Mean percent stenosis	Range percent stenosis
Iliac	1	12			100
Femoral	86	5.7 ± 0.40	1–15	84 ± 2	60–100
Popliteal	19	2.40 ± 0.30	1–6	86 ± 3	75–100
Tibioperoneal					
Trunk	38	2.6 ± 0.2	1–6	85 ± 1	70–100
Posterior tibial	7	2.6 ± 0.6	1–5	79 ± 2	70–90
Peroneal	16	2.4 ± 0.3	1–4	82 ± 2	75–99
Anterior tibial	45	3.4 ± 0.6	1–20	82 ± 1	60–100
Total	106	2.9 ± 0.3	1–20	83 ± 0.7	60–100
Total	212	4 ± 0.2	1–20	83 ± 0.7	60–100

Table 16.4 Lesion lengths by location

	<3 cm	4–6 cm	>7 cm
Above knee	45 (42%)	30 (28%)	31 (30%)
Below knee	77 (72%)	24 (23%)	5 (5%)
Total	122 (58%)	54 (25%)	36 (17%)

Table 16.5 Procedural details

Parameters	No. of patients.
Approaches:	
Ipsilateral femoral	141
Contralateral femoral	5
Popliteal	4
Bilateral	20
Atherectomy associated with:	
Femoral lesion dilatation	14
Popliteal lesion dilatation	2
Distal lesion dilatation	3

calcified, and 63% were located at important bifurcations or collateral branch origins. Fifty percent of the lesions were located below the knee. The length of the lesions varied from 1 to 20 cm; 17% of the treated lesions were longer than 7 cm, 25% were between 4 and 6 cm, and 58% were smaller than 3 cm. The lesions at the femoral level were significantly longer than those in other segments (5.70 ± 0.40 cm vs 2.97 ± 0.30 cm) ($p<0.001$). The maximum number of lesions treated in one patient was four.

There was no difference between the male and the female population regarding the characteristics or location of the lesions, but the average number of treated lesions was lower in males (1.35 lesion per patient) than in females (1.53 per patient). The approach techniques used and incidence of concomitant procedures are listed in Table 16.5. One lesion in an anterior tibial stenosis was excluded when a guide wire failed to pass successfully. Rotational ablation alone was used to treat 16 patients (19%) at the femoral level, 9 (47%) at the popliteal level, and 92 (87%) at the distal artery level (Figures 16.2–16.5). Adjunctive dilatation was necessary in 70 patients (81%) at the femoral level, 10 (53%) at the popliteal level, and 14 (13%) at the distal leg artery level (Figure 16.6).

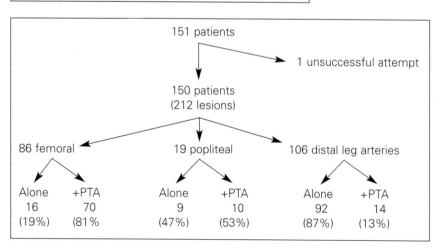

Figure 16.2

Treatment with Rotablator alone and with adjunctive balloon dilatation by vessel segment. PTA, percutaneous transluminal angioplasty.

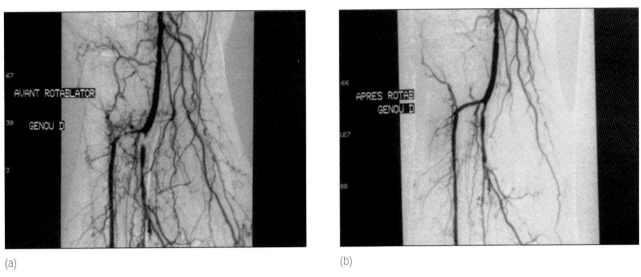

(a)

(b)

Figure 16.3

(a) Multiple, severe anterior tibial and peroneal stenoses. (b) The result after Rotablator therapy is excellent.

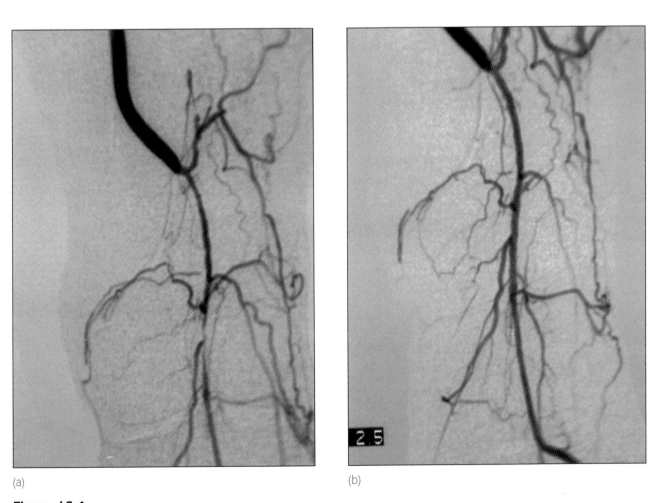

(a)

(b)

Figure 16.4

(a) A very tight stenosis exists distal to a femoropopliteal bypass graft. (b) Satisfactory outflow has been re-established with the Rotablator.

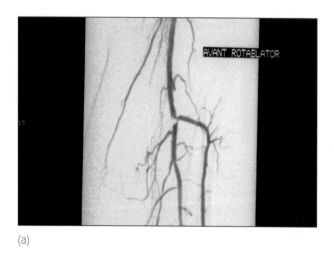

(a)   (b)

Figure 16.5
(a) A severe lesion at a bifurcation. (b) Results after Rotablator.

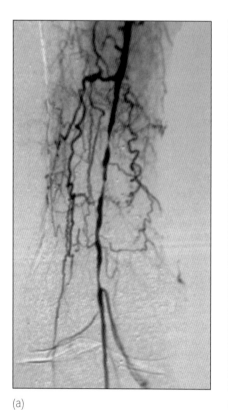
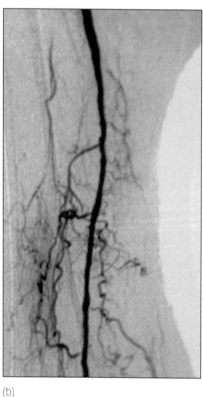
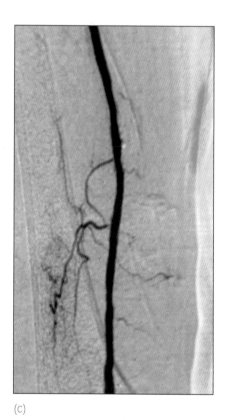

(a)   (b)   (c)

Figure 16.6
(a) Lesions in the superficial femoral artery and in the popliteal artery. (b) Results after Rotablator. (c) Results after balloon angioplasty.

Procedural success

Seven procedures failed subsequent to intra-procedural complications (see below). Therefore, the immediate technical success by lesion was 97% (95% by patient). Figure 16.7 summarizes the percentage stenosis before and after

Rotablator and following adjunctive dilatation at the femoral, popliteal, and distal arterial levels. Residual stenosis after Rotablator was higher at the femoropopliteal levels (44%) than in the distal segment ($p < 0.01$), due to the burr:vessel diameter ratio, which was $80.8 \pm 1.6\%$ at the distal level but only $61.1 \pm 2.6\%$ at the femoropopliteal levels ($p < 0.001$).

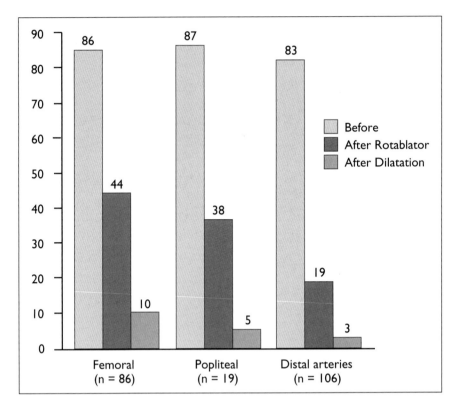

Figure 16.7
Percent stenosis before and after Rotablator and after adjunctive balloon dilatation.

Complications

There were 37 intra-procedural complications (25%) related to the Rotablator treatment (Table 16.6). Among these, arterial spasm (17 cases; [11%]) comprised the majority of these events. It occurred more frequently in the distal arteries (15; [88%]) than in the femoropopliteal segment ($p < 0.02$), but it was successfully treated in most patients (16/17). Twelve thromboses (8%) were encountered; 8 were successfully treated by fibrinolysis. Dissections and perforations occurred rarely (3%), as did distal embolism (2 cases; [1.3%], one of which was successfully treated by aspiration). Two instances of no-reflow phenomena were observed and treated.

Table 16.6 Complications according to lesion location (above and below knee)

	Above knee	Below knee	No. cured/ No. total
Ablation site:			
Spasm	2	15	16/17
Thrombosis	6	6	8/12
Dissection	1	2	3/3
Perforation	0	1	0/1
Distal emboli	1	1	1/2
No reflow	2	0	2/2
Total	12	25	30/37

In the immediate postoperative period, there were 7 (5%) cases of hemoglobinuria and 2 cases (1.3%) of transitory renal insufficiency; these resolved within 24 hours without any consequences.

Follow-up

The mean observation period for this population was 14.4 ± 1 months (range 1–51). A total of 125 patients were available for ≥4 month follow-up evaluation (this cohort did not differ significantly in gender, age, risk factors, or location/type of lesions from the initial population). Of these, 114 patients underwent angiography at 4 months in addition to clinical evaluation and Doppler examination. Of the remaining 11 patients, 4 patients were lost to follow-up, 3 died, and 4 were excluded because they had stent implantation. In these 114 patients, 163 lesions (77% of original treatment group) were re-examined: 123 (76%) were patent with a residual percent stenosis of $17 \pm 1.1\%$, and 40 arteries (24%) showed restenosis (≥50% luminal narrowing) of $82 \pm 2.1\%$, as shown in Table 16.7; the restenosis rate was highest at the femoral level. Restenosis was more frequent for all lesions longer than 7 cm ($p < 0.001$) (Table 16.8) and at both the femoropopliteal level (55% vs 19% of <7 cm; $p < 0.03$) and the distal segment (80% vs 18%; $p < 0.01$).

Table 16.7 Number and location of restenosed and patent arteries in follow-up period ($n = 163$)

	Restenosed			Patent			
	No.	Percent stenosis	Mean length	No.	Percent stenosis	Mean length	Percent restenosis
Femoral	19	80	6.5 ± 0.8	34	20	4.9 ± 0.5	36%
Popliteal	1	90	2	14	18	2.1 ± 0.3	7%
Distal	20	84	4.9 ± 1.2	75	15	2.4 ± 0.2	21%
All	40	82 ± 2.1	5.6 ± 0.7	123	17 ± 1.1	3 ± 0.2	24%

Table 16.8 Relationship of restenosis to lesion length

Mean length	Femoral and popliteal			Distal artery		
	Restenosed	Patent	Percent	Restenosed	Patent	Percent
>7 cm	11	9	55	4	1	80
	$p<0.001$	$p<0.03$			$p<0.01$	
<7 cm	9	39	19	16	74	18

Discussion

The mechanism of rotational ablation differs completely from that of balloon dilatation. In the latter, compression of the lesion promotes rupture of the atherosclerotic plaque and stretches the arterial wall. The Rotablator, on the other hand, does not crack the plaque or deform the vessel wall, as is shown by radiological, histological, angioscopic, and ultrasound studies.[2–4] Rather, the Rotablator has an abrasive action that removes the obstructing material, preferentially ablating rigid, calcified atherosclerotic tissue while leaving healthy elastic tissue intact.[4–5] This differential cutting produces a lumen that is smooth and polished in appearance. Despite the device's preference for inelastic tissue, however, the endothelium adjacent to a lesion can suffer damage during progression of the burr. The same situation is encountered with a balloon whose length is greater than the stenosis; both may alter the endothelium on either side of a stenosis. As opposed to balloon treatment, however, the Rotablator rarely injures the media,[2] an event that has been reported to be the impetus for intimal hyperplasia and restenosis. Whereas it is simple to select a balloon sized to match the lesion and artery, it is not so for rotational atherectomy. Using large-diameter introducers (>9F) to accommodate the percutaneous introduction of burrs >3 mm would significantly increase the rate of access site complications. Dorros et al.,[6] for example, used burrs up to 4.5 mm requiring a 14F introducer for renal arteries; however, their incidence of local and systemic complications were considerable (e.g., 23% hematoma, 5% perforation, 63% hemoglobinuria). From our own experience and these early reports, we now treat only arteries <6 mm in diameter using up to a 3-mm burr; this gives us residual stenosis of <50%.

This interdiction against rotational ablation in arteries >6 mm has necessarily limited our experience with the Rotablator at the iliac level. In the one iliac artery we have treated, the vessel was very calcified and had 12 cm of old thrombus. Even though a hydrophilic guide wire passed the lesion, the balloon could not be advanced. In this case, we used the 3-mm Rotablator to debulk the lesion, producing a channel to facilitate balloon dilatation. In our experience, adjunctive dilatation is necessary at the femoral level to obtain satisfactory immediate results. This is not the case at the distal segment, where we have usually been able to introduce a burr equal to at least 80% of the arterial diameter. This burr : artery diameter ratio may explain our lower restenosis rate at the distal level (21%) compared to the higher rate in the SFA (36%) and, in particular, when balloon angioplasty did not follow Rotablator ablation.

At present, our series is too limited to offer conclusive proof, but it would seem that the use of adjunctive balloon dilatation might reduce the restenosis rate at the femoral level. Such an observation has been made at the coronary level by Bertrand et al.[7] in a collaborative study of 129 patients treated with the Rotablator and balloon dilatation. They found an average restenosis rate of 37.8% overall, but in patients treated with the Rotablator alone, the rate was 46%, as opposed to only 30% when complementary balloon angioplasty was used.

The same effect may occur at the peripheral level, but we have not studied this possibility. Insofar as determining an optimum technique for rotational ablation, we have used three treatment protocols:

1 beginning the procedure with small burrs and increasing the size until an optimal result is reached, with the burr size closely approaching that of the arterial diameter

2 initially using a single large burr equal to 75–80% of the arterial diameter

3 simply debulking the lesion using a small burr to remove inelastic material, then dilating the vessel at low pressure with a balloon that matches the diameter of the artery.

Only for treatment of distal arteries have we developed a preference among these. We believe that it is advisable to use incrementally sized burrs that approach at least 80% of the artery's diameter. This avoids the need for balloon dilatation and reduces the risk of dissection.

The same opinion does not apply, however, to the femoropopliteal arteries or those with diameters >3 mm. In these larger-bore arteries, it would appear preferable to routinely complete the procedure with balloon dilatation to ensure residual stenosis of no more than 20% in order to limit the incidence of restenosis.

Unlike balloon angioplasty, the Rotablator appears to be particularly well suited to deal with calcified and/or eccentric lesions and stenoses at bifurcations or in tortuous arteries. Further, the Rotablator may be useful for the treatment of severe, extensive lesions; by reducing the plaque burden, balloon dilatation may be applied with less risk of dissection. One situation in which the Rotablator must not be used is in the presence of thrombus; chronic thrombus tends to deflect away from the rotating burr, leading to suboptimal results.

In terms of outcome, our procedural success with Rotablator therapy in the limb arteries has been high (97%); other investigators have reported similar results in the 92–95% range.[4,6,8,9] However, the published results of a multicenter trial (CRAG) of the Rotablator found only a 77% angiographic success in 107 lesions treated in 72 patients.[10] This is not surprising when one considers that only half as many patients were treated by several physicians in three centers as represented in our single-center study. Clearly, the inevitable learning curve and operator inexperience with the technique probably contributed to these somewhat poorer procedural results. Moreover, their patient population had more advanced disease (56% limb-threatening ischemia vs 24%), and the lesions treated were twice as long (9 cm average vs 4 cm).

Given that the Rotablator would often be applied in complex lesions unsuitable to other interventions, the complications inherent to the procedure seem acceptable, and most can be easily treated. Overall, in our study, no particular complication was statistically linked to gender, age, or lesion location. However, the frequency of complications at the ablation site seemed to be influenced by the length of the treated lesion (<6 cm: 15%; >6 cm: 85%). The most frequent complication we have encountered is arterial spasm (11%), which occurs more often in the distal arteries and for 2 or 3 cm proximal to the treatment site. Of particular note is the fact that the incidence of spasm appears to be related to operator experience. Indeed, spasms occurred at a rate of 14% during our first 50 procedures, decreasing to 8% over the next 50 cases, and finally ending at 2% ($p < 0.05$).

Although some operators have postulated that arterial spasm may be caused by vibrations transmitted to the guide wire during rotation or to the liberation of vasoconstrictive substances contained within the plaque, endothelium, or blood cells, we are of the opinion that is dependent upon technique. In our experience, spasm appears most frequently when a too-large burr is used, the rotation sequences are too long, or the rotation speed is too fast or too slow. Also, spasm will occur if the burr becomes entrapped in the wall or the drive shaft is deflected by a bent guide wire (the rotation drive shaft irritates the adjacent arterial wall).

To prevent spasm, all patients are placed on vasodilators the day before the treatment. During the procedure, we routinely inject molsidomine and nitrates intra-arterially. If a spasm occurs, the same drugs are reinjected. If this medical treatment fails, low-pressure balloon dilatation is performed, which usually relieves the spasm in most arteries.

Our acute thrombosis rate has been low (5.6%), almost half that reported in the multicenter trial.[10] Moreover, most of these have been successfully treated either by thrombolysis, thromboaspiration, or thromboembolectomy. A number of factors may predispose to thrombosis: a residual stenosis, an intimal flap, elastic recoil, dissection, lengthy lesion, or vasopasm. Once the artery is reopened, low-pressure balloon dilatation may be attempted. The incidence of dissection, perforation, or angiographically visible flaps has been rare (<2%), and these were encountered at the beginning of our experience. Because these complications are caused by the guide wire or the burr, they can be circumvented by cautions wire manipulation to prevent subintimal incursion and by prudently selecting the burr, avoiding a too-large diameter for the vessel.

Although the Rotablator produces fine particles (5–180 μm) that are disseminated in the peripheral circulation,[2,5] we have observed only 2 cases (1.3%) of distal embolism from particulate migration, and thromboaspiration was effective in treating one case. Other authors have experienced this complication at a much higher rate. Ahn et al.,[8] for example, encountered emboli in 20% of their cases, but these were coincident to long lesion treatment with large burrs (4–4.5 mm). Not surprisingly, the CRAG trial reported a 10% incidence of emboli for the same reasons. Hemolysis, another complication related to rotational atherectomy, appears more or less constant with this technique, due to destruction of the red blood cells by the burr rotation. The intensity of this response is proportional to the ablation time, size of the burr, and length of the treated lesion. According to a study we performed following 54 patients at time intervals up to 24 hours postatherectomy, we saw an increase in free hemoglobin, a drop in haptoglobin, and a rise in lactic dehydrogenase within the first 5 min following the procedure. The phenomenon was transitory, reversible, and usually without attendant complications, but, in 2 of our cases, there was a slight transitory renal failure that resolved within 48 hours. Our 5% rate of hemoglobinuria is again less than half that reported in the CRAG trial (13%).

One other complication we encountered in 2 cases was slow flow or no reflow, a phenomenon seen in coronary angioplasty when the contrast agent ceases to flow, although no thrombus, flap, or spasm is visible. Several mechanisms have been proposed for this, from capillary obstruction by atherosclerotic or thrombotic embolism to interstitial edema. In the case of the Rotablator, however, cavitation may produce micro-bubbles that temporarily block outflow.[11] Indeed, in our cases, stagnation of the contrast medium downstream in the popliteal artery followed successful atherectomy in the SFA. The phenomenon disappeared 2–3 min after the injection of molsidomine and nitroglycerine. No distal embolism was visible after contrast medium washing. As compared to the CRAG trial, our overall 25% complication rate is half what they observed, and the greater part of our complications (46%) was due to spasm, a sequela the CRAG report did not even mention. This difference is particularly noteworthy when one considers that 21 of the 79 atherectomized limbs (27%) in their cohort required urgent or emergent surgical therapy, including two amputations. We have encountered nothing like this in our experience, and it is important to recognize that the CRAG trial was testing the gamut of Rotablator burrs in extremely long lesions (40 cm) requiring up to 35 min of rotation time! In these circumstances, neither their results nor their complication rates are surprising. Early in our experience, we recognized that protracted rotational ablation was inadvisable, and we restricted the rotation time whenever possible.

Regarding our follow-up results, we have amassed angiographic data on 91% of our patients who were 4 months post-treatment. These data have shown that the restenosis rate is relatively low (24% overall), considering the severity of the initial pathology. This is comparable to the 66% primary patency at 6 months reported by Ahn et al.[8] Both the site of the lesion and the length of the segment treated influenced restenosis. For lesions > 7 cm, the rate was very high, and complications were four times as frequent in lesions < 6 cm. This relationship between lesion length and restenosis is, however, not unique to rotational ablation. Other authors have reported a similar correlation for balloon angioplasty.[12] Supported by these statistics, we feel that Rotablator therapy should be limited to lesions ≤ 6 cm.

If restenosis does occur, repeat treatment should be carried out without hesitation, either with the same procedure or a different technique. In our experience, this produces marked improvement in the secondary patency. This early re-intervention is possible only if regular follow-up is maintained to facilitate early diagnosis, thus avoiding or at least postponing surgery.

It is difficult to compare the results of one technique with those of another because the lesions treated are often different. Certainly, in terms of procedural success, the Rotablator is comparable to other atherectomy techniques[4,8] and balloon angioplasty.[12] However, perhaps the advantage of rotational ablation lies in its ability to enlarge the treatment potential for percutaneous interventions as a whole.

Certain lesions cannot be treated by balloon dilatation alone, so the Rotablator is an important auxiliary technique that enhances our interventional capabilities overall. Further, the Rotablator allows percutaneous treatment of other lesions that until now had been impossible to treat non-surgically or posed higher risks with other endovascular or surgical techniques. Moreover, the potential to treat runoff vessels using this method should improve the long-term patency of ilio–femoro–popliteal bypasses and proximal angioplasties.

Other techniques may make such claims as well. Lasers, either excimer or holmium, would also be capable of treating long, eccentric, calcified, ostial, or bifurcation lesions.[13,14] However, the complication rate appears to be no lower, particularly for spasms in excimer-treated arteries, and the costs of a laser are far greater than an atherectomy device. The holmium laser can be used in the presence of thrombus, which is an advantage over the Rotablator, but, here again, the expense of the laser versus the cost of thrombolytic therapy preliminary to Rotablator therapy is unquestionably greater.

Directional atherectomy using the Simpson device may be preferred to the Rotablator in certain cases of ostial or bifurcation lesions and in short eccentric lesions. Its manipulation is more taxing and particularly difficult in tortuous arteries. Moreover, the risks are greater, particularly at the distal level, and the restenosis rate is high.[15]

The Transluminal Extraction Catheter (TECR) could compete with the Rotablator in certain disease pathologies, most notably for the treatment of focal stenoses and bypass lesions where thromboses are likely to be encountered. However, the device does not perform well in calcified vessels.[16]

The Rotarex catheter at the femoropopliteal level could also compete with the Rotablator but it is not proved that it is as effective for very calcified lesions.

In our experience, rotational ablation has taken a pre-eminent position in the treatment of distal leg arteries. Its low complication and restenosis rates have encouraged us to broaden its applications. The main limitation remains its cost; the catheters are expensive, and, when multiple burrs are needed, the procedural costs can rise. Without this drawback, it is probable that a far greater number of angioplasties would be preceded by rotational atherectomy. In our center, fully 15% of our procedures are today performed with this device, which attests to its importance. However, this enthusiasm must be tempered by the necessity for sound theoretical and practical knowledge of the device before approaching complex lesions.

References

1   Henry M, Amor M, Ethevenot G et al. Percutaneous peripheral rotational ablation using the Rotablator: immediate and mid-term results. Single center experience concerning 146 lesions treated. *Int Angiol* 1993; **12**: 213–44.

2   Ahn SS, Auth DC, Marcus DR et al. Removal of focal atheromatous lesions by angioscopically guided high speed rotational atherectomy: preliminary experimental observations. *J Vasc Surg* 1988; **7**: 292–300.

3   Ahn SS. Angioscopic controlled atherectomy. In: White GH, White RA (eds), *Angioscopy vascular and coronary applications.* Chicago: Year Book Medical Publishers, 1988: 114–22.

4   Ahn SS, Eton D. The Rotablator-high-speed rotary atherectomy: indications, technique, results, and complications. In: Ann SS, Moore WS (eds), *Endovascular surgery*, 2nd edn. Philadelphia: WB Saunders, 1992: 295–307.

5   McLean GK. Percutaneous peripheral atherectomy. *J Vasc Intervent Radiol* 1993; **4**: 465–80.

6   Dorros G, Iyer S, Zaitoun R et al. Acute angiographic and clinical outcome of high speed percutaneous rotational atherectomy (Rotablator). *Cathet Cardiovasc Diagn* 1991; **22**: 157–66.

7   Bertrand ME, Lablanche JM, Leroy F et al. Percutaneous transluminal coronary rotary ablation with Rotablator (European experience). *Am J Cardiol* 1992; **69**: 470–4.

8   Ahn SS, Eton D, Yeatman LR et al. Intraoperative peripheral rotary atherectomy: early and late clinical results. *Ann Vasc Surg* 1992; **6**: 272–80.

9   White CJ, Ramee SR, Escobar A et al. High speed rotational ablation (Rotablator) for unfavorable lesions in peripheral arteries. *Cathet Cardiovasc Diagn* 1993; **30**: 115–19.

10 The Collaborative Rotablator Atherectomy Group (CRAG). Peripheral atherectomy with the Rotablator: a multicenter report. *J Vasc Surg* 1994; **19**: 509–15.

11 Zotz RJ, Erbel R, Philipp A et al. High speed rotational angioplasty induced echo contrast in vivo and in vitro optical analysis. *Cathet Cardiovasc Diagn* 1992; **26**: 98–109.

12 Capek P, McLean GK, Berkowitz HD. Femoropopliteal angioplasty: factors influencing long-term success. *Circulation* 1991; **83**(Suppl I): I-70–I-80.

13 Litvack F, Grundfest WS, Adler L et al. Percutaneous excimer-laser and excimer-laser-assisted angioplasty of the lower extremities: results of intial clinical trial. *Radiology* 1989; **17**: 331–5.

14 McCarthy WJ, Vogelzang RL, Nemcek AA et al. Excimer laser-assisted femoral angioplasty: early results. *J Vasc Surg* 1991; **13**: 607–14.

15 Hinohara T, Selmon MR, Robertson GC et al. Directional atherectomy: new approaches for treatment of obstructive coronary and peripheral vascular disease. *Circulation* 1990; **81**(Suppl III):II-79-III-91.

16 Wholey MH, Levitt RG, Fein-Millar D. The transluminal endarterectomy catheter: indications, techniques, results, and complications. In: Ann SS, Moore WS (eds), *Endovascular surgery*, 2nd edn. Philadelphia: WB Saunders, 1992: 308–15.

17

A new rotational thrombectomy and atherectomy catheter: the Rotarex system

Isabelle Henry, Michel Henry and Michèle Hugel

Introduction

Balloon percutaneous transluminal angioplasty (PTA) has a major role in the treatment of coronary and peripheral significant stenoses and is now the first treatment to be proposed. Nevertheless this technique alone has some limitations in its application to some specific subgroups of complex lesions, such as calcified, ulcerated, eccentric, long lesions and thrombotic lesions with the risk of embolization. There is also the problem of restenosis, with a restenosis rate which can be high in some locations (e.g. femoropopliteal arteries, small vessels, ostial lesions, bifurcational lesions, long lesions, diabetic patients, etc.).

Several techniques have been proposed to reduce the restenosis rate and to treat some lesions not amenable to balloon angioplasty alone, such as stenting and debulking techniques with atherectomy devices. Atherectomy is defined as excision and removal of obstructive tissue, a concept first introduced by Simpson et al.[1-3]

The amount of plaque burden in the artery correlates with the restenosis rate. So, by creating a large, smooth lumen and by preventing elastic recoil, rather than increasing luminal diameter by arterial stretching and plaque fracture, as with balloon angioplasty, debulking could yield better clinical outcomes and short- and long-term patency rates.

The first directional atherectomy procedure was performed in 1985 by Simpson et al. in a superficial femoral artery using a peripheral atherectomy device. This initial experience demonstrated the safety of directional atherectomy for peripheral vascular disease.[4] It was approved by the US Food and Drug Administration (FDA) in 1987. This device was then adapted for coronary procedures and the directional coronary atherectomy (DCA) device was approved by the FDA in 1990 as the first non-balloon percutaneous coronary interventional device. In contrast to DCA, which relies on excision and tissue removal,

the transluminal extraction-endarterectomy catheter (TEC) (Interventional Technologies, Inc., San Diego, CA) was designed by Stack to cut and aspirate atheroma and debris. In 1989, this device was approved by the FDA for peripheral vascular disease, and in 1992 for revascularization of saphenous vein bypass grafts and native coronary arteries. Other devices have been proposed, e.g. the Rotablator,[5] the Simpson Atherotrack TM,[6] the Pullback Atherectomy Catheter[7] and, more recently, the Rotarex system.

The purpose of this chapter is to present the first clinical experiences with the Rotarex catheter. This device was first used by Schmitt et al.[8] working in the Department of Internal Medicine, University Hospital, Basel, as a thrombectomy device. We report the first clinical study of this catheter as an atherectomy device.

Rotarex system

Description – equipment and mechanism of action (Figures 17.1–17.4)

The system has three components:

- the Rotarex catheter (Straub Rotarex, patent pending, Straub Medical, Wangs, Switzerland);
- a 40 W D.C. electric motor drive;
- an electronic control unit.

Inside the whole length of the 8F polyurethane catheter rotates a coated stainless steel spiral, which glides over a 0.020 inch guide wire (Schneider Europe, Bülach, Switzerland). The catheter head consists of two cylinders that fit over each other. The outer rotating cylinder is fixed to the spiral; the inner one is attached to the catheter shaft. Each cylinder has two oval slits. The blunt tip of the outer cylinder is perforated for the guide wire. Catheter and motor drive are connected by a magnetic clutch. The motor rotates the spiral at 40 000 rpm, resulting in 80 000 cuts/minute. The high frequency of revolution creates a negative pressure at the catheter head of 5.8 kPa (43.5 mmHg). When the catheter is activated, soft and solid occlusion material is caught in the slits, transported by the spiral to the proximal sideport and discharged into a plastic bag. No additional suction is required. The transport of the occlusion material is done exclusively by the rotating spiral. The catheter is for one-time use, while the motor drive and the connecting cable to the electronic control unit can be sterilized.

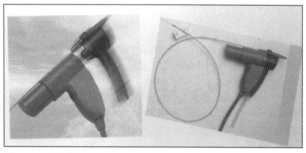

Figure 17.1
The Straub Rotarex catheter attached to the motor drive.

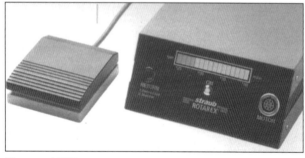

Figure 17.2
Electronic control unit.

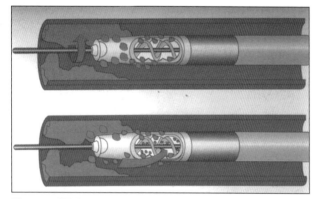

Figure 17.3
Schematic draining of the catheter head.

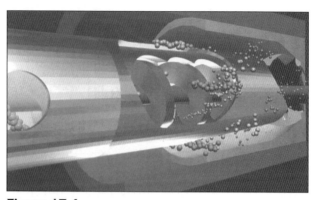

Figure 17.4
The rotating outer cylinder glides over the inner fixed cylinder with its oval slits. The guide wire runs inside the transport spiral, which is attached to the tip of the perforated head of the outer cylinder.

Preclinical studies

The catheter was tested in an arterial model made of silicon tubing and in fresh bovine carotid arteries. Translucent silicone tubing of 4, 6 and 8 mm inner diameter and length 15–30 cm served as an arterial model, allowing observation and video documentation of the catheter function. The tubes were bendable to test the behavior of the catheter at various angles. The tubing was filled with occlusion material of different consistencies: (1) bovine blood that was allowed to coagulate for 48 hours or 2 weeks and stored at 4°C; (2) stamp cylinders of 'black pudding', a mixture of thrombus, muscle, fat and connective tissue, 4, 6 and 8 mm thick, and 15 mm long, simulating organized thrombus; (3) strips of bovine arteries (3 cm long, 1 mm broad) sutured intraluminally to the vessel wall, imitating intimal flaps. The tubing was clamped at one end and connected to an infusion line on the other, where a mixture of saline and glycerol could be infused under a continuous pressure of 120 mmHg. In this infusion tube an 8F sheath (Cook, Bjaerverskov, Denmark) was introduced, a 0.020 inch Teflon-coated guide wire threaded through the occlusion material and the catheter advanced.

In a second test series ($n = 72$), the silicon tubing was replaced by fresh bovine carotid arteries with an average length of 20 cm and a diameter of 6–7 mm. The side branches were ligated and the arteries filled with the above-mentioned occlusion material. During catheter activation, tube and arteries were either kept straight or bent at different angles up to 50°. Occlusion of the arteries was achieved by tightening a 5 mm wide rubber band around the vessel, completely interrupting the flow of perfusate. The occlusion was passed with the catheter over the wire. All tests were recorded on video. The time of catheter activation was recorded, the volume of aspirated fluid measured and the fluid passed through different filters for analysis of particle size. The arteries were cut open and examined visually and histologically for remnants of occlusion material and possible intimal damage.

Results

The catheter removed 48-hour-old thrombi in silicone tubing of 4 and 6 mm diameter completely and regularly; the maximum working diameter was 8 mm. On average, 1 cm of thrombus was aspirated within 2 seconds. Thrombi stored in the refrigerator for 2 weeks often showed adherence to the wall of the tubing, but could also be easily aspirated, leaving occasionally a thin residual layer attached to the inner curvature if the tube was bent. Occlusion material of higher and inhomogenous consistency, such as muscle, fat and connective tissue, was caught readily in the catheter head and transported to the outside by the spiral. Fluid was aspirated at a rate of 1.5 ml/second. While fresh thrombus was completely homogenized, more solid material was cut into particles of 100–500 μm. Strips of bovine arteries, sutured intraluminally to the vessel wall to imitate intimal flaps, were cut and fragmented, leaving only small stumps at the suture site. Bovine arteries filled with thrombi or 'black pudding' could be cleared of the occlusion material without remnants. No intimal damage was noticed on visual examination or after staining. When the arteries were compressed to complete occlusion by a rubber band, the catheter drilled a lumen corresponding to its shaft size. When tubing or arteries were bent, the catheter followed the guide wire smoothly. No perforation was noticed. The catheter needs fluid (blood) for lubrication. Under experimental conditions the temperature of the catheter head rose by 1.5°C after rotating for 4 minutes at 40 000 rpm in a tube of 3 mm diameter perfused with a saline-glycerol solution (80 ml/minute) at room temperature.

Clinical studies as thrombectomy devices

Based on the results of the preclinical tests, the institutional review board of the Department of Internal Medicine, University Hospital, Basel, accepted the protocol of a pilot study for the evaluation of the device for the treatment of thrombotic occlusions in femoropopliteal arteries in humans.

Ten patients (eight women and two men; 58–87 years of age, mean age 70.6 ± 10.1) with acute or subacute occlusion of the femoropopliteal artery with an estimated age < 4 weeks and patent proximal segments of lower leg vessels, were included in the study. All patients were informed in detail about the procedure and gave their written consent. Patients with aneurysms of the popliteal artery, severe coagulation disturbances or a history of adverse reactions to contrast media were excluded.

Seven patients suffered from critical ischemia (rest pain) and three from peripheral arterial occlusive disease (PAOD) stage II (intermittent claudication). The estimated age of the lesions was between 2 and 28 days. The mean length of the occluded segments was 5.8 cm (range 2–15 cm).

The diagnosis was established by clinical examination, oscillography, Doppler pressure recordings, duplex sonography[9] and digital subtraction arteriography. Laboratory examinations included hemoglobin, free plasma arteriography, hematocrit and coagulation parameters, both before, immediately after and 24 hours after thrombectomy. Non-invasive examinations (oscillography, Doppler pressure recordings, duplex sonography) were performed after 48 hours and after 3 months. Antegrade arteriography was performed via the common femoral artery to determine the length of occlusion and to document the collateral circulation and the peripheral runoff.

Using the road-map technique, the occlusion was passed with a Teflon-coated 0.020 inch guide wire and its flexible tip placed in the distal popliteal artery. An 8F sheath was introduced and 5000 U of heparin injected. The thrombectomy catheter was threaded over the guide wire. One centimeter proximal to the upper end of the occlusion, the catheter was activated by a foot switch and advanced through the occlusion in gentle forward and backward movements under fluoroscopic control. The continuous suction of blood and occlusion material into the reservoir bag was observed. After the catheter had passed the occlusion it was withdrawn in the proximal femoral artery and angiography was repeated via the side port of the sheath. Depending on the result, thrombectomy was either terminated, repeated or completed by PTA. The number and the duration of catheter passes, and the volume of aspirated fluid, were recorded. Extracted occlusion material was examinated histologically.

Results

Thrombectomy was technically successful in all patients. A mean of 2.4 catheter passes (range 2–3) were required to recanalize the occluded segment, and 2.8 seconds on average were needed to reopen 1 cm of occlusion. Blood and detritus were aspirated at 1.1 ml/second; the total aspirated volume ranged from 20 to 90 ml, depending on the length and consistency of the lesion. In nine patients, an underlying residual stenosis was treated by PTA after the thrombectomy. Forty-eight hours after the intervention no patient suffered from critical ischemia: eight patients were classified as PAOD stage I, and two patients as stage II. The ankle–brachial index (ABI) improved from 0.41 ± 0.18 (range 0.13–0.65) preinterventionally to 0.88 ± 0.15 (range 0.64–1.11) after the intervention ($p < 0.0005$). Three months after the intervention the mean ABI was 0.84 ± 0.20 (range 0.52–1.07).

All patients received either oral anticoagulation or antiplatelet drugs and were assessed by duplex sonography 48 hours and 3 months after the intervention. The treated arterial segment remained patent in eight patients. Two patients had a reocclusion within 2 weeks after the intervention. In a 60-year-old woman with an occlusion 3 cm long in a smoothly outlined superficial femoral artery of 5 mm diameter and with three patent lower leg vessels, fresh thrombus was removed with the Rotarex catheter in two passes of 7 seconds. Complete vessel patency was restored, no peripheral embolism occurred and additional PTA was not considered to be indicated. As usual, the patient received 5000 U of heparin during the intervention and oral anticoagulation afterwards. After 48 hours duplex sonography revealed a reocclusion. At that time coagulation parameters were not in the therapeutic range, which might have contributed to the rethrombosis. The ABI, which improved from 0.61 to 0.71 after the intervention, remained at this level. The patient was classified as PAOD stage II without the need for a reintervention. The second patient was a 78-year-old diabetic woman with a history of claudication of several years, rest pain for 12 days and a 15 cm long occlusion of the popliteal artery with poor lower leg outflow. Thrombectomy was primarily successful and complete vessel patency was restored after additional PTA. The ABI rose from 0.65 to 0.95 and duplex sonography showed a residual stenosis of < 50% diameter reduction. One week after hospital discharge the patient complained of recurrence of intermittent claudication and a reocclusion was documented. Since the patient was clinically in PAOD stage II, no further intervention was performed. Reduced outflow due to pre-existing lower leg artery occlusions was considered as a possible cause for rethrombosis.

No patient had signs of mechanical damage to red blood cells. There was no increase in free plasma hemoglobin, nor relevant changes in hemoglobin and hematocrit after thrombectomy. Histologic examination of the aspirate showed mostly fresh thrombotic material and small components of fibrotic intima with sclerotic fragments. No serious complication occurred. In one patient a small embolus was detected angiographically within the proximal posterior tibial artery and lysed successfully by 100 000 U of urokinase.

Clinical study as atherectomy device – authors' personal experience

A second pilot study for the evaluation of the device for the treatment of chronic atherosclerotic stenoses or in-stent restenoses in femoropopliteal arteries in humans was conducted in our catheterization lab.

Population

Twenty-one patients (17 men and four women; 44–86 years of age, mean age 69.0 ± 11.9) with 26 lesions (tight chronic

atherosclerotic stenoses or restenoses) of the femoro-popliteal artery or tibioperoneal trunk, were included in the study.

All patients were informed in detail about the procedure and gave their written consent. Patients with aneurysms of the popliteal artery, severe coagulation disturbances or a history of adverse reactions to contrast media were excluded.

Cardiovascular risk factors of these patients were: diabetes 3/21 (14.3%), high blood pressure 19/21 (90.5%), dyslipidemia 15/21 (71.4%), tobacco 11/21 (52.4%). A history of coronary artery disease was present in 3/21 (14.3%) and previous peripheral transluminal angioplasty in 12/21 (57.1%). None of the patients had a history of femoropopliteal or distal bypass surgery.

All the patients suffered from intermittent claudication and were in class IIb of Fontaine's classification. None of them suffered from critical ischemia (rest pain). The estimated age of claudication varied between 2 months and 1 year.

Pre- and post-procedure assessment

Diagnosis was established by clinical examination, duplex sonography[9] and digital subtraction arteriography.

Duplex sonography was performed before, 24 hours and 6 months after the intervention. An arteriography was performed via the common femoral artery in all patients before the procedure to determine the characteristics of the lesions, to document the collateral circulation, the peripheral runoff and to decide the method of approach.

Laboratory examinations included hemoglobin, hematocrit and coagulation parameters, both before and 24 hours after atherectomy.

Characteristics of the lesions

The characteristics of the lesions are summarized in Table 17.1.

The mean arterial diameter of the artery was 5.4 ± 0.8 mm (range 3–6 mm) and the mean pre-intervention minimal lumen diameter (MLD) was 1.4 ± 0.6 mm (range 0–1.5 mm). The mean percentage diameter of the stenosis was: 83.5 ± 7.9% (range 70–100%) and the mean lesion length 31.1 ± 35.0 mm (range 10–150 mm). The majority of the patients had a good runoff (three distal leg vessel patency, seven patients; two distal leg vessel patency, 11 patients; one distal leg vessel patency, two patients).

Table 17.1	Lesion characteristics				
Characteristics	No. patients		No. patients		No. patients
Location					
Femoral	19	Upper part	4		
		Middle part	9		
		Low part	6		
Femoropopliteal	6				
Tibioperoneal trunk	1				
Etiology					
De novo	15				
Restenosis	11	Post-PTA	2		
		Instent restenosis	9	Expander	7
				Palmaz	1
				Optimed	1
Characteristics					
Calcifications	12				
Eccentricity	10				
Collaterals	5				
Ulceration	1				

PTA, Percutaneous transluminal angioplasty

Technique

Adjunctive medical therapy

Adjunctive medical therapy for debulking with the Rotarex system is similar to PTA, including preprocedural aspirin (160 mg/day starting at least 1 day prior the debulking procedure) and intraprocedural heparin (5000 U IV). Molsidomine was administered at the discretion of the operator to minimize vasospasm. The vascular sheath was removed immediately after the procedure. Heparin was given as enoxaparin (40 mg twice daily subcutaneously) for 24–72 hours at the discretion of the operator, depending on the difficulties and the result of the procedure. Other platelet antagonists such as dipyridamole, dextran, sulfinpyrazone and anti-GIIb-IIIa inhibitors [abciximab (ReoPro)] were never prescribed. All patients received aspirin 160 mg/day continuously after the procedure and clopidogrel 75 mg/day for 1 month if a stent was placed.

Technique of debulking

We used the ipsilateral antegrade approach in most of the cases (19/21) and the contralateral retrograde approach in two cases to treat lesions of the upper part of the superficial femoral artery (SFA). An 8F sheath was introduced in the femoral artery. In case of a stenosis, it was crossed with a Teflon-coated 0.020 inch guide wire and its flexible tip placed in the distal popliteal artery. In case of an occlusion, the lesion was first recanalized by a 0.035 inch hydrophilic guide wire, then exchanged for a 0.020 inch guide wire through a 4F catheter. The atherectomy catheter was threaded over the guide wire. One centimeter proximal to the upper end of the stenosis or occlusion, the catheter was activated by a foot switch and advanced through the lesion in gentle forward and backward movements under fluoroscopic control. The continuous suction of blood and occlusion material into the reservoir bag was observed. After the catheter had passed the lesion it was withdrawn in the proximal femoral artery and angiography was repeated via the side port of the sheath. Depending on the result, atherectomy was either terminated, repeated or completed by PTA, with or without stent. The number of catheter passes and the volume of aspirated fluid were recorded.

Optimal atherectomy

The end of the Rotarex procedure was based on angiographic appearance and was at the discretion of the operator.

A technical success is defined as a post-procedural residual stenosis < 30% at angiography or a pressure gradient < 5 mmHg. In contrast to PTA, which often leaves moderate residual stenosis (20–50%) that requires stenting to enhance the result, the goal of optimal atherectomy was to create the largest possible lumen without complications, with a final residual stenosis < 30%, to avoid angioplasty and stenting.

Optimal atherectomy could be achieved as follows: by debulking alone if the control angiogram demonstrates a residual stenosis < 30%, debulking followed by PTA ± stenting if the angiogram demonstrated a residual stenosis > 30% after debulking. PTA was performed using a balloon:artery ratio of 1:1.2 and inflation pressure of 4–6 atm. The 'ideal' residual stenosis is unknown. In our study, we attempted to achieve a residual stenosis of < 30%.

Results

Immediate angiographic results

Technical success. Atherectomy was technically successful in all patients and all lesions. One occlusion was first recanalized by a Terumo guide wire before the atherectomy with the Rotarex system. One very tight stenosis needed to perform an angioplasty with a small diameter balloon to enlarge the lumen before the Rotarex system could cross the lesion. A mean of 4.6 catheter passes (range 3–8) were required to enlarge the arterial lumen. Results in terms of MLD and percentage residual diameter stenosis after atherectomy with the Rotarex are shown in Table 17.2.

Blood and detritus were aspirated at 1.1 ml/second; the total aspirated volume ranged from 40 to 110 ml, depending on the length and consistency of the lesion.

In 19/26 lesions (73.1%), an underlying post-atherectomy significant residual stenosis (> 30%) was present and treated by PTA alone in 15/19 lesions (78.9%) and with PTA + stent in 4/19 lesions (21.1%). The mean residual stenosis after Rotarex was 36.8 ± 15.1% (range 5–55).

Six stents were placed for significant residual stenosis (n = 4) or residual dissection (n = 2). The different types were: JoMed (JoMed France SARL, Voisins le Bretonneaux) one patient; Optimed (Optimed Medizinische Instrumente GmbH, Ettlingen, Germany, four patients; Smart (Cordis Corp, Warren NJ), one patient. The type of stent placed depended on the location, the diameter and the length of the lesion. Final results after Rotarex and PTA + stent procedure are shown in Table 17.2.

Angiographic complications

The overall incidence of angiographic complications after the Rotarex procedure was 6/26 (23.1%).

Dissection and abrupt closure. A small non-occlusive dissection, not compromising the arterial flow, occurred in 15.4% of cases (4/26 lesions) after the atherectomy procedure. It was treated by PTA (three cases – 75%), and stent (one case–25%) without further revascularization. No abrupt closure was observed.

Distal embolization and No-Reflow. Distal embolization causing abrupt cutoff of the target vessel distal to the original

Table 17.2   Angiographic results

	Mean arterial diameter (mm)	Minimal lumen diameter (mm)	Mean stenosis (%)
Before atherectomy	5.4 ± 0.8	1.4 ± 0.6	83.5 ± 7.9
After atherectomy	5.3 ± 0.9	3.2 ± 0.4	36.8 ± 15.1
After procedure (PTA + stent)	5.4 ± 0.7	5.2 ± 0.8	2 ± 3.5

PTA, Percutaneous transluminal angioplasty.

target lesion has been seen in one case and treated successfully by thrombosuction. No emergency bypass was needed. This type of macroembolization was probably due to dislodgment of thrombus or friable plaque from the target lesion, or release or incomplete capture of tissue stored in the collection chamber of the device.

Perforation. Artery perforation was observed in one case (3.8%) in a tibioperoneal trunk and treated with a covered JoMed stent after unsuccessful prolonged balloon inflations.

Vasospasm. No severe vasospasm was observed after Rotarex.

Side branch occlusion. No side branch occlusion occurred.

Clinical outcomes

A clinical success at 24 hours was observed in all patients (100%) with no major clinical complications, no vascular injury requiring blood transfusion or vascular repair.

All patients were classified as class 1 of Fontaine's classification. The ABI improved from 0.53 ± 0.12 (range 0.13–0.65) pre-interventionally to 0.91 ± 0.13 (range 0.64–1.11) post-intervention (P < 0.0005).

All treated arterial segments remained patent with good results and no significant residual stenosis, except in one patient whose residual stenosis was evaluated to 50% and treated medically.

No patient had signs of hemolysis. There were no relevant changes in hemoglobin and hematocrit after thrombectomy. Results are shown in Table 17.3.

Table 17.3

	Hematocrit (%)	Hemoglobin (g/dl)
Before	40.0 ± 4.1	13.5 ± 1.4
After	38.0 ± 4.3	12.7 ± 1.5

Follow-up

Three months after intervention, the mean ABI was 0.84 ± 0.20 (range 0.52–1.07).

Restenosis and late outcome. Three restenoses were observed. Two at 6 months: 2/21 patients, 2/26 lesions (two in-stent restenosis: one Expander and one Optimed).

One patient treated by Rotarex and PTA alone for a severe long in-stent restenosis (90% in diameter stenosis, 100 mm in length. Optimed stent), had an occlusion of the left SFA at 4 months treated by femoropopliteal bypass surgery.

The other patient was also treated by Rotarex and PTA alone for a severe in-stent restenosis (90% diameter stenosis, 30 mm in length, Expander stent (Bolton, Vandœuvre-les-Nancy, France) of the low part of the left SFA, developed an occlusion at 6 months which was treated medically.

The third restenosis occurred at 9 months in a patient who had been treated for a de novo lesion (75% diameter stenosis, 10 cm in length) in the mid part of a small left SFA (maximum lumen diameter 3 mm). This restenosis was treated by femoropopliteal bypass surgery at 9 months.

At a mean follow-up of 9.6 ± 2.7 months all patients were asymptomatic and in class I of Fontaine's classification.

Discussion

In the last decade, great efforts have been made to provide an alternative to time-consuming local fibrinolysis and surgical thrombectomy in the treatment of arterial thrombosis. Percutaneous aspiration thrombectomy through thin-walled, straight catheters is still a common, readily available, simple and cost-effective technique for the removal of fresh thrombi.[10] Its restriction to loose, i.e. not adherent, thrombi, the necessity of usually several passes, and the risk of plaque avulsion and antegrade dissection have, however, led to the construction of more sophisticated devices.[11]

Devices to debulk arteries with severe chronic atherosclerotic stenoses prior to angioplasty and stenting have been developed. The expectancy was to decrease post-angioplasty residual stenoses and restenosis rates.

The experience with the first catheter equipped with a fast-rotating, coaxially driven cam (Trac-Wright, formerly Kensey) was disappointing. The device was, however, the predecessor of several generations of rotational catheters,[12,13] which can be roughly classified into two types of devices:

- those using recirculation, e.g. pulverization of thrombi by a hydrodynamic vortex created either by a high-speed impeller[14–17] or the Venturi effect;[18–20]

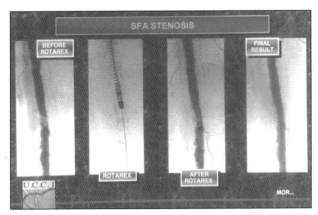

Figure 17.5
Tight calcified superficial femoral artery (SFA) stenosis. Angioplasty after Rotarex.

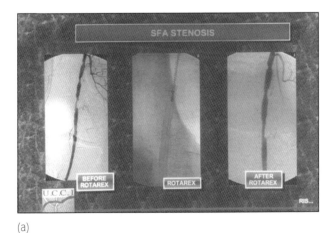

(a)

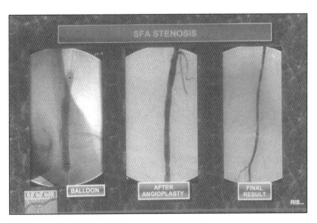

(b)

Figure 17.6
In-stent restenosis treated with (a) Rotarex and (b) angioplasty.

- non-circulation catheters with concomitant suction, using either a rotating recessed propeller[21,22] or rotating cutting blades[23,24] and aspiration via a roller pump or any other suction modality.[25]

These devices are effective in clearing fresh thrombi, especially in arterial and hemodialysis grafts; however, their effectiveness decreases with the age of thrombi and their adherence to the vessel wall. Since many occlusions are 'acute on chronic' thromboses, a thrombectomy device should have the potential to remove not only fresh but also underlying organized thrombi. Furthermore, it should track over a guide wire in order to prevent vessel perforation. Finally, it should transport the occlusion material to the outside without the risk of peripheral embolization.

The new Rotarex catheter described here meets many of these requirements: its constriction is relatively simple, using only one lumen for the spiral and coaxial guide wire. No extra channels for suction, lubrication or cooling are needed. The transport of the occlusion material is done exclusively by the spiral. Some devices are easily obstructed by sticky occlusion material, especially by fibrin, which has to be transported through a narrow catheter over a distance of 80–100 cm. In the new catheter, this drawback was eliminated by a special coating of the spiral and by adjusting the rotational speed to 40 000 rpm. As with all rotating devices, heat caused by friction can be a problem.[26] The new device needs blood for lubrication. Therefore, it should not be advanced continuously in an occlusion, but in gentle forward and backward movements, allowing the uninterrupted aspiration of blood and avoidance of running dry. Provided these precautions were observed, no undue warming of the catheter was noted. The average time for thrombectomy or atherectomy in these two pilot studies was short and did not exceed 90 seconds for occlusions up to 15 cm in length or long severe stenoses.

Blood loss during thrombectomy or atherectomy is generally low, amounting to 80–90 ml/minute, depending on the composition of the occlusion material that has to be transported and the blood available in the artery.

A useful parameter for the assessment of the efficacy of a thrombectomy catheter is the radial force coefficient, i.e. the ratio of the lumen recanalized by thrombectomy to the catheter diameter. For this new catheter, the coefficient is 2 in vitro, meaning that the catheter with a diameter of approximately 3 mm clears a thrombus of 6 mm. In vivo the radial expansion coefficient depends on the composition of the occlusion material. It is about 2 in fresh thrombi but drops to 1 in solid material, which means that the reopened or debulked lumen corresponds to the diameter of the catheter head. Experimental data suggest use of the catheter for the treatment of obstructed vessels with a diameter up to 8 mm. These studies showed its feasibility and efficacy in superficial femoral or popliteal arteries of 5–7 mm diameter. Its applicability in larger vessels, such as pelvic arteries, vena cava or pulmonary arteries, needs to be validated in further trials.

Compared with other thrombectomy or atherectomy devices, the potential of the Rotarex catheter to remove not only fresh loose thrombus but also solid, organized occlusion material must be considered as an advantage. With fresh thrombi we may expect to remove all the material, but with organized occlusion it remains, in most cases, a residual stenosis, so we have to treat either by PTA alone or PTA + stent.

The catheter can also treat calcified plaques but seems less efficient than the Rotablation atherectomy catheter (Rotablator), in particular in small distal peripheral arteries.[5] Therefore, adjunctive PTA after thrombectomy or atherectomy is often necessary to eliminate residual stenosis.

We expect that debulking prior to angioplasty can avoid stenting in peripheral arteries and decrease the restenosis rate at follow-up, but we have no proof and further large-scale randomized studies are needed.

As shown in arterial models, the wire-guided catheter removes thrombus or atherosclerotic material without intimal abrasion, severe arterial dissection or perforation if the original caliber of the artery is larger than the catheter head. Consequently, the catheter in the 8F version is not suitable for thrombectomy or atherectomy in vessels distal to the popliteal artery. For use in small vessels, a 5F version is in preparation.

Hemolysis occurs in recirculation catheters without aspiration, but its clinical effect seems minimal.[27] In these small studies no change in hemoglobin or hematocrit was noticed after thrombectomy or atherectomy.

Except for a small embolus in a posterior tibial artery after thrombectomy, which was removed by focal fibrinolysis, and one in a distal leg artery after atherectomy, treated successfully by thrombosuction, no relevant complications occurred. It can be assumed that the negative pressure built up by the catheter system is sufficient to avoid peripheral embolization.

As expected from the preclinical tests, the catheter was easy to handle and helped to save considerable time by shortening thrombectomy to few minutes, so avoiding lengthy procedures such as local fibrinolysis or surgical intervention.

The potential benefit of debulking could be to reduce the restenosis rate [we observed only three cases of restenosis in the 26 lesions treated (11.5%)] and treatment of some difficult lesions not well treated by PTA alone.

Indications for treatment with the Rotarex system could be:

- as a thrombectomy device
  thrombotic lesions
  acute and subacute occlusions
- as an atherectomy device
  in-stent restenosis
  ulcerated, embolic, eccentric, ostial, long lesions (either stenosis or occlusion)
  bifurcated lesions
  calcified lesions (but the Rotablator, whose safety and efficacy has been well documented, could be better for this type of lesion, and particularly in small vessels).

Due to the efficacy and safety, the potential benefit of such a debulking device for the treatment of peripheral stenoses or occlusions has to be well evaluated. The immediate, mid- and long-term results of this technique compared with those obtained with conventional therapy (PTA + stent) in larger multicenter randomized series, show that use of this device greatly increases the duration and cost-effectiveness of the procedure.

Theoretical advantages of debulking techniques are tissue removal, the stepwise controlled approach and reduced mechanical trauma to the vessel wall (less 'overstretching'). Its limitations are specific complications (possibility of stent damage, perforation, dissection), duration of the procedure, costs and the possible need of specific medications (e.g. ticlopidine, clopidogrel).

Conclusions

The Rotarex system is a thrombectomy and atherectomy catheter which is easy to handle. Its feasibility has already been published for the treatment of acute and subacute occlusions. This study is the first one of the treatment of chronic arterial occlusive disease using the Rotarex system. It appears feasible and safe in arteries > 4–5 mm in diameter.

Immediate and mid-term results are promising with a low restenosis rate. Indications for this device have to be determined but it seems that long lesions and in-stent restenosis could be better treated with this device than with PTA alone.

Larger randomized studies (atherectomy versus conventional angioplasty) are needed to evaluate if atherectomy before angioplasty could avoid stenting in arteries < 6 mm in diameter, reduce the restenosis rate and improve the clinical outcome.

References

1   Simpson JB, Johnson DE, Thapliyal HV et al. Transluminal atherectomy: a new approach to the treatment of atherosclerotic vascular disease. *Circulation* 1985; **72** (suppl III): III-111–III-146 (abstract).

2   Simpson JB, Robertson GC, Selmon MR. Percutaneous coronary atherectomy. *J Am Coll Cardiol* 1988; **11** (suppl A): 110A (abstract).

3   Simpson JB. Future interventional techniques. In: (Califf RM, Mark DB, Wagner GS, eds) *Acute Coronary Care in the Thrombolytic Era.* Year Book Medical Publishers: Chicago 1988, 392–404.

4   Simpson JB, Selmon MR, Robertson GC et al. Transluminal atherectomy for occlusive peripheral vascular disease. *Am J Cardiol* 1988; **61**:96G–101G.

5   Henry M, Amor M, Ethevenot G et al. Percutaneous peripheral rotational ablation using the Rotablator: immediate and mid-term results. Single center experience concerning 146 lesions treated. *Int Angiol* 1993; **12**:231–44.

6   Hoshino S, Midorikawa H. Clinical results of directional peripheral atherectomy. *Nippon Geka Gakkai Zasshi* 1996; **97**:568–73.

7   White CJ. Peripheral atherectomy with the Pullback Atherectomy Catheter: procedural safety and efficacy in a multicenter trial. PAC Investigators. *J Endovas Surg* 1998; **5**:9–17.

8   Schmitt HE, Jäger KA, Jacob AL et al. A new rotational thrombectomy catheter: system design and first clinical experiences. *Cardiovasc Intervent Radiol* 1999; **22**:504–9.

9   Jäger K, Frauchiger B, Eichlisberger R. Ultrasonographic investigation of the peripheral arteries. In: Tooke JE, Lowe GDO eds. *A Textbook of Vascular Medicine.* Oxford University Press: New York, 1996: 84–89.

    Wagner H-J, Starck E. Acute embolic occlusions of the infrainguinal arteries: percutaneous aspiration embolectomy in 102 patients. *Radiology* 1992; **182**:403–7.

10 Brossmann J, Müller-Hülsbeck S, Heler M. Perkutane Thrombektomie und mechanische Thrombolyse. *Fortschr Rontgenstr* 1998; **169**:344–54.

11 Kensey KR, Nash JE, Abrahams C et al. Recanalization of obstructed arteries with a flexible, rotating tip catheter. *Radiology* 1987; **165**:387–9.

12 Triller J, Do DD, Maddern G et al. Femoropopliteal artery occlusion: clinical experience with the Kensey catheter. *Radiology* 1992; **182**:257–61.

13 Bildsoe MC, Moradian GP, Hunter DW et al. Mechanical clot dissolution: a new concept. *Radiology* 1989; **171**:231–3.

14 Pozza CH Gomes MR, Qian Z et al. Evaluation of the newly developed Amplatz maceration and aspiration thrombectomy device using in vitro and in vivo models. *AJR* 1994; **162**:139.

15 Uflacker R. Mechanical thrombectomy in acute and subacute thrombosis with the use of the Amplatz device: arterial and venous application. *J Vasc Intervent Radiol* 1997; **8**:923–32.

16 Rilinger N, Görich J, Scharrer-Pamler R et al. Short-term results with use of the Amplatz thrombectomy device in the treatment of acute lower limb occlusions. *J Vasc Intervent Radiol* 1997; **8**:343–8.

17 Reekers JA, Kromhout, JG, Van der Waal K. Catheter for percutaneous thrombectomy: first clinical experience. *Radiology* 1993; **188**:871–4.

18 Bücker A, Schmitz-Rode T, Vorwerk D et al. Comparative in vitro study of two percutaneous hydrodynamic thrombectomy systems. *J Vasc Intervent Radiol* 1996; **7**:445–9.

19 Henry M, Amor M, Henry I. The hydrolyser catheter: our clinical experience about 50 cases. Presented at the 8th International Course of Peripheral Vascular Intervention, Paris, 1997; 101–9.

20 Guenther RW, Vorwerk D. A new aspiration thrombectomy catheter with propeller tipped rotating wire: in vitro study. *J Intervent Radiol* 1990; **1**:17–20.

21 Guenther RW, Vorwerk D. Aspiration catheter for percutaneous thrombectomy: clinical results. *Radiology* 1990; **175**:271–3.

22 Yedlicka JW, Carlson JE, Hunter DW et al. Thrombectomy with the transluminal endarterectomy catheter (TEC) system. *J Vasc Intervent Radiol* 1991; **2**:343–7.

23 Rillinger N, Görich J, Scharrer-Palmer R et al. Percutaneous transluminal rotational atherectomy in the treatment of peripheral vascular disease using transluminal endarterectomy catheter (TEC): initial results and angiographic follow-up. *Cardiovasc Intervent Radiol* 1997; **20**:263–7.

24 Müller-Hülsbeck S, Schwarzenberg H, Bangard C et al. Saugpumpenunterstützte Aspirationsthrombektomie: in vitro Vergleich mit einem. Thrombusfragmentierungsverfahren. *Fortschr Rontgenstr* 1998; **162**:191–4.

25 Gehani AA, Rees MR. Can rotational atherectomy cause thermal tissue damage? A study of the potential heating and thermal tissue effects of a rotational atherectomy device. *Cardiovasc Intervent Radiol* 1998; **21**:481–6.

26 Nazarian GK, Qian Z, Coleman CC et al. Hemolytic effect of the Amplatz thrombectomy device. *J Vasc Intervent Radiol* 1994; **55**:155–60.

18

Open subintimal angioplasty of the superficial femoral and distal arteries

P Balas and Christos Klonaris

Introduction

The pioneer work on percutaneous recanalization of occluded peripheral arteries of Dotter and Judkins[1] and on arterial dilation of the stenosed arteries by balloon angioplasty of Gruntzig and Hoff[2] have opened the field of endovascular therapies, which at present are applied by interventionist radiologists, cardiologists, medical angiologists and vascular surgeons. Over the years, various methods and techniques of endovascular procedures have been developed and have been applied with satisfactory results in short-term and long-term follow-up.[3–10]

Bolia et al[11] developed the technique of subintimal angioplasty of the superficial femoral artery and distal arteries, and reported satisfactory long-term results in patients with critical limb ischemia.[12]

However, percutaneous subintimal angioplasty is difficult or impossible to perform when there is severe stenosis or occlusion of the distal external iliac and common femoral arteries and also when there is occlusion at the origin of the superficial femoral artery (SFA). In these cases, in order to overcome this difficulty, we have developed the invasive approach to open subintimal angioplasty.

Technique

Under local or general anesthesia, a subinguinal incision is made to expose the common femoral artery to the superficial femoral and profunda femoris arteries, which are then surrounded by elastic loops. A 5-mm-long arteriotomy in the SFA is opened on the anterior aspect at its origin; the edges are retracted with 6-0 Prolene stitches. Carefully, the underlying atheromatous core is partially dissected to create a small subintimal channel (Figure 18.1). A hydrophilic-coated guidewire with a straight floppy tip (Glidewire, Boston Scientific/Vascular, Natick, MA, USA) is inserted into this channel and advanced slowly under fluoroscopic guidance for ≥10 cm.

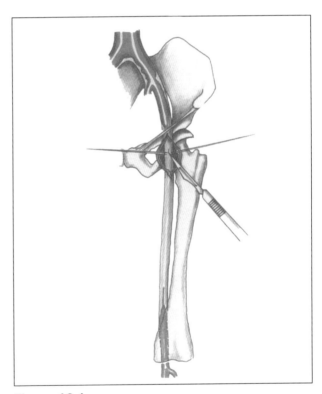

Figure 18.1
Small incision through the adventitia on the anterior aspect of the occluded SFA origin.

After insertion and advancement of the wire, a 5F or 6F sheath is introduced. A 5F guide catheter is advanced over the wire, leaving the tip of the wire free to dissect the atheromatous core from the adventitia (Figures 18.2 and 18.3). At this point, 5000–7500 units of unfractionated heparin are given intravenously. As the wire progresses down the artery, small amounts of dye are injected to check for proper advancement

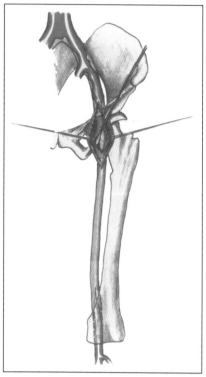

Figure 18.2
Dissection of the atheromatous plaque to create a subintimal channel.

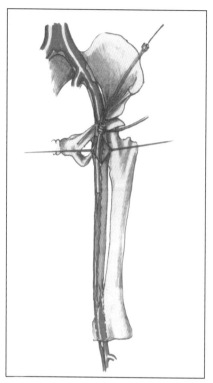

Figure 18.3
Guide catheter is inserted over the guidewire to facilitate the subintimal dissection, leaving the tip of the wire free to advance the dissection.

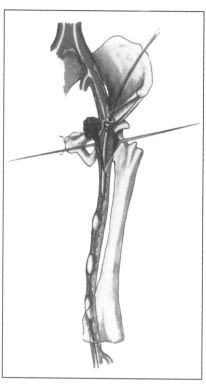

Figure 18.4
Progressive balloon dilation up the artery expands the subintimal channel.

or any extravasation. By manipulating the catheter and the wire, the distal open arterial segment, usually the popliteal, is reached. Following this maneuver, the wire is advanced free or with the support of the guide catheter into one of the distal arteries. The catheter is then removed, and an arteriogram is taken to assess the developed subintimal false lumen and to exclude any gross extravasation.

Using a balloon catheter (4 or 6 mm × 40 mm) passed to the distal aspect of the lesion, the subintimal space–neolumen is dilated sequentially up the artery (Figure 18.4). At the proximal aspect, the sheath is withdrawn to allow dilation. Before removing the sheath completely, an arteriogram is performed to verify that the false lumen is satisfactory. If not, additional dilations are done with a larger balloon.

After development of the false lumen, any stenotic or occluded trifurcation vessels are dilated with smaller balloons. Papaverine (80 mg) or nitroglycerin (100–200 μg) may be injected intra-arterially to relieve distal spasm. In some cases, fluoroscopy at this point may show extravasated dye moving cephalad, giving the impression of dye flowing into the accompanying vein or veins. This represents filling of the vein or veins through the arterial and venous vasa vasorum and typically disappears after a few minutes.

After satisfactory dilation, the sheath is removed, and the

balloon is withdrawn so that its distal half is within the artery and the proximal portion extends out of the arteriotomy. A final inflation is performed, and the balloon is removed. After obtaining satisfactory backflow, the wire is removed and the origin of the SFA is clamped.

Once the endovascular component is completed, the arteriotomy is extended cephalad to the common femoral artery, and endarterectomy of the common femoral, profunda and even of the external iliac arteries is performed, starting from the origin of the SFA (Figure 18.5). The proximal part of the atheromatous core in the SFA is trimmed carefully and usually tacked down with 6-0 Prolene suture. A patch of Dacron or bovine pericardium (Vascuguard, Bio-Vascular, Inc., St Paul, MN, USA) is fashioned for closure of the arteriotomy. One end of the patch is carefully sutured at the opening of the SFA, which has been dilated to secure a satisfactory entrance into the false arterial lumen (Figures 18.6–18.8).

Before closing the wound, a drain is placed, which allows postoperative heparinization to commence immediately. An activated clotting time is taken; if >200 s, a small amount of protamine sulfate is injected intravenously. Low molecular weight heparin is given for 1 week, and the drain is removed after 12–24 h. After discharge, clopidogrel is prescribed for a month, and aspirin is to be taken indefinitely.

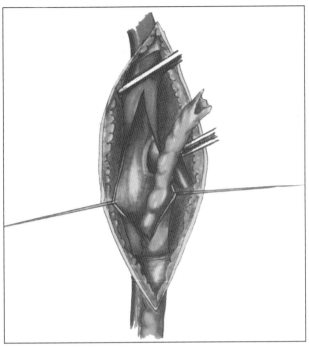

Figure 18.5
The arteriotomy is extended proximally, opening the common femoral artery, through which an endarterectomy is performed.

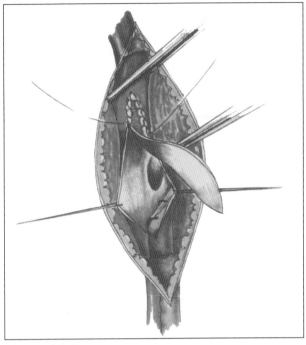

Figure 18.6
After removal of the atheromatous plaque from the common femoral artery, its end is trimmed at the SFA origin and tacked down with interrupted 6-0 Prolene suture.

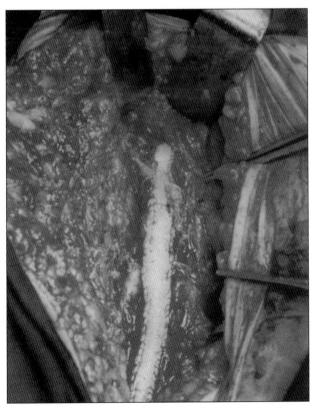

Figure 18.7
With a patch graft, the arteriotomy is closed.

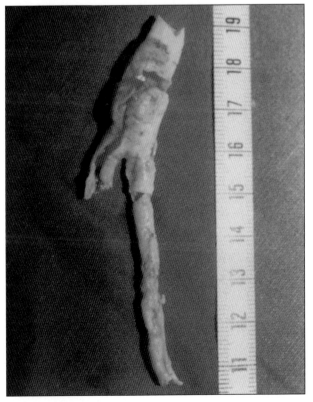

Figure 18.8
The excised atheromatous plaque from the common, superficial and profunda femoris arteries.

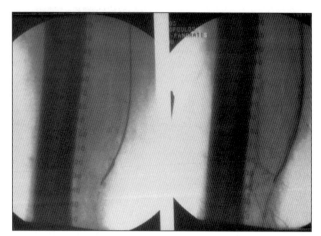

Figure 18.9

Imaging of the guide catheter which is advanced over the guide-wire into the dissected subintimal space opacified after injection of dye.

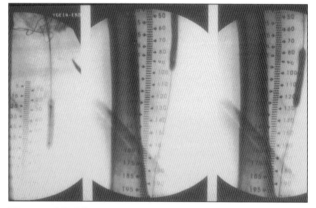

Figure 18.10

Under fluoroscopy, the neolumen is dilated sequentially up the artery.

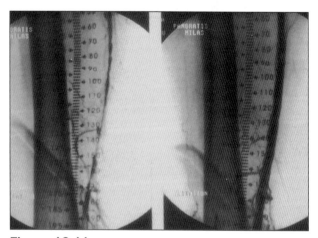

Figure 18.11

Arteriography before (left) and after (right) the complete dilation of the neolumen.

Discussion

In patients with complete occlusion of the SFA and associated proximal and distal lesions, conventional revascularization to ameliorate symptoms and ward off impending tissue loss can require lengthy incisions and placement of venous or prosthetic bypasses. Subintimal angioplasty offers a less invasive means of restoring distal bloodflow by establishing an alternative channel within the vessel rather than externally bypassing the obstructions. Although the percutaneous delivery of this technique is the least invasive approach and can be performed under local anesthesia by any interventionist (radiologist, cardiologist, or vascular surgeon), it is limited in its application. If the occlusion begins at the origin of the SFA, blunt dissection with the wire and development of the cleavage plane between the atheromatous core and the adventitia may be difficult or entirely impossible (Figures 18.9–18.11).

Also, this approach is very difficult, dangerous or impossible to perform in the presence of severe stenosis or occlusion of the distal part of the external iliac and common femoral arteries.

Open subintimal angioplasty, on the other hand, circumvents this obstacle by creating the subintimal channel surgically, but this has to be done by a vascular surgeon and, sometimes, under general anesthesia. Advantageously, the open approach does allow other procedures to be performed through this single femoral incision. For example, balloon dilation of homolateral common and external iliac lesions can be done via the arteriotomy. In addition, complete endarterectomy of the common femoral, profunda and external iliac arteries is feasible.

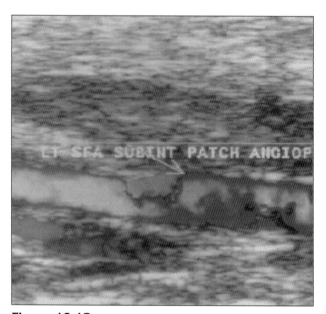

Figure 18.12

Triplex ultrasonography 2 years after subintimal angioplasty. The patched common femoral artery and the first part of the subintimal neolumen of the SFA.

We have employed this technique with good success in several patients with complex and lengthy lower limb lesions. In most cases, biplanar arteriography at 6–12 months has shown an excellent subintimal conduit similar to that of the normal lumen (Figures 18.12–18.14). An alternative approach put forth by Moll[13] uses a ring cutter for remote endarterectomy through a single femoral incision; the distal intimal edge is stented to prevent distal dissection and occlusion. Bray[14] and others[15] took this procedure one step further by relining the endarterectomized segment with various types of endoprostheses. The preliminary results seem to be satisfactory.

In conclusion, open subintimal angioplasty is a simple minimally invasive alternative treatment for complete SFA occlusion; however, more patient experience with longer follow-up has to be amassed to evaluate the durability of the patency of the false arterial lumen.

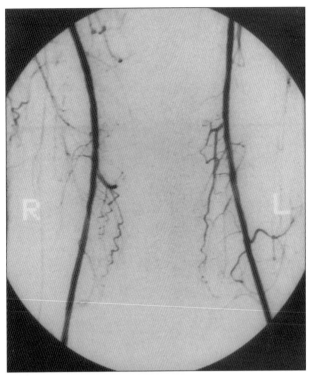

Figure 18.14
Arteriogram taken 2 years after the procedures. Complete patency of both SFAs.

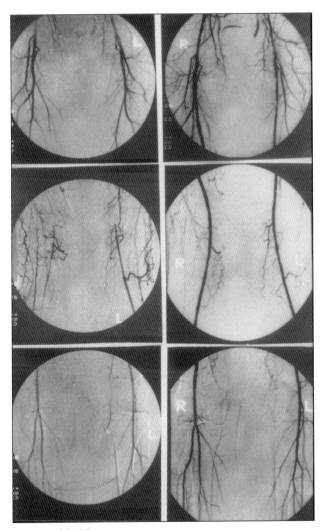

Figure 18.13
Complete occlusion of the entire right SFA and part occlusion of the left. An open subintimal angioplasty was performed on the right SFA and balloon dilation on the left.

Acknowledgement

Reproduction permission was granted by Alliance Communications Group to reproduce part of the text and the figures 18.1, 18.4, 18.5, 18.6, 18.9 and 18.10 from the article: Balas, Pangratis, Ioannou, Milas, Klonaris, Massouridou. Open subintimal angioplasty of the superficial femoral and distal arteries. *J Endovasc Ther* 2000; **7**: 68–71.

References

1   Dotter CT, Judkins MP. Transluminal treatment of atherosclerotic obstruction: description of a new technique and a preliminary report of its application. *Circulation* 1974; **30**: 654–70.

2   Gruntzig A, Hoff H. Percutaneous Rekanalization chronischer arterieller Verschlusse mit einem neuen dilatation Katheter: Modification der Dotter Technik. *Dtsch Med Wochenschr* 1974; **99**: 2502–5.

3   Zeitler E, Richter EI, Roth FJ, Schoop W. Results of percutaneous transluminal angioplasty. *Radiology* 1983; **146**: 57–60.

4   Ahn SS, Moore WS. *Endovascular Surgery* Philadelphia: WB Saunders, 1992.

5   Diethrich EB. Guest Editor of the issue on endovascular surgery. *Int Angiol* 1993; **12**: 195–290.

6 Diethrich EB. Endovascular intervention suite design. In: White RA, Fogarty JT, eds. *Peripheral Endovascular Interventions*. St Louis: Mosby-Year Book, 1996: 133–142.

7 White RA, Fogarty TJ. *Peripheral Endovascular Interventions*. St Louis: Mosby-Year Book, 1996.

8 Henry M, Amor M. Stenting of femoral and popliteal arteries. In: Henry M, Amor M, Diethrich EB, Katzen BT, eds. *Endovascular Therapy Course Coronary and Peripheral. Proceedings of Eighth International Course of Peripheral Vascular Intervention*. Europa Organization, Paris: 1997.

9 Cleveland TJ, Gaines PA, Cumberland DC. Limb salvage: indications, techniques, results. In: Henry M, Amor M, Diethrich EB, Katzen BT, eds. *Endovascular Therapy Course Coronary and Peripheral. Proceedings of Eighth International Course of Peripheral Vascular Intervention*. Europa Organization, Paris: 1997.

10 Criado FJ. Endovascular surgery: back to basics. *Int Angiol* 1997; **16**: 81–2.

11 Bolia A, Sayers RD, Thompson MM, Bell PRF. Subintimal and intraluminal angioplasty recanalization of occluded crural arteries by percutaneous balloon angioplasty. *Eur J Vasc Surg* 1994; **8**: 214–19.

12 Bolia A, Bell PR. Femoro-popliteal and crural artery recanalization using subintimal angioplasty. *Semin Vasc Surg* 1995; **8**: 253–64.

13 Bray A. Superficial femoral endarterectomy with intra-arterial PTFE grafting. *J Endovasc Surg* 1995; **2**: 297–301.

14 Marc van Sambeek RHM, Hagenaars T, Gussenhoven EJ et al. Vascular response in the femoropopliteal segment after implantation of an ePTFE balloon-expandable endovascular graft: an intravascular ultrasound study. *J Endovasc Surg* 2000; **7**: 204–12.

15 Teijink JAW, Ho GH, Heijmen RH, Moll FL. Remote endarterectomy with the Mollring Cutter. The Enduring endolining experience. *EndoCardiovascular Multimedia Magazine* 2000; **4**: 131–6.

19

Percutaneous peripheral atherectomy

Manuel Maynar and Zhong Qian

Percutaneous atherectomy is a technique designed to mechanically debulk intraluminal atheroma and create a smooth luminal surface in atherosclerotic arteries using a catheter-based device. Theoretically, atherectomy appears to be attractive because it actually removes obstructing atheromatous material rather than merely stretches, cracks, or displaces it, as opposed to balloon angioplasty. However, atherectomy has never been a treatment of choice in the management of the peripheral vascular diseases, because the long-term efficacy remains questionable. Currently, percutaneous atherectomy is primarily used as a complementary technique to other therapies, such as balloon angioplasty, stent placement, and fibrinolysis.

The atherectomy can be classified into two categories. Extirpative atherectomy is characterized by cutting or shaving atheromatous material and instantaneously removing the excised debris from the vessel lumen with a collecting system. The commonly used extirpative devices are Simpson AtheroCath and Transluminal Extraction Catheter. Ablative atherectomy, on the contrary, is characterized by pulverizing, evaporating or grinding atheroma with a high-speed rotational device. With ablative atherectomy, atheromatous material is instantaneously fragmented into small particles that either embolize distally or are cleared by the reticuloendothelial system. Ablative devices include the Auth Rotablator and the

Trac-Wright Catheter. Since the 1990s, various atherectomy devices have been used clinically and experimentally; this chapter focuses on a number of the commonly used devices that have been approved by the US Food and Drug Administration and on their clinical applications. For the scientific perspective, several investigative devices are also described.

AtheroCath directional atherectomy catheter

The AtheroCath catheter, also known as the Simpson catheter, developed in 1985 (Devices for Vascular Intervention, Redwood City, CA, USA),[1] was available in two types: AtheroCath (a fixed-wire device) and AtheroTrac (an over-the-wire catheter). After having undergone multiple refinements and modifications during the past decade, the AtheroCath continues to be manufactured by Guidant (Menlo Park, CA, USA) and is available in four versions: AtheroCath GTO, AtheroCath-Bantam, AtheroCath Sca-Ex, and Sca-Ex/Shortcutter (Figure 19.1a–d). The fifth version, the so-called Flexi-Cut catheter, was developed in 2000, with a lower profile, lower friction, less stiffness, and higher cutter efficiency (Figure 19.1e). The features of each version are

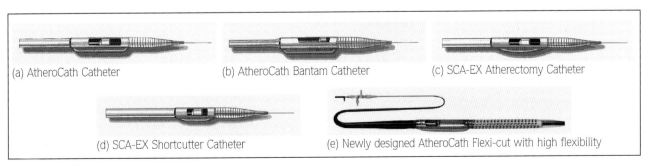

(a) AtheroCath Catheter (b) AtheroCath Bantam Catheter (c) SCA-EX Atherectomy Catheter

(d) SCA-EX Shortcutter Catheter (e) Newly designed AtheroCath Flexi-cut with high flexibility

Figure 19.1
Currently available five versions of the AtheroCath.

Table 19.1 AtheroCath summary

Features	SCA-EX	GTO	Bantam	Flexi-Cut
Guiding catheter	10F	10F	9F	8F
Device sizing	Housing dependent	Housing dependent	Housing dependent	Housing dependent
Housing size	5–7F	5–7F	5–7F	6F (with three balloon sizes)
Cutter window length	5mm and 9mm	9mm	9mm	9mm
Cutter window arc	117°	117°	117°	127°
Cutter material	Stainless steel	Stainless steel	Stainless steel	Titanium nitride-coated stainless steel
Nosecone shape	Conical	Conical	Conical	Cylindrical with dam
Torque response	1.5:1	1:1	1.5:1	1:1
Working length	125cm	125cm	125cm	134cm
Shelf-life	6 months	6 months	2 years	2 years

summarized in Table 19.1. The basic design of the device consists of a cylindrical metal housing attached to the end of the shaft (Figure 19.2). The housing has a 5-mm to 20-mm window with an opposing balloon. Atherectomy is achieved by pushing this open window against the atherosclerotic plaque with an eccentrically placed balloon. The trapped plaque is then excised and pushed by a high-speed rotating cutter into the distal collecting chamber. This mechanism permits restoration of the vessel lumen to a diameter larger than the catheter's size due to its expansion ratio.

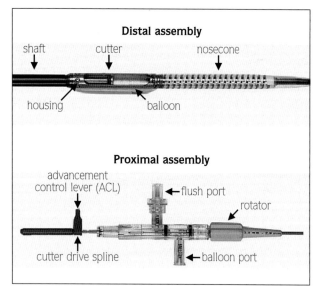

Figure 19.2
Close-up views of the distal and proximal parts of the AtheroCath.

Indications and contraindications

Peripheral applications of the AtheroCath have been focused on the iliac, superficial femoral and popliteal stenotic lesions, which have one of these features:[2–8]

1. Discrete stenosis with intermittent claudication for at least a 3-month period
2. Short (less than 5 cm), focal and eccentric atheroma
3. Focal intimal hyperplasia and ulcerative plaque
4. Lesions associated with 'blue toe syndrome'
5. Excision of tissue or biopsy for histologic study
6. Intimal flap
7. Debulk total occlusion
8. Bypass graft stenosis, anastomotic stenosis, intrastent stenosis associated with fibrointimal hyperplasia

In addition, the use of this device can be extended to the management of hemodialysis failure in selected cases and of retained valve leaflets on in situ bypass graft. Contraindications for the use of the AtheroCath include acute angle of entry into the artery, acute ischemia, trash foot syndrome, morbid obesity, heavily calcified lesions, and those applied to angioplasty of the lower extremities. In order to avoid vascular perforation, care should be taken if a stenosis is close to a side-branch or near a vessel bifurcation, or if the vessel is tortuous.

Procedure

Because of its design, the AtheroCath must be introduced through a check-flow sheath using an ipsilateral approach. The puncture should be performed as horizontally as possible to avoid kinking of the sheath, which would make passage of the device difficult. A retrograde approach should be used in the case of the iliac and renal arteries, and an antegrade access is usually adopted if the femoral, popliteal and tibioperoneal arteries are attempted. In the case of dialysis fistula, the approach may be made either on the cephalic vein or directly on the prosthetic graft. After access is established, the patient is systematically given 8000–10 000 IU of heparin. Vasodilators may be used, particularly during atherectomy of the popliteal or tibioperoneal arteries. A digital subtraction angiogram should be obtained in at least two planes to localize the lesion and to study its morphologic characteristics. Real-time fluoroscopic road-mapping guidance can facilitate precise position of the resection window. The use of intravascular ultrasound (IVUS) before, during and after atherectomy allows a more precise evaluation of post-treatment results. With careful manipulation of the steerable leading wire, the device is advanced using road mapping to cross the lesion. Once the window has been positioned against the atheromatous plaque, the balloon is inflated to 30 lb/in^2, forcing the plaque into the window. The rotating cutter blade, driven by a hand-held battery-powered motor, is activated and slowly advanced to shave the atheromatous plaque protruding into the window. While the cutter blade is held down, the motor is stopped and the atheromatous material is stored in the distal collecting compartment. After each cut, the balloon is deflated and the system can be rotated by 30–60° to reposition the window for removal of additional atheroma. The procedure can be repeated until the circumferential atheroma is completely excised. The endpoint of the procedure should leave less than 20% residual stenosis. When the balloon is deflated or the catheter is withdrawn, the cutter blade should always be held against the distal end of the metal housing to prevent escape of resected atheromatous materials, which would cause distal embolization.

Technical considerations

1. It is very important to select the proper size of device to ensure optimization of extraction of atheromatous materials. The best match is one in which the working diameter (of the metal housing plus the inflated positioning balloon) is at least equal to the diameter of the normal arterial segment adjacent to the stenotic lesion.

2. An appropriate-length sheath should be introduced as close to parallel as possible into the common femoral artery in order to facilitate the AtheroCath introduction.

3. Excessive residual stenosis may be associated with the high risk of restenosis. Residual stenosis should not exceed 20%. Multiple passes of the atherectomy catheter are frequently necessary to achieve maximum removal of atheromatous plaque.

4. In case of stenotic bypass graft associated with thrombosis, thrombolytic therapy should be initiated before the atherectomy procedure.

5. Whenever the AtheroCath is being advanced, rotated or withdrawn, the cutter should be fully extended into the housing to avoid embolization of tissue and the balloon must be deflated.

6. To eliminate postprocedural hematomas at the entry site due in part to the larger vascular sheath, the effects of heparin may be reversed with protamine, and the sheath is removed when the activated clotting time is less than 160 s. In order to reduce time to hemostasis at the puncture site and reduce time to ambulation in the patients, several hemostatic closure devices have been used, including Angio-seal (St Jude Medical, St Paul, MN, USA), Vaso-seal (Datascope, Montvale, NJ, USA), and Perclose (Perclose, Inc. Redwood City, CA, USA).

Complications and limitations

Complications associated with the AtheroCath are relatively few (5–21%),[9–12] minor and manageable, including entry-site hematomas, distal embolization, thrombosis at treated site, and pseudoaneurysm. Its main drawback is prolonged procedure time. It is not suitable for atherectomy in long or diffuse lesions or in the tortuous arteries.

Clinical results

The first report on peripheral application with the AtheroCath was published in 1988.[9] Since then, the AtheroCath catheter has seldom been utilized in the larger vessels (i.e. the common iliac artery), because the working diameter of the device plus the inflated balloon is usually smaller than these vessels' calibers. Most of the peripheral applications with directional atherectomy were reported in the external iliac artery or below. Technical success has been reported in all experienced hands.[13–17] However, a wide discrepancy of the mid- or long-term patencies has been observed based on the published literature. Maynar et al claimed 87% patency after 18 months,[18] which is echoed by other investigators. Maquin et al and Kim et al reported 86% and 94% patency rates at 12 months respectively.[17,19] On the other hand, Dorros and colleagues observed only 45% patency at 6 months following the atherectomy. Katzen et al also found extremely disappointing results of 2-year follow-up. In their series, there was a 63% recurrence rate when patients were studied at 24 months.[13] Although some studies indicate that deep vessel wall excision may aggravate occurrence of restenosis,[20–22] other investigators have not found a correlation between restenosis and medial layer retrieval.[23,24] Kuntz et al observed a reverse relationship, where there is a lower recurrence rate with deep vessel layer excision.[25] It seems to be difficult to explain why the discrepancy is so wide, since there have been relatively few scientific publications addressing this issue in depth.

The role of directional atherectomy with AtheroCath in the management of peripheral vascular disease, especially in comparison with well-established techniques (i.e. balloon angioplasty), has been sought since the advent of this technique. It was not clear until 1996, when Tielbeek and co-workers published a prospective randomized study to carefully compare directional atherectomy with AtheroCath to balloon angioplasty in the femoropopliteal artery.[26] In their study, the primary angiographic patency and secondary patency rates seemed to be higher with balloon angioplasty (67% and 80%) than with directional atherectomy (44% and 65%) at 2 years of follow-up. However, the differences showed a lack of statistical significance. At the present time, directional atherectomy has not yet proven to be superior to balloon angioplasty in terms of long-term patency rate. Given the higher cost of peripheral atherectomy and longer procedure time compared to conventional balloon angioplasty, the AtheroCath should not replace balloon angioplasty for the management of short peripheral stenotic lesions.

Rotablator rotational atherectomy system

The Rotablator (Boston Scientific Corporation, Natick, MA, USA) also known as the Auth rotational atherectomy device, was first introduced in 1987[27] and has been approved for peripheral and coronary applications by the US Food and Drug Administration. The device consists of an oval-shaped abrasive burr rotated at high speed over a wire (Figure 19.3). The diamond chips (20–30 μm) are embedded on the surface of the front half of the burr and create millions of microscopic divots at high speed, offering the potential for restoring patency of occluded vessels by boring out the atheromatous lesion and creating a polished intraluminal surface with no intimal flaps. The burr, ranging from 1.25 to 6 mm in diameter, is attached to a flexible helical shaft driven by an air turbine at up to 190 000 rev/min. The rotational shaft is sheathed within a 4F Teflon catheter; thus, the only rotating part that is exposed to the vessel wall is the anterior aspect of the abrasive tip. Rotational speed is controlled by compressed air pressure, which is regulated by dial on the control panel. The turbine also pumps sterile saline into the plastic sheath to lubricate and cool the system. A 0.009-inch guidewire with a platinum tip helps to maintain the intraluminal position of the burr during the procedure. The guidewire is lodged in the central hollow channel of the catheter and fixed in a stationary position during rotation of the drive shaft and remains in position following withdrawal of the device. Recently, the device has been further refined. The system allows multiple catheters with various burr sizes to be easily connected and disconnected from a single advancer, making the exchange of incremental burrs during a procedure easy (Figure 19.4).

The mechanism of atheromatous ablation with the device is based on the principles of differential cutting and orthogonal displacement of friction. Differential cutting preferentially removes inelastic materials such as fibrous, calcified and fatty atheromatous tissue, while sparing healthy elastic tissue. Orthogonal displacement of friction generated by the burr permits easy advancement of the device through a tortuous vessel without damage to normal intima and media. In addition, the Rotablator neither stretches the arterial wall nor displaces atheromatous plaque. Barotrauma associated with balloon inflation is thereby eliminated. One of the most appealing features of this device is exceptional smoothness in the recanalized lumen. The design of the device specifically addresses the pathology of the organized and calcified lesions. As with most other atherectomy devices, there is no expansion ratio, so that satisfactory removal of atheromatous material usually requires the use of burrs in sequential fashion (Figure 19.5). One legitimate concern regarding the use of an abrasive mechanism is the resultant particles as a potential source of distal embolization. However, most investigators have found the vast majority of these particles to be in the 2–10-μm range,[28–30] which is small enough to pass through the capillary bed and be captured by the reticuloendothelial system.

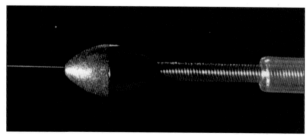

Figure 19.3
Close-up enlargement of the Rotablator burr as it tracks over its 0.009-inch guidewire. Hundreds of microscopic diamond chips are embedded in the burr. When the burr rotates, each chip scoops out a microscopic amount of plaque.

Indications and contraindications

In general, patient selection criteria for the use of this device are similar to the inclusion criteria for percutaneous transluminal angioplasty (PTA). Candidates should have symptomatic peripheral vascular disease; gangrene, non-healing ulcers, rest

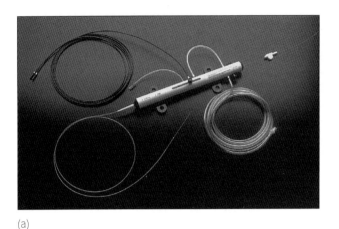

(a)

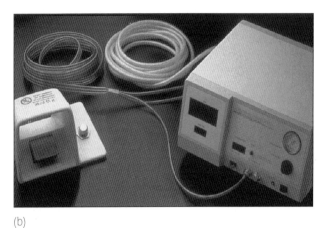

(b)

Figure 19.4

The Rotablator system showing the burr advancer unit, guidewire, sheath and burr (a), a small console to control and monitor the burr revolutions/min, and an air source (b).

pain, and severe claudication. Use of the Rotablator is particularly indicated in the following situations:

1. Heavily calcified or organized atheroma resistant to balloon angioplasty, especially in diabetic patients with claudication or limb-threatening ischemia
2. Long and diffuse stenosis or occlusion of the superficial femoral, popliteal or tibial arteries
3. Eccentric atheromatous lesions, preferentially ablated by the device
4. Occlusive lesion amenable treatment only if it is traversed with a central guidewire

Atherectomy with the Rotablator should not be performed when a dissection is evident on an angiogram. It would make the dissection worse and result in abrupt closure and vessel perforation.

Procedure

After diagnostic angiography, the Rotablator is introduced through a guiding catheter, which usually has a diameter 0.004 inch larger than the burr. Once the guiding catheter is

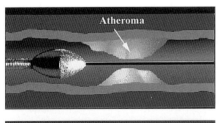
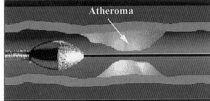

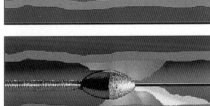
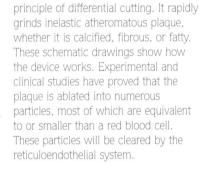

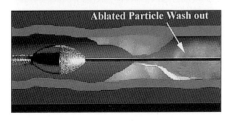
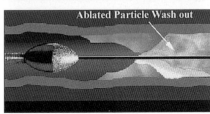

Figure 19.5

The Rotablator functions on the principle of differential cutting. It rapidly grinds inelastic atheromatous plaque, whether it is calcified, fibrous, or fatty. These schematic drawings show how the device works. Experimental and clinical studies have proved that the plaque is ablated into numerous particles, most of which are equivalent to or smaller than a red blood cell. These particles will be cleared by the reticuloendothelial system.

seated just proximal to the lesion, a 0.035-inch central guidewire is inserted across the lesions into the distal segment. The guidewire should not be forced, but turned gently in multiple directions in order to seek the residual lumen. If the lumen cannot be found, a combination of guidewire manipulation and thrombolytic therapy is often sufficient to allow passage of the guidewire across the occlusion. Once the guidewire has crossed the lesion, a 5F straight catheter with an end-hole is advanced distally over the wire approximately 5–10 cm below the inferior aspect of the lesion. With the guiding catheter positioned proximal to the occlusion and the 5F catheter traversing the lesion, the access guidewire is exchanged for the 0.009-inch stiff exchange guidewire that accompanied the Rotablator device. While the change wire is positioned across the lesion, the 5F catheter is removed and the Rotablator is then advanced over the wire that also stabilizes the device during the procedure. Atherectomy is accomplished under fluoroscopic guidance by slowly advancing the device through the lesion while the burr is activated by depressing a foot pedal switch. The optimal burr spinning speed is 160 000–190 000 rev/min to ensure a smooth intraluminal surface. The activated device should be advanced slowly, but evenly, over the wire in a to-and-fro fashion. Audio feedback as the device passes through the lesion is helpful. Calcified lesions produce a high-pitched tone as the device ablates the lesions. Softer organized thrombus gives a lower-pitched tone. When calcified material is encountered, the device should be used in pulsed fashion. Constant normal saline drip irrigation accompanies application. After the initial successful passage of the first burr, the diameter of the abrasive tip can be increased until the stenosis or occlusion is reduced to less than 25% of the normal luminal diameter of the native vessel. In order to minimize early thrombosis, heparinization should be maintained with partial thrombin time (PTT) between 50 and 90 s following the procedure for 24–48 h. Aspirin should be given before and after the procedure.

Technical considerations

1. A gradual increase in burr size is necessary for treatment of long (more than 10 mm) or diffuse lesions to avoid massive ablated particle burden.
2. If the speed of the burr is suddenly decreased or resistance is encountered during atherectomy, the burr should be slightly withdrawn and readvanced.
3. Adjunctive balloon angioplasty may be performed to improved luminal gains if the residual (more than 50%) stenosis remains after atherectomy.
4. In case of total occlusive lesion, infusion of thrombolytic agent can be performed in combination with guidewire manipulation to allow passage of the central guidewire across the occlusion.

5. During atherectomy, excessive pushing force should be avoided to prevent vessel perforation resulting from alteration of burr slope, especially in severe tortuous vessels. The activated Rotablator must be advanced gently but evenly in a to-and-fro fashion.
6. Intermittent injection of contrast medium during atherectomy facilitates identification of the margins of the lesion and burr-working status.

Complications and limitations

Complications have been noted when the Rotablator is used, including early thrombosis,[31] arterial spasm[32,33] and distal embolism,[31,34] as well as hemoglobinuria and hemoglobinemia,[31,32,34] which are apparently caused by hemolysis resulting from the high-speed rotation of the burr. The degree of hemolysis is believed to be associated with the activation time of the device and the size of the burr used for atherectomy. Limiting the activation time and selecting reasonable, smaller burr sizes have been recommended to minimize hemolysis caused by the high-speed Rotablator.[35] A large particle burden downstream may constitute a potential problem of distal embolization, although most of the particles are microscopic and clinically insignificant. In order to minimize the risk of distal embolism, retrograde passage of the device has been proposed for patients with vascular lesions above the knee.[31] The particulate matter can then be flushed out from the treated arterial segment before the flow is restored. This method is not applicable for the management of occlusive lesions below the popliteal artery. Vessel perforation has also been reported and may be related to rapid advancement of the device.[31,32] A slow advancement of the device is recommended. The main limitation of the Rotablator is that it is unable to bore through organized thrombus or rubbery atherosclerotic intima.[35]

Clinical results

Despite encouraging initial technical (89–95%) and clinical (72–92%) success reported by several authors from multi-institutional investigations,[31–34,36,37] a poor mid- or long-term outcome of primary patency has limited its wide application.[31] The results from a multicenter study including 72 patients showed that the cumulating primary patency was 47% at 6 months, 31% at 12 months, and 18.6% at 24 months; the secondary patency rates were 83% at 1 month, 60% at 6 months, 45% at 12 months, and 30% at 24 months.[31]

The Rotablator is presently not the choice for the treatment of peripheral arterial occlusive lesions, because of its relatively high complications and disappointing long-term outcome. The use of this device is only reserved for some very selective cases, such as highly calcified lesions resistant to balloon angioplasty or in the case of other interventional techniques failing to demonstrate a dramatic improvement of local flow.

Transluminal extraction catheter

The transluminal extraction catheter (TEC, Interventional Technologies, Inc., San Diego, CA, USA), developed in the late 1980s, is a forward-cutting atherectomy device. The system is somewhat complicated in design compared to other devices. It includes a semiflexible and torque-controlled catheter, a low-speed (750 rev/min) rotational cutting unit mounted on the distal tip of the catheter, an attached 30-ml vacuum bottle, a specialized guidewire, and a battery-powered drive unit (Figure 19.6). The device is mounted over a compatible 0.014-inch ball-tipped steerable wire with a 0.020-inch ball on the tip (Figure 19.7), which must be passed through the lesion before the cutting head can be advanced. The two triangular cutter blades (Figure 19.8) on the cone-shaped tip of a hollow catheter driven by a battery-powered motor shave off the surface of the atheromatous plaque, while the excised materials are continuously aspirated by the vacuum effect, thereby reducing the risk of distal embolization. Unlike with the Simpson catheter, a larger amount of atheromatous materials can be immediately removed from the system. However, the TEC provides no expansion ratio and therefore must be employed on a one-to-one basis. Peripheral TEC catheters are available in several sizes: 5–10, 12 and 14F, with a cutter diameter ranging from 2.0 to 4.7 mm (Figure 19.9). The working length of the catheter is 113 cm.

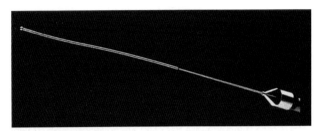

Figure 19.7
The unique TEC guidewire combines optimal flexibility and steerability. Note that there is a 0.020-inch ball on the tip of the wire.

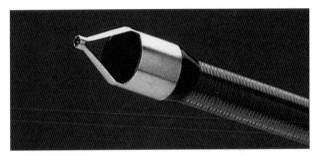

Figure 19.8
Microtome-sharp TEC blades cut plaque circumferentially. Slow and controlled rotational speed allows clean cuts and eliminates damaging frictional heat caused by high-speed devices.

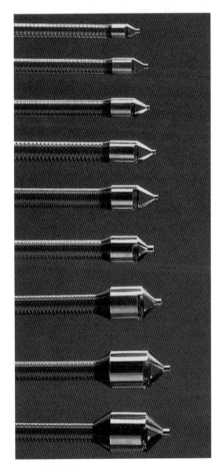

Figure 19.9
TEC catheters are available in a wide range of sizes.

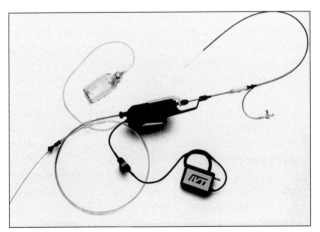

Figure 19.6
Components of the TEC peripheral atherectomy device.

Indications and contraindications

The TEC was designed for use in atherosclerotic stenosis or occlusions of arteries or grafts.[38–40] Insights from percutaneous hagioscope and IVUs prove that the TEC is also able to remove intraluminal thrombus.[41] There is no restriction on the number, length or severity of lesions, as long as the 0.014-inch leading guidewire can be advanced across the lesion. However, the optimal outcomes are usually obtained in patients with short or asymmetric atherosclerotic stenoses.[42] In total occlusions or long stenotic lesions, atherectomy with the TEC system can be performed as an adjunctive technique before balloon angioplasty to achieve maximum lumen gain.[39,43] The device can also be used for restoring patency of failing hemodialysis access and for thrombectomy.[41]

The use of the TEC is contraindicated whenever the guidewire cannot be positioned across the obstruction. The outside diameter of the selected TEC system should never exceed the intraluminal diameter of the native vessel or graft immediately proximal or distal to the lesion(s).

Procedure

The TEC catheter is introduced over a 0.014-inch ball-tipped guidewire into the target vessel through an introducer sheath. One should avoid sharp angulation or kinking of the sheath to facilitate passage of the device. Patients should be heparinized with an intravenous injection of 5000 IU heparin. Intravascular injection of 100–200 μg nitroglycerin is recommended if the lesion is below the knee. The guidewire must be advanced to be beyond the leading part of the lesion. The cutting head then follows the wire to the segment proximal to the trailing part of the lesion. The device is slowly advanced while activated by the motorized drive unit. The flow into the vacuum bottle should be monitored continuously. The vacuum bottle is immediately changed when it is full. The post-atherectomy site is evaluated by removing the TEC device while holding the guidewire in position and injecting contrast medium through the sheath. If a large lumen is desirable, the device is replaced with one of larger diameter and the procedure is repeated. Adjunctive balloon angioplasty is usually required to achieve symptomatic relief for patients with femoropopliteal lesions.

Technical considerations

1. Because the catheter creates a channel with a diameter equal to that of itself, the catheter should never be chosen with any diameter larger than the intraluminal diameter of the native vessel or graft immediately proximal or distal to the lesion(s).
2. Although there is no absolute restriction on the number, length or severity of the lesions, the treated vessel(s) must be crossed by the 0.014-inch leading guidewire.
3. In severe stenosis, atherectomy should start with a smaller-size cutter, and then the cutter should be upsized.
4. Activation time of the TEC should be strictly limited to the duration of passage through the targeted lesion, in order to minimize extra blood loss.

Complications and limitations

The rate of procedure-related complications is relatively low in experienced hands. Most of these complications manifest as puncture-site hematoma, thrombosis at the treated vessel, dissection and intimal flaps, which can be managed by percutaneous techniques, such as thrombectomy and stent placement. Restenosis and reocclusion remain major constraints on TEC atherectomy. Heavily calcified lesions do not respond well to TEC atherectomy.

Clinical results

Initial clinical experience with the TEC device was mostly reported from a single institute.[39,40,44,45] The higher technical success rates (88–100%) and immediate clinical improvement (90–96%) generated the early universal enthusiasm for physical removal of atheromatous material. More recently, 83.8% of cumulative clinical patency and 79.1% of angiographic patency were reported at 6-month follow-up.[44] However, long-term results and prospective studies are not available to determine its role in the management of peripheral atherosclerotic lesions. Evidently, there has been an increase in the use of adjunctive techniques, such as balloon angioplasty and directional atherectomy, to achieve the optimal lumen gain. Clinical data showed that 30–50% residual stenosis remained in 54% of cases following atherectomy with the TEC, and required additional balloon angioplasty.[44] Therefore, it is difficult to determine the true value of the TEC in the management of occlusive arterial lesions. Recent experience with the TEC has revealed that intravascular lumen created by the device is often not as optimal as initially expected. In a randomized trial comparing the TEC and the TEC plus balloon angioplasty with balloon angioplasty alone, no significant difference was found on the cross-sectional area of atheroma, monitored by IVUS imaging, among the three groups. The authors concluded that the luminal gain after the procedure primarily resulted from balloon dilation.[45]

Trac-Wright catheter

The Trac-Wright catheter (Dow Corning, Miami Lakes, FL, USA), also known as the Kensey catheter, was developed in 1987. Manufacture of this device has been discontinued. However, the concept of the Trac-Wright catheter is still being utilized in the development of newly emerging devices (e.g. the Aegis Vortex System), which will be described in the next section. It is worthwhile mentioning it here for historical reasons only. The device consists of a flexible polyurethane catheter and a blunt spinning cam driven by a power unit at speeds of up to 100 000 rev/min (Figure 19.10). It was designed to ablate atheromatous tissues into microparticles by a powerful fluid vortex generated by the high-speed spinning cam. Three theoretical features seem to make the device attractive: (1) the activated catheter tends to travel the path of least resistance due to fluid jets and vibration; (2) the device is able to selectively micropulverize fibrous or atheromatous material without damage to viscoelastic tissue such as the vessel wall; and (3) powerful micropulverization by a combination of mechanical and hydrodynamic effects minimizes the risk of distal embolization. A high-pressure fluid-irrigating system is used to dilute particulate density in the distal circulation, to cool and lubricate the device, to allow the addition of medications locally, and to monitor atherectomy status by injection of contrast medium. The Trac-Wright catheter can only be advanced to the target vessel through a guiding catheter, because it does not have a central channel for a wire passage. The sizes of the devices range from 5F to 10F.

Procedure

After ipsilateral femoral arterial access is established either in antegrade or in retrograde fashion, depending on the level of

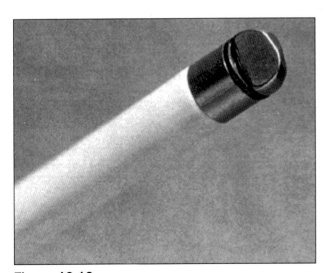

Figure 19.10
Close-up view of the rotating cam of the Trac-Wright catheter.

the lesion, the Trac-Wright catheter is introduced through the sheath. Irrigating solution can be constituted of normal saline, non-ionic contrast medium and urokinase, delivered with a flow rate of 20–30 ml/min at 100 lb/in². The initial rotation speed of the device should be maintained at about 20 000 rev/min until the lesion is in direct contact with the tip. The speed is then increased to the regular operational level (60 000–90 000 rev/min), while the catheter is slowly advanced at 1 mm/s to give the spinning cam sufficient time to pulverize the atherosclerotic plaque. It is recommended that the catheter should pass through the proximal segment of the occluded artery several times before the leading end of the occlusion is reached. Following complete penetration of the occlusion, the spinning speed should slow down to 20 000 rev/min, and the catheter is slowly removed. Since the Trac-Wright catheter offers no expansion ratio, adjunctive balloon dilation is almost always needed to achieve adequate luminal gain. If the device does not penetrate the leading end of the occlusion, recanalization may be further accomplished by a combination of steerable guidewire manipulation and balloon angioplasty.

Complications and limitations

Complications are frequently seen following application of the device. The initial conceptual advantages of the Trac-Wright catheter have not yet been corroborated by clinical observations. Overall complications range from 15% to 37%, including vessel perforation, dissections and distal embolization.[45–47] Because of its size limitation, the Trac-Wright catheter has been restricted to use as a mechanical adjunct to balloon angioplasty for long occlusion or thrombolytic therapy.[48] Because of its higher complication rates and lower patency rates, it is not surprising that the Trac-Wright catheter is no longer marketed.

Emerging technologies

A couple of new designs have undergone preclinical studies and are currently under clinical investigation. Although their scientific value is still unknown, their potential 'niche' in the treatment of arterial occlusive lesions is worth our attention.

Redha-Cut atherectomy catheter system

The first clinical results with the Redha-Cut catheter (Sherine Med AG Utzenstorf, Switzerland) were published in 1994.[49]

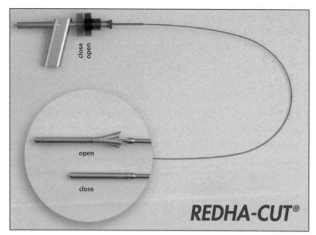

Figure 19.11
Redha-Cut® atherectomy catheter system. Note the positions of the handle controlling the cutting blades' functional status

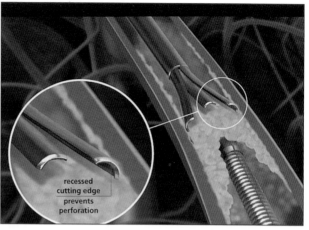

Figure 19.12
The recessed cutting edge minimizes the risk of vascular perforation during atherectomy.

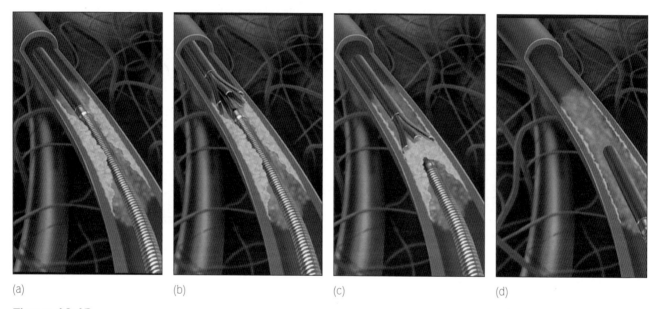

(a)   (b)   (c)   (d)

Figure 19.13
The mechanism of atherectomy with the Redha-Cut catheter system. (a) The tip of the Redha-Cut catheter is traversed through a stenotic lesion. (b) While the cutting blade portion of the catheter is positioned distal to the leading end of the lesion, the blades are opened by pushing the blade controller. (c) Atherectomy is achieved by pulling the catheter with the opened blades to excise atheroma by one blade length only. The blades are then closed and the catheter is withdrawn. (d) Repeated procedures are usually required to obtain satisfactory results.

The device is constructed with an 8F flexible stainless steel catheter and a hollow blunt-tipped cylinder on the tip of the catheter. There are two cutting blades in the cylinder, which can be opened and closed like an umbrella by sliding the cylinder in a back-and-forth motion (Figure 19.11). The cutting blade edges are slightly recessed to avoid the risk of vascular perforation (Figure 19.12). The device is an over-the-wire system and can be advanced across the lesion either over a 0.012-inch guidewire or through a guiding catheter. Atherectomy is achieved by pulling back the opened cutting blades to trap atheromatous plaque, closing the blades to retain it within the cylinder, and withdrawing the catheter to bring it out (Figure 19.13). The procedure usually needs to be repeated several times until satisfactory results are obtained.

Preliminary clinical experience with the Redha-Cut device has mostly been gathered from a single group in Switzerland.[49–51] A high technical success rate (100%) was reported in a series of 93 symptomatic femoropopliteal lesions treated with the Redha-Cut.[51] The intra-arterial luminal stenosis was significantly reduced from a pre-procedural

$74 \pm 2.3\%$ to a post-procedural $26 \pm 2.0\%$ (Figure 19.14). There was neither vessel perforation nor early thrombosis in this series. Minor complications were noted in four patients, including distal embolism ($n = 4$) and pseudoaneurysm at the entry site ($n = 2$), which were successfully treated with aspiration embolectomy and ultrasound-guided compression, respectively. The mid-term results were impressively higher: 6-month cumulative patency rates were 97% in primary lesions and 62% in recurrent lesions; and 12-month cumulative patency rates were 81% in primary lesions and 41% in recurrent lesions.[51] Its long-term benefit should be further examined before the Redha-Cut can be clinically accepted.

TriActiv™ Balloon Protected Vortex Extraction System

The TriActiv™ Balloon Protected Vortex Extraction (Kensey Nash Corporation, Exton, PA, USA) is a newly developed device for treatment of cardiovascular disease with distal protection. The system consists of a coaxial assembly including a 5F vortex catheter with a high-speed blunt spinning cam (150 000 rev/min), a specialized guidewire with a protection balloon (Figure 19.15) isolating the treated segment of the vessel, and a pump-extraction unit (Figure 19.16) providing

constant aspiration of the debris from the treated vessel. Once the system is advanced proximal to the trailing end of the lesion, the guidewire with the low-profile balloon is carefully traversed across the lesion. The balloon is then inflated to block the leading end of the target vessel to avoid distal embolism during the vortex treatment. The vortex catheter is advanced and activated through the target vessel with a gentle back-and-forth motion to remove thrombotic and atheromatous material. During vortex treatment, fluid is pumped into the isolated segment through the coaxial system. Injected fluid and macerated debris are continually removed from the isolated segment by a peristaltic vacuum action in the system. As soon as acceptable results are confirmed by angiograms,

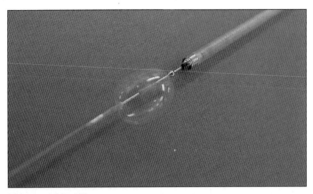

Figure 19.15
Close-up view of the distal protection guidewire balloon.

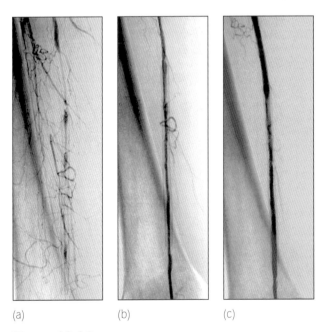

(a)   (b)   (c)

Figure 19.14
A patient with severe claudication and multiple previous interventions. (a) An angiogram shows a severe stenosis proximal to a Wallstent in the distal femoral artery and a moderate stenosis within the stent. (b) Atherectomy with an 8F Redha-Cut catheter is performed to debulk the atheromatous plaque without additional balloon angioplasty. (c) After two cutting cycles, a satisfactory result is obtained.

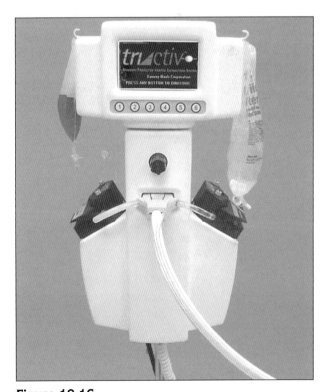

Figure 19.16
The pump-extraction unit.

the balloon is deflated and the system is withdrawn. Adjunct therapy, such as percutaneous transluminal coronary angioplasty, or stenting, can then be performed, also under the protection of the distal balloon. A flush catheter is provided to remove any remaining debris from the vessel before the balloon is finally deflated and removed.

At the present time, TriActiv is primarily used in vein bypass grafts. A clinical trial is underway to determine its safety and efficacy in vascular occlusive lesions. A peripheral version is under development (Figure 19.17).

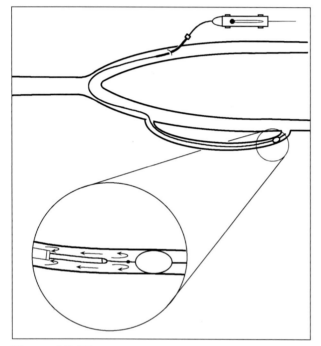

Figure 19.17
Schematic drawing of the mechanism of atherectomy with the TriActiv™ peripheral system.

References

1   Simpson JB, Johnson DE, Thapliyal HV et al. Transluminal atherectomy: a new approach to the treatment of atherosclerotic vascular disease. *Circulation* 1985; **72**(suppl II): II–146.

2   Castaneda F, Moradian G, Hunter DW et al. Percutaneous intravascular biopsy using a Simpson atherectomy catheter: technique note. *Cardiovasc Interv Radiol* 1990; **12**: 342–3.

3   Dolmatch BL, Rholl KS, Moskowitz LB et al. Blue toe syndrome: treatment with percutaneous atherectomy. *Radiology* 1989; **172**: 799–804.

4   Dorros G, Lewin RF, Sachdev N et al. Percutaneous atherectomy of occlusive peripheral vascular disease: stenosis and/or occlusions. *Cathet Cardiovasc Diagn* 1989; **18**: 1–6.

5   Gray RJ, Dolmatch BL, Buick MK. Directional atherectomy treatment for hemodialysis access: early results. *J Vasc Interv Radiol* 1992; **3**: 497–503.

6   Maynar M, Reyes R, Cabrera V et al. Percutaneous atherectomy as an alternative treatment for postangioplasty obstructive intimal flaps. *Radiology* 1989; **170**: 1029–31.

7   Vorwerk D, Guenther RW. Removal of intimal hyperplasia in vascular endoprostheses by atherectomy and balloon dilatation. *Am J Radiol* 1990; **154**: 617–19.

8   Zemel G, Katzen BT, Dake MD et al. Directional atherectomy in the treatment of stenotic dialysis access fistula. *J Vasc Interv Radiol* 1990; **1**: 35–8.

9   Simpson JB, Selmon MR, Robertson GC et al. Transluminal atherectomy for occlusive peripheral vascular disease. *Am J Cardiol* 1988; **61**: 96G–101G.

10 Hinohara T, Selmon MR, Robertson GC et al. Directional atherectomy: new approaches for treatment of obstructive coronary and peripheral vascular disease. *Circulation* 1990; **81**(suppl IV): 79–91.

11 Wildenhaim PM, Wholey MH, Jarmolowski CR, Hill KL. Long-term follow-up and comparison with percutaneous transluminal angioplasty. *Cardiovasc Interv Radiol* 1994; **17**: 305–11.

12 Savader SJ, Venbrux AC, Mitchell SE et al. Percutaneous transluminal atherectomy of the superficial femoral and popliteal arteries: long-term results in 48 patients. *Cardiovasc Interv Radiol* 1994; **17**: 312–18.

13 Katzen BT, Becker GJ, Benenati JF et al. Long-term follow-up of directional atherectomy in the femoral and popliteal arteries. *J Vasc Interv Radiol* 1992; **3**: 38–9 (abst).

14 von Pölnitz A, Nerlich A, Berger H et al. Percutaneous peripheral atherectomy: angiographic and clinical follow-up of 60 patients. *J Am Coll Cardiol* 1990; **15**: 682–8.

15 Dorros G, Iyer S, Lewin R et al. Angiographic follow-up and clinical outcome of 126 patients after percutaneous directional atherectomy (Simpson AtheroCath) for occlusive peripheral vascular disease. *Cathet Cardiovasc Diagn* 1991; **22**: 79–84.

16 Craor RA, Whitlow P. Atherectomy for directional atherectomy for peripheral vascular disease: two-year patency and factors influencing patency. *J Am Coll Cardiol* 1991; **17**: 106A.

17 Kim D, Gianturco LE, Porter DA et al. Peripheral directional atherectomy: 4-year experience. *Radiology* 1992; **183**: 773–8.

18 Maynar M, Reyes R, Cabrera P et al. Percutaneous atherectomy of iliac arteries. *Semin Intervent Radiol* 1988; **5**: 253–5.

19 Maquin PR, Rousseau HP, Levade M et al. Peripheral atherectomy with the Simpson catheter: midterm results. *Radiology* 1991; **181**: 294 (abstr).

20 Nobuyyoshi M, Kimura T, Ohishi H et al. Restenosis after percutaneous transluminal coronary angioplasty: pathological observation in 20 patients. *Am Coll Cardiol* 1991; **17**: 344–9.

21 Adelman AG, Cohen EA, Kimball BP et al. A comparison of directional atherectomy with balloon angioplasty for lesions of the left anterior descending coronary artery. *N Engl J Med* 1993; **329**: 228–33.

22 Gonschior P, Gerauser F, Gonschior GM et al. Experimental directional atherectomy injury in arterial vessels: impact of trauma depth on cellular response. *Am Heart J* 1995; **129**: 1067–77.

23 Garratt KN, Holmes DR, Bell MR et al. Restenosis after directional coronary atherectomy: differences between primary atheromatous and restenosis lesions and influence of subintimal tissue resection. *J Am Coll Cardiol* 1990; **16**: 1665–71.

24 Umans VAWM, Robert A, Foley D et al. Clinical histologic and quantitative angiographic predictors of restenosis after directional coronary atherectomy: a multivariate analysis of the renarrowing process and late outcome. *J Am Coll Cardiol* 1994; **23**: 39–58.

25 Kuntz RE, Hinohara T, Safian RD et al. Restenosis after directional coronary atherectomy: effects of luminal diameter and deep wall excision. *Circulation* 1992; **86**: 1394–9.

26 Tielbeek AV, Vroegindeweij D, Buth J, Landman GHM. Comparison of balloon angioplasty and Simpson atherectomy for lesions in the femoropopliteal artery: angiographic and clinical results of a prospective randomized trial. *J Vasc Interv Radiol* 1996; **7**: 837–44.

27 Richie JL, Hansen D, Intlekofer MJ et al. Rotational approaches to atherectomy and thrombectomy. *Z Kardiol* 1987; **76**: 56–65.

28 Zacca NM, Rainzner AE, Short HD et al. First in-vivo human experience with a recently developed rotational atherectomy device. *Circulation* 1987; **76**:(suppl IV): 46 (abstr).

29 Zacca NM, Rainzner AE, Noon GP et al. Short-term follow-up of patients treated with a currently developed rotational atherectomy device and in vivo assessment of the particles generated. *Circulation* 1987; **76**(suppl IV): 48 (abstr).

30 Ahn SS, Auth D, Marcus DR et al. Removal of focal atheromatous lesions by angioscopically guided high-speed rotational atherectomy. *J Vasc Surg* 1988; **7**: 292–300.

31 The Collaborative Rotablator Atherectomy Group. Peripheral atherectomy with Rotablator: a multicenter report. *J Vasc Surg* 1994; **19**: 509–15.

32 Dorros G, Iyer S, Zaitoun R et al. Acute angiographic and clinical outcome of high speed percutaneous rotational atherectomy (Rotablator). *Cathet Cardiovasc Diagn* 1991; **22**: 157–66.

33 Henry M, Amor M, Ethevenot G et al. Percutaneous peripheral atherectomy using the Rotablator: a single center experience. *J Endovasc Surg* 1995; **2**: 51–66.

34 Ahn SS, Yeatman LR, Deutsch LS et al. Intraoperative peripheral rotary atherectomy: early and late clinical results. *Ann Vasc Surg* 1992; **6**: 272–80.

35 Ahn SS. The Rotablator high-speed rotary atherectomy: indications, technique, results and complications. In: Moore WS, Ahn SS, eds. *Endovascular Surgery*. Philadelphia: WB Saunders, 1989: 327–35.

36 White CJ, Ramee SR, Escobar A et al. High speed rotational ablation (Rotablator) for unfavorable lesions in peripheral arteries. *Cathet Cardiovasc Diagn* 1993; **30**: 115–19.

37 Myers KA, Denton MJ. Infrainguinal atherectomy using the Auth Rotablator: patency rates and clinical success for 36 procedures. *J Endovasc Surg* 1995; **2**: 67.

38 Stack RS, Quigley PJ, Sketch MHJ et al. Treatment of coronary artery disease with the transluminal extraction–endodarterectomy catheter: initial results of a multicenter study. *Circulation* 1989; **80**(suppl II): II 583.

39 Wholey MH, Jarmolowski CR. New reperfusion device: the Kensey catheter, the atherolytic reperfusion wire device, and the transluminal extraction catheter. *Radiology* 1989; **172**: 947–52.

40 Wholey MH, Jarmolowski CR, Fein DL et al. Multicenter trial with the transluminal endarterectomy catheter in 200 patients with peripheral vascular occlusive disease. *Radiology* 1989; **173**(suppl): 267 (abstr).

41 Yedlicka JWJ, Carlson JE, Hunter DW et al. Thrombectomy with the transluminal endarterectomy catheter (TEC) system: experimental study and case report. *J Vasc Interv Radiol* 1991; **2**: 343–7.

42 Ahn SS, Concepcion B. Current status of atherectomy for peripheral arterial occlusive disease. *World J Surg* 1996; **20**: 635–43.

43 Myers KA, Denton MJ, Devine TJ. Infrainguinal atherectomy using the transluminal endarterectomy catheter: patency rates and clinical success for 144 procedures. *J Endovasc Surg* 1994; **1**: 61–70.

44 Rilinger N, Görich J, Scharrer-Pamler R et al. Percutaneous transluminal rotational atherectomy in the treatment of peripheral vascular disease using a transluminal endoatherectomy catheter (TEC): initial results and angiographic follow-up. *Cardiovasc Interv Radiol* 1997; **20**: 263–7.

45 Wholey MH, Smith JA, Godlewski P, Nagurka M. Recanalization of total arterial occlusions with the Kensey dynamic angioplasty catheter. *Radiology* 1989; **172**: 95–8.

46 Cull DL, Feinberg RL, Wheeler JR et al. Experience with laser-assisted balloon angioplasty and a rotary angioplasty instrument: lessons learned. *J Vasc Surg* 1991; **14**: 332–9.

47 Triller J, Do DD, Maddern G, Mahler F. Femoropopliteal artery occlusion: clinical experience with the Kensey catheter. *Radiology* 1992; **182**: 257–61.

48 McLean GK. Percutaneous peripheral atherectomy. *J Vasc Interv Radiol* 1993; **4**: 465–80.

49 Redha F, Do DD, Mahler F et al. Initial clinical results in the treatment of peripheral arterial occlusive diseases using new percutaneous atherectomy equipment (REDHA-CUT). *Swiss Surg* 1996; **2**: 102–4.

50 Baumgartner I, Redha F, Baumgartner RW et al. Ultrasonic–pathologic comparison of postangioplasty myointimal hyperplasia and primary atheroma of the superficial femoral artery. *Ultrasound Med Biol* 1996; **22**: 815–21.

51 Do DD, Triller J, Baumgartner I et al. A new approach to plaque removal: the Redha-Cut Device. *J Invas Cardiol* 1998; **10**: 578–82.

20

Cutting balloon angioplasty in peripheral vascular diseases

Sanjay Tyagi

Introduction

Balloon angioplasty is an established revacularization procedure for coronary and non-coronary vascular stenosis at various locations in the body. However, conventional balloon dilatation results in application of force in a random manner to the components of the stenosis. This circumferential shear stress often causes irregular intimal tear, splits, and stretches. Vessel wall trauma can cause dissection, intimal proliferative response, and restenosis.[1] Elastic recoil also limits response to balloon angioplasty. Some lesions, either in native vessels or grafts, may be difficult to dilate with conventional balloon angioplasty. This may be as a result of the simultaneous presence of atherosclerosis, fibrosis, and calcification. To overcome these limitations, Barth et al.[2] designed a hybrid device, a cutting balloon (CB), that has tiny, razor-sharp blades mounted on the surface of the balloon. It is designed to minimize the vessel wall trauma that is traditionally associated with conventional balloon angioplasty.

Vascular use of a CB has been explored mainly in coronary arteries. Initial studies suggests its usefulness in the treatment of concentric lesions, aorto-ostial lesions, small vessels, and long diffuse lesions.[1,3] Long-term effectiveness of balloon angioplasty is limited by restenosis. The pathogenesis of restenosis is mainly intimal hyperplastic reaction in response to vessel injury. CB angioplasty has been proposed to reduce restenosis by inflicting less barotrauma to the vessel.[4]

CB offers a simple and effective option for treatment of in-stent restenosis in coronary arteries. Initial reports suggest that it may achieve a better result than conventional PTCA, by making the tissue more amenable to being pushed outward through the stent struts.[1,5,6] This hypothesis needs to be confirmed in large studies. Experience in peripheral arteries with CB angioplasty is presently limited; however, its use is being explored in a number of situations.

Device description and mechanism of cutting balloon angioplasty

The CB (Inter Ventional Technologies Inc, San Diego, CA) features a non-compliant balloon with three or four Atherotomes™ (microsurgical blades), depending on balloon diameter, mounted longitudinally on the outer surface. The Atherotomes are microtome grade blades, approximately five times sharper than the surgical scalpel blades. When the CB is inflated, the Atherotomes are exposed. As inflation continues and the balloon expands, the blades concentrate the dilation force upon an extremely small area along the entire length of the atherotome. The hoop strength of the vessel is overcome and cut occurs along the line of the Atherotome (Figure 20.1). These incisions facilitate dilatation of the target lesion with less

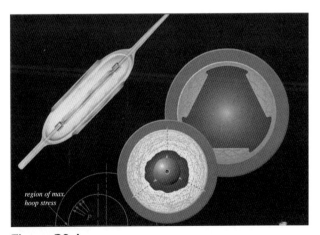

Figure 20.1
Illustration of cutting balloon with Atherotomes™ (blades) and mechanism of microsurgical dilatation.

dilating force, thus minimizing trauma to the vessel. The concentration of dilating force enables a more resistant stenosis to be overcome.

The device currently available has been designed for coronary use and has a diameter of 3–4 mm: soon, peripheral CB with diameter up to 10 mm will be available. The device available is a rapid exchange system. It consists of an inflation shaft, which connects the inflation port to the balloon. At approximately 27 cm from the distal tip, there is a guide-wire port leading into the guide-wire lumen, which forms the distal tip of the catheter and is coaxial with the balloon. The guide-wire lumen permits passage of an 0.014-inch diameter guide wire. It is recommended that an 8F or large lumen 7F guiding catheter is used for CB angioplasty.

Technical aspects of CB angioplasty

To obtain an optimal result with the CB, it is best to slightly oversize the balloon (1.1–1.2:1, balloon to artery). The CB has a special fold manufactured into the balloon to protect the three or four blades from being exposed; therefore, only a negative prep should be used. No air or fluid should be introduced into the CB until the first inflation of the lesion. The metal blades on the CB make it stiffer and somewhat larger than the regular balloons. For successful advancement of the balloon across the lesion, the guiding catheter should be coaxial and should provide a strong back-up. The guide wire should be stiff to allow a CB to be advanced smoothly to the stenotic area. In a tortuous/angled vessel or in a diffuse tight stenosis, a shorter 10 mm balloon would provide better trackability and crossability. Balloon pressure should be increased gradually stepwise (1 atm/s) up to 6 atm to reach nominal size. If an indentation is still noted, pressure is gradually increased to 8 atm. If further inflations are needed, a slow inflation technique should be used to prevent the balloon from being cut by the blades. If the lesion is longer than the length of the CB, inflate the distal portion of the lesion first and move proximal with further inflations. This minimizes risk of dissection.

Clinical experience

Peripheral artery stenosis due to aortoarteritis

Stenotic lesions in aortoarteritis often require high inflation pressure (>10 atm), for dilatation and residual stenosis is not uncommon.[7] This is because the stenosis is caused by dense

transmural fibrosis. We evaluated the use of a CB in dilating stenotic arterial lesions at various sites in this condition. Eighteen stenotic lesions (≥ 75%) – 14 in renal, 2 in carotids, 1 in subclavian, and 1 in axillary artery – in 14 patients aged 10–45 years (mean 15.4 ± 7.1 years), were treated by CB. Fifteen of these lesions were *de novo* and 3 had in-stent restenosis.

A cutting balloon, 4 mm in diameter and Atherotome length of 10–15 mm, was passed through an 8F guiding catheter or a 7F sheath over a 0.014-inch diameter, extra-support guide wire. The femoral approach was used in 12 patients and a high-brachial approach in 2 patients with severe caudal angulation of renal artery. The balloon could be negotiated through stenosis with ease in all patients. On inflation of the balloon at 6–8 atm pressure, 'waist' on the CB could be eliminated in 16/18 (88.9%) lesions. Adjunctive balloon angioplasty using a 5–6 mm balloon was performed in 13 lesions. The stenosis decreased from 87.9 ± 11.4% (mean ± SD) to 34.9 ± 9.5% (mean ± SD) after CB and further reduced to 9.5 ± 8.4% ($p < 0.001$) after further dilatation/stent implantation. There was no complication. Follow-up restudy performed after 3–6 months in 12 lesions showed restenosis in 2 patients (18.7%); one of these also had stent implantation. Both of these patients underwent redilatation. Failure to abolish 'waist' of CB in two patients could be due to the inability of the 0.177 mm working height of the blade to reach the dense fibrosis in the media and adventitia through markedly thickened intima, which is often the pathology.[8] The CB was found to be especially effective in dilating in-stent renal artery restenosis. Complete abolition of 'waist' could be achieved at low pressure (5–6 atm) in both the children. The angiogram shows good dilatation with smooth lumen (Figure 20.2). Recent studies have shown that in-stent restenosis results from smooth muscle cell proliferation,[9] which can be easily sliced by CB. Axillary artery stenosis could be abolished by CB angioplasty at 6 atm and did not require further dilation or stent implantation (Figure 20.3).

Our initial experience suggests that CB angioplasty is safe and permits dilatation at lower pressure in a number of patients; however, larger-diameter CBs are required to cut through dense fibrosis to achieve complete dilatation.

CB angioplasty for resistant venous stenosis of a hemodialysis fistula

A venous stenosis in a hemodialysis shunt is often resistant to high-pressure balloon dilatation. This could be due to dense fibrous strands incorporated in the venous neointimal layer or

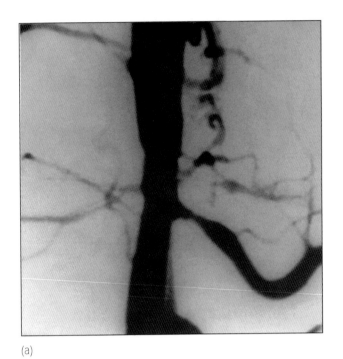

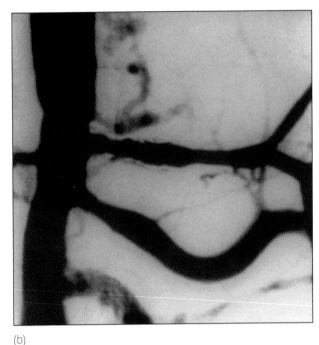

(a)

(b)

Figure 20.2
(a) Severe in-stent restenosis of the proximal segment of the upper left renal artery in a young girl. (b) Good dilatation of stenosed segment after 4 × 10 mm cutting balloon angioplasty.

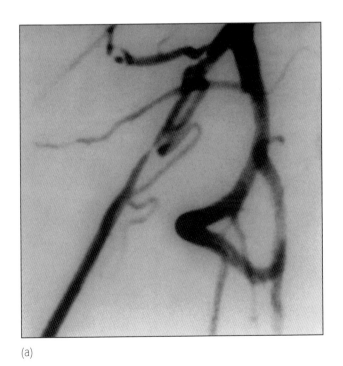

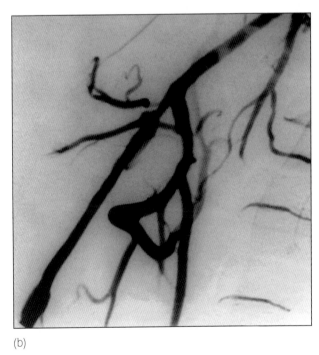

(a)

(b)

Figure 20.3
(a) Severe stenosis of axillary artery in a young boy. (b) Good dilatation of stenosed segment after 4 × 10 mm cutting balloon angioplasty.

be caused by scar tissue developing from recurrent puncture trauma to the venous wall in hemodialysis shunts. Vorwerk et al.[10] performed CB angioplasty in 19 stenosed hemodialysis fistulas and grafts. In 7 patients, CB angioplasty was followed by conventional balloon angioplasty. The balloon expanded completely in all patients and no balloon waist remained. The degree of stenosis decreased from $65 \pm 15\%$ (mean $\pm$ SD) to $14 \pm 9\%$ (mean $\pm$ SD). CB increased the technical success of balloon dilatation of hemodialysis fistulas and grafts.

Other situations

Experimental studies have shown the usefulness of CBs in the treatment of branch pulmonary artery stenosis.[11] Recently, a case report described the successful use of CB for treatment of severe *peripheral pulmonary stenosis* in a $2\frac{1}{2}$-year-old child.[12]

In addition to these reported usages, currently available CB may be useful in the treatment of infrapopliteal stenosis that has a high restenosis rate following conventional balloon angioplasty.

Conclusion

CB angioplasty in peripheral arteries is safe, easy to use, and has potential to improve the efficacy of balloon angioplasty in resistant stenotic lesions. However, the maximum available diameter of 4-mm CB limits the use of this balloon to small arteries and veins. The role of this technique in improving the long-term patency of peripheral arteries is still unknown. Future development of larger-diameter cutting balloons and further studies will clarify the place of this technique in peripheral angioplasty.

References

1   Yamaguchi T, Nakamura M, Nishida T et al. Update on cutting balloon angioplasty. *J Interven Cardiol* 1998; 11(Suppl. 1): S114–19.

2   Barath P, Fishbein MC, Vari S, Forrester JS. Cutting balloon: a novel approach to percutaneous angioplasty. *Am J Cardiol* 1991; **68**: 1249–52.

3   Voigt B, Pfitzer P, Weismueller P et al. Cutting balloon angioplasty: an alternate way in the treatment of complex coronary lesions. *J Am Coll Cardiol* 2000; **35**(Suppl A): 1062–78.

4   Inoue T, Sakai Y, Hoshi K et al. Lower expression of neutrophil adhesion molecule indicates less vessel wall injury and might explain lower restenosis rate after cutting balloon angioplasty. *Circulation* 1998; **97**: 2511–18.

5   Kurbaan AS, Foale RA, Sigwart U. Cutting balloon angioplasty for in-stent restenosis. *Cathet Cardiovasc Intervent* 2000; **50**: 480–3.

6   Albiero R, Nishida T, Karvouni E et al. Cutting balloon angioplasty for in stent restenosis. *Cathet Cardiovasc Interv* 2000; **50**: 452–9.

7   Tyagi S, Verma PK, Gambhir DS et al. Early and long term results of balloon angioplasty in aortoarteritis (Takayasu disease): comparison with atherosclerosis. *Cardiovasc Intervent Radiol* 1998; **21**: 219.

8   Hotchi M. Pathological studies on Takayasu arteritis. *Heart Vessels* 1992; Suppl. 7: 11–17.

9   Kearney M, Pieczek A, Haley L et al. Histopathology of in-stent restenosis in patients with peripheral artery disease. *Circulation* 1997; **95**: 1998–2002.

10 Vorwerk D, Adam G, Muller-Leisse C, Guenther RW. Hemodialysis fistulas and grafts: use of cutting balloon to dilate venous stenosis. *Radiology* 1996; **201**: 864–7.

11 Magee AG, Wax D, Saiki Y et al. Experimental branch pulmonary artery stenosis angioplasty using a novel cutting balloon. *Can J Cardiol* 1998; **14**: 1037–41.

12 Schneider MD, Zartner PA, Magee AG. Images in cardiology: cutting balloon for treatment of severe peripheral pulmonary stenosis in a child. *Heart* 1999; **82**: 108.

21

Chronic total occlusions: new therapeutic approaches

Philip A Morales and Richard R Heuser

Introduction

The prevalence of peripheral vascular disease ranges from 1 to 6% in the general population. This dramatically increases in patients with established coronary artery disease.[1] Screening for peripheral vascular disease, therefore, becomes an important step in completing the evaluation of patients with established or suspected coronary artery disease. The ankle–brachial index (ABI) and segmental blood pressure measurements with pulse volume recordings are standard screening tools.[2] However, the sensitivity of detecting distal aortic or common iliac artery disease is low with ABI measurements whether the lesion is a simple stenosis or is chronically occluded. In addition, segmental blood pressure measurements with pulse volume recordings can help localize the level of arterial disease but cannot distinguish between stenoses or chronic occlusions. Magnetic resonance angiography (MRA)[3] or ultra-fast computed tomography (CT)[4] angiography increase the sensitivity of diagnosing peripheral vascular disease, in particular, total occlusions. Despite these advances in detecting peripheral vascular disease, invasive arteriography is still the diagnostic standard for establishing the diagnosis and the extent of peripheral vascular disease (i.e., stenosis vs occlusions).

Surgical vs percutaneous interventions

With the increasing use of peripheral stents or endovascular grafts in clinical practice, guidelines have been formed to help direct physicians determine the appropriate choice of therapy (i.e. percutaneous vs surgical intervention). Recent guidelines for interventions of the distal abdominal aorta and lower extremity vessels classified the severity of peripheral vascular disease into four different categories (Table 21.1).[1] Category 1 lesions are suitable for percutaneous intervention alone. Category 2 lesions are suitable for percutaneous intervention in conjunction with surgical intervention. Category 3 lesions can be treated by percutaneous intervention but may have a lower rate of initial technical success or long-term benefit compared with surgical intervention. Category 4 lesions are more suitable with surgical interventions, whereas the percutaneous approach has a limited role. Although these are not strict guidelines, new technical advances and therapeutic approaches in percutaneous interventions have blurred the lines (or boundaries) between these predefined categories. Surgical interventions, considered the standard of choice for treatment for certain peripheral vascular lesions (e.g., aortoiliac occlusions, long superficial femoral occlusions, infrapopliteal occlusions), are now being replaced by percutaneous interventions as a strong viable option. This chapter discusses new therapeutic approaches to the treatment of chronic total occlusions in the peripheral arteries.

Histology

The pathohistology of chronic coronary occlusions has been well described.[5] The general aspects of chronic peripheral occlusions are not vastly different. They are usually characterized by two histological components. The first is a lumen-obstructing atherosclerotic plaque; the second is an overlying occlusive thrombus. The thrombus may vary in size, age, and stage of organization. Fresh thrombus, as seen in acute occlusions, is associated with a high recanalization success because it is easily penetrated by a guide wire. With chronic occlusions, the thrombus reorganizes to form loose or dense fibrotic tissue, and eventually it will be calcified and make reopening vessels more difficult.

Table 21.1 Morphological stratification of peripheral lesions by category

Category	Location
	Aorta:
1	• Short stenosis length of infrarenal aorta < 2 cm
2	• Medium stenosis length 2–4 cm
3	• Long segment stenosis length > 4 cm
	• Aortic stenosis with atheroembolic disease
	• Medium stenosis length 2–4 cm with moderate–severe atherosclerosis of aorta
4	• Aortic occlusion
	• Aortic stenosis associated with an abdominal aortic aneurysm
	Iliac:
1	• Concentric and noncalcified stenosis length < 3 cm
2	• Stenosis length 3–5 cm
	• Calcified or eccentric stenosis length < 3 cm
3	• Stenosis length 5–10 cm
	• Occlusion length < 5 cm after thrombolytic therapy
4	• Stenosis length > 10 cm
	• Occlusion length > 5 cm after thrombolytic therapy
	• Extensive bilateral aortoiliac disease
	• Iliac stenosis with an abdominal aortic aneurysm
	Femoropopliteal:
1	• Single stenosis length up to 5 cm not at the superficial femoral artery (SFA) origin or distal popliteal
	• Single occlusion length up to 3 cm not involving the SFA or distal popliteal
2	• Single stenosis length 5–10 cm not involving distal popliteal artery
	• Single occlusion length 3–10 cm not involving distal popliteal artery
	• Heavily calcified stenosis length up to 5 cm
	• Multiple lesions, length < 3 cm, either stenoses or occlusions
	• Single or multiple lesions with no continuous tibial runoff to improve inflow for distal surgical bypass
3	• Single occlusion length 3–10 cm, involving distal popliteal artery
	• Multiple focal lesions, length 3–5 cm (heavily calcified)
	• Single lesion length > 10 cm, either stenosis or occlusion
4	• Complete common and/or superficial femoral occlusions
	• Complete popliteal and proximal trifurcation occlusions
	• Severe diffuse disease with multiple lesions and no intervening normal vascular segments
	Infrapopliteal:
1	• Single focal stenosis length up to 1 cm of tibial or peroneal vessels
2	• Multiple focal stenosis lengths up to 1 cm of tibial or peroneal vessels
	• One or two focal stenosis length up to 1 cm of tibial trifurcation
	• Tibial or peroneal stenosis dilated in combination with femoropopliteal bypass
3	• Moderate stenosis length 1–4 cm or occlusion length 1–2 cm of tibial or peroneal vessels
	• Extensive stenosis of tibial trifurcation
4	• Tibial or peroneal occlusion length > 2 cm
	• Diffusely diseased tibial or peroneal vessels

Source: Pentecost et al.[1]

Rationale for treatment

The rationale for revascularizing chronic coronary occlusions has long been debated.[6] Much like coronary occlusions, peripheral occlusions need to be treated with the purpose of improving clinical symptoms (i.e., exertional claudication) and decreasing the need for vascular bypass surgery. A further incentive is reduced likelihood of developing critical limb ischemia and the threat of amputation. As a result of decreasing the need for vascular bypass surgery, saphenous veins can be spared for future use (i.e., coronary artery bypass surgery).

Conventional means of treatment

Success in revascularizing total occlusions is hampered by the inability to cross the lesion. Acute or subacute total occlusions tend to fair better with conventional means compared with chronic occlusions. For example, thrombolysis or fibrinolysis is an important adjunct therapy to angioplasty and/or stenting when treating acute occlusions. Thrombolysis has less of an impact on chronic occlusion and only serves to prolong the procedure and increase the risk of serious bleeding complications.[7] Hydrophilic wires (e.g., Terumo) have considerable success in crossing chronic occlusion but run the risk of distal perforation.

PIER – percutaneous intentional extraluminal (subintimal) recanalization

One method of treating long superficial femoral artery occlusions, described by Bolia et al.,[8] predates the stent era. It is a simple and alternative method worth describing. The method described as percutaneous intentional extraluminal recanalization (subintimal angioplasty) for obvious reasons usually requires an antegrade approach to the common femoral artery. Once access is obtained, a guide wire and guiding catheter are advanced through the femoral artery and then positioned in the stump of the superficial femoral artery just cranial of the occlusion. By pushing the catheter slowly forward and with minimal rotation, after initial resistance the catheter will suddenly jump forwards a few millimeters. The tip of the catheter has now entered the extraluminal space. This situation is commonly known as subintimal dissection. Alternatively, the proximal superficial femoral artery and, subsequently, the occlusion can be entered with a curved-tip guide wire.

Now with the catheters in the extraluminal space, a standard 0.035-inch angled guide wire (e.g. Terumo) is pushed down until it forms into a large loop configuration. With this loop the extraluminal space is explored distally. The catheter can support the wire-loop, but the loop must always be ahead to make the subintimal dissection. By pushing the loop and the catheter towards the distal patent part of the vessel, a suddenly decreased resistance can be felt and the wire seems to move down freely. After bringing the catheter down and removing the wire, the intraluminal alignment of the catheter should be checked by contrast injection. To prevent damage to the first major collateral artery, the site of re-entry must not be too distal. After the re-entry into the true patent distal lumen is confirmed with contrast, heparin can be given. The new lumen is now dilated in a standard fashion with an appropriate-sized balloon catheter, eventually with prolonged dilation times up to 3 min to improve initial results.

New devices

Laser

The idea of using laser energy to vaporize atherosclerotic material within the vessel lumen dates back to early 1980s and was initially met with great enthusiasm.[5] However, early results were fraught with disastrous complications such as perforations and this enthusiasm for laser angioplasty waned. Over the years, various types of laser catheters have been developed for angioplasty. Some of these laser catheters have proved ineffective (i.e. the argon laser, metal tips, or sapphire laser) or, quite simply, never made it into clinical practice (i.e., 'smart laser,' angioscopically guided laser).[5] Now with improvements in catheter design and the use of the saline infusion technique, there has been a renewed interest in laser angioplasty.

Currently, the excimer laser wire is the focus of attention as a valuable alternative or adjunct to conventional means for chronic occlusion angioplasty. In contrast to earlier laser systems that depended on continuous-wave irradiation, the excimer laser is a pulsed-wave system that induces photoablation during an athermic process. Photoablation is simply the disruption of chemical bonds at very high-energy densities with short interaction times. The system uses xenon chloride 308 nm as the source of energy. At this wavelength, the ablation of the irradiated tissue is no longer a consequence of a photochemical disruption of molecular chains. It is predominantly a local, very fast micro explosion provoked by an extremely high temperature rise of the irradiated volume with energy densities of about 3–6 J/cm.[2] As a result of the excimer laser beam's small penetration depth and the extremely short pulse duration in comparison to the pulse repetition rate used, the thermal damage induced by the excimer laser is minimal even when high-energy densities are used.

Results

Scheinert et al. recently published results from a large series of patients who underwent excimer-laser-assisted revascularization for chronic superficial femoral artery occlusions.[9] With a total number of 318 patients (411 limbs or lesions) being treated with excimer-laser-assisted angioplasty, the primary success rate for revascularization was 83.2% (342/411 cases). A secondary attempt was performed in 44 cases, including using the retrograde popliteal approach in 39 cases. The total technical success rate was 90.5% (372/411 cases). Relevant interventional complications were acute reocclusion (1.0%), perforation (2.2%), and embolization/distal thrombosis (3.9%). Postinterventionally, 219 patients (68.8%) were in clinical category 0 (Rutherford classification); 53 patients (16.6%) were in category 1, and 26 patients (8.2%) were in category 2. Restenosis was detected in more than

50% of the cases; however, using secondary interventions, in the majority of the patients reobstructions were treatable on an outpatient basis. As a result, the clinical benefit was maintained in 75.1% of the patients after 1 year.

Lumend Frontrunner™ CTO catheter

Designed to cross total occlusions and recently approved for clinical use in coronary arteries only, the Lumend Frontrunner™ CTO catheter (Lumend, Inc., Redwood, CA) consists of a 3.0 or 4.0 mm distal tip (straight or spherical), a 4F catheter shaft (135 cm long), and a hand-held distal tip control device at the proximal end of the catheter. The distal tip of the Frontrunner™ catheter is operator-controlled and can be opened or closed, much like the distal tip of bioptomes used for percutaneous endomyocardial biopsies. The catheter makes blunt micro-dissections, separating atherosclerotic plaques, and creates a passage through the occlusion. Whitlow et al.[10] has reported so far the largest series of patients (n = 100) with chronic total occlusions who underwent treatment using the Frontrunner™ catheter. These patients had earlier failed the use of conventional means in crossing total occlusions prior to the use of the Frontrunner™ catheter. Of the 100 patients, the lesion was successfully engaged in 79% of the cases and guide-wire placement beyond the lesion allowing stent placement had a success rate of 71% (56/79). These early and encouraging results will hopefully lead to further developments that may one day have applications in treating chronic occlusion in the peripheral arteries.

MollRing Cutter®

This is a remote endarterectomy device designed to transect the distal end of an atheromatous core in chronic occlusions. The MollRing Cutter® (Vascular Architects, Inc., San Jose, CA) consist of stainless steel double ring cutters and a hypotube with angled interior blades. The ring diameters come in many sizes, from 5 mm (for femoral arteries) to 10 mm (for iliac arteries). A detailed description of the device and the technique in using the device can be seen in a review by Teijink et al.[11]

Safe-Cross™ TO RF Guidewire System

This 'forward-looking' fiberoptic guide-wire system is based on the principle of low-coherence interferometry that has been extensively described.[12] In general, a light source is divided into two beams, a reference arm and a sample arm. The light in the reference arm is reflected at a determinable path length and, for measurement purposes, the path length can be changed. Light in the sample arm is also reflected or scattered by the material present in the sample. The reflections and backscattered light are combined at the coupler and if the path lengths of the two arms are within the coherence length of the light, the beams will recorrelate or interfere with one another. The detector measures the interference intensity. Since the reference path length is known and adjustable, the intensity profile of scattered light from a sample arm can be determined as a function of the reference arm path length. The resolution of the system is largely dependent on the coherence length of the light. Since the coherence length is inversely proportional to the bandwidth, a broadband source is desirable. Resolution of approximately 10 μm can be obtained with commercially available sources and components.[13]

OCR system

The optical coherence reflectometry (OCR) system consists of an optical interferometer, a demodulation-computer unit and monitor, fiberoptic cables, and a light source (Figure 21.1). The Safe-Cross™ TO RF Guidewire System (Intraluminal Therapeutics, Carlsbad, CA) consists of an OCR system, optical guide wire, and catheter (Figure 21.2). The optical interferometer operates in an A-scan mode to detect the distance to the normal arterial wall interface through plaque or thrombus. No real imaging is attempted with the optical guide wire: rather, the optical fiber in the guide wire illuminates the tissue in front of the distal tip of the guide wire and collects the backscattered light; hence, the derived nomenclature of optical coherence reflectometry.[14]

The backscattered light is analyzed through the low-coherence interferometer, producing a signal tracing that is displayed and updated every half-second on an OCR monitor. The signal tracing is monitored through a series of algorithms to determine if the normal arterial wall interface is within the field of view. If the normal arterial wall is detected, a visual indication of a red bar across the top portion of the signal tracing is displayed to the operator and the relative distance to the arterial wall is shown. If the normal arterial wall is not in the field of view, a green bar is displayed, indicating the guide wire can be advanced. This simple method allows the interventional cardiologist to safely navigate through the total occlusion within the arterial vessel.

The Safe-Cross™ RF TO guide wire is equipped with radiofrequency energy that is delivered at the tip of the wire to facilitate crossing occlusions. The radiofrequency energy ablates through the atherosclerotic plaques. As an added safety feature, the radiofrequency energy cannot be applied and becomes automatically disabled when the guide wire identifies an arterial wall. Early experience with the guide wire has been initially successful with chronic coronary occlusions.[15]

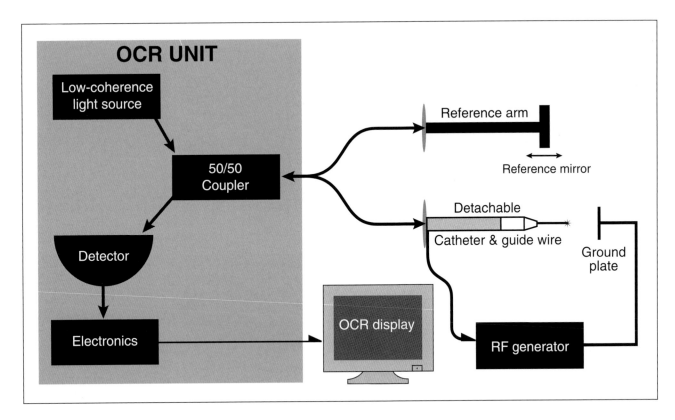

Figure 21.1
Schematic diagram of the optical coherence reflectometry (OCR) system.

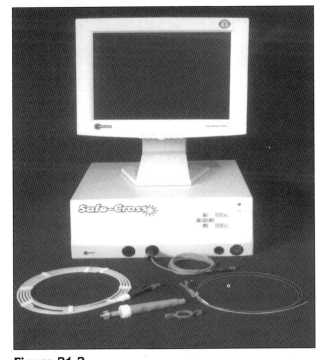

Figure 21.2
The console and guide-wire control system.

GRIP trial

The Safe-Cross™ RF TO guide wire is part of a clinical investigation trial named GRIP, which is an acronym for Guided Radio Frequency in Peripheral Total Occlusions. The main purpose of this clinical trial is to determine and establish the safety and efficacy of the Safe-Cross™ RF TO guide wire system in crossing peripheral total occlusions in symptomatic patients with peripheral vascular disease (Figures 21.3–21.5). The primary end point is device success, which is defined as successful advancement of the assigned wire across the total occlusion and achievement of distal intraluminal wire position. Secondary end points are:

1. clinical success, defined as device success with no procedural events, defined as perforation, dissection, or distal embolization
2. final peripheral flow, as determined by the ABI
3. time to successful crossing of lesion.

This small multicenter pilot trial is ongoing in the United States.

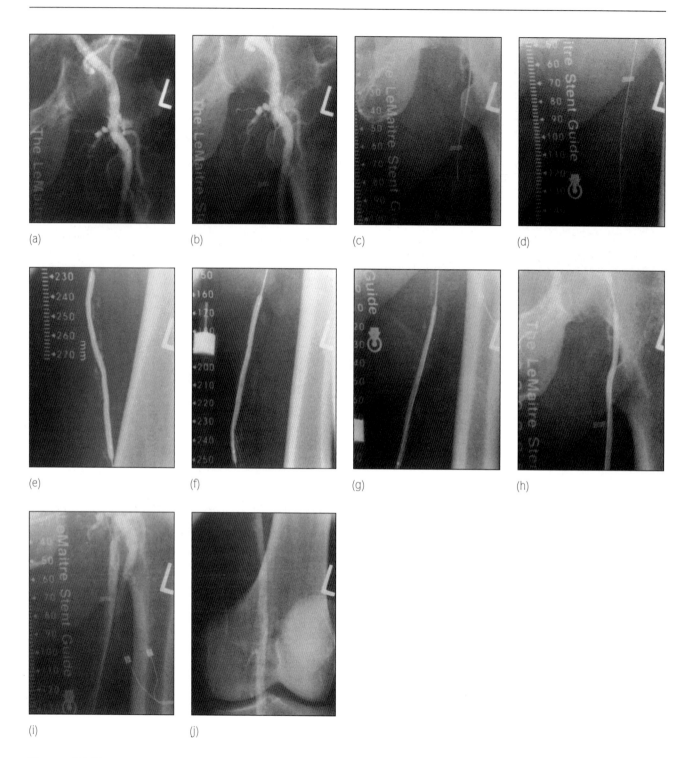

Figure 21.3

(a) Left superficial femoral artery (SFA) occlusion near the femoral bifurcation. (b) Safe-Cross™ guidewire tip across the initial part of the left SFA occlusion. (c) Safe-Cross™ guidewire tip further advanced distally in the left SFA occlusion. (d) Further advancement of the Safe-Cross™ guidewire in the distal left SFA. (e–h) Successive balloon angioplasties along the length of the SFA (from distal SFA to SFA origin). (i) Post-angioplasty angiogram confirming a patent left SFA. (j) Post-angioplasty angiogram confirming a patent left popliteal artery.

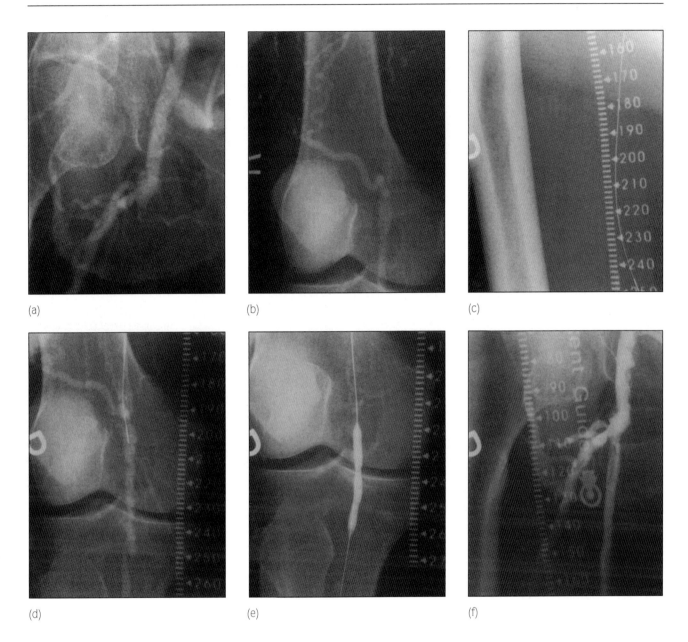

(a)   (b)   (c)

(d)   (e)   (f)

Figure 21.4
(a) Right superficial femoral artery (SFA) occlusion at the femoral bifurcation. (b) Distal end of the right SFA occlusion with right popliteal artery filling in via collateral vessels. (c) Safe-Cross™ guidewire tip across the right SFA occlusion and positioned in the distal right SFA. (d) Safe-Cross™ guidewire tip completely across the right SFA occlusion and positioned in the right popliteal artery. (e) Balloon angioplasty of the distal portion of the right total occlusion. (f) Post-angioplasty angiogram confirming a patent right SFA.

Conclusion

Since the development of percutaneous interventions, treating peripheral vascular disease with balloon angioplasty and/or stenting have rapidly become the choice of therapy where initial and long-term results are comparable to surgical outcomes. Chronic total occlusions of the peripheral vessels remain a therapeutic challenge that once was treated by surgical means alone. Technologies such as 'fiberoptic' guide wires with optical coherence reflectometry and radiofrequency ablation capabilities and excimer laser angioplasty make it possible to successfully treat chronic occlusions via the percutaneous approach. Add future applications with drug delivery, systemic or local (i.e., coated stents), and restenosis will hopefully one day become a trivial issue, especially with superficial femoral arterial occlusions. As new technologies evolve, it may be possible to treat almost all chronic occlusions in the peripheral arteries non-surgically.

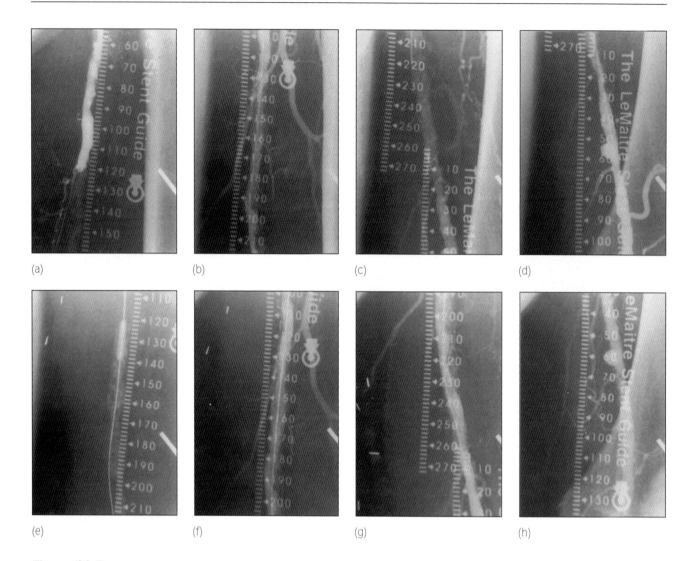

(a)   (b)   (c)   (d)

(e)   (f)   (g)   (h)

Figure 21.5
(a) Total occlusion at mid-level of left superficial femoral artery (SFA) (ruler marker 122). (b) Safe-Cross™ guidewire tip across the total occlusion (positioned between ruler markers 200 and 210). (c) Safe-Cross™ guidewire tip (ruler marker 220) advanced further into the left SFA occlusion. (d) Angiogram through the glide catheter confirming the catheter's intraluminal position in the left popliteal artery. Safe-Cross™ guidewire was removed for angiogram. (e) Balloon angioplasty at the original site of the left SFA occlusion. (f) Post-angioplasty angiogram confirming a patent mid-level left SFA. (g–h) Post-angioplasty angiograms confirming a patent left distal SFA and popliteal artery.

References

1   Pentecost MJ, Criqui MH, Dorros G et al. Guidelines for peripheral percutaneous transluminal angioplasty of the abdominal aorta and lower extremity vessels. *Circulation* 1994; **89**: 511–31.

2   Hirsh A, Criqui MH, Treat-Jacobson D et al. Peripheral arterial disease detection, awareness, and treatment in primary care. *JAMA* 2001; **286**: 1317–24.

3   Carpenter JP, Owen RS, Baum RA et al. Magnetic resonance angiography of the peripheral runoff vessels. *J Vasc Surg* 1992; **16**: 807–15.

4   Kramer SC, Gorich J, Aschoff AJ et al. Diagnostic value of spiral-CT angiography in comparison with digital subtraction angiography before and after peripheral vascular intervention. *Angiology* 1998; **49**: 599–606.

5   Meier B. Chronic total occlusion. In: Topol EJ (ed.), *Textbook of interventional cardiology*, 3rd edn. Philadelphia: WB Saunders, 1999: 280–96.

6   Puma JA, Sketch MHJ, Tcheng JE et al. Percutaneous revascularization of chronic total occlusions: an overview. *J Am Coll Cardiol* 1995; **26**: 1–11.

7   Olin JW, Graor RA. Thrombolytic therapy in the treatment of peripheral arterial occlusions. *Ann Emerg Med* 1988; **17**: 1210–15.

8   Bolia A, Miles KA, Brennan J et al. Percutaneous transluminal angioplasty of occlusions of the femoral and popliteal arteries by subintimal dissection. *Cardiovasc Intervent Radiol* 1990; **13**: 357–63.

9   Scheinert D, Laird JR, Schroeder M et al. Excimer Laser-assisted recanalization of long chronic superficial femoral artery occlusions. *J Endovasc Ther* 2001; **8**: 156–66.

10 Whitlow PL, Selmon M, O'Neill W et al. Treatment of uncrossable chronic total occlusions with the Frontrunner: multicenter experience. *J Am Coll Cardiol* 2002; **39**: (Suppl. A) 5.

11 Teijink JA, van den Berg JC, Moll FL. A minimally invasive technique in occlusive disease of the superficial femoral artery: remote endarterectomy using the MollRing Cutter. *Ann Vasc Surg* 2001; **15**: 594–8.

12 Mandel L, Wolf E. *Optical coherence and quantum optics.* Cambridge: Cambridge University Press, 1995: 147–59.

13 Newton S. Technology trends in optical reflectometry. *Photonic Spectra* 1991; 118–26.

14 Neet JM, Winston TR, Hedrick AD et al. Navigating a guide wire through total occlusions: clinical experience. In: Anderson RR, Bartels KE, Bass LS et al. (eds.), *Lasers in surgery: advanced characterization therapeutics, and systems X, Pro SPIE* 2000; **3907**: 536–43.

15 Morales PA, Heuser RR. Chronic total occlusions: experience with fiber-optic guidance technology – optical coherence reflectometry. *J Interven Cardiol* 2001; **14**: 611–16.

22

Thrombolysis in peripheral vascular diseases

Krishna Kandarpa and Luis H Melendez Morales

Until recently surgery was the only means of treating limb ischemia secondary to peripheral arterial occlusion. Acute lower limb ischemia (ALLI) has been considered a surgical emergency as mortality and rates of limb loss are closely associated to delay in treatment.[1,2] Treatment algorithms are aimed at reestablishing reperfusion to salvageable limbs: embolectomy/thrombectomy for critical ischemia, angiography and percutaneous therapy for viable limbs with no critical ischemia, and amputation for irreversible ischemia.[3] Despite this aggressive surgical approach, 10–18%[4,5] of patients lose their limb, and 5–18% of patients die.[5,6] Drawbacks in balloon thromboembolectomy, i.e. endothelial damage plus the inability to clear small vessels of thrombus, plus the inherent complications in surgical revascularization, have raised interest in catheter-directed thrombolytic therapy (CDTT) for peripheral arterial occlusion (PAO).[7–9]

CDTT is aimed at removing thromboemboli to restore arterial patency by infusion of concentrated lytic agents (plasminogen activators)[10] directly into the thrombus within the affected vessel. It is preferred over intravenous infusion due to higher success and lower complication rates.[11] CDTT rapidly restores blood flow to the ischemic limb and serves to uncover underlying lesions, which can then be treated percutaneously and/or surgically. By locally infusing the lytic agent, the risks of bleeding complications associated with lytic therapy are decreased, as the amount of drug used and its systemic effects are reduced. In addition, the initial trial of lytic therapy rarely compromises the timing or result of subsequent surgical procedure.[12] In fact, as a result of successful lytic therapy, the extent of required surgery may decrease, and an improvement in the outcome, including amputation-free survival, may be expected.[6,12]

Patient selection

Selective intravascular thrombolytic therapy is aimed at reestablishing blood flow in patients with thrombotic or embolic arterial occlusion, with best results in acute (less than 14 days' duration) cases.[7,13–15] CDTT is indicated in patients with new-onset claudication or limb-threatening ischemia, either acute or chronic, resulting from thrombotic or embolic arterial occlusion.[7,12,14,16,22–25]

Patients should be selectively chosen to minimize risks of bleeding, systemic embolization, and reperfusion syndrome.[12,16,17–21] Absolute contraindications to lytic therapy include: (7,13–15) active or recent internal bleeding within the last 10 days, recent cerebrovascular accident within the last 6–12 months or recent transient ischemic attack (TIA) within the previous 2 months, recent (within the previous 3 months) craniotomy or spinal surgery, known intracardiac neoplasm. Relative contraindications include recent major surgery (10–14 days), history of gastrointestinal bleeding, recent trauma, coagulopathy, organ biopsy, cardiopulmonary resuscitation, trauma, pregnancy or postpartum status, diabetic hemorrhagic retinopathy, uncontrolled hypertension (systolic blood pressure > 180 mmHg or diastolic blood pressure > 110 mmHg), bacterial endocarditis, hepatic failure, and renal failure.[20] Patients who have undergone recent vascular surgery should have a waiting period of 1 week to 10 days to allow for wound healing. Certain grafts such as Dacron may require up to 3 months to seal properly before initiating CDTT.[26] If lytic therapy is required before this period, local infusion should be initiated carefully and the patient closely monitored for signs of local bleeding, at which time the infusion should be terminated.

Another group of patients who require special consideration are those with intracardiac thrombi. Protruding or mobile intracardiac thrombi are at a higher risk of embolizing during lytic therapy,[21] and such patients should be excluded from CDTT. When these findings are not present, the rate of embolic stroke is less than 1%.[21] However, prelysis echocardiogram is considered unnecessary since the risk of subsequent embolization is considered to be low.[13]

Reperfusion syndrome refers to the consequences of rapid restoration of blood flow to a severely ischemic limb.[27,28] The most serious consequences are cardiac dysfunction resulting from severe systemic acidemia and hyperkalemia caused by the washout of metabolites from necrotic tissue, and renal failure from myoglobinuria. McNamara et al.[12] reported 25% amputation rate and one death from reperfusion syndrome in patients with irreversible acute limb ischemia. The same study demonstrated no deaths, and 0 and 8% amputation rates in patients with viable or threatened limbs, respectively. Therefore, it is this group of patients who are good candidates for lytic therapy.

Procedural considerations

Patient preparation and monitoring

As is the usual practice, informed consent should always be obtained from the patient or guardian. This should include all the risks and benefits clearly explained. The possibilities of other additional procedures, such as angioplasty and stent, should be included in the written consent.

Initial laboratory evaluation should include a complete blood cell count to evaluate for pre-procedure levels of hemoglobin and hematocrit; platelet count; blood urea nitrogen and creatinine levels to assess renal function; and prothrombin time and partial thromboplastin time to evaluate initial coagulation parameters, even though it has been proven that activated clotting time (ACT) should be used to assess response to heparin.[29] It has been proven that the routine assessment of parameters that reflect the systemic lytic state – (e.g. fibrinogen, fibrin degradation products (FDP), plasminogen levels) – is of limited use in predicting possible hemorrhagic complications.[19,21,30,31] Still, extremely low levels of fibrinogen tend to correlate with bleeding complications.[31]

Technique

The goal of treatment is to lyse thrombus as rapidly as possible to prevent bleeding complications. To achieve this goal, several techniques have been developed, which include initial intrathrombus lacing, and pulse-spray (forced periodic) infusion. These techniques appear to minimize infusion times and shorten duration of treatment.[32–34]

Initial angiography should be performed to map out the location and extent of the thrombus. Previous angiograms and non-invasive vascular studies should be reviewed and the shortest approach achieved to minimize catheter manipulations. A vascular sheath should be used to facilitate catheter exchanges and minimize arterial trauma. Puncture of the axillary artery should be avoided to prevent compression of the brachial plexus in case hematoma formation at the puncture site occurs. If an arm approach is unavoidable, a high brachial artery approach should be used.

The occluded vessel should be selectively catheterized and the entire length of the thrombus crossed (guide-wire traversal test). Failure to cross the thrombus probably signifies that the thrombus is chronic and harder to lyse.[33] At this point the catheter should be left just proximal to the thrombus and a short trial of infusion started. In many cases the thrombus will soften and be crossed successfully.

After crossing the thrombus, an infusion catheter is placed into the thrombus along its entire length to ensure that it is all optimally bathed with plasminogen activator. An intrathrombic dose of lytic agent is given as a pulsed spray to saturate the thrombus, and the low-dose infusion is started.[32,34] The infusion is continued until all the thrombus is lysed, or until it is considered safe. The goal of treatment is to lyse the entire thrombus, as residual thrombus is highly thrombogenic.

The ideal catheter should have side holes at different lengths to cover the entire thrombus and be used for both pulsed-spray and continuous infusion. Angiodynamics (Glen Falls, NY) has a pulse-spray catheter with pressure-responsive side-slit orifices and an end hole, which is occluded by a 0.035-inch tip-occluding wire. It comes in 4F and 5F sizes. The McNamara coaxial catheter infusion set (Cook Inc., Indianapolis, IN) has a 3F inner catheter, which allows the infusion length to be varied as thrombolysis progresses. The Mewissen multi-side-hole over the wire infusion catheter (5F) can be used either alone or in combination with a coaxially placed 0.035-inch Katzen infusion wire (Medi-Tech/Boston Scientific, Watertown, MA), which works similarly to the McNamara catheter. Other 3F end-hole catheters that can be used include the Sos infusion wire (Bard, Billerica, MA) and the Cragg Convertible Wire (Medi-Tech).

Monitoring

The patient should be admitted to an intensive care or step-down unit setting to ensure adequate monitoring. Laboratory evaluation ensures that the patient is adequately anticoagulated and that there is no occult bleeding. Urine output should also be closely monitored, assessing for acute renal failure and occult bleeding (a Foley catheter should be inserted prior to the procedure). Fibrinogen levels are not followed routinely by us.

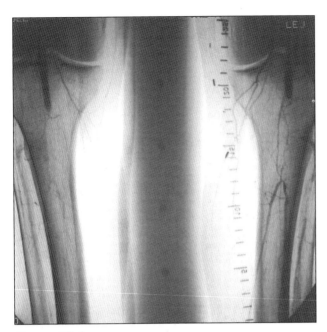

Figure 22.1a

A 45-year-old man admitted with acute bilateral feet pain at rest secondary to emboli from a central source. A day after the initial angiogram, which shows occlusion of the popliteal arteries bilaterally, both common femoral arteries were punctured in an antegrade fashion and 5 french (5F) multi-side-hole catheters were placed through hemostatic introduction sheaths into the thrombosed popliteal arteries. A total of 5 mg of recombinant tissue plasminogen activator (rt-PA) was given, utilizing the pulse-spray technique into each leg. Subsequently, a drip of rt-PA at 0.5 mg/h was started bilaterally. The patient was also fully anticoagulated.

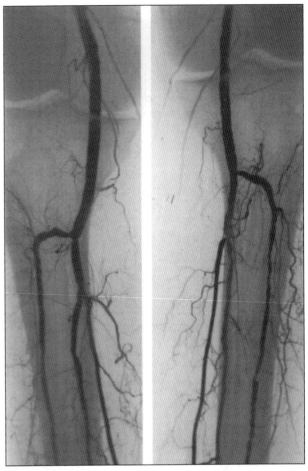

Figure 22.1b

At 16 hour post-initiation of rt-PA infusion. Follow-up arteriogram shows bilateral resolution of thrombosis with patent three-vessel run-off bilaterally. At this point, the procedure was terminated.

Upon termination of treatment, both infusion catheter and wire or inner coaxial catheters are removed and the sheath left in place (with heparinized saline to KVO) until coagulation parameters return to normal. Systemic anticoagulation can be restarted approximately 4–5 hours after the sheath has been removed.

Results

Initial results

Positive clinical and lysis outcome can be expected in about 85–95% of cases treated with urokinase (UK) with a time duration of about 24 hours.[14,19,36–39] Presently urokinase has been removed from the market by the US Food and Drug Administration (FDA) due to a theoretical risk of contamination during manufacturing.[36] Currently available agents include altepase, or recombinant tissue plasminogen activator (rt-PA); reteplase, or recombinant plasminogen activator (r-PA); and streptokinase. The most used and currently studied is rt-PA. It has been found that duration of infusions is generally shorter with rt-PA and much longer with streptokinase.[7,22,37–39] Recent studies have shown equal efficacy and no significant difference in rates of intracranial hemorrhage between rt-PA and UK.[5,13] In addition, it has been found that by decreasing the duration of infusion and using the lowest possible effective dose of rt-PA, bleeding complications can be kept to a minimum.[40] Furthermore, the STILE (surgery vs thrombolysis in the lower extremity) study found that both rt-PA and UK were similar in safety and efficacy.[5]

Streptokinase use has decreased significantly in the past years due to its inherent problems. It is a bacterial protein; therefore, people with prior streptococcal infections might develop hypersensitivity reactions to the medication during treatment due to the presence of antibodies to it. Antibodies may also decrease the bioavailability of the agent.[41] In addition, people treated with streptokinase may develop antibodies, resulting in delay if retreatment was needed.[42]

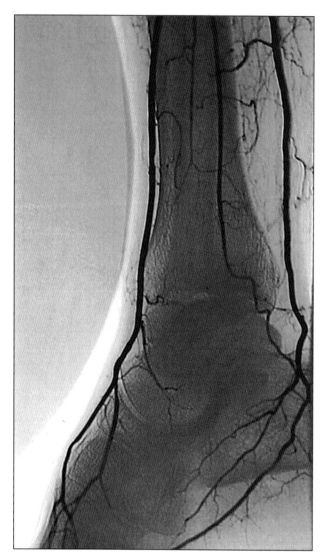 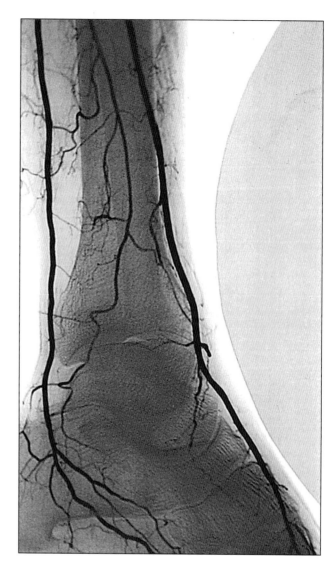

Figure 22.1c

Reteplase (Retavase; Centocor, Malvern, PA), a genetically altered form of rt-PA (currently approved by the FDA for use in acute myocardial infarction), has been used for the treatment of pulmonary emboli.[43] Recently Davidian et al. reported on their initial positive experience using reteplase for acute lower extremity arterial occlusions.[44]

Long-term results

Long-term patency is improved if underlying lesions are treated promptly with either percutaneous and/or surgical procedures, regardless of vessel or conduit.[12,14,23,45] If thrombolysis fails, then surgical procedures (graft revision and/or thrombectomy) also tend to do poorly.[22,45]

Suprainguinal conduits tend to have a longer patency than infrainguinal conduits.[12,45] In addition, vein grafts also tend to do better than synthetic grafts.[23] Still, Durham et al.[45] found that surgically treated occluded suprainguinal grafts tend to do better than when lysed. The best results suggest that grafts that have been treated with thrombolysis followed by a definitive revascularization procedure – percutaneous transluminal angioplasty (PTA) or surgery – have an 85% patency after 2 years.[23] This is comparable to failing (stenosing) grafts that have been successfully repaired surgically (patch angioplasty)[46] and superior to graft replacement. There is also a reported 2-year cumulative patency rate of 81% after intra-arterial thrombolysis.[47] In addition, Ouriel et al.[6] showed a significant improvement in event-free survival in patients treated with thrombolysis (with or without subsequent surgery) compared with those treated surgically.

Recent literature

Early studies dealing with the use of intra-arterial thrombolytic therapy were retrospective and often did not recognize variables relevant to the selection of appropriate therapy. Only recently have prospective studies been conducted dealing with the respective roles of thrombolytic therapy versus surgery in the treatment of occlusive lower extremity ischemia. These studies showed how both treatment options can be complementary to each other and clarified some issues dealing with intra-arterial thrombolytic therapy of lower extremity ischemia.

Ouriel et al.[6] studied 114 patients who suffered of limb-threatening lower extremity ischemia of less than 7 days' duration. Patients were divided into those going straight into surgery vs those who received a trial of intra-arterial lytic therapy with urokinase before subsequent surgical revascularization. The primary end point of the study was patient survival and limb salvage. Results of patients in the latter group were analyzed on an-intent-to-treat basis.[48] In the study, 70% of patients had successful thrombolysis. In addition, even though the cumulative limb-salvage rates were similar in both groups at 82% after 12 months, the cumulative survival rates were significantly higher in those given thrombolysis (84% vs 58%, $p = 0.001$). This finding was mostly due to the frequency of in-hospital cardiopulmonary complications in the surgical group (49%) vs the thrombolysis group (58%, $p = 0.01$). In addition, the thrombolysis group required fewer interventions than the surgical group. The authors concluded that thrombolytic therapy offered a safe and effective alternative to surgery in the initial treatment of acute, limb-threatening arterial occlusion.

The STILE trial[5] was a multicenter prospective randomized trial comparing surgery with thrombolytic therapy for nonembolic, lower extremity arterial occlusion. Patients included had lower limb ischemia of equal or less than 6 months' duration and were randomized into three groups:

- surgery
- intra-arterial thrombolysis with urokinase
- intra-arterial thrombolysis with rt-PA

The results of urokinase and rt-PA were similar and were combined. Overall, the study showed no significant difference on mortality, amputation, or major morbidity between surgery and lysis groups.

Secondary end points of the trial included 'outcome based on duration of ischemia.' It was concluded that patients who suffer from acute lower limb ischemia respond better to intra-arterial thrombolytic therapy and that those with chronic ischemia had better outcomes with surgery.

The TOPAS trial[49] had a primary objective to compare the safety and efficacy of intra-arterial thrombolytic therapy (using urokinase) and surgery for patients with acute arterial occlusion of less than 14 days' duration. Phase I studied the best dose of recombinant urokinase to give the best results in the 4-hour angiogram. Also, safety and changes in hemostatic parameters were determined. The optimal dose was found to be 4000 U/min. Phase II[50] compared this optimal dose of recombinant urokinase (r-urokinase) with surgery. It was determined that lytic therapy can reduce the need for invasive procedures during the first 6 months and 30% of patients were spared an open surgical procedure. In addition, that graft occlusions were more likely to lyse than native arteries. At 6 months there was no significant difference in the frequency of deaths or major amputations between surgery and lysis.

A cost-analysis[51] based on Ouriel's original data[6] showed no significant difference in cost between surgery and lytic therapy.

Since urokinase has been removed from the market there has been much confusion among the community as to what thrombolytic agent to use. As previously stated, presently, rt-PA and reteplase are the most commonly used agents. Valji[40] recently reviewed the current protocols for the use of these agents. However, it was concluded that prospective clinical trials need to be conducted to find the 'safest and most effective protocols for use of these agents'.[40]

Venous thrombolysis

Until recently, the treatment of acute deep venous thrombosis (DVT) of the lower extremities has focused on relieving symptoms and decreasing the risk of pulmonary embolism. Typically, patients have been treated with intravenous infusion of heparin and subsequent oral anticoagulation with warfarin with good results.[52] Lately low-molecular-weight heparins have been tried, particularly on an outpatient basis.[53] No studies are yet available regarding the complete resolution of DVT or prevention of chronic vein thrombosis with this therapy.

Treatment of DVT with conventional therapy has shown that less than 10% of patients had complete resolution of thrombus and that, despite adequate anticoagulation, over 40% of patients had thrombus propagation.[54] Many of the patients in this group developed post-thrombotic syndrome (PTS), which consists of persistent leg pain and edema, hyperpigmentation, and even skin ulceration and venous claudication.

Late sequelae of DVT may be reduced by early thrombus regression.[55] Several studies[55–59] concluded that systemic thrombolytic therapy was beneficial to patients with DVT, particularly in the acute state (less than 7 days).[59] However, systemic infusion of thrombolytic therapy presents with increased risks of bleeding complications and less efficacy than local intrathrombus infusion.

Catheter-directed thrombolytic therapy is indicated for patients with symptoms of DVT (acute leg edema and pain) of less than 14 days' duration and with documented iliofemoral DVT. Its application has been described previously.[60] Treatment progression is monitored every 8–12 hours to document progression of lysis and stopped once the thrombus is completely resolved or there is no improvement. Use of prophylactic inferior vena cava (IVC) filters is debatable and considered generally unnecessary. Subsequent interventions (angioplasty and/or stent) may be performed after the treatment is completed. Systemic anticoagulation through the introducer sheath is initiated until oral anticoagulation takes effect.

Since UK is presently off the market, several studies have reported the use of rt-PA[61–68] in venous thrombolysis. A comparison between the use of rt-PA and UK[69] demonstrated complete lysis in 27% of patients treated with rt-PA vs 50% of patients treated with UK.

The US venous thrombolysis national multicenter registry has collected data on 473 symptomatic patients with lower extremity DVT treated with urokinase and analysis on 287 of these patients with 6-month follow-up was published.[70] Overall, they found that 83% of patients had over 50% lysis of their DVT with complete thrombolysis in 31% of patients. This depended mainly on placing the catheter within the clot. The overall patency rate after 1 year was 60%, with 79% patency when complete lysis was achieved. Semba, on the other hand[60] had a 1-year patency rate of 90% among patients free of malignancy. Patients with extrinsic compression of the iliac vein had extremely good results. He also reported no major complications such as pulmonary embolism, hemorrhagic stroke, or death. The venous registry[70] on the other hand, reported 11% major bleeding rate, 6 pulmonary emboli (1 fatal), and 1 death from intracranial hemorrhage. Still more data are needed to prove the long-term efficacy of venous thrombolysis, hopefully, the national venous registry will provide the data.

References

1   Baxter-Smith D, Ashton F, Slaney G. Peripheral arterial embolism: a 20-year review. J Cardiovasc Surg 1988; **29**: 453.

2   Linton RR. Peripheral arterial embolism: a discussion of the post-embolic vascular changes and their relation to the restoration of circulation in peripheral embolism. N Eng J Med 1941; **224**: 189.

3   Mackey WC. Peripheral embolization and thrombosis. In: Strandness DE Jr, van Berda A (eds), Vascular diseases: surgical and interventional therapy. New York: Churchill Livingstone, 1994: 341–54.

4   McPhail NV, Frastesi SJ, Barber GG et al. Management of acute thromboembolic limb ischemia. Surgery 1983; **93**: 381–5.

5   The STILE investigators. Results of a prospective randomized trials evaluating surgery versus thrombolysis for ischemia of the lower extremities. Ann Surg 1994; **220**: 251–68.

6   Ouriel K, Shortell CK, De Weese JA et al. A comparison of thrombolytic therapy with operative revascularization in the initial treatment of acute peripheral arterial ischemia. J Vasc Surg 1994; **19**: 1021–30.

7   McNamara TO, Fisher JR. Thrombolysis in peripheral arterial and graft occlusions: improved results using high dose urokinase. AJR 1985; **144**: 764–75.

8   Belli AM. Thrombolysis in the peripheral vascular system. Cardvasc Intervent Radiol 1998; **21**: 95–101.

9   Bowles CR, Olcott C, Pakter RL, Lombard C, Mehigan JT, Walter JF. Diffuse arterial narrowing as a result of intimal proliferation: a delayed complication of embolectomy with the Fogarty balloon catheter. J Vasc Surg 1988; **7**: 487–94.

10 Dotter CT, Rosch J, Seaman AJ. Selective clot lysis with low-dose streptokinase. Radiology 1974; **111**: 31–7.

11 McNicol GB, Reid W, Bain WH, Douglas AS. Treatment of peripheral arterial occlusions by streptokinase perfusion. Br Med J 1963; **1**: 1508–12.

12 McNamara TO, Bomberger RA. Factors affecting initial and six month patency rates after intra-arterial thrombolysis with high dose urokinase. Am J Surg 1986; **152**: 709–12.

13 The International Working Group. Thrombolysis in the management of lower limb peripheral arterial occlusion: a consensus document. Am J Cardiol 1998; **81**: 207–18.

14 McNamara TO. Thrombolysis as an alternative initial therapy for the acutely ischemic limb. Semin Vasc Surg 1992; **5**: 89–98.

15 Huetl EA, Soulen MC. Thrombolysis of lower extremity embolic occlusions: a study of the results of the STAR registry. JVIR 1995; **197**: 141–5.

16 Luppatelli L, Barzi F, Corneli P, Lemmi A, Mosca S. Selective thrombolysis with low-dose urokinase in chronic atherosclerotic occlusions. Cardiovasc Intervent Radiol 1988; **11**: 123–6.

17 Wholey MH, Maynar MA, Wholey MH et al. Comparison of thrombolytic therapy of lower-extremity acute, subacute, and chronic arterial occlusions. Cath Cardiovasc Diagn 1998; **44**: 159–69.

18 Graor RA, Olin J, Bartholomeu JR, Ruschhaupt WF, Young JR. Efficacy and safety of intraarterial local infusion of streptokinase, urokinase, or tissue plasminogen activator for peripheral arterial occlusion: a retrospective review. J Vasc Med Biol 1990; **2**: 310–15.

19 Woo KS, White HD. Comparative tolerability profiles of thrombolytic agents: a review. Drug Safety 1993; **8**: 19–29.

20 Braithwaite BD, Davies B, Birch PA, Heather BP, Earnshaw JJ. Management of acute leg ischemia in the elderly. Br J Surg 1998; **85**: 217–20.

21 McNamara TO, Goodwin SC, Kandarpa K. Complications associated with thrombolysis. Semin Intervent Radiol 1994; **2**: 134–44.

22 Gardiner GA et al. Thrombolysis of occluded femoropopliteal grafts. AJR 1986; **147**: 621–6.

23 Sulhvan KL et al. Efficacy of thrombolysis in infrainguinal bypass grafts. Circulation 1991; **83**:(suppl 1): 1-99–1-105.

24 Belkin M et al. Intra-arterial fibrinolytic therapy. Arch Surg 1986; **121**: 769–73.

25 Motarjeme A. Thrombolytic therapy in arterial occlusion and graft thrombosis. Semin Vasc Surg 1989; **2**: 155–78.

26 Van Breda A. Thrombolytic therapy of peripheral vascular occlusions. In: Kim D, Orron DE (eds) Peripheral vascular imaging and interventions. St. Louis: Mosby, 1992: 429–39.

27 Haimovici H. Arterial embolism with acute massive ischemic myopathy and myoglobinuria. *Surgery* 1960; **47**: 739–47.

28 Beyersdorf F, Matheis G, Kruger S et al. Avoiding reperfusion injury after revascularization: experimental observations and recommendations for clinical application. *J Vasc Surg* 1989; **9**: 757–66.

29 Ogilby JD, Kopelman HA, Klein LW, Agarwal JB. Adequate heparinization during PTCA: assessment using activated clotting times. *Cath Cardiovasc Diagn* 1989; **18**: 206–9.

30 Gardiner GA, Sullivan KL. Complications of regional thrombolytic therapy. In: Kadir S (ed.), *Current practice of interventional radiology*. Philadelphia: BC Decker 1991: 87–91.

31 Marder VJ. Relevance of changes in blood fibrinolytic and coagulation parameters during thrombolytic therapy. *Am J Med* 1987; **83**(2A): 15–19.

32 Sullivan KL, Gardiner GA, Shapiro MJ, Bonn J, Levin DC. Acceleration of thrombolysis with a high-dose transthrombus bolus technique. *Radiology* 1989; **173**: 805–8.

33 Meyerovitz MF, Goldhaber SZ, Reagan K et al. Recombinant tissue-type plasminogen activator versus urokinase in peripheral arterial and graft occlusions: a randomized trial. *Radiology* 1990; **175**: 75–8.

34 Kandarpa K, Chopra PS, Aruni JE et al. Intraarterial thrombolysis of lower extremity occlusions: a prospective, randomized comparison of forced periodic infusion and conventional slow continuous infusion. *Radiology* 1993; **188**: 861–7.

35 Luppatelli L et al. Selective thrombolysis with low-dose urokinase in chronic atherosclerotic occlusions. *Cardiovasc Intervent Radiol* 1988; **11**: 213–26.

36 Food and Drug Administration. Important drug warning. Center for Biologics Evaluation and Research. Urokinase. Dated July 1999.

37 Graor RA et al. Efficacy and safety of intraarterial local infusion of streptokinase, urokinase, or tissue plasminogen activator for peripheral arterial occlusion: a retrospective review. *J Vasc Med Biol* 1990; **2**: 310–15.

38 Katzen BT, van Breda A. Low-dose streptokinase in the treatment of arterial occlusion. *AJR* 1981; **136**: 1171–8.

39 Van Breda A et al. Relative cost-effectiveness of urokinase versus streptokinase in the treatment of peripheral vascular disease. *JVIR* 1991; **2**: 77–87.

40 Valji K. Evolving strategies for thrombolytic therapy of peripheral vascular occlusion. *JVIR* 2000; **11**: 411–20.

41 Van Breda A, Katzen BT, Deutsch AS. Urokinase versus streptokinase in local thrombolysis. *Radiology* 1987; **165**: 109–11.

42 Marder V, Sherry S. Thrombolytic therapy: current status. *N Engl J Med* 1988; **318**: 1512–20.

43 Tebbe U, Graf A, Kamke W et al. Hemodynamic effects of double bolus reteplase versus alteplase infusion in massive pulmonary embolism. *Am Heart J* 1999; **138**: 39–44.

44 Davidian MM, Powell A, Benenati JF, Katzen BT, Becker GJ, Zemel G. Initial results of reteplase in the treatment of acute lower extremity arterial occlusions. *JVIR* 2000; **11**: 289–294.

45 Durham JD, Rutheford RB. Assessment of long-term efficacy of fibrinolytic therapy in the ischemic extremity. *Semin Intervent Radiol* 1992; **9**: 166–73.

46 Cohen JR et al. Recognition and management of impending graft failure. *Arch Surg* 1986; **121**: 758–9.

47 Lammer J et al. Intraarterial fibrinolysis: long term results. *Radiology* 1986; **161**: 159–63.

48 Ouriel K, Shortell CK, Azodo MVU et al. Acute peripheral arterial occlusion: predictors of success in catheter-directed thrombolytic therapy. *Radiology* 1994; **193**: 561–6.

49 Ouriel K, Veith FJ, Sasahara AA. Thrombolysis or peripheral arterial surgery (TOPAS): Phase I results. *J Vasc Surg* 1996; **23**: 64–73.

50 Ouriel K, Veith FJ, Sasahara AA. A comparison of recombinant urokinase with vascular surgery as initial treatment of acute arterial occlusions in legs. *N Engl J Med* 1998; **338**: 1105–11.

51 Ouriel K, Kolassa M, DeWeese JA, Green RM. Economic implications of thrombolysis or operation as the initial treatment modality in acute peripheral arterial occlusion. *Surgery* 1995; **118**: 810–14.

52 Hirsh J, Hoak J. Management of deep venous thrombosis and pulmonary embolism. *Circulation* 1996; **93**: 2212–45.

53 Hull RD, Raskob GE, Rosenblum D et al. Treatment of proximal vein thrombosis with SQ low molecular weight heparin versus IV heparin. *Arch Intern Med* 1997; **157**: 289–94.

54 Krupski WC, Bass A et al. Propagation of deep venous thrombosis identified by duplex ultrasonography. *J Vasc Surg* 1990; **12**: 467–75.

55 Bredding HK. Treatment of deep vein thrombosis: Is thrombosis regression a desirable endpoint? *Sem Thromb Hemost* 1997; **23**: 179–83.

56 Goldhaber SZ, Buring JE et al. Pooled analyses of randomized trials of streptokinase and heparin in phlemographically documented acute deep venous thrombosis. *Am J Med* 1984; **76**: 393–7.

57 Goldhaber SZ, Meyerovitz MF et al. Randomized controlled trials of tissue plasminogen activator in proximal deep venous thrombosis. *Am J Med* 1990; **88**: 235–40.

58 Comerota AJ, Aldridge BC. Thrombolytic therapy for deep venous thrombosis: a critical review. *Can J Surg* 1993; **36**: 359–64.

59 Eichlisberger R, Frauchiger B et al. Late sequela of deep venous thrombosis: a 13-year follow-up of 223 patients. *Vasa* 1994; **23**: 234–43.

60 Semba CP, Dake MD. Iliofemoral deep venous thrombosis: aggressive therapy with catheter directed thrombolysis. *Radiology* 1994; **191**: 487–94.

61 Comerota AJ. Local fibrinolytic therapy of iliac vein thrombosis. *Int J Angiology* 1996; **5**: S41–6.

62 Buelens V, Vandenbosch G et al. Cockett's syndrome: initial experience wth percutaneous treatment in 6 patients. *J Belge Radiol* 1996; **79**: 132–5.

63 Armon MP, Whitaker SC, Tennant WG. Catheter-directed thrombolysis of iliofemoral deep vein thrombosis: a new approach via the posterior tibial vein. *Eur J Vasc Endovasc Surg* 1997; **13**: 413–6.

64 Comerota AJ, Aldridge SC et al. A strategy of aggressive regional therapy for acute iliofemoral venous thrombosis with contemporary venous thrombectomy or catheter-directed thrombolysis. *J Vasc Surg* 1994; **20**: 244–54

65 Grossman C, McPherson S. Safety and efficacy of catheter-directed thrombolysis for iliofemoral venous thrombosis. *AJR* 1999; **172**: 667–72.

66 Verhaege R, Stockx L et al. Catheter-directed lysis of iliofemoral vein thrombosis with use of rt-PA. *Eur J Radiol* 1997; **7**: 996–1001.

67 Palombo F, Porta C et al. Loco-regional thrombolysis in deep venous thrombosis. *Phlebologie* 1993; **46**: 293–302.

68 Chang R, Horne MK III et al. Pulse-spray treatment of subclavian and jugular venous thrombi with recombinant tissue plasminogen activator. *JVIR* 1996; **7**: 845–51.

69 Schweizer J, Elix H et al. Comparative results of thrombolysis treatment with rt-PA and urokinase: a pilot study. *Vasa* 1998; **27**: 167–71.

70 Mewissen MW, Seabrook GR et al. Catheter-directed thrombolysis for lower extremity deep venous thrombosis: a report of a National Multicenter Registry. *Radiology* 1999; **211**: 39–49.

71 Kandarpa K. Catheter-directed thrombolysis of peripheral arterial occlusions and deep venous thrombosis. *Thromb Haemost* 1999; **82**: 987–96.

23

Catheter-directed thrombolysis for lower extremity deep vein thrombosis

Mark W Mewissen

Introduction

The therapeutic goals for treating the patient with acute deep vein thrombosis (DVT) include preventing pulmonary embolus, restoration of unobstructed bloodflow through the thrombosed segment, prevention of recurrent thrombosis and preservation of venous valve function. Success in achieving these clinical goals will minimize the morbidity and mortality of pulmonary embolism and will also diminish the sequelae of the post-thrombotic syndrome (PTS). As shown by Johnson, it is the combination of reflux and obstruction that correlates with the severity of PTS, as opposed to either alone.[1] Up to two-thirds of the patients with iliofemoral DVT will develop edema and pain, with 5% developing ulcers in spite of adequate anticoagulation.[2]

The standard of care at the moment includes systemic anticoagulation with heparin followed by coumarin therapy.[3] Such a regimen, however, does not promote lysis to reduce the thrombus load nor does it contribute to restoration of venous valvular function. Anticoagulation alone, therefore, does not protect the limb from PTS, which can occur months to years following the acute thrombotic event.[2]

Thrombolysis is a potentially attractive form of therapy, since it provides the opportunity for promptly restoring venous patency and preserving venous valve function. This therapy provides the potential for preventing the long-term sequelae of DVT. There is published evidence that thrombolytic agents, even administered systemically, are superior to standard anticoagulation therapy in achieving early lysis of thrombus. In a pooled analysis of 13 randomized studies, Comerota and Aldridge found that only 4% of patients treated with heparin had significant or complete lysis compared to 45% of patients randomized to systemic streptokinase therapy.[4] Similarly, in reviewing pooled data from six trials judged to have proper randomization, systemic thrombolysis was 3.7 times more effective in producing some degree of lysis than was heparin.[5] In spite of these results, progress was hindered, probably because of the use of systemic administration, where the drug does not reach the thrombus in sufficient concentration to provide optimal results.

The report by Semba and Dake in 1994 provided the first insight into the potential role of catheter-directed thrombolytic (CDT) techniques.[6] They reported complete lysis in 72% of the patients with concomitant resolution of symptoms. Only one patient suffered a bleeding complication of heme-positive stools. After the drug was discontinued, there were no significant adverse sequelae. Delivering the thrombolytic agent directly into the thrombus offers significant advantages over systemic therapy, which may fail to reach and penetrate an occluded venous segment. Because thrombolytic agents activate plasminogen within the thrombus, delivery of the drug to that site enhances its effectiveness. By focusing the delivery of higher concentrations of drug, lysis rates can be improved, the duration of treatment can be reduced, and complications associated with the exposure of the patient to systemic thrombolytic therapy may be reduced. The progress of CDT can be monitored by direct imaging techniques, and lesions potentially contributing to the thrombosis can be identified. These defects, such as stenosis of the common iliac vein, can be treated by balloon angioplasty with or without the placement of endovascular stents (Figure 23.1).

The abrupt removal of urokinase in the USA in 1999 has had a swift and profound effect on the management of venous (and arterial) thromboses. Currently, the agents of choice for non-coronary lytic therapy therapy are alteplase (rt-PA) and retaplase (r-PA). Their optimal dose, use of concomitant heparin, and the technique of catheter-directed treatment are undergoing evaluation.

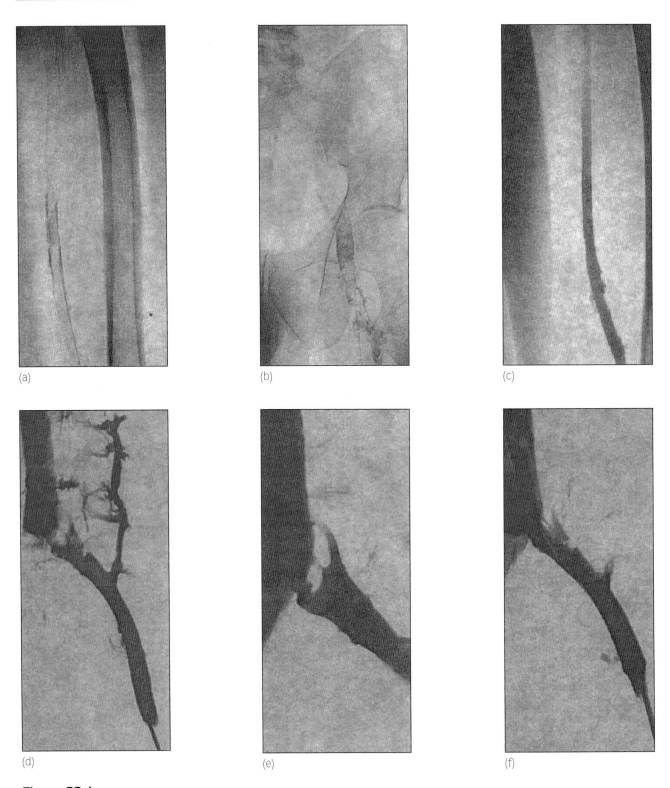

(a)

(b)

(c)

(d)

(e)

(f)

Figure 23.1

Forty-five-year-old man who presented with a 1-week history of worsening pain and swelling of the left lower extremity. Duplex study revealed DVT extending from the popliteal vein to the common iliac vein. Following catheterization of the left posterior tibial vein at the ankle under ultrasound guidance, the non-invasive studies are confirmed at venography: there is thrombosis of the superficial femoral, common femoral, and external and common iliac veins (a, b). Following administration of 20 units of retavase over 20 h directly into the thrombus with a 5F coaxial infusing system, there is complete lysis demonstrated in all previously thrombosed vein (c, d). Note uncovered stenosis in proximal common iliac vein (e), successfully treated with a self-expanding stent (f). At 6 months of follow-up, the deep veins remain patent and the patient is asymptomatic.

Technique of catheter-directed thrombolysis

With the patient prone on the angiographic table, we prefer the ipsilateral popliteal venous approach, because it is often difficult to penetrate an occluded superficial femoral vein from the internal jugular vein or the contralateral common femoral vein, due to venous valves that may prevent safe catheter and guidewire manipulations. Should the popliteal vein be thrombosed, the ipsilateral posterior tibial vein is cannulated. The venous access site should be accessed under ultrasound guidance with a small-gauge echogenic needle. A 5F short sheath is then introduced, via which all subsequent catheters can be exchanged. Following baseline venography obtained via the venous sheath, the occluded venous segment is crossed with a straight-tip 5F catheter and a 0.035-inch curved-tip glide wire. Venography is then repeated to confirm intraluminal passage of the catheter, which is then exchanged for a 5F infusing coaxial system, consisting of a proximal multi-sidehole catheter and a distal infusing wire. It is critical to position the system directly into the thrombus, to maximize plasminogen activation at the site of obstruction. Before 1999, urokinase therapy was initiated at 150 000–200 000 units/h, evenly split between the infusing ports. Currently, anecdotal experience with retaplase and alteplase would suggest that one unit per hour for the former and 0.5 mg/h for the latter is a safe and effective strategy. Intravenous heparin is concomitantly administered via the popliteal (or tibial) sheath at a rate of 500–1000 units/h following a 5000–unit bolus of heparin. Patients are monitored in the intensive care unit or a step-down unit, like those receiving thombolytic treatment for acute PE or an arterial occlusion. Because the duration of therapy may be in excess of 24 h, it is not necessary to frequently assess the progress of lysis. The frequency of follow-up venograms should be every 12 h, primarily to reposition the infusion devices into the remaining thrombus. Gentle thrombus maceration with a 6-mm balloon angioplasty catheter may be helpful, particularly in the superficial femoral vein, where focal narrowings are at times encountered, probably representing sites of organized thrombus. Typically, unless a complication would dictate otherwise, lytic therapy should be continued until complete lysis is achieved, unless no discernable progress is venographically demonstrated from the previous venogram obtained 12 h previously. Since the grade of thrombolysis has been shown in the Registry to be a strong predictor of continued patency, it is critical that a complete lysis venogram be achieved. Lesions uncovered in the iliac venous segments should probably be treated with stents, although the long-term benefits of such devices are not known. However, if left untreated, there appears to be a significant risk of early rethrombosis.

Results of the venous registry

Clearly, the initial report by Semba and Dake suggested that CDT can be effective in achieving significant lysis of thrombus and may be associated with low complication rates. This experience stimulated the development of a multicenter study with enrollment of almost 500 patients within over 50 Northern American centers.[7] Complete data with follow-up of at least 6 months were available on nearly 300 patients, 70% of whom had iliofemoral DVT (IFDVT). Treatment duration averaged more than 48 h with close to 7 million units of urokinase being administered in those with direct intrathrombus delivery. One-third of the patients received adjunctive stenting for residual narrowing, but close to 40% in the IFVT group and close to half of those with left-sided involvement. The difference between the pre- and post-lytic thrombus scores divided by the pre-lytic score resulted in a percentage of thrombolysis achieved, which was then classified into three groups for analysis: grade I, <50% lysis; grade II, >50% lysis; and grade III, 100% or complete lysis (Table 23.1). Grade II and III lysis were achieved in over 80% of cases. Complete lysis was achieved in close to one-third.

The degree of lysis was found to be a significant predictor of early and continued patency (Figure 23.2). Seventy-five per cent

Table 23.1   Example of pre- and post-lysis thrombus scores and calculation of lysis grade in a patient with Iliofemoral DVT

	IVC	CIV	EIV	CFV	pSFV	dSFV	PopV	Score
Pre-lysis	0	2	2	2	2	0	0	8
Post-lysis	0	0	0	1	1	0	0	2

Thrombus score: 0: patent; 1: partially occluded; 2: complete occlusion.

Venous segments: IVC, inferior vena cava; CIV, common iliac vein; EIV, external iliac vein; CFV, common femoral vein; pSFV, proximal superficial femoral vein; dSFV, distal superficial femoral vein; PopV, popliteal vein.

Pre-lysis venographic evaluation of a patient with iliofemoral DVT, extending into the proximal superficial femoral vein. Following lysis, residual partially occluding thrombus remains in the common femoral and proximal superficial veins. The lysis grade is calculated as follows: (8–2)/8 = 0.75, resulting in grade II lytic grade.

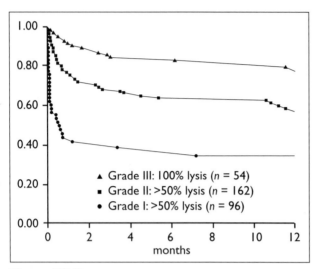

Figure 23.2
Patency curves following thrombolysis with respect to lytic grades.

of limbs with complete lysis remained patent at 1 year, compared to only 32% for limbs with insignificant lysis (<50%). In general, acute DVT (<10 days) predicted a better lysis grade when compared to chronic DVT (>10 days), although significant lysis could be achieved in patients with chronic IFDVT. When isolated FPDVT was present for more than 10 days, none achieved complete lysis. Reflux at 6-months of follow-up was less than 30% in those with complete lysis, around 45% in those with >50% lysis, but over 60% in those with <50% initial lysis, again showing the greater protective effect of complete clot removal. Longer follow-up, including those who still had incomplete data at 6 months, should provide more definitive recommendations based on careful subgroup analysis and functional evaluation. There were only two deaths in the entire study (0.4%), one from intracranial hemorrhage and one of the six patients who suffered a PE (1.2%).

Because the Registry was not designed to be a controlled trial, no restrictions were imposed on patient enrollment, such as duration of symptoms, location of thrombus, prior history of DVT or technique of thrombolysis. Therefore, patients with a variety of these features were prospectively enrolled. This may help explain a relatively low overall yield of complete lysis (31%). However, when the patients are analyzed by subgroups, several important observations can be made. For example, for a patient with acute IFDVT and no prior history of previous DVT, when CDT was performed via the popliteal vein (without a pedal infusion), complete lysis occurred 65% of the time and the 1-year patency was 96%. At the other extreme, complete lysis never occurred in any patients with chronic FPDVT. Analysis of groups with particular combinations of features provides a useful perspective of what can be expected from CDT in different settings and can serve as a guide to patient selection for this potentially effective form of treatment (although the groups are not always numerous enough for statistical comparison).

Based on health-related quality of life (HRQOL) evaluation, Camerota et al recently reported on the benefits of catheter lysis in patients entered in the venous registry with IFDVT.[8] After lytic treatment, patients reported better overall physical functioning, less stigma, less health distress, and fewer post-thrombotic symptoms, compared with similar patients treated with anticoagulation alone. Successful lysis was directly correlated with improved HRQOL, with patients who were classified as lytic failures having similar outcomes to patients treated with heparin alone.

Patient selection for lower extremity DVT

Patients with acute IFDVT and a life-expectancy not hampered by fatal illness are likely to suffer from severe post-thrombotic sequelae and should benefit most from lytic therapy. Any patient who presents with phlegmasia cerulea dolens, irrespective of age or underlying disease, should be considered for treatment unless a contraindication is obvious. Final analysis of the Venous Registry data will hopefully identify variables that will impact upon late outcome, and help better define patients who will most benefit from lytic therapy.

Conclusion

CDT can safely and effectively dissolve thrombus from the deep veins of identifiable groups of patients with symptomatic lower limb DVT. The best results can be expected in patients with acute symptoms without a prior history of DVT, who are treated with CDT without systemic infusion. The long-term benefits of this form of therapy are not yet known and cannot be conclusively derived from this study. The Registry data should help in the design of the protocol of a controlled trial comparing CDT and anticoagulation which will be necessary to validate the long-term benefits of CDT and its application for the prevention of the post-thrombotic syndrome.

References

1   Johnson BF, Manzo RA, Bergelin RO, Srandness DE Jr. Relationship between changes in the deep venous system and the development of the post-thrombotic syndrome after an acute episode of lower limb deep venous thrombosis: a one-to-six year follow-up. *J Vasc Surg* 1995; **21**: 307.

2   Strandness DE, Langlois Y, Cramer M et al. Long-term sequelae of acute venous thrombosis. *JAMA* 1983; **250**: 1289–92.

3   Hull RD, Raskob GE, Rosenbloom D et al. Heparin for 5 days as compared with 10 days in the initial treatment of proximal venous thrombosis. *N Engl J Med* 1990; **322**(18):1260–4.

4   Comerota A, Aldridge SC. Thrombolytic therapy for deep venous thrombosis: a clinical review. *Can J Surg* 1993; **36**: 359–64.

5   Goldhaber SZ, Buring JE, Lipchick RJ et al. Pooled analysis of randomized trials of streptokinase and heparin in phlebographically documented acute deep venous thrombosis. *Am J Med* 1984; **76**: 393–7.

6   Semba CP, Dake MD. Catheter directed thrombolysis for iliofemoral venous thrombosis. *Radiology* 1994; **191**: 487–94.

7   Mewissen MW, Seabrook GR, Meissner MH et al. Catheter-directed thrombolysis for lower extremity deep venous thrombosis: Report of a National Multicenter Registry. *Radiology* 1999; **211**: 39–49.

8   Camerota AJ, Throm RC, Mathias SD et al. Catheter-directed thrombolysis for iliofemoral deep vein thrombosis improves health-related quality of life. *Vasc Surg* 2000; **32**:130–7.

24

Drug-eluting stents for peripheral applications

Philip A Morales and Richard R Heuser

Introduction

Stents have significantly changed the field of interventional therapy. They are becoming more widely used in everyday clinical practice. Whereas endovascular stent–grafts in the aortoiliac vessels help maintain immediate and long-term patency rates that are comparable to that of surgery,[1–3] the same cannot be said for femoropopliteal vessels. Stents in femoropopliteal vessels do not significantly improve the long-term patency rates when compared to angioplasty alone.[4–6] The usual indications for stenting in the femoropopliteal vessels are therefore left for suboptimal balloon angioplasty results with residual stenosis or flow-limiting dissections. Still, the long-term success of stenting is hampered by in-stent restenosis. This becomes a major clinical problem, as the increasing use of stents will only increase the incidence of in-stent restenosis. Also the treatment of in-stent restenosis can be, despite progress in radiation therapy, technically challenging and costly.

In-stent restenosis is marked by exaggerated and uncontrolled neointimal hyperplasia.[7–8] It is considered as a component of the general vascular response to injury. Catheter-induced injury consists in denuding of the intima and stretching of the media and adventitia. The wound-healing reaction starts with an inflammatory phase, characterized by platelets, growth factor, and smooth muscle cell activation. Next, the granulation phase is characterized by smooth muscle cell and fibroblast migration and proliferation into the injured area. Finally, the remodelling phase is characterized by maturation of the neointima, proteoglycan, and collagen synthesis, which replaces early fibronectin as major components of extracellular matrix.

In-stent restenosis is associated with diabetes mellitus,[9] vessel size,[10] lesion length, extent of disease, number of stents, and minimal stent diameter or area. Over the years, treating restenosis has focused on optimizing stent characteristics and placement technique. Systemic pharmacological therapy has not been successful in totally eliminating restenosis.[11] One explanation for repeated failure of clinical drug studies could be that these agents when given systemically cannot reach sufficient levels in the injured (treated) arteries. Local drug delivery can offer advantages not readily available through systemic drug delivery. The active drug, coated on a stent, can be applied to the vessel at the precise site and at the time of vessel injury (i.e. angioplasty and/or stenting). Higher tissue concentration of the drug is possible through local drug delivery. There would be reduced risk of remote systemic toxicity given the minimal systemic release of the drug.

Potential candidates for local drug delivery

Ideally, the potential candidate or drug should effectively inhibit the multiple components of the complex restenosis process. Several pharmacological agents with antiproliferative properties have failed to inhibit restenosis after intervention.[12] Table 24.1 lists the potential agents for local drug delivery. Even though there is a wide variety of potential agents, some have not shown convincing preclinical results that may lead to further testing in clinical trials. The potential agents that are being tested in randomized clinical trials are actinomycin, rapamycin, and paclitaxel. Although the majority of drug-eluting stent trials deal with the treatment of coronary artery disease, one trial named SIROCCO (SIROlimus-Coated Cordis SMART™ nitinol self-expandable stent for the treatment of Obstructive superficial femoral artery disease) deals with the treatment of superficial femoral arteries.

Table 24.1 List of potential candidates for local drug delivery

Antineoplastic:
- Paclitaxel (Taxol®)
- Taxol derivative (QP-2)
- Actinomycin D
- Vincristine
- Methotrexate
- Angiopectin
- Mitomycin
- BCP 678
- Antisense c-muy
- Abbott ABT 578

Migration inhibitor/ECM modulators:
- Halofuginone
- Propyl hydroxylase inhibitor
- C-proteinase inhibitor
- Metalloproteinase inhibitors
- Batimastat

Antithrombus:
- Hirudin and Iloprost
- Heparin
- Abciximab

Immunosuppressants:
- Sirolimus (rapamycin)
- Tacrolimus (FK506)
- Tranilast
- Dexamethasone
- Methylprednisolone
- Interferon gamma 1b
- Leflunomide
- Cyclosporin

Enhance healing/promote endothelial function:
- VEGF
- 17-ß-estradiol
- Tkase inhibition
- BCP 671
- HMG CoA reductase inhibitor

Actinomycin D (Cosmegen®)

Actinomycin D is an antibiotic produced by various species of *Streptomyces* and is used for its antiproliferative properties in the treatment of various malignant neoplasms (e.g., Wilms' tumor, rhabdomyosarcomas, carcinoma of testis and uterus). It inhibits the proliferation of cells by forming a stable complex with double-strand DNA and inhibiting DNA-primed RNA synthesis.

There is no current published research documenting the use of antinomycin D for the treatment of coronary artery disease and restenosis. In 2001, a phase one, randomized clinical trial named ACTION (ACTinomycin-eluting stent Improves Outcomes by reducing Neointimal hyperplasia) was started to evaluate the safety and performance of the Multi-link tetra-D stent system. The enrollment is 360 patients randomized to receive an actinomycin D coated stent (high dose $10\,\mu g/cm^2$; low dose $2.5\,\mu g/cm^2$) or a non-coated stent for treatment of de-novo lesions in native coronary arteries with a vessel caliber of 3.0–4.0 mm. Six-month angiographic follow-up is expected to be completed in 2002 and a 12-month clinical follow-up is expected to be completed at the end of 2002.

Rapamycin (Sirolimus; Rapamune®)

Rapamycin has its roots in Easter Island where an actinomycete, *Streptomyces hygroscopicus*; was found to produce a macrolide

antibiotic with potent antifungal, immunosuppressive, and antimitotic properties. After its immunosuppressive properties had been established it was given the pharmacopoeial name sirolimus. Since 1999, sirolimus has been used as an anti-rejection drug in organ-transplant recipients, particularly renal transplant recipients. It is a naturally occurring macrocyclic lactone that inhibits cytokine-mediated and growth-factor-mediated proliferation of lymphocytes and smooth muscle cells. Sirolimus blocks G1 to S cell cycle progression by interacting with a specific target protein (mTOR – mammalian Target of Rapamycin) and inhibits its activation. The inhibition of mTOR suppresses cytokine-driven T-cell proliferation. Sirolimus also prevents proliferation and migration of smooth muscle cells. Preclinical efficacy studies demonstrated a 35–50% reduction in in-stent neointimal hyperplasia for the sirolimus-coated stents compared with bare metal stents at 28 days in the porcine and rabbit model.[13]

Paclitaxel (Taxol®)

Paclitaxel was originally isolated from the bark of the Pacific yew tree. It is an antineoplastic agent that is currently used to treat several types of cancer, most commonly breast and ovarian cancer. It is a diterpenoid with a characteristic taxane skeleton of 20 carbon atoms and has a molecular weight of 853.9Da. Its pharmacological action is through formation of numerous decentralized and unorganized microtubules. This enhances the assembly of extraordinarily stable microtubules, interrupting proliferation, migration, and signal transduction. Unlike other antiproliferative agents of the colchicine type, which inhibit microtubuli assembly, paclitaxel shifts the microtubule equilibrium towards microtubule assembly. It is highly lipophilic, which promotes a rapid cellular uptake, and has a long-lasting effect in the cell due to structural alteration of the cytoskeleton.

Preliminary studies have shown that paclitaxel may prevent or attenuate restenosis.[14,15] In a rat balloon injury model, intraperitoneal administration of paclitaxel reduced neointimal area. Paclitaxel-eluting stents have been studied using different types of stents and different animal models.[16,17] These studies reveal a significant, dose-dependent inhibition of neointimal hyperplasia. Furthermore, the tissue response in paclitaxel-treated vessels includes incomplete healing, few smooth muscle cells, late persistence of macrophages, and dense fibrin with little collagen as well as signs of positive remodelling of the stented segment.

Some of the current clinical trials using a paclitaxel-eluting stent include the ASPECT (Asian Paclitaxel Eluting stent Clinical Trial), ELUTES (European evaLUation of pacliTaxel Eluting Stent), and TAXUS I-IV (Paclitaxel-eluting NIR stent trial).[18] These current trials are mainly in the treatment of coronary artery disease. There are no current trials that deal with the treatment of peripheral vessels, particularly superficial femoral arteries.

Clinical trials using drug-eluting stents

RAVEL

The RAVEL (RAndomized, double-blind study with the sirolimus-eluting BX VElocity™ balloon expandable stent in the treatment of patients with de novo native coronary artery Lesions) trial is a multicenter, prospective trial comparing a bare metal stent to a drug-coated stent.[19] A total of 238 patients were randomized to a single sirolimus-coated stent ($140 \mu g/cm^2$) vs a bare metal BX Velocity™ stent. At 6 months follow-up, the degree of neointimal proliferation, manifested as the mean late lumen loss, was significantly lower in the sirolimus-stent group compared to the bare-stent group. The restenosis rate of the sirolimus-stent group was zero. There were no episodes of stent thrombosis. For the follow-up period of up to 1 year, the overall rate of major cardiac events was 5.8% in the sirolimus-stent group compared to 28.8% in the bare-stent group. Interestingly, the restenosis rate in the bare-stent group was 26.6%.

SIRIUS

The SIRIUS (a multicenter, randomized, double-blind study of the SIRollmUS-coated BX Velocity™ balloon-expandable stent in the treatment of patients with de-novo coronary artery lesions) trial is a prospective clinical trial being conducted in the United States. A total of 1100 patients with de-novo coronary artery lesion were randomized to either treatment with sirolimus-coated stent or bare-metal BX Velocity stent. The primary end point of the SIRIUS trial is target vessel failure at 9 months. Secondary end points are core laboratory analysis of angiographic and intravascular ultrasound (IVUS) data to determine treatment effects on neointimal hyperplasia and in-stent restenosis.

SIROCCO

The SIROCCO trial is a multicenter, double-blind, randomized, prospective feasibility trial. Thirty-six patients with obstructive superficial femoral artery disease were randomized to either a sirolimus-coated stent or a bare-metal SMART™ stent. At 6 months follow-up, the restenosis rate of the treated group was zero and there was no target lesion revascularization.

TAXUS I–IV[19]

The TAXUS I trial is a 61 patient, randomized, double-blind, multicenter feasibility trial to evaluate the safety of a slow-release paclitaxel-coated ($1.0 \mu g/mm^2$) NIR® coronary stent. Six-month angiographic and IVUS follow-up demonstrated a 50% reduction in late loss index for the paclitaxel-coated stent group compared with the bare-stent group. The TAXUS II trial is a 532 patient, double-blind, randomized, multicenter study that will evaluate the safety and performance of a slow- and moderate-release paclitaxel-coated stent in de-novo lesions. The TAXUS III–ISR trial is a feasibility study that will evaluate the safety of the paclitaxel-coated stent in the treatment of in-stent restenosis. The TAXUS IV trial is a 1600 patient pivotal, randomized, double-blind trial designed to study the safety and efficacy of moderate-release paclitaxel-coated stents in de-novo and in-stent restenosis lesions.

Conclusion

Restenosis continues to be the 'Achilles heel' of percutaneous interventions. Drug-eluting stents represent a new and exciting approach to reduce the incidence of restenosis. It is a simple modification of a technology that still has not proven its efficacy in treating superficial femoral arteries. Planned and ongoing clinical trials will help determine their full potential, especially in the treatment of long lesions, small distal vessels, chronic total occlusions, and multilevel disease in the peripheral vessels. Future direction of drug-eluting stents includes further study with the different classes of drugs that are potential agents for the inhibition of restenosis to the combination of biodegradability with drug delivery, or local gene therapy (e.g., local expression of proliferation regulatory genes; transfer of cytotoxic genes, VEGF).

References

1   Henry M, Amor M, Ethevenot G et al. Percutaneous endoluminal treatment of iliac occlusions: long-term follow-up in 105 patients. *J Endovasc Surg* 1998; **5**: 228–35.

2   Vorwerk D, Gunther RW, Schurmann K et al. Primary stent placement for chronic iliac artery occlusions: follow-up results in 103 patients. *Radiology* 1995; **194**: 745–9.

3   Sullivan TM, Childs MB, Bacharach JM et al. Percutaneous transluminal angioplasty and primary stenting of the iliac arteries in 288 patients. *J Vasc Surg* 1997; **25**: 829–39.

4   Do-dai-Do, Triller J, Walpoth BH et al. A comparison study of self-expandable stents vs. balloon angioplasty alone in femoropopliteal artery occlusions. *Cardiovasc Intervent Radiol* 1992: **15**: 306–12.

5   Rosenfield K, Schainfeld R, Pieczek A et al. Restenosis of endovascular stents from stent compression. *J Am Coll Cardiol* 1997; **29**: 238–38.

6   Strecker EP, Hagen B, Liermann D et al. Iliac and femoropopliteal occlusive disease treated with flexible tantalum stents. *Cardiovasc Intervent Radiol* 1993; **16**: 158–64.

7   Kearny M, Pieczek A, Haley L et al. Histopathology of in-stent restenosis in patients with peripheral artery disease. *Circulation* 1997; **95**: 1998–2002.

8   Komatsu R, Ueda M, Naruko T et al. Neointimal tissue response at sites of coronary stenting in humans: macroscopic, histological, and immunohistochemical analyses. *Circulation* 1998; **98**: 224–33.

9   Sobel BE. Acceleration of restenosis by diabetes: pathogenetic implications. *Circulation* 2001; **103**: 1185–7.

10   Mintz GS, Popma JJ, Pichard AD et al. Intravascular ultrasound predictors of restenosis after percutaneous transcatheter coronary revascularization. *J Am Coll Cardiol* 1996; **27**: 1678–87.

11   Lefkovits J, Topol EJ. Pharmacological approaches for the prevention of restenosis after percutaneous coronary intervention. *Prog Cardiovasc Dis* 1997; **40**: 141–58.

12   de Feyter PJ, Vos J, Rensing BJ. Anti-restenosis trials. *Curr Inter Cardiol Rep* 2000; **2**: 326–31.

13   Suzuki T, Kopia G, Hayashi S-I et al. Stent-based delivery of sirolimus reduces neointimal formation in a porcine coronary model. *Circulation* 2001; **104**: 1188–93.

14   Sollott SJ, Cheng L, Pauly RR et al. Taxol inhibits neointimal smooth muscle cell accumulation after angioplasty in the rat. *J Clin Invest* 1995; **95**: 1869–76.

15   Axel DT, Kunert W, Goggelmann C et al. Paclitaxel inhibits arterial smooth muscle cell proliferation and migration in vitro and in vivo using local drug delivery. *Circulation* 1997; **96**: 636–45.

16   Farb A, Heller PF, Shroff S et al. Pathological analysis of delivery of paclitaxel via a polymer-coated stent. *Circulation* 2001; **104**: 473–9.

17   Heldman AW, Cheng L, Jenkins GM et al. Paclitaxel stent coating inhibits neointimal hyperplasia at 4 weeks in a porcine model of coronary restenosis. *Circulation* 2001; **103**: 2289–95.

18   Hiatt BL, Ikeno F, Yeung AC. Drug-eluting stents for the prevention of restenosis: in quest for the Holy Grail. *Catheter Cardiovasc Interv* 2002; **55**: 409–17.

19   Morice MC, Serruys PW, Sousa JE et al. A Randomized comparison of a sirolimus-eluting stent with a standard stent for coronary revascularization. *N Engl J Med* 2002; **346**: 1773–80.

25

PTFE-covered stents

Richard R Heuser

Treatment for heart disease has changed considerably over the last several decades. One of the most important advances has been the advent of catheter-based techniques that allow minimally invasive solutions for treating ischemic heart disease. After Charles Dotter introduced transluminal angioplasty in the 1960s, coronary angioplasty was pioneered by Andreas Gruentzig following development of his balloon catheter in 1974. More recently, stents and covered stents have proven to be important adjuncts to Gruentzig's original procedure.

Dilatation of an artery with balloon angioplasty may injure the arterial lumen and produce a rough, irregular surface with small areas of dissection. The current theory of restenosis suggests a myoproliferative response to this injury causes subsequent intimal hyperplasia and a rapid cellular proliferation that leads to stenosis. Stenting may prevent injury to the lumen and reduce the potential for hyperplasia and restenosis; the likelihood of plaque disruption and embolization may also be decreased.

The introduction of stents has impacted the fields of cardiology and vascular surgery substantially by expanding therapeutic options for the treatment of cardiac and blood vessel disease. Stenting has been used with great success to improve luminal diameter and restore flow in occluded arteries; results have proved far superior to those seen with laser and atherectomy procedures. When compared with coronary balloon angioplasty, coronary stenting has been shown to reduce angiographic and clinical restenosis rates in patients with de-novo lesions in a single coronary artery[1–5] and/or vein graft.[6] A meta-analysis of the BENESTENT, STRESS, and START trials indicates that stenting reduced restenosis by 31% as compared to angioplasty ($p < 0.0001$) and decreased the risk of further need for a revascularization procedure by 35% ($p < 0.001$).[5] The mechanism by which a stent reduces restenosis is thought to be its ability to safely enlarge the vessel lumen at the obstructive coronary lesion

[2,7,8] and prevent acute coronary recoil and late-term vascular contraction.[9]

Although stents have reduced restenosis as compared to angioplasty, they have not obliterated the problem. The role of covered stents (also known as endoluminal grafts) as a treatment modality for both occlusive and aneurysmal disease is under study worldwide. The use of endovascular grafts for treatment of abdominal aortic aneurysms (AAAs) was introduced by Parodi in 1991,[10] and since that time, a number of investigators have described the successful use of covered stents or endoluminal grafting in these procedures. Comparison of open repair and endovascular intervention in the general population indicates that endovascular treatment of AAAs is associated with significant reductions in blood loss and transfusions.[11,12]

Covered stents may offer a measure of protection against intimal hyperplasia and restenosis because their internal surface inhibits neointimal formation. Much of the work to date has employed polytetrafluoroethylene (PTFE) tube grafts fixated by Palmaz stents. In the 1930s, researchers at Dupont were studying chlorofluorocarbons and inadvertently developed PTFE, which is much better known by the tradename Teflon®. PTFE does not attract oils, fats, or proteins, and it stands up to some of the most corrosive chemicals we know. The latter property made it ideal for use in the atomic bomb, where it protected gaskets and other mechanisms from uranium hexafluoride. In 1969, Bob Gore, of W.L. Gore and Associates, discovered that PTFE could be stretched to form a strong material and expanded its uses under the tradename Gore-Tex®. PTFE material is a natural for grafts and stent coverings; it is inert, biocompatible, resists corrosion, and conforms to a variety of shapes. The inhibition of neointimal formation with PTFE is related to the electronegativity and porosity of the expanded polymer.

Since 1995, when our group first noted the importance of providing complete PTFE coverage in an endoluminal graft used to exclude an aneurysm in an aortocoronary saphenous vein graft,[13] a variety of investigators have made similar observations about PTFE's success in reducing intimal hyperplasia and restenosis in coronary and peripheral interventions.[14–17] Whereas many investigators have fashioned covered stents themselves, there are several commercial grafts available or coming to market.

The commercial devices we are seeing today are lower in profile and easier to deliver than the prototypes used in the mid to late 1990s. In general, these new PTFE-covered devices incorporate self-expanding stents, which are well suited for use in large vessels, but can be difficult to place accurately in small vessels. One stent–graft system (JoMed, Helsingbord, Sweden) designed for use in the coronaries comprises a balloon expandable stent, which can be placed directly at the site of the lesion. The graft itself is constructed using a 'sandwich' technology – ultrathin PTFE is placed between two stents. The material stays fixed longitudinally as the graft is expanded so that stent–graft shortening is minimized and complete PTFE coverage is provided. The design of the JoMed device represents a considerable advance over the early prototype devices. Likewise, a new device by SciMed (Symbiot, SciMed/Boston Scientific, Maple Grove, MN), which has not yet been approved in the United States, incorporates a self-expanding nitinol stent and uses a similar PTFE 'sandwich' that minimizes shortening. The device is deployed distal rather than proximal to the lesion, with the idea that this may reduce the risk of embolic phenomena. As yet, this theory has not been proven in actual practice.

Recently, Stoerger and colleagues have reported their results with 70 JoMed grafts in 62 patients with degenerated saphenous vein grafts.[18] Acute technical success was 99%, and the binary restenosis rate was 22%. The authors concluded that the grafts were a safe and effective treatment; however, restenosis rates were similar to those obtained with conventional stents in these difficult lesions – this despite the use of aspirin and ticlopidine in all patients and the addition of glycoprotein (GP) IIb/IIIa inhibitors in 26 patients. Clearly, the relative effectiveness of covered stents in these lesions will require further study.

Our own experience with covered stents includes their use in saphenous vein grafts, enlarging aneurysms and pseudoaneurysms, as well in the exclusion of arteriovenous fistulas. In general, our results have been encouraging, but we have yet to determine the long-term success of these interventions. Results of the STents And Radiation Therapy (START) trial ($n = 476$) – the largest in-stent radiation trial ever – indicate that beta-radiation may play an important role in reducing in-stent restenosis without the risk of acute or chronic thrombosis. Studying combination therapies that incorporate multiple modalities for preventing restenosis is a logical next step for research in percutaneous intervention strategies.

References

1   Nobuyoshi M, Kimura T, Nosaka H et al. Restenosis after successful percutaneous transluminal angioplasty: serial angiographic follow-up of 229 patients. J Am Coll Cardiol 1988; 12: 616–23.

2   Hirshfeld JW Jr, Schwartz JS, Jugo R et al. Restenosis after coronary angioplasty: a multivariate statistical model to relate lesion and procedure variables to restenosis. J Am Coll Cardiol 1991; 18: 647–56.

3   Fischman DL, Leon M, Baim D et al. A randomized comparison of coronary-stent placement and balloon angioplasty in the treatment of coronary artery disease. Stent Restenosis Study Investigators. N Engl J Med 1994; 331: 496–501.

4   Serruys PW, de Jaegere P, Kiemenij F et al. A comparison of balloon-expandable stent implantation with balloon angioplasty in patients with coronary artery disease. Benestent Study group. N Engl J Med 1994; 331: 489–95

5   Masotti M, Serra A, Betriu A. Stents and de novo coronary lesions. Meta-analysis. Rev Esp Cardiol 1997; 50 (suppl):3–9.

6   Savage MP, Douglas JS, Fischman DL et al. Stent placement compared with balloon angioplasty for obstructed coronary bypass grafts. Saphenous Vein De Novo Trial Investigators. N Engl J Med 1997; 337: 740–7.

7   Kuntz RE, Safian RD, Levine MJ et al. Novel approach to the analysis of restenosis after the use of three new coronary devices. J Am Coll Cardiol 1993; 19: 1493–9.

8   Kuntz RE, Gibson CM, Nobuyoshi M et al. Generalized model of restenosis after conventional balloon angioplasty, stenting, and directional atherectomy. J Am Coll Cardiol 1993; 21: 15–25.

9   Mintz GS, Popma JJ, Hong MK et al. Intravascular ultrasound to discern device specific effects and mechanisms of restenosis. Am J Cardiol 1996; 78:18–22.

10   Parodi JC, Palmaz JC, Barone HD. Transfemoral intraluminal graft implantation for abdominal aortic aneurysm. Ann Vasc Surg 1991; 5: 491–9.

11   May J, White GH, Yu W et al. Concurrent comparison of endoluminal versus open repair in the treatment of abdominal aortic aneurysm: analysis of 303 patients by life table method. J Vasc Surg 1998; 27: 213–20.

12   Zarins KZ, Rodney AW, Schwarten D et al. AneuRx stent graft versus open surgical repair of abdominal aortic aneurysm: multicenter prospective clinical trial. J Vasc Surg 1999; 29: 292–308.

13   Heuser RR, Reynolds GT, Papazoglou C, Diethrich EB. Endoluminal grafting for percutaneous aneurysm exclusion in an aortocoronary saphenous vein graft: the first clinical experience. J Endovasc Surg 1995; 2: 81–8.

14   Marin ML, Veith FJ, Cynamon J et al. Effect of polytetrafluoroethylene covering of Palmaz stents on the development of intimal hyperplasia in human iliac arteries. J Vasc Interv Radiol 1996; 7:651–6.

15   Heuser RR, Woodfield S, Lopez A. Obliteration of a coronary artery aneurysm with a PTFE-covered stent: endoluminal graft for coronary disease revisited. Cathet Cardiovasc Interv 1999; 64:113–6.

16   Lukito G, Vandergoten P, Jaspers L, Dendale P, Benit E. Six months clinical angiographic, and IVUS follow-up after PTFE graft stent implantation in native coronary arteries. *Acta Cardiol* 2000; **55**:255–60.

17   Baldus S, Koster R, Elsner M et al. Treatment of aorto-coronary vein graft lesions with membrane-covered stents: a multicenter surveillance trial. *Circulation* 2000; **102**: 2024–7.

18   Stoerger H, Haase J, Hofmann M, Schwarz F. Implantation of coronary PTFE-grafts in degenerated saphenous vein grafts: acute and intermediate term results [abstract]. *Circulation* 2000; **102** (suppl): 2642.

26

Foreign body and stent retrieval

Dieter Liermann and Johannes Kirchner

Foreign body retrieval

Incidence

Owing to the increasing number of interventional procedures, intravascular foreign bodies frequently occur as a serious iatrogenic complication.[1] Both the nature of intravascular foreign bodies and the available devices to retrieve them have changed substantially since the first report by Turner and Sommers[2] on an embolized intravenous catheter and the first report of Thomas et al[3] on the non-surgical removal of a broken steel spring guide. Some studies estimate the incidence of foreign bodies after angiography, cardiac catheterization or pacing and intensive care monitoring to be 0.1–0.2%.[4] Thus the embolization of intravascular catheter fragments has become a well-known complication, and the removal of catheter tips or guidewire emboli is a common challenge for the interventional radiologist.[5]

Foreign bodies could be either fragments of catheters or guidewires, dislodged coils or stents. The most common cause for an intravascular embolized foreign body during the angiographic examination seems to be the puncture needle injury of polyethylene catheters or tapped guidewires, e.g. an accidentally cut strip of the indwelling wire. The breakage of a catheter or the detachment from the connector are less frequent.

Indications

Today it is agreed that the removal of embolized intravascular foreign bodies is essential to prevent complications such as:

- Thrombosis (with arterial or pulmonary embolization)
- Infection (septicemia, endocarditis)
- Vascular perforation

This holds true in particular for centrally located foreign bodies. The remaining intravascular foreign body is a potential source of morbidity and mortality.[6] One cause of this seems to be the high percentage of bacterial contamination in angiographic catheters. Thus Fisher and Ferreyro[7] reported a 71% incidence of serious morbidity or death in patients from whom embolized catheter fragments had not been removed. Bernhardt et al[8] reported on 62 patients with embolized catheter fragments. In this group, 34 patients underwent percutaneous foreign body removal, and the other 28 patients were only observed. None of the former developed any complications, but 17 of the 28 non-treated patients died.

Materials

Several techniques and tools for intravascular foreign body removal have been described. Devices used for intravascular foreign body removal are:

- Curved catheters (Pigtail, Sidewinder, Judkins)
- Loop snares
- Forceps
- Baskets

The different devices will be described in the following, with regard to their special indications.

Curved catheter

Some authors suggest the pigtail catheter as the first instrument with which to start foreign body retrieval.[9] First and foremost curved catheters have been used to pull foreign

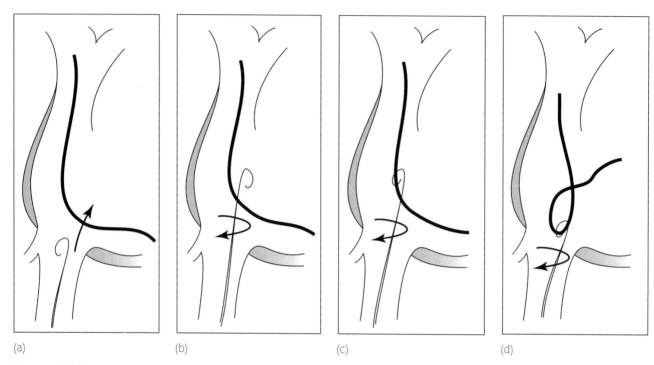

(a)　　　　　(b)　　　　　(c)　　　　　(d)

Figure 26.1

Retrieval of an intravascular foreign body with the help of a pigtail catheter. (a,b) The pigtail catheter is localized close to the intravascular foreign body and is then (c) looped around the fragment by means of gentle rotation and (d) withdrawn to the sheath.

bodies like catheter fragments from the right atrium, ventricle or pulmonal artery into the inferior vena cava (or other less vulnerable locations), where they can be trapped by a snare or forceps.[4,10] Nevertheless, the complete extraction of foreign bodies using the pigtail catheter alone is also possible.[9] In such cases, the use of a long introducing sheath is necessary. The pigtail catheter engages the fragment along its shaft and is then looped around the fragment. During gentle rotation of the pigtail catheter, the fragment is knotted and withdrawn slowly into the sheath (Figure 26.1).

Loop snares

Besides the pigtail catheter, loop snares seem to be the cheapest tool for retrieval of vascular foreign bodies. Snare techniques were originally described for transcolonoscopic removal of colonic polyps[11] and first used for the vascular approach by Curry.[12] Snare devices can be easily made from an open multipurpose catheter and a long (for example 190 cm) 0.46-mm (0.0018-inch) guidewire.[13] The wire is folded in its end section and retrogradely introduced in a catheter. The configuration results in a loop orientated either in the same axis as the introducer catheter or at a right angle to the axis (Figure 26.2). The

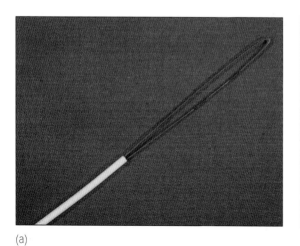

(a)　　　　　(b)

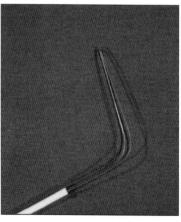

Figure 26.2

Different configurations of self-made snare loops with loops orientated either in the same axis (a) or at a right angle (b) to the introducer catheter.

latter is also called a gooseneck snare. The formation of a loop in the plane perpendicular to the axial direction of the guiding catheter is helpful for trapping catheter fragments, especially in tubular vascular structures.[4] Other variants are shaped like the heart or formed by use of catheters with sideholes (Welter loop). At first, the introducer catheter, together with the loop, is directed to the immediate neighborhood of the foreign body. The foreign body is then encircled by the loop and the catheter is advanced to close the loop. As a result, the foreign body is grasped. We emphasize the following: to close the loop it is better to advance the introducer catheter than to retrieve the wire, because the latter could result in removal of the not securely grasped foreign body and further embolization. Finally, the grasped foreign body, loop and introducer catheter are withdrawn to the sheath and removed together.

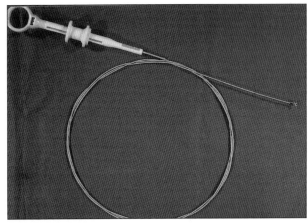

Figure 26.3
Bivalvar forceps with opened branches.

Forceps

Forceps proven in foreign body removal from the urogenital tract, the bronchial system or the esophagus may also be used in the vessels. Thus, even the first reported retrieval of a foreign body (broken segment of a steel spring guide) from the vascular system (right atrium) was performed by Thomas using such a device.[3] Several different types of forceps exist that are potentially suitable to retrieve intravascular foreign bodies. Single-tooth ('rat tooth'), multiple-tooth ('alligator tooth'), bronchoscopic three- and four-pronged as well as bivalvar, round-edged forceps (Figure 26.3) have been described.[4] All these forceps show poor flexibility and can only be directed securely over a small distance (Figure 26.4). Use in curved vessels is dangerous and can result in vascular damage and perforation. Therefore, foreign bodies should first be directed to a suitable position by means of a curved catheter.

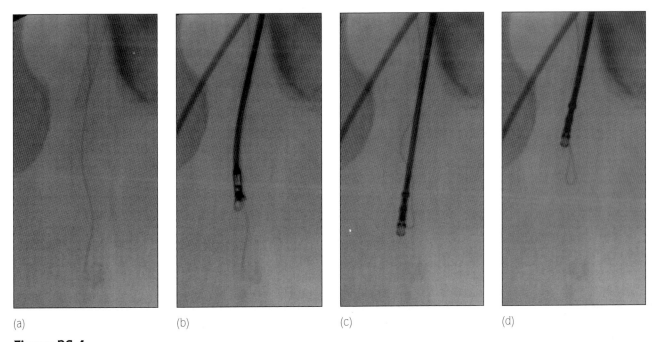

(a) (b) (c) (d)

Figure 26.4
(a) Approximately 10-cm-long cut strip of tapped guidewire embolized to the superficial femoral artery (SFA). An 8F sheath has already been introduced antegrade to the SFA. (b) A bivalvar, round-edged forceps with opened branches is directed towards the distal end of the intravascular foreign body. (c,d) After grasping the catheter fragment by closing the branches, the forceps is slowly withdrawn to the sheath.

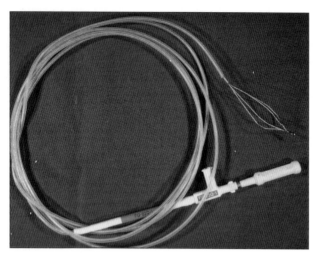

Figure 26.5
Fife wire helical stone extractor with opened loop basket.

Baskets

The use of baskets is only suitable when at least one end of the foreign body is free in the lumen of the vessel. A basket consists of 4–6 helical wires, expanding outside the catheter. As well as special baskets designed for intravascular use, the common helical bile duct (Figure 26.5) or ureteric stone baskets can also be used in the vessels. The size of the basket is chosen with regard to the vessel diameter. Especially in large vessels (vena cava), only large baskets may be used,[14] because the end of a foreign body is close to the vessel wall and can only be grasped if the basket reaches the periphery of the vessel. To avoid damage of the vessel wall, only the closed, catheter-covered basket should be moved in a longitudinal direction in the vessel. First it is advanced close to the foreign body. In the following, the catheter is withdrawn until the basket expands. The opened basket is then slowly rotated to embrace the foreign body. To close the basket around the foreign body, the catheter is advanced over the helical wires and the whole couple is withdrawn to the sheath. If the maneuver fails it can be helpful to bring the foreign body in a more suitable position by means of other tools, e.g. a curved catheter.

Results

Besides numerous case reports dealing with special aspects, there exist only a few sample studies demonstrating the benefit of the techniques in a comparably small number of patients[7,15–23] and reviews.[4,6,7,10,24–26] Most authors report encouraging results in the non-surgical removal of vascular foreign bodies. Egglin et al,[1] regarding an own group of 32 cases of intravascular foreign bodies, reported that the removal was successful in 97%. In most cases the preformed goose-neck snare facilitated the procedure, but other devices (forceps, basket) were necessary in 25% of the cases. The benefit of the self-made loop catheter as a primary approach to retrieve catheter tips or guidewires was also reported by Kappenberger et al[18] in a group of 12 patients. In a study on 21 patients, Cho et al[15] demonstrated the benefit of the non-surgical retrieval of intravascular catheter fragments ($n = 11$) as well as the possibility of unknotting intravascular catheters ($n = 9$). The overall success rate in both groups was 95%, but one embolization to the lung periphery occurred. Uflacker et al[20] performed foreign body retrieval in 20 patients with a success rate of 95%. Similar results were reported by Yang et al,[21] who retrieved 11 of 12 foreign bodies successfully, although they preferred the basket retriever. The results of Dondelinger et al,[16] who performed foreign body removal in 12 patients over an 11-year period, are somewhat outstanding, showing a success rate of 100%. The same authors demonstrate a review of 176 cases from the literature showing overall success in 90% of all reported cases.

Conclusion

The percutaneous non-surgical removal of foreign bodies is now a well-established principle. Various techniques enable us to retrieve foreign bodies from the great vessels and the heart in nearly all cases. Nevertheless, some locations remain difficult, notably the peripheral vessels of the lower extremity.

Stent retrieval

Vascular stents are increasingly used to restore patency and improve suboptimal results after percutaneous transluminal angioplasty (PTA). Commonly, the stent placement is terminal, but sometimes it seems to be necessary to retrieve stents from the vascular system due to misplacement or migration of the stent. Stent dislodgement is an unwelcome but increasingly observed complication. In the venous system it results in embolization into the right cavities or the pulmonary artery, which is one of the most feared complications of the venous application.[7,27] Stent dislodgement in the arteries tends to occur when negotiating a tortuous and irregularly calcified artery with a balloon-mounted stent.[28] Furthermore the implantation of permanent metallic stents sometimes seems to be inappropriate, and temporary stenting is preferred, which calls for a practicable and safe method of stent removal. Here, therapy of a dissection after PTA in the region of the popliteal artery warrants first mention.

Techniques to retrieve a dislodged or misplaced stent, especially stents of the coronaries, have been described recently,[27,29–35] but there are only a few reports dealing with temporary stenting.[36,37]

The use of forceps in retrieving dislodged coronary stents is common. Eeckhout et al[24] used a 5F Alligator Forceps catheter (Cook OB/Gyn., Spencer, IN, USA), which was introduced through an 8F coronary guiding catheter.

Bogart and Jung[13] described a two-wire technique for retrieving coronary stents. To avoid moving the dislodged stent during positioning of the snare device, the author used an additional stiff angioplasty wire positioned beside the initial stent guidewire.

Loop devices have also been used in the coronaries. Elsner et al[31] reported on four cases of misplaced intracoronary stents which were successfully retrieved using a 2-mm closed-loop nitinol device. Kobayashi et al[32] used a nitinol goose-neck snare to retrieve an unexpanded Palmaz–Schatz stent from the left main coronary artery.

The largest sample study during a 5-year period dealing with misplaced or migrated stents was reported by Slonim et al from Stanford University.[33] The authors reported on 17 venous and 10 arterial stents which were successfully retrieved by means of various techniques in 26 cases (96%). Most often (13 cases) the stents had to be repositioned and deployed in a stable alternative position, e.g. in the iliac artery. In 11 cases the stents could be removed through the sheath. In the cases of venous stents, retrieval from the right atrium and subsequent deployment into the right external iliac vein was described by Bartorelli et al.[27]

Temporary stenting

It is not the aim of this chapter to describe the pros and cons of temporary stenting. It should be mentioned that an essential factor in stent retrieval is the appropriate flexibility of the stent material, allowing the stent to be deformed and pulled into the sheath without damage to the vessel wall. Owing to positive experiences in joint-spanning locations, we recommended high-flexibility tantalum stents (Strecker Stent) for temporary insertion and retrieval. For these purposes, we used a commercially available polyp forceps of 7F or 9F, which was gradually pushed through the stented area. The arms of such forceps are rounded on the outside and the tip, avoiding vascular damage, but have a sharp hook on the inside. In an open condition these hooks can snare in the mesh of the stent. The arms of the forceps are then closed again and the stent is carefully withdrawn into the sheath. In a study on 10 patients, it was possible in all cases to retrieve the stent. When using the stable Terumo® (Corporation, Tokyo, Japan) sheath, we always managed to pull the stent–forceps combination completely into the sheath.

References

1   Egglin TK, Dickey KW, Rosenblatt M, Pollak JS. Retrieval of intravascular foreign bodies: experiences in 32 cases. *Am J Roentgenol* 1995; **164**: 1259–64.

2   Turner DC, Sommers SG. Accidental passage of a polyethylene catheter from a cubital vein to right atrium: fatal case. *N Engl J Med* 1954; **251**: 744–5.

3   Thomas J, Sinclair Smith B, Bloomfield D. Nonsurgical retrieval of a broken segment of steel spring guide from the right atrium and inferior vena cava. *Circulation* 1964; **30**: 106–8.

4   Yedlicka JW, Qian Z, Castaneda-Zuniga WR. Intravascular foreign body removal. In: Castaneda-Zuniga WR, ed. *Interventional Radiology*, Williams and Wilkins, Baltimore, 1992; 967–83.

5   Zollikofer C, Nath PH, Castaneda-Zuniga WR et al. Nonsurgical removal of intravascular foreign bodies. *ROFO* 1979; **130**: 590–3.

6   Gerlock AJ, Mirfakhraee M. Retrieval of intravascular foreign bodies. *J Thorac Imaging* 1987; **2**: 52–60.

7   Fisher RG, Ferreyro R. Evaluation of current techniques for nonsurgical removal of intravascular iatrogenic foreign bodies. *Am J Roentgenol* 1978; **130**: 541–8.

8   Bernhardt LC, Wegner GP, Mendenhall JT. Intravenous catheter embolization to the pulmonary artery. *Chest* 1970; **57**: 329–38.

9   Auge JM, Oriol A, Serra C, Crexells C. The use of pigtail catheters for retrieval of foreign bodies from the cardiovascular system. *Cathet Cardiovasc Diagn* 1984; **10**: 625–8.

10 Mathias K. Perkutane transvasale Fremdkörperextraktion. In: Günther RW, Thelen M, eds. *Interventionelle Radiologie*. Stuttgart: Thieme, 1996: 374–81.

11 Hubert JW, Krone RJ, Shatz BA. Susman N. An improved snare system for the nonsurgical retrieval of intravascular foreign bodies. *Cathet Cardiovasc Diagn* 1980; **6**: 405–11.

12 Curry JL. Recovery of detached intravascular catheter or guide wire fragments. A proposed method. *Am J Roentgenol* 1969; **105**: 894–6.

13 Bogart DB, Jung SC. Dislodged stent: a simple retrieval technique. *Catheter Cardiovasc Intervent* 1999; **47** 323–4.

14 Clouse ME, Costello P, O'Leary DH. Removal of intravascular foreign bodies using modified Grollman catheter and Dormia basket. *J Can Assoc Radiol* 1984; **35**: 305–7.

15 Cho SR, Tisnado J, Beachley MC et al. Percutaneous unknotting of intravascular catheters and retrieval of catheter fragments. *Am J Roentgenol* 1983; **141**: 397–402.

16 Dondelinger RF, Lepoutre B, Kurdziel JC. Percutaneous vascular foreign body retrieval: experience of an 11-year period. *Eur J Radiol* 1991; **12**: 4–10.

17 Dotter CT, Rösch J, Bilbao MC. Transluminal extraction of catheter and guide wire fragments from heart and great vessels: 29 collected cases. *Am J Roentgenol* 1971; **111**: 467–71.

18 Kappenberger L, Tartini R, Steinbrunn W. Transluminal removal of intravascular foreign bodies. *Schweiz Med Wochenschr* 1985; **115**: 258–60.

19 Rossi P, Passariello R, Simonetti G. Intravascular iatrogenic foreign body retrieval. Experience in 13 cases. *Ann Radiol (Paris)* 1980; **23**: 286–90.

20 Uflacker R, Lima S, Melichar AC. Intravascular foreign bodies: percutaneous retrieval. *Radiology* 1986; **160**: 731–5.

21 Yang FS, Ohta HJ, Lin JC et al. Non-surgical retrieval of intravascular foreign body: experience of 12 cases. *Eur J Radiol* 1994; **18**: 1–5.

22 Ando K, Sano A, Kigami Y et al. Angiographic retrieval of foreign bodies in pulmonary artery: a report of three cases. *Radiat Med* 1993; **11**: 69–74.

23 El Feghaly M, Soula P, Rousseau H et al. Endovascular retrieval of two migrated venous stents by means of balloon catheters. *J Vasc Surg* 1998; **28**: 541–6.

24 Feldman T. Retrieval techniques for dislodged stents. *Catheter Cardiovasc Intervent* 1999; **47**: 325–6.

25 Kuffer G, Gebauer A, Antes G, Rath M. Percutaneous transluminal removal of embolised catheter fragments. *ROFO* 1981; **135**: 691–4.

26 Rubinstein ZJ, Morag B, Itzchak Y. Percutaneous removal of intravascular foreign bodies. *Cardiovasc Intervent Radiol* 1982; **5**: 64–8.

27 Bartorelli AL, Fabbiocchi F, Montorsi P et al. Successful transcatheter management of Palmaz Stent embolization after superior vena cava stenting. *Cathet Cardiovasc Diagn* 1995; **34**: 162–6.

28 Meisel SR, Di Leo J, Rajakaruna M et al. A technique to retrieve stents dislodged in the coronary artery followed by fixation in the iliac artery by means of balloon angioplasty and peripheral stent deployment. *Cathet Cardiovasc Diagn* 2000; **49**: 77–81.

29 Bogart DB, Earnest JB, Miller JT. Foreign body retrieval using a simple snare device. *Cathet Cardiovasc Diagn* 1990; **19**: 248–50.

30 Eeckhout E, Stauffer JC, Goy JJ. Retrieval of a migrated coronary stent by means of an alligator forceps catheter. *Cathet Cardiovasc Diagn* 1993; **30**: 166–8.

31 Elsner M, Pfeifer A, Kasper W. Intracoronary loss of balloon-mounted stents: successful retrieval with a 2mm – 'microsnare' – device. *Cathet Cardiovasc Diagn* 1996; **39**: 271–6.

32 Kobayashi Y, Nonogi H, Miyazaki S et al. Successful retrieval of unexpanded Palmaz–Schatz stent from left main coronary artery. *Cathet Cardiovasc Diagn* 1996; **38**: 402–4.

33 Slonim SM, Dake MD, Razavi MK et al. Management of misplaced or migrated endovascular stents. *J Vasc Intervent Radiol* 1999; **10**: 851–9.

34 Irie T, Furui S, Yamauchi T et al. Relocatable Gianturco expandable metallic stents. *Radiology* 1991; **178**: 575–8.

35 Liermann D, Zegelman M. Extraction of misplaced or occluded endovascular stents. In: Liermann D, ed. *Stents – State of the Art and Future Developments*. Morin Heights: Polyscience Publishers, 1995: 371–8.

36 Liermann D. Temporary stenting. In: Liermann D, ed. *Stents – State of the Art and Future Developments*. Morin Heights: Polyscience Publishers, 1995: 329–38.

37 Liermann D, Kirchner J. *Angiographische Diagnostik und Therapie*. Stuttgart: Thieme, 1997.

27

Aortoiliac artery angioplasty and stenting

Christopher J White and Stephen R Ramee

Introduction

It is important in the initial assessment of patients with peripheral vascular occlusive disease to remember that there is a significant association of coronary artery disease, and that coronary artery disease is the major cause of mortality in these patients.[1,2] A complete cardiovascular assessment of the patient with aortoiliac occlusive disease should be performed, given the high incidence of associated atherosclerotic diseases. Appropriate assessment of these patients includes a complete carotid, abdominal, and lower extremity vascular examination as well as appropriate screening and assessment for coronary artery disease. A non-invasive cardiac stress test is appropriate to assess the risk of suspected coronary artery disease.

Patients with aortoiliac occlusive disease may be asymptomatic or present with a full range of symptoms from mild claudication to limb-threatening ischemia. The severity of symptoms will depend upon the severity of the occlusive lesion, the presence of collateral circulation, and the presence of multilevel vascular disease. With isolated terminal aorta stenoses, generally both legs are equally affected, although disparities in collateral circulation may render one limb more ischemic than the other.

The initial assessment should include a physical examination for signs of peripheral ischemia, distal embolization, and the status of the peripheral pulses. A rest and exercise ankle–brachial index (ABI) should be performed. A mild impairment in the resting ABI may be dramatically exaggerated with exercise. Segmental ABIs with pulse volume recordings will indicate the presence or absence of multilevel occlusive disease. Another very helpful test in the pre-procedural assessment of these patients is the duplex (Doppler and ultrasound) examination. The duplex scan will provide information regarding the presence or absence of abdominal aortic aneursymal disease and indicate the severity of occlusive

lesions. If there is doubt as to the presence of aneurysmal disease an abdominal computed tomagraphic (CT) scan or magnetic resonance (MR) image should be performed.

Aortoiliac angiography

Vascular access may be obtained from either the upper extremity (radial, brachial, or axillary approach) or via a femoral (ipsilateral or contralateral) artery. Whenever possible, we prefer to use the ipsilateral femoral artery for access. Using a standard Seldinger technique, access is obtained in the common femoral artery (the mid-level of the femoral head is a useful marker for this vessel) and a 4–6 Fr vascular sheath is placed to ensure access. A soft, steerable, 0.035-inch Wholey guide wire (Malinckrodt, St Louis, MO) is an excellent wire for crossing occlusive aortoiliac lesions. If this wire fails, we next choose an angled Glidewire (Terumo, BSC, Watertown, MA) taking care not to pass the wire subintimally across the lesion. Once the wire is across the lesion, a pigtail catheter is advanced to the level of the renal arteries (L1 or L2) and above the level of the occlusive disease. The Glidewire is then exchanged for an Amplatz (Cook, Bloomington, IL) extra-stiff 0.035-inch guide wire. It is important that once retrograde access across the aortoiliac lesion is gained, care is taken not to lose it during catheter exchanges.

A diagnostic aortogram, showing inflow and outflow of the target lesion, and runoff angiography to visualize the lower extremity circulation is performed. A 'working view' of the lesion is obtained to serve as a 'road map'. Bony landmarks or an external radiopaque ruler are helpful to guide intervention. When performing the diagnostic aortogram it is important to image the renal arteries and any collateral circulation in the pelvis. Occasionally, it is necessary to perform additional selective or angulated views of the terminal aorta and common iliac arteries to define the extent of the stenosis.

Aortoiliac balloon angioplasty

After the target lesion has been imaged it is important that an accurate assessment of the reference vessel diameter be made. This can be done with quantitative angiography (taking care to image an appropriate reference object to calibrate for any magnification errors) or intravascular ultrasound (IVUS). The duplex scan or abdominal contrast CT scan may also offer good estimates of luminal diameter of the target vessels. In our experience, visual estimation of vessel diameters in these large vessels is inaccurate and can lead to procedural complications, if an oversized balloon is chosen.

Aspirin (325 mg) is given once a day several days prior to the procedure. After access has been obtained and prior to the intervention, we routinely administer 2500–5000 IU of heparin. From the ipsilateral retrograde femoral approach, we prefer to cross the lesion with an atraumatic guide wire, a soft, steerable, 0.035-inch Wholey wire. If a complete diagnostic angiogram showing inflow and outflow from the lesion has not been previously obtained, a baseline angiogram of the lesion is performed with a pigtail catheter in the best view to show the lesion. An extra-stiff guidewire (0.035-inch or 0.038-inch Amplatz wire is then advanced through the pigtail catheter above the lesion and the pigtail catheter is removed. The lesion is then dilated with a balloon, sized 1:1 with the reference vessel diameter. It is important to quantitatively measure the diameter of these large vessels, as large errors in estimation are possible. The balloon catheter is inflated to the lowest pressure that will fully expand the balloon. The pigtail catheter is then readvanced above the dilated lesion and angiography is performed to assess the result. The residual stenosis should be less than 30%. The presence of a potentially flow-limiting dissection should be looked for. At this time, a pressure gradient across the lesion should also be measured between the pigtail catheter in the aorta and access sheath below the lesion. The gradient should be ≤5 mmHg following successful dilation. If a suboptimal angioplasty result has been obtained, the option at this time is to proceed with stent placement or to repeat the balloon inflation to either higher pressure or for longer duration.

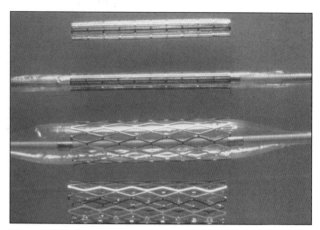

Figure 27.1
Photograph of the Palmaz 308 stent.

lower profile and are less likely to embolize from the balloon catheter. The premounted stent is advanced within the sheath to the lesion site; this technique avoids the risk of the stent being snagged on the irregular surface of the pre-dilated lesion and minimizes the risk of stent embolization. Using bony landmarks or an external radiopaque ruler as a guide for stent placement, the sheath is then pulled back to uncover the stent. Contrast injections through the delivery sheath can be performed to confirm accurate stent placement. The stent is deployed by fully inflating the balloon to a minimum of 6 atmospheres to ensure full inflation of the balloon and adequate deployment of the stent.

It is important to assess the adequacy of stent deployment. Angiographically there should be a slight 'step-up and step-down' apparent. Intravascular ultrasound may also be used to visualize the adequacy of stent deployment (Figure 27.2). A simultaneous pressure gradient between the distal catheter and the access sheath should be measured to confirm that the pressure gradient across the lesion is ≤5 mmHg. To deploy the stent at higher pressures, the deployment balloon is positioned so that the distal shoulder of the balloon is within the distal margins of the stent. This minimizes the chance of a distal dissection occurring during high pressure inflation. The pigtail catheter is then readvanced over the guide wire and final angiography and pressure gradient measurements are performed (Figure 27.3).

Aortoiliac stent placment

Balloon expandable stent

When deploying a balloon expandable stent (Figure 27.1), we prefer to use a long sheath (usually 20–30 cm long), which can be advanced across the lesion. Premounted stents have a

Self-expanding stent

It is generally recommended that a self-expanding stent with a nominal diameter ≥1 mm larger than the reference diameter and ≥1 cm longer than the lesion is placed. A long delivery sheath is not required as stent embolization is prevented by the constraining sheath. The stent is advanced over an extra-stiff guide wire (already in the aorta following

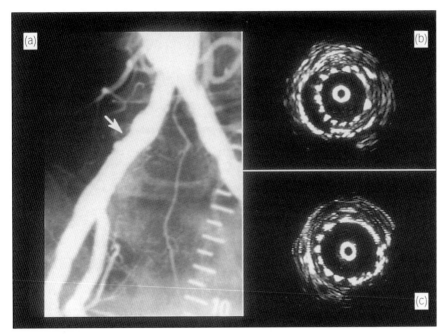

Figure 27.2
(a) angiography of a right common iliac stent deployment. (b) intravascular ultrasound (IVUS) image of suboptimally expanded stent (8-mm balloon). (c) IVUS image after using a larger balloon (9 mm). There was no difference detectable on angiograpy alone.

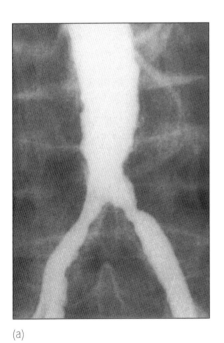

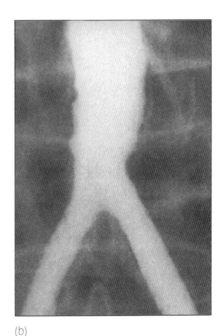

(a)   (b)

Figure 27. 3
(a) Baseline angiography of bilateral common iliac stenosis. (b) Bilateral ostial stent (Palmaz 308) deployment.

angiography) to several centimeters above the lesion and approximately 25% of the stent is uncovered by retracting the constraining sheath. The stent may be withdrawn, but not advanced once it has begun to be deployed. To be sure that the distal segment of the lesion will be covered by the stent, compare the bony landmarks or an external radiopaque ruler with the diagnostic 'road-map' angiogram of the lesion, and complete the deployment. The predilation balloon is then readvanced within the stent and inflated to ensure full balloon expansion, which further apposes the stent against the vessel

wall. The pigtail catheter is then advanced over the wire and above the stented lesion for final angiography (Figure 27.4). A simultaneous pressure gradient between the pigtail catheter and the access sheath should be measured to confirm that the pressure gradient across the lesion is ≤5 mmHg.

Whenever possible, it is desirable to keep the inflated balloon within the stent to avoid injury to non-stented segments of the vessel wall. If the balloon is longer than the stent, then it should be withdrawn so that its distal end is within the stent. Should a dissection occur, it will be proximal

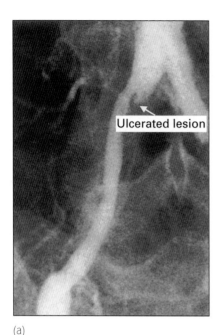

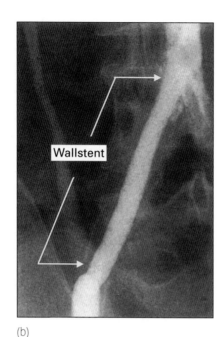

(a)

(b)

Figure 27.4

(a) Baseline angiography showing an ulcerated segment of a long right common iliac stenosis. (b) Angiography after placement of a Wallstent.

to the stent and correctable with the placement of a second stent without having to recross the deployed stent. It is important to remember that stents will shorten further with balloon expansion, so that when positioning the stent, it is ideal to center the lesion on the stent.

Following stent deployment, the balloon catheter is removed, taking care to keep the guide wire above the lesion and through the stent. The diagnostic pigtail catheter may then be re-advanced through the stent and completion angiography performed. Simultaneous pressure recordings from above and below the lesion should confirm that the baseline gradient has been abolished. The target should be a zero gradient in large arteries. If there is any doubt as to the adequacy of stent implantation, intravascular ultrasound may be used to confirm stent apposition to the vessel wall.

One final note of caution is appropriate regarding angioplasty and stent placement in external iliac arteries. These arteries are particularly delicate and prone to rupture with oversized balloons. Care must be taken not to use oversize balloons in the external iliac arteries.

Patient aftercare

The vascular sheath is removed when the activated clotting time (ACT) falls to <160 s (usually within 2 h). When compressing the ipsilateral femoral access site, which is distal to the stent deployment, care should be taken not to occlude flow which may lead to stent thrombosis. Alternatively, one can use a femoral access site closure device. Patients are continued on oral aspirin (325 mg per day) indefinitely. Clopidogrel is not routinely administered, but may be used at the discretion of the attending physician. Prior to hospital discharge (18–24 h following the procedure) ABIs and duplex scanning may be performed to establish a post-treatment baseline. Patients are followed up in the clinic at 1, 2, and 6 months, and at 6-month intervals thereafter with non-invasive testing to document continued patency.

Clinical outcomes of abdominal aorta intervention

Distal abdominal aortic disease has been conventionally treated with endarterectomy or bypass grafting.[3,4] Frequently, distal aortic occlusive disease accompanies occlusive disease of the common or external iliac arteries. The potential advantages of a percutaneous technique compared to an aortoiliac reconstruction are significant in that there is no requirement for general anesthesia or an abdominal incision, and percutaneous therapy is associated with a shorter hospital stay and lower morbidity.[5] While axillofemoral extra-anatomic bypass offers a lower risk surgical alternative for patients with terminal aorta occlusive disease and severe co-morbidities, it has the disadvantages of a lower patency rate than direct surgical bypass of the lesions and requires that surgical intervention of a normal vessel be performed to achieve inflow.

Since 1980, balloon angioplasty has been used successfully, although not extensively, in the terminal aorta.[6] An extension of this strategy has been the use of endovascular stents in the treatment of infrarenal aortic stenoses. While balloon dilation of these lesions has been reported to be effective,[6–8] the placement of stents offers a more definitive treatment with a larger acute gain in luminal diameter, scaffolding of the lumen to prevent embolization of debris, and an enhanced long-term patency compared to balloon angioplasty alone.[3–5,9–12]

Ballard and co-workers[11] reported the successful use of a Wallstent placed from the axillary artery approach to successfully recanalize a total occlusion of the terminal aorta and bilateral iliac arteries in a patient who was not considered a candidate for thrombolysis or surgical bypass due to severe co-morbidities. They described the advantages of using a Wallstent in this case due to its length in covering long lesions and flexibility. Martinez and co-workers reported excellent late follow-up (mean 48 months) in 24 patients treated with infrarenal aortic stents. They reported no in-stent restenosis.[10]

Stents are an attractive therapeutic option for the management of large artery occlusive disease to maintain or improve the arterial lumenal patency after balloon angioplasty. The utility of stents for aortic stenoses has not been demonstrated in randomized trials, however the initial clinical results are encouraging.

Clinical outcomes of aortoiliac stent grafts

It is estimated that 100 000 abdominal aortic aneurysms (AAA) are diagnosed each year and approximately 40 000 require surgical correction. The incidence of AAA appears to have been rising over the past several decades. Men are affected more commonly than women and AAA is the tenth leading cause of death in men. It is generally accepted that there is clinical benefit in electively repairing aneurysms larger than 5.0 cm, and in patients with hypertension and chronic obstructive lung disease aneurysms larger than 3.0 cm should be repaired.[13] In low-risk patients, the operative mortality for AAA repair is estimated to be 5% compared with greater than 10% in higher risk patients. The experience with covered stent grafts to exclude abdominal aortic and aortoiliac aneurysms is still early, requiring surgical vascular access to introduce large diameter devices.

Several AAA stent grafts have received Food and Drug Administration (FDA) approval for clinical use. Using a modular bifurcated stent graft system with nitinol and polytetrafluoroethylene (PTFE) components (Excluder, Gore, Sunnyvale, CA) Matusumara and colleagues reported on a prospective randomized trial in 334 patients with AAA ≥5.5 cm in diameter, comparing the stent graft procedure with conventional surgery.[14] They found no difference in survival rate between the two procedures. The 30-day mortality rate was 0% for the surgery group and 1% for the stent graft group ($P = NS$). Cardiac, pulmonary and bleeding complications occurred more frequently in the surgical group ($P < 0.001$). Endoleaks were present in 17% at 1 year and in 20% at 2 years (Table 27.1). At 2 years, 14% of the stent graft aneurysms were enlarging by 5 mm or more. Aneurysm reintervention was necessary in 14% of patients with stent graft repair in the first 2 years. The use of stent grafts for AAA repair offers a less morbid procedure than surgery, but is associated with a higher frequency of late failure requiring a commitment to long-term surveillance, which is not

Table 27.1 Classification of aorta stent graft endoleaks

- Type I: A separation of the graft from the vessel wall at the proximal or distal attachment site
- Type II: Filling of the aneurysm sac with retrograde flow from mesenteric arteries
- Type III: A tear in the fabric of the graft
- Type IV: Contrast blush through the porous fabric of the graft

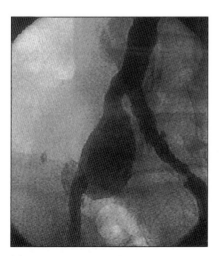
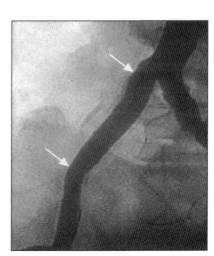

(a)   (b)

Figure 27.5
(a) Right common iliac aneurysm. (b) Angiography following stent graft which has sealed the aneurysm.

necessary with conventional surgery.

The use of endovascular stent grafts to treat long-segment aortoiliac occlusive disease has been reported by Marin and co-workers in 42 patients with limb-threatening ischemia.[15] The stent grafts were hand-made and were constructed using Palmaz stents and 6-mm PTFE thin-walled grafts. Surgical exposure of the femoral access site was obtained and the lesion crossed with a guide wire. The stent was sewn to the proximal end of the graft and deployed with balloon inflation at the inflow site to the lesion. The distal end of the graft was surgically anastomosed at the outflow site. Procedural success was obtained in 91% (39 of 43) of arteries. The 18-month patency rate was 89% and the 2-year limb salvage rate was 94%.

Clinical outcomes of iliac artery intervention

Iliac artery intervention represents an important skill for the cardiovascular interventionist to master, not only to relieve patients' lower extremity symptoms, but also to preserve vascular access for what may be lifesaving cardiovascular therapies, such as coronary angioplasty, management of an arterial access site complications, or insertion of an intra-aortic counterpulsation balloon.

Accepted indications for iliac intervention include lifestyle limiting or progressive claudication, ischemic pain at rest, non-healing ischemic ulcerations, and gangrene. It is important that the angiographic anatomy of the inflow vessels and outflow vessels be demonstrated prior to performing intervention (Tables 27.2 and 27.3).

The clinical benefit of percutaneous transluminal

Table 27.4 Patency after iliac PTA by clinical and lesion variables[22]

	1-year %	3-year %	5-year %
ST/CL/GR	81	70	63
ST/LS/GR	65	48	38
OC/CL/PR	61	43	33
OC/LS/PR	56	17	10

CL, claudication; LS, limb-threatening ischemia; ST, stenosis; OC, occlusion; GR, good runoff; PR, poor runoff.

angioplasty (PTA) versus medical therapy in iliac and femoral lesions has been demonstrated in a randomized trial with end points that included relief of symptoms, improvement in walking distance, and continued patency of the affected artery.[16] A favorable procedural result is more likely with stenoses than with occlusions, with aortoiliac than with femoropopliteal or tibioperoneal disease, and in patients with claudication rather than limb salvage situations (Table 27.4).[7,17–19] The primary success rate of angioplasty for selected iliac artery stenoses should be >90% with an expected 5-year patency rate of between 80% and 85% while iliac occlusions have a lower expected procedural success rate (33–85%).[20,21]

The long-term patency of iliac vessels treated with balloon angioplasty is influenced by both clinical and anatomic variables.[22] Restenosis rates tend to be lower in non-diabetic male patients with claudication and discrete non-occlusive stenoses with good distal runoff. Conversely, restenosis is more likely to occur in diabetic female patients with rest pain, and diffuse and lengthy occlusive lesions with poor distal runoff.

Traditional surgical therapy for iliac obstructive lesions includes aortoiliac and aortofemoral bypass, and these are reported to have a 74–95% 5-year patency which is comparable to balloon angioplasty. Ameli and coworkers[23] reported their results for a series of 105 consecutive patients undergoing aortofemoral bypass of which 58% were treated for claudication. The operative mortality was 5.7%, the early graft failure rate was 5.7%, and the 2-year patency was 92.8%.

A randomized trial comparing PTA to bypass surgery for 157 iliac lesions was reported by Wilson et al.[24] They found no significant difference between PTA and surgery for death, amputations, or loss of patency at 3 years (Figure 27.6). They also found no significant difference in the hemodynamic (ankle–brachial index) result of a successful procedure between the surgery group and PTA group at 3 years (Table 27.5).

Endovascular stents have dramatically improved the success rates for PTA of the iliac arteries.[25–34] Owing to the large diameter of the iliac vessels, the risk of thrombosis or restenosis after iliac placement of metallic stents is quite low.

Table 27.2 Ideal iliac PTA lesions

- Stenotic lesion
- Non-calcified
- Discrete (≤3 cm)
- Patent runoff vessels (≥2)
- Non-diabetic patients

Table 27.3 Contraindications (relative) to iliac baloon angioplasty

- Occlusion
- Long lesions (≥5 cm)
- Aortoiliac aneurysm
- Atheroembolic disease
- Extensive bilateral aortoiliac disease

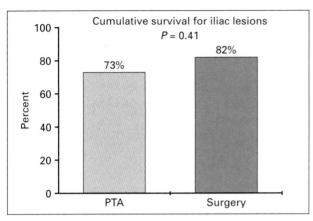

Figure 27.6
Bar graph of the 3-year event-free survival of percutaneous transluminal angioplasty (PTA) versus surgery for iliac lesions.[24]

Table 27.5 Ankle–brachial index in randomized iliac lesions ($P = NS$ for all)[24]			
	Baseline	*Post-treatment*	*At 3 years*
PTA	0.50 ± .01	0.78 ± .04	0.80 ± .07
Surgery	0.50 ± .02	0.82 ± .03	0.78 ± .05
PTA, percutaneous transluminal angioplasty.			

Stents may be placed 'primarily' in an iliac lesion, regardless of the balloon angioplasty result, or they may be used 'provisionally' for a suboptimal angioplasty result. The balloon expandable stents have greater radial force and allow greater precision for placement, which is particularly useful in ostial lesions. Self-expanding stents are more longitudinally flexible and can be delivered more easily from the contralateral femoral access site. The self-expanding stents also allow for normal vessel tapering and are particularly suited to longer lesions in which the proximal vessel may be several millimeters larger than the distal vessel.

The overall clinical benefit of iliac stent placement has been demonstrated using a meta-analysis of more than 2000 patients from eight reported angioplasty (PTA) series and six stent series.[35] The patients who received iliac stents had a statistically higher procedural success rate and a 43% reduction in late (4-year) failures for patients treated with stents compared to those treated with balloon angioplasty alone.

Clinical results for provisional iliac stent placement with the Palmaz stent in 184 iliac lesions demonstrated a 91% procedural success rate and a 6-month patency rate of 99%.[36] Long-term follow-up of these iliac lesions demonstrated a 4-year primary patency rate of 86% and a secondary patency rate of 95%.[36] Results for provisional iliac stent placement with the self-expanding Wallstent have demonstrated patency rates at 1 year of 95%, 2 years of 88%, and 4 years of 82% in 118 treated lesions.[37]

A relatively small randomized trial comparing PTA with provisional stenting (stent placement for unsatisfactory balloon angioplasty results) to primary stenting in iliac arteries demonstrated that pressure gradients across the lesions after primary stent placement (5.8 ± 4.7 mmHg) were significantly lower than after PTA alone (8.9 ± 6.8 mmHg) but not after provisional stenting (5.9 ± 3.6 mmHg).[38] The primary technical success rate, defined as a post-procedural gradient less than 10 mmHg, revealed no difference between the two treatment strategies (primary stent = 81% vs PTA plus provisional stenting = 89%). By using provisional stenting, the authors avoided stent placement in 63% of the lesions, and still achieved an equivalent acute hemodynamic result compared to primary stenting. Longer term follow-up will be necessary to evaluate the feasibility and safety of this approach and the impact of provisional stenting on late patency.

Primary placement of Palmaz balloon expandable stents has been evaluated in a multicenter trial for iliac placement in 486 patients followed for up to 4 years (mean 13.3 ± 11 months after surgery).[39] Using a life-table analysis, clinical benefit was present in 91% at 1 year, 84% at 2 years, and 69% of the patients at 43 months of follow-up. The angiographic patency rate of the iliac stents was 92%. Complications occurred in 10% and were predominantly related to the arterial access site. Five patients suffered thrombosis of the stent of which four were recanalized with thrombolysis and balloon angioplasty. A preliminary report from a European randomized trial of primary iliac (Palmaz) stent placement versus balloon angioplasty demonstrated a 4-year patency of 92% for the stent group versus a 74% patency for the balloon angioplasty group (Table 27.6).[40]

Iliac stent placement may also be used as an adjunctive procedure to surgical bypass procedures. Clinical results for iliac angioplasty with or without stent placement to preserve

Table 27.6 Randomized trial of iliac percutaneous transluminal angioplasty (PTA) vs stents[40]					
Procedure	*Technical success (%)*	*Hemodynamic success (%)*	*Clinical success (%)*	*Complication rate (%)*	*Patency 4-year (%)*
Stent (N = 123)	98.4	97.6	97.6	4.1	91.6
PTA (N = 124)	91.9	91.9	89.5	6.5	74.3

inflow for a femoro-femoral bypass over a 14-year period in 70 consecutive patients have been very encouraging.[41] It was found that the patients requiring treatment of the in-flow iliac artery with angioplasty or stent placement did just as well as those without iliac artery disease at 7 years after surgery. These results suggest that percutaneous intervention can provide adequate long-term inflow for femoro-femoral bypass as an alternative to aortofemoral bypass in patients at increased risk for major surgery.

Conclusion

The use of percutaneous therapy in aortoiliac disease has dramatically changed the standard of care by which patients are currently treated. It is distinctly unusual in hospitals with qualified interventionalists for a patient to undergo aortofemoral bypass surgery for aortoiliac occlusive disease if a percutaneous approach is feasible. With the maturation and development of aneurysm exclusion devices (stent grafts) it is likely that the requirement for a major surgical procedure to correct infrarenal aortic aneurysmal disease will become an infrequent occurrence. It is the nature of surgical procedures to change. And while many surgeons feel that their specialty and livelihood are threatened by percutaneous interventions, they must accept the fact that there will be a relentless progression towards less invasive, less morbid procedures in the future.

Acknowledgment

The authors would like to express their appreciation to Mr James O'Meara for his assistance in the preparation of the figures and tables.

References

1   Hertzer NR, Beven EG, Youn JR et al. Coronary artery disease in peripheral vascular patients: a classification of 1000 coronary angiograms and results of surgical management. *Ann Surg* 1984; **199**: 223–23.

2   Jamieson WRE, Janusz MT, Miyagishima RT, Gerein AN. Influence of ischemic heart disease on early and late mortality after surgery for peripheral occlusive vascular disease. *Circulation* 1982; **66**(suppl I): 92–7.

3   Marin ML, Veith FJ, Cynamon J et al. Transfemoral endovascular stented graft treatment of aorto-iliac and femoropopliteal occlusive disease for limb salvage. *Am J Surg* 1994; **168**: 156–62.

4   Williams JB, Watts, PW, Nguyen VA, Peterson CL. Balloon angioplasty with intraluminal stenting as the initial treatment modality in aorto-iliac occlusive disease. *Am J Surg* 1994; **168**: 202–4.

5   Diethrich EB, Santiago O, Gustafson G, Heuser RR. Preliminary observations on the use of the Palmaz stent in the distal portion of the aorta. *Am Heart J* 1993; **125**: 490–501.

6   Charlbois N, Saint Geoges G, Hudon G. Percutaneous transluminal angioplasty of the lower abdominal aorta. *Am J Radiol* 1991; **146**: 369–71.

7   Tegtmeyer CJ, Hartwell GD, Selby JB et al. Results and complications of angioplasty in aortoiliac disease. *Circulation* 1991; **83**(suppl I): 53–60.

8   Iyer SS, Hall P, Dorros G. Brachial approach to management of an abdominal aortic occlusion with prolonged lysis and subsequent angioplasty. *Cath Cardiovasc Diagn* 1991; **23**: 290–3.

9   Long AL, Gaux JC, Raynaud A. Infrarenal aortic stents: Initial clinical experience and angiographic follow-up. *Cardiovasc Intervent Radiol* 1993; **16**: 203–8.

10   Martinez R, Rodriguez-Lopez J, Diethrich EB. Stenting for abdominal aortic occlusive disease. Long-term results. *Tex Heart Inst J* 1997; **24**: 15–22.

11   Ballard JL, Taylor FC, Sparks SR, Killen JD. Stenting without thrombolysis for aortoiliac occlusive disease: Experience in 14 high-risk patients. *Ann Vasc Surg* 1995; **9**: 453–8.

12   Roeren T, Post K, Richter et al. Stent angioplasty of the infrarenal aorta and aortic bifurcation. Clinical and angiographic results in a prospective study. *Radiologe* 1994; **34**: 504–10.

13   Cronenwett JL. Infrainguinal occlusive disease. *Semin Vasc Surg* 1995; **8**: 284–8.

14   Matsumura JS, Brewster DC, Makaroun MS et al. A multicenter controlled clinical trial of open versus endovascular treatment of abdominal aortic aneurysm. *J Vasc Surg* 2003; **37**: 262–71.

15   Marin ML, Veith FJ, Sanchez LA et al. Endovascular repair of aortoiliac occlusive disease. *World J Surg* 1996; **20**: 679–86.

16   Whyman MR, Kerracher EMG, Gillespie IN et al. Randomised controlled trial of percutaneous transluminal angioplasty for intermittent claudication. *Eur J Vasc Surg* 1996; **12**: 167–72.

17   O'Keeffe ST, Woods BO, Beckmann CF. Percutaneous transluminal angioplasty of the peripheral arteries. *Cardiol Clin* 1991; **9**: 519–21.

18   Wilson SE, Sheppard B. Results of percutaneous transluminal angioplasty for peripheral vascular occlusive disease. *Ann Vasc Surg* 1990; **4**: 94–7.

19   Reidy JF. Angioplasty in peripheral vascular disease. *Postgrad Med J* 1987; **63**: 435–8.

20   Gallino A, Mahler F, Probst P, Nachbur B. Percutaneous transluminal angioplasty of the arteries of the lower limbs: a 5 year follow-up. *Circulation* 1984; **70**: 619–23.

21   Cassarella WJ. Noncoronary angioplasty. *Curr Prob Cardiol* 1986; **11**: 141–74.

22   Johnston KW. Balloon angioplasty: Predictive factors for long-term success. *Semin Vasc Surg* 1989; **3**: 117–22.

23   Ameli FM, Stein M, Provan JL et al. Predictors of surgical outcome in patients undergoing aortobifemoral bypass reconstruction. *J Cardiovasc Surg* 1990; **30**: 333–9.

24   Wilson SE, Wolf GL, Cross AP. Percutaneous transluminal angioplasty versus operation for peripheral arteriosclerosis: Report of a prospective randomized trial in a selected group of patients. *J Vasc Surg* 1989; **9**: 1–9.

25   Becker GJ, Palmaz JC, Rees CR et al. Angioplasty-induced

dissections in human iliac arteries: management with Palmaz balloon-expandable intraluminal stents. *Radiology* 1990; **176**: 31–8.

26 Katzen BT, Becker GJ. Intravascular stents: status of development and clinical application. *Surg Clin North Am* 1992; **72**: 941–57.

27 Palmaz JC, Richter GM, Noeldge G et al. Intraluminal stents in atherosclerotic iliac artery stenosis: preliminary report of a multicenter study. *Radiology* 1988; **168**: 727–31.

28 Palmaz JC, Garcia OJ, Schatz RA et al. Placement of balloon-expandable intraluminal stents in iliac arteries: first 171 procedures. *Radiology* 1990; **174**: 969–75.

29 Sullivan TM, Childs MB, Bacharach JM et al. Percutaneous transluminal angioplasty and primary stenting of the iliac arteries in 288 patients. *J Vasc Surg* 1997; **25**: 829–39.

30 Murphy KD, Encarnacion CE, Le VA, Palmaz JC. Iliac artery stent placement with the Palmaz stent: Follow-up study. *J Vasc Intervent Radiol* 1995; **6**: 321–9.

31 Sapoval MR, Chatellier G, Long AL et al. Self-expandable stents for treatment of iliac artery obstructive lesions: Long-term success and prognostic factors. *Am J Radiol* 1996; **166**: 1173–9.

32 Laborde JC, Palmaz JC, Rivera FJ et al. Influence of anatomic distribution of atherosclerosis on the outcome of revascularization with iliac stent placement. *J Vasc Intervent Radiol* 1995; **6**: 513–21.

33 Kichikawa K, Uchida H, Yoshioka T et al. Iliac artery stenosis and occlusion: Preliminary results of treatment with Gianturco expandable metallic stents. *Radiology* 1990; **177**: 799–802.

34 Rees CR, Palmaz JC, Garcia O et al. Angioplasty and stenting of completely occluded iliac arteries. *Radiology* 1989; **172**: 953–9.

35 Bosch JL, Hunink MGM. Meta-analysis of the results of percutaneous transluminal angioplasty and stent placement for aortoiliac occlusive disease. *Radiology* 1997; **204**: 87–96.

36 Henry M, Amor M, Thevenot G et al. Palmaz stent placement in iliac and femoropopliteal arteries: Primary and secondary patency in 310 patients with 2–4 year follow up. *Radiology* 1995; **197**: 167–74.

37 Vorwerk D, Gunther RW, Schurmann K, Wendt G. Aortic and iliac stenosis: Follow-up results of stent placement after insufficient balloon angioplasty in 118 cases. *Radiology* 1996; **198**: 45–8.

38 Tetteroo E, Haaring C, van der Graaf Y et al. Intraarterial pressure gradients after randomized angioplasty or stenting of iliac artery lesions. Dutch Iliac Stent Trial Study Group. *Cardiovasc Intervent Radiol* 1996; **19**: 411–17.

39 Palmaz JC, Laborde JC, Rivera FJ et al. Stenting of the iliac arteries with the Palmaz stent: experience from a multicenter trial. *Cardiovasc Intervent Radiol* 1992; **15**: 291–7.

40 Richter GM, Noeldge G, Roeren T et al. First long-term results of a randomized multicenter trial: iliac balloon-expandable stent placement versus regular percutaneous transluminal angioplasty. In: Lierman D (ed.), *State of the art and future developments*. Morin Heights, Canada: Polyscience, 1995: 30–5.

41 Perler BA, Williams GM. Does donor iliac artery percutaneous transluminal angioplasty or stent placement influence the results of femorofemoral bypass? Analysis of 70 consecutive cases with long-term follow up. *J Vasc Surg* 1996; **24**: 363–70.

28

Iliac occlusions

Isabelle Henry and Michel Henry

Introduction

Historically, reconstructive vascular surgery has been the cornerstone of treatment for symptomatic aortoiliac occlusive diseases. Aortobifemoral bypass gives good results with a 5-year patency rate of approximately 85% and a 10-year patency rate of 70%.[1] Indications for surgery are well-established severe claudication and limb-threatening ischemia. But larger indications are impossible because of the significant morbidity and mortality associated with surgical procedures.[2,3] In a meta-analysis of studies published after 1975 the aggregated operative mortality was 3.3% and the aggregated systemic morbidity was 8.3%.[2]

With improvement in technology, percutaneous transluminal angioplasty (PTA), such as balloon angioplasty and endovascular stenting, are proving to be effective and have become increasingly popular and the treatment of choice.

These lower-risk procedures have allowed a blurring of the traditional indications for treatment and a broadening of the indications for endovascular procedures based on this very low-procedural complication rate with percutaneous interventions. Now, patients with vascular claudication who do not respond to a medication and walking program may experience low-risk symptomatic relief.[4]

Angioplasty has now become the standard method of treatment for iliac stenoses and has long-term results that seriously challenge surgery.

In 1989, Becker et al.[5] analyzed 2697 angioplasties that were reported in the literature and reported a 72% patency rate at 5 years. Van Andel et al.[6] reported a 92% patency at 7 years, and Tegtmeyer et al.[7] a primary patency rate of 92%. In a randomized study of surgery vs angioplasty, Wilson[8] found no significant differences in the patency at 3 years. The implantation of endoprostheses seems to yield excellent results[9–10] and limits the complications of angioplasty.

However, percutaneous transluminal recanalizations of iliac occlusions have been more controversial. The first published series showed poor results and high complication rates.[11–13] However, recent papers have shown encouraging results,[14–18] reporting a low rate of complications and good long-term results that are comparable to surgery.

The management of iliac lesions evolved in three stages: the first stage was the development of balloon angioplasty with its own set of complications; the second stage was the development of endoprostheses, which has increased its indications and limited the complications; the third, current, stage is the development of stent grafts and covered stents which enable the implantation of a real internal bypass graft via the percutaneous approach – this opens up a new field of applications for long arterial lesions and all aneurysmal diseases.

However, the respective indications of each stent are still to be discussed as well as the primary stenting interest and direct stenting to avoid embolic complications.

The complexity of lesions and operator experience should be considered in the treatment decision. If an iliac stenosis is generally easy to treat, an iliac occlusion may be difficult to recanalize. An operator with limited experience, for example, should not treat a chronic iliac ostial occlusion in a patient with mild-to-moderate claudication, because of the risks of complications with this procedure. The highest level of expertise may be needed to solve all the problems we may encounter in treating the patient with safety and efficiency.

We have to discuss not only the approach methods but also the use of thrombolysis, catheter thrombectomy and stenting.

Percutaneous interventions should have a low complication rate, and be repeatable; now they may be carried out on an outpatient basis.[4]

Materials and methods

Population

A total of 173 lesions in 155 patients with acute or chronic iliac occlusions were treated by various percutaneous interventional techniques – i.e. fibrinolysis, mechanical thrombectomy, thromboaspiration, angioplasty, or stent implantation – either applied separately or in combination: 142 males and 13 females with a mean age of 56.9 ± 10.6 years (range: 33–80) were enrolled in the study. Based on Fontaine's classification, 120 patients were in stage IIb, 26 in stage III, and 9 in stage IV. The mean ABI (ankle – brachial index) was 0.38 ± 0.14 before treatment.

The occlusion was located in the common iliac artery (CIA) in 106 cases and in the external iliac artery (EIA) in 67 cases (total iliac artery occlusion involving CIA and EIA in 20 patients). The mean lesion length was 60.6 ± 22.5 mm in the CIA and 73.6 ± 31.7 mm in the EIA. The mean arterial diameter was 7.8 ± 1.1 mm in the EIA and 7.3 ± 1.2 mm in EIA. A total of 24 CIA and 12 EIA were very calcified.

Risk factors

- Hypertension ($n = 74$)
- Diabetes mellitus ($n = 23$)
- Dyslipidemia ($n = 52$)
- Smokers ($n = 108$).

Initial non-invasive work-up

Prior to diagnostic and interventional procedures, the patients underwent clinical and non-invasive assessment of their vascular disease. Doppler ultrasound pressures of distal leg arteries were measured and the ABI was calculated. A treadmill test was also required in patients presenting with chronic ischemia. A study of $TCPO_2$ was carried out for critical ischemia. Prior to angioplasty, it is essential to carefully perform a color Doppler ultrasound so as to identify the type and extent of the lesion, the presence and extent of calcification, as well as the underlying and collateral arterial circulation. This is important in selecting the interventional procedure and the type of endoprosthesis to be implanted.

In certain cases, Doppler ultrasound detects an aneurysmal disease which so far has gone unnoticed. This raises the issue of the indication of other examinations such as spiral computed tomography (CT) scans or magnetic resonance imaging (MRI).

In patients with generalized arterial diseases, a search for the associated lesions is always indispensable (coronary, renal, carotid, vertebral, and mesenteric arteries) and the additional investigation is selected in accordance with the patient's condition and the urgency of ischemia.

Angiography

Prior to the interventional procedure, all our patients underwent angiography, including frontal and oblique views of the lower limbs as well as frontal and lateral views of the abdomen. This angiography remains essential prior to determining the interventional gesture and results in a better identification of the lesion, its extent, and the arterial circulation upstream and downstream. It equally supports the technique selected, the approach site, and the possible use of an endoprosthesis (type, diameter, length).

Determining the onset of thrombosis

By carefully interviewing all of our patients, we tried to determine the onset of thrombosis and the therapeutic approach required, as well as the need for fibrinolysis, the age of the thrombosis (at least 3 months old), or the need for a mechanical recanalization in the case of an older thrombosis. Acute or sudden onset of an ischemic condition and the aggravation of a persisting claudication are indicative of a recent ischemia. A total of 89 patients were diagnosed with an occlusion less than 3 months old, and 84 had older occlusions.

Iliac recanalization techniques

Percutaneous treatment of iliac occlusion may be completed via several different leg approaches (ipsilateral, contralateral, bilateral femoral) but also via arm access occasionally or popliteal access in rare indications.

The choice of access site is dependent on several factors

- technique of recanalization
- onset of occlusion
- stent used
- operator preference.

Mechanical recanalization

Mechanical recanalization with hydrophilic guide wire was carried out for occlusions more than 3 months old. In our series several approaches were used.

Ipsilateral femoral approach. This approach was used whenever the common femoral artery (CFA) could be punctured ($n = 104$).

The puncture of the CFA was best performed after fluoroscopic localization of the bony femoral head. A 7F or 8F sheath, preferably a long sheath (23 cm), was then placed. This sheath will accept most balloons and stents. A 6F sheath may be used if the iliac artery is small. A straight or curved 0.035-inch hydrophilic guide wire placed in a hydrophilic 5F catheter was carefully advanced through the occlusion. False passage was likely but the correct positioning in the aortic lumen (and not in the wall) was checked by injecting contrast medium. Detection of the false passage may be more difficult if the guide wire butts against fibrous or calcified plaques and has a subintimal course at this point and then crosses into the true aortic lumen. This could lead to an extensive dissection. It is therefore essential to recognize the exact subintimal location of the guide to avoid performing an angioplasty or placement of a prosthesis in the wrong channel, which would generally lead to catastrophic complications.

Contralateral femoral approach. This approach has been used either *per primum* or when the ipsilateral approach failed or could not be used (*n* = 93). We usually place a 7 or 8F introducer at the contralateral femoral level. Catheters such as the Sidewinder (Cordis, Raden, the Netherlands), Simmons (Cordis), Motarjeme, or 'cane' type (Mallinckrodt Medical, Bondoufle, France), as well as catheters for the selective catheterization of the intimal mammary artery, usually made it easy to go over to the other side.

The same hydrophilic guide wires or catheters were utilized. It was important to have a good support to achieve an appropriate 'push' to enter the thrombosis. When the recanalization was performed it was very important to ensure that the guide wire was actually located in the arterial lumen. Ideally, it should be placed in the introducer located on the side of the lesion, either directly or recovered with a snare and extracted through the introducer. Then, the ipsilateral approach could be used to facilitate the implantation of endoprostheses (notably covered ones). Quite often, we used the contralateral approach, and ensured the correct position of the guide wire by angiography. While implanting the endoprostheses, the hydrophilic guide wire was replaced by a stiff AMPLATZ-type guide wire (Boston-Scimed, Natick, MA) on which a Cordis type 8F cross introducer was fitted – if the thrombosis was located at the common iliac level – or a long 40 cm 8F Arrow-Flex® introducer (Arrow International, Weesp, the Netherlands) – if the thrombosis started at a distance from the aortoiliac bifurcation – which has the advantage of being reinforced and does not bend at the bifurcation. Many 'flexible' sheaths will kink at the significant angulation of the aortic bifurcation and should not be used. Braided sheaths are recommended for use with this contralateral approach.

Contralateral angioplasty and stenting are completed in a manner similar to that used with the ipsilateral approach. In choosing a stent, detailed knowledge of the stent's ability to traverse the bifurcation is necessary. Self-expanding stents should pass easily. Flexible balloon expandable stents may also be easily implanted, but implantation of rigid stents such as Palmaz stents could be limited, depending on the bifurcation angle. Nevertheless, braided introducers facilitate the passage of these stents.

Bilateral approach – kissing technique. A bilateral approach was used in the case of distal aortic or bilateral iliac lesions (*n* = 42). A kissing technique may be needed to prevent compromise of the contralateral vessel from stent encroachment or to decrease the possibility of embolization into the contralateral limb.

Brachial approach. The need for arm access is less common. This approach was useful when significant common femoral plaque was present or in the case of total bilateral iliac occlusion (*n* = 8). The brachial approach may be complicated, because these patients often have elongated tortuous aortic arches. We used a long 6 or 7F sheath (80–90 cm) with the same guide wire as for the other approach methods. In 7 cases this approach was completed via the bilateral femoral approach to implant a prosthesis following iliac recanalization.

Popliteal approach. This approach was successfully used in 3 cases of occlusion of the external iliac and common femoral arteries when the contralateral approach could not be used owing to tortuous iliac arteries.

Fibrinolysis

A total of 38 patients were treated by fibrinolysis in accordance with MacNamara's protocol (4000 U/min urokinase for 2 hours followed by 2000 U/min during the following hours, and angiography was repeated after 24 hours to check for the re-opening of the vessel). Fibrinolysis lasted from 6 to 24 hours, the catheter was in contact with the thrombus via the contralateral approach. Re-opening of the artery was achieved in 33 cases (87%). We experienced 5 failures, and the artery was recanalized using the hydrophilic guide wire. Thrombolysis may decrease the risk for embolization as well as shortening the lesion that needs treatment.

Mechanical thrombectomy and thromboaspiration

A mechanical thrombectomy using a Hydrolyser (Cordis) was performed in 5 cases (fresh thrombus), resulting in re-opening the artery. Thromboaspiration was performed in 14 cases, which probably prevented distal embolisms. A total success was obtained in 12 patients, a partial success in 2 being completed by fibrinolysis. While performing this technique, a tourniquet was used at the femoral level to avoid distal embolisms.

Laser recanalization

In 8 cases, an Excimer laser fiber (Spectranetics, Nieuwegen, the Netherlands) was used to recanalize the artery, following failure of the hydrophilic guide wire. It was successful in 6 cases.

Angioplasty

Following arterial recanalization, the guide wire was left in place in the arterial lumen. Preangioplasty angiography was done with distal runoff evaluation to recognize significant embolization and to treat it and to assess the vessel size (external iliac artery 5–8 mm; common iliac artery 7–10 mm) and extent of calcifications. In certain cases, it may be difficult to determine the size of the balloon or endoprosthesis. The diameter of the contralateral artery was then taken as a reference. Endovascular ultrasound may also help for the arterial diameter evaluation and to evaluate the lesion characteristics. For reasons of cost, we limited this technique to 12 patients.

In most of the cases, balloon angioplasty was performed with a balloon size equal to that of the artery.

When an endoprosthesis was implanted, the predilatation was carried out with a slightly smaller balloon, as recommended by Vorwerk et al.,[16,17] because it is best not to overdilate the artery.

In the case of significant calcification, it is better to predilate with a non-compliant, conservatively sized balloon. If the vessel is not significantly calcified, predilatation may or may not be done depending on operator experience and preference. Balloon expandable stents should always be protected by a sheath to allow for passage through the lesion. Predilatation is done: as the balloon deflates, the sheath is advanced past the area of stenosis. Re-advancing the sheath in this manner allows for protection of the stent from dislodgement during placement.[4] With self-expanding stents, which are protected, this maneuver is not necessary. Final balloon dilatation is completed with an appropriately sized balloon.

Hemodynamic evaluation may be carried out by advancing the sheath through the stent or placing a catheter. By using a pullback maneuver, the gradient pressure may be measured. An endovascular ultrasound examination may also be performed to appreciate the expansion of the stent and the final result. Then, a final angiography is performed, with evaluation of the runoff vessels to assess for embolization.

When a bilateral procedure with kissing technique is performed, both balloon expandable and self-expanding stents should be deployed simultaneously. Simultaneous balloon inflation and deflation is important to allow for equal stent expansion.[4]

The placement of a stent at aortic bifurcation is an important consideration.[4] Recent animal data have shown that the practice of placing kissing stents high in the aorta and 'raising the bifurcation' may not be desirable. This technique significantly alters the hemodynamics at the bifurcation and may increase the risk for restenosis.[19] For Scheinert et al.,[20] to ensure an optimal reconstruction of the aortic bifurcation, stents are deliberately placed in the aortic lumen somewhat beyond the assumed bifurcation. Furthermore, this technique may contribute to a reduction of embolic complications because dislodgement of thrombotic material or plaque displacement may be prevented by stent struts. Aortic stent deployment should always be completed before the iliac arteries are stented. Attempting to place the aortic stent after iliac stent deployment often leads to incomplete plaque coverage and an unsatisfactory result.[4] The role of the internal iliac arteries (IIAs) has to be considered, especially in male patients. When performing iliac angioplasty it is often necessary to cross these arteries, with a risk of occlusion. It is preferable to leave one of the internal iliac vessels patent and, in the case of ostial IIA stenosis, to perform an angioplasty of this lesion. We have treated 18 lesions at this level with stenting in 16 cases.

Choice of the endoprosthesis

At the start of our experience a stent was not systematically implanted to treat iliac occlusions and we used provisional stenting for inadequate PTA (dissection, residual stenosis). However, because of the positive results obtained at the iliac level we now routinely stent total occlusions at this level.

Among the 155 recanalized iliac arteries, 132 were treated with stents. A direct stenting was performed in 23 cases. Several type of stents may be implanted:

- Non-covered stents
  1 Balloon-expandable stents
  Palmaz stents (Figure 28.1)
  Medtronic. AVE
  VIP Medtronic
  Corinthian (Cordis)
  Angiodynamics
  MegaLink (Guidant)
  Intrastent (Intratherapeutics)
  2 Nitinol self-expanding stents
  Sinus Optimed (Optimed)
  Expander (Boston Medical)
  Symphony (Boston)
  Intracoil (Intratherapeutics)
  Smart (Cordis)
- Covered stents
  Cragg Endopro (Boston) (Figure 28.2)
  Corvita (Boston) (Figure 28.3)
  Wallgraft (Boston)
  Hemobahn (Gore)
  Jomed stent (Jomed) .

Table 28.1 Stent indications, depending on lesion location

	Palmaz	Palmaz Long Medium	Palmaz Corinthian	INTRASTENT MegaLink AVE VIP	Wallstent	Optimed Memotherm	IntraCoil	Expander	SMART	Symphony	Z Stent	Covered stents
CIA	+++	+++	+++	+++	+++	+++	++	+++	+++	+++	+++	+++
EIA	+	++	++	++	+++	+++	+++	+++	+++	++	+++	+++
IIA	+++	+	+++	+++	−	+	−	−	+	−	−	−

CIA, common iliac artery; EIA, external iliac artery; IIA, internal iliac artery.
0 to +++: no indication to good indication.

Table 28.2 Stent indications

	Palmaz	Palmaz Long Medium	Palmaz Corinthian	INTRASTENT MegaLink AVE VIP	Wallstent	Optimed Memotherm	IntraCoil	Expander	SMART	Symphony	Z Stent	Covered stents
Tortuous arteries	−	−	+	+	+++	++	+++	++	+++	+	+++	+++
Calcifications	+++	+++	+++	++	+	++	−	++	++	+++	+	++
Joint	−	−	−	−	+++	++	+++	++	++	−	++	+
Length >8 cm	−	−	−	−	+	+++	+	++	+++	+	+++	+++
Ostium	+++	+++	+++	+++	−	++	−	++	++	++	++	+
Collateral branches	+	+	+	+	+	+	+++	+	+	+	++	−
Contralateral approach	+	+	++	++	+++	+++	+++	+++	+++	++	+++	++

0 to +++: no indication to good indication.

The choice of the stent depends on the location, the length, the characteristics of the lesion, the approach method, and the operator experience. Tables 28.1 and 28.2 show the stent indications depending on lesion location, lesion morphology, and approach way.

For short lesions, any stent may be used. For long lesions, covered stents could be preferred but, more recently, various self-expanding nitinol stents have given excellent long-term results.[21–23] All stents are not equivalent, and it is important to have several different types in a cath-lab to choose the best stent suited to the lesion.

Patient follow-up and adjunct therapy

Twenty-four hours after the procedure, the patient underwent a duplex scan. At 6 months a duplex scan was repeated and angiography was performed; subsequently, the patients were followed up by regular duplex scans. Angiography was performed only when restenosis was suspected. The patients were also administered ticlopidine (250 mg/day) or clopidogrel (75 mg/day), and aspirin (100 mg/day) for 1 month and then only aspirin (160–300 mg/day). In cases where stents were not implanted, only aspirin was administered.

Results

Initial results

The initial results are shown in Table 28.3. Among our 173 lesions, 155 were recanalized, resulting in an immediate success rate of 90%. The age of the thrombosis seems to be the important and determining factor of success. All our patients, except those presenting with an occlusion less than 3 months old, were successfully recanalized (88/89, i.e. 99%). We were able to recanalize only 67 out of 84 chronic

Table 28.3   Initial results

- Immediate success rate: 155/173   (90%)
- Factors of success
  - Onset of thrombosis
    - < 3 months   88/89   (99%)
    - ≥ 3 months   67/84   (80%)
  - Site $p<0.0001$
    - CIA and CIA + EIA   95/106   (90%)
    - EIA   60/67   (90%)
  - Length of occlusion   N.S.
    - < 60 mm   51/52   (98%)
    - ≥ 60 mm   104/121   (86%)
    - Calcification $p<0.02$
      - Calcified   23/26   (64%)
      - Non calcified   132/137   (96%)
      - Abi: 0.38±0.14→0.85±0.30   ($p<0.001$) $p<0.0001$

occlusions that were more than 3 months old (80%) ($p < 0.0001$). Most failures were due to old and highly calcified lesions.

No significant differences were observed in our results in terms of:

- Site

  External iliac occlusions: success was achieved in 60 out of 67 (90%)

  Common iliac occlusions: with or without occlusion of the EIA success was achieved in 95 out of 106 (90%)
- Gender

Significant differences were observed, depending on lesion length and calcification. Short lesions (< 60 mm) were recanalized in the majority of the cases (98%). It was the same for non-calcified lesions (96%). The ABI values increased from 0.38 ± 0.14 to 0.85 ± 0.30 ($p < 0.001$). Clinical improvement of one of more stages occurred in 143 patients (92%). In the patients ($n = 12$) who had no clinical benefit from the intervention, a poor runoff or an occlusion of the superficial femoral or popliteal were seen. Surgical revascularization was performed in these cases.

Table 28.4 summarizes the type of stents implanted to treat 132 lesions (CIA = 86, EIA = 46). Table 28.5 summarizes the stents' results, in terms of lesion length and arterial diameter.

Complications

Six peripheral embolisms were observed immediately after the procedures during angiographic control. In 4 of them, the occlusion was less than 3 months old; 4 were successfully treated by thromboaspiration and 2 by surgical embolectomy

Table 28.4   Type of stents implanted

- 132 lesions stented
  - CIA: 86
  - EIA: 46
- Type of stents
  - Non-covered stents: 109 lesions – 138 stents
    - Palmaz: 101
    - Nitinol self-expanding: 33
      - Sinus Optimed: 22
      - Expander: 7
      - Symphony: 1
      - Vascucoil: 1
      - Smart: 2
    - VIP Medtronic: 4
  - Covered stents: 23 lesions – 30 stents
    - Cragg endopro: 24
    - Corvita: 5
    - Wallgraft: 1

(Fogarty). Nine patients had thromboses within 24 hours: they were treated surgically. We observed 1 arterial rupture immediately treated with a covered stent (PASSAGER). Three minor hematomas (which did not require a surgical procedure) and 1 false aneurysm (treated surgically) also occurred. Presently, the local complications have been reduced thanks to the use of puncture site closure devices (ANGIOSEAL, PROSTAR PLUS, PERCLOSE).

Patient follow-up

Follow-up ranged from 1 to 11 months (mean: 30 ± 2.5 months). Primary (PI) and secondary (PII) patencies were computed in accordance with Rutherford and Becker's

Table 28.5   Stents results

	Number of stented arteries	Mean lesion length (mm)	Mean stented lesion length (mm)	Mean art Ø (mm)	Mean stent Ø (mm)
CIA	46	60.6±22.5	60.1±22.1	7.8±1.1	7.8±0.7
EIA	86	73.6±31.7	70.2±29.1	7.3±1.2	7.4±1

Table 28.6   8-year follow-up – all lesions (173)

	Number of lesions	PI (%)	PII (%)
All lesions	173	66	77
CIA	106	66 ⎤ N.S.	80 ⎤ N.S.
EIA	67	67 ⎦	72 ⎦
<3 months	89	68 ⎤ N.S.	86 ⎤ p<0.01
≥3 months	84	63 ⎦	67 ⎦
Length <6cm	52	78 ⎤ p<0.01	90 ⎤ p<0.001
Length >6cm	121	61 ⎦	71 ⎦
Ø <8 mm	80	67 ⎤ N.S.	76 ⎤ N.S.
Ø ≥8 mm	93	65 ⎦	78 ⎦
Calcified	36	50 ⎤ p<0.01	53 ⎤ p<0.008&
Non-calcified	137	70 ⎦	83 ⎦
Good run off	98	71 ⎤ N.S.	80 ⎤ N.S.
Poor run off	75	58 ⎦	7 ⎦

Table 28.7   8-year follow-up – recanalized patients (155)

	Number of lesions	PI (%)	PII (%)
All lesions	155	73	86
CIA	95	74 ⎤ N.S.	90 ⎤ p<0.05
EIA	60	75 ⎦	80 ⎦
<3 months	88	69 ⎤ N.S.	87 ⎤ N.S.
≥3 months	67	79 ⎦	84 ⎦
Length <6cm	51	80 ⎤ N.S.	92 ⎤ N.S.
Length >6cm	104	71 ⎦	83 ⎦
Ø <8 mm	75	71 ⎤ N.S.	81 ⎤ N.S.
Ø ≥8 mm	80	76 ⎦	90 ⎦
Calcified	23	78 ⎤ N.S.	82 ⎤ N.S.
Non-calcified	132	72 ⎦	86 ⎦
Good run off	89	79 ⎤ p<0.04	88 ⎤ N.S.
Poor run off	66	66 ⎦	83 ⎦

criteria[24] for all the lesions (173) (Table 28.6) and for recanalized lesions (155) (Table 28.7). Given the limited number of occlusions found over the whole iliac artery (20 cases), they have been listed together with the common iliac occlusions. During the follow-up we observed:

- 9 total thromboses: 4 before 6 months treated surgically and 5 after 6 months treated by new PTA ($n = 2$) or surgically ($n = 3$).2
- 10 restenoses: 5 before 6 months treated with success by new PTA and stent and 5 after 6 months treated also by new PTA and stent.

For all the lesions: PI at 8 years follow-up is 66% – 66% for the CIA and 67% for the EIA – and PII is 77%, 80%, and 72%, respectively (non-significant difference).

PII appear significantly different for lesions more than 3 months old and less than 3 months old: 86 vs 67% ($p < 0.01$). No significant difference was observed with respect to gender or lesion diameter. Length of the occlusion has important impacts on primary and secondary patency rates. PI is 78% in occlusions less than 6 cm long and 61% in occlusions more than 6 cm long ($p < 0.01$) and for PII it is

90% and 71%, respectively ($p < 0.001$). Calcifications also have important impacts on PI and PII, but we observed no significant difference depending on the runoff.

If we compute PI and PII at 8 years follow-up, by considering only recanalized lesions, PI comes to 73% and PII is 86%. There was no significant difference for PI at the level of the common iliac and external iliac arteries, 74% vs 75%; however, the difference became significant for PII [90% vs 80% ($p < 0.05$)]. No significant difference was observed in primary and secondary patency rates with respect to occlusion age, lesion diameter, length of the lesion, calcifications, and runoff. The results in patients treated with stents or with angioplasty alone are difficult to compare (Table 28.8). At the start of our experience, the stents were only implanted to treat a complication, but now they are routinely implanted in the case of occlusion. It is also difficult to compare the results with regard to the type of prostheses. However, we observed a significant difference between stented and non-stented lesions (PI = 76% vs 61%, PII = 87 vs 74% – $p < 0.03$). This difference appeared for CIA and EIA lesions. Covered stents seem to give no benefit for iliac occlusion in comparison with non-covered stents. Specific indications should be discussed in the future.

Table 28.8	Long-term follow-up – stented arteries		

	Number of lesions	PI (%)	PII (%)
All lesions			
• Stented	132	76 ⎤ p<0.03	87 ⎤ p<0.03
• Non-stented	23	61 ⎦	74 ⎦
• Covered stents	23	73 ⎤ N.S.	84 ⎤ N.S.
• Non-covered stents	109	81 ⎦	91 ⎦
CIA			
• Stented	86	77 ⎤ p<0.001	90 ⎤ p<0.003
• Non-stented	9	52 ⎦	78 ⎦
• Covered stents	15	68 ⎤ p<0.02	84 ⎤ p<0.02
• Non-covered stents	71	83 ⎦	94 ⎦
EIA			
• Stents	46	77 ⎤ p<0.05	82 ⎤ p<0.06
• Non-stents	14	64 ⎦	71 ⎦
• Covered stents	8	85 ⎤ N.S.	85 ⎤ N.S.
• Non-covered stents	38	79 ⎦	84 ⎦

Discussion

Interventional management of iliac occlusions remains a debated issue. The first results published in the literature were far from encouraging. In 1979, Tegtmeyer et al.[25] reported the first success and suggested that angioplasty could be used to treat iliac occlusions. In 1980, Motarjeme et al.[26] were only able to recanalize two patients out of 8 (25%). In 1982, Ring et al.[11] had a low primary patency rate of 40% in 10 patients and a high complication rate (20%). They reported three major drawbacks of the PTA of iliac occlusions:

1. failure to pass the occlusion,
2. failure to create a sufficient channel, and
3. danger of embolization.

In 1984, Pilla et al.[27] considered the PTA of iliac arteries to be a useful therapeutic modality and an alternative to surgery.

Subsequently, larger series were published and they reported satisfactory results and suggested angioplasty to be the treatment of choice in the case of iliac occlusions. High technical success rates were achieved: 78% for

Colapinto et al.[18] and Gupta et al.,[28] 82% for Johnston et al.,[13] 81% for Vorwerk et al.,[17] and 98% for Blum et al.[15] This has been made possible because of improved material, a better knowledge of the various approaches, and the experience of the operator. It is now reasonable to expect a technical success rate of 90%, regardless of the occlusion length. For example, Vorwerk,[17] who only obtained a success rate of 71% in his first 50 patients, secured 93% with his following series of 50 patients.

In our cohort of patients, the age of the occlusion, the length of the lesion, and the presence of important calcification seem to be the determining factors of immediate success. One of the major complications that was sometimes encountered was the false passage of the guide wire into the wall, leading to long dissections. Long occlusions and very calcified plaques were the determining factors in technical failures. The subintimal passage must be immediately diagnosed because a balloon angioplasty or the implantation of an endoprosthesis in a false channel would create severe complications or early thromboses.[17] It is important to point out that, usually, a recanalization failure does not result in complications or an aggravation of the patient's condition. The patient can be referred for surgery at a later date without an emergency.

Another complication may be encountered during iliac occlusion recanalization: a vessel wall perforation or rupture, which may be catastrophic in the iliac artery if it is not quickly recognized and treated because of high flow into the retroperitoneum. This situation may lead to death. Inflation of a balloon, large enough to occlude the abdominal aorta, can stop the hemorrhage before referring the patient to the surgeon or placing a covered stent. For more local perforations, prolonged balloon inflation (at least 20 min) at the site, along with residual of anticoagulation, will often suffice.[4]

Different recanalization techniques have been reported and can be discussed. Recanalization using a hydrophilic guide wire seems the most popular technique now; recanalization with a laser is an alternative in the case of failure or to clean up the artery.[29] Fibrinolysis has been recommended by many authors.[30–35] Auster et al.[31] first treated iliac occlusions with fibrinolysis. Rees et al.[30] and Kichikawa et al.[34] combined thrombolysis, PTA, and stent implantation and achieved a high primary patency rate (80–100%). In a series of 42 patients, Hausseger et al.[33] concluded that additional fibrinolysis helps improve the results of mechanical passage of an occluded segment.

Rominger et al.[35] recommended overnight lysis after mechanical passage of the occlusion to prevent embolization. Blum et al.[15] reported 98% technical success (46/47 patients) with a rotational angioplasty device; lytic therapy was performed for 2–36 hours, but it is uncertain what percentage of their patients had a chronic occlusion.

Fibrinolysis remains a topical issue. We performed fibrinolysis in recent occlusions to transform an occlusion into an easier-to-treat stenotic lesion. In older occlusions or in the event of failure, the addition of fibrinolysis may help by softening the thrombus to facilitate mechanical recanalization, which could be the only option in patients in whom mechanical passage has not yet been achievable.[17] However, fibrinolysis treatment for all types of occlusion is not justified because of its high cost and the inherent risks of the technique. Moreover, it does not limit the risk of distal embolization. The new procedures of mechanical thrombectomy (Hydrolyser, AngioJet) should help recanalize recent occlusions. They can be used alone or supplemented by thromboaspiration or a fibrinolysis.[36,37]

The main complication of the techniques for iliac occlusion that remains is distal embolism. Colapinto et al.[18] reported 2 perforations and 2 embolic events (4%) requiring surgery. Ring et al.[11] reported two embolizations in 5 successful procedures. Gupta et al.[28] had a major complication rate of 18% with embolization in 4 patients. Blum et al.[15] reported major and minor complications in 15% of their cases. Peripheral embolism occurred in 3 patients (7%) after fibrinolysis. Vorwerk et al.[17] despite primary stenting, observed 5 peripheral embolisms (4.8%). They suggested that embolization occurs when the post-dilatation of the stent is performed with a balloon. It squeezes the occlusive material out of the proximal end of the stent, which they found can be avoided by not overdilating the balloon.

In our series, we observed 6 peripheral embolisms; however, a primary stenting or fibrinolysis were not used in many cases. It seems clear to us that no technique can prevent this complication. Debris from embolization of large, chronic thrombus may lead to large vessel closure and acute limb-threatening ischemia. Fortunately, in many instances, it can be satisfactorily dealt with via an interventional technique, thromboaspiration, or fibrinolysis.

Occasionally, the debris may be pinned against the vessel wall with a self-expanding stent to allow for restoration of flow in the case of profound ischemia.[4] Surgery was used as the last resort when other procedures failed. It would be worthwhile to point out that a number of distal embolisms occur on the opposite side of the occlusion following recanalization of the initial part of the CIA. To avoid this, we used the 'kissing' technique to block the flow into the opposite iliac artery, which also avoided a prolapse of atheromatous thrombus during balloon inflation.

The issue of endoprosthesis implantation is discussed below. Implantation can be performed in three different ways:

1. The endoprosthesis can be implanted only in the case of a complication or a suboptimal result.[15]
2. It can be used as first intention without predilatation (direct stenting) so as to limit distal embolic complications; prosthesis dilatation is performed after its implantation.[17,38] However, we observed that this technique did not prevent all distal embolisms[17] and, in our series, in which most of the

endoprostheses were implanted after predilatation, the embolic complications were not high.

3. Endoprostheses can be proposed as a first intention to limit the complications and to reduce the restenosis rate. Richter's study[9] showed that the long-term patency benefits could be derived through the primary stenting with a Palmaz stent in iliac occlusions. In a non-randomized study,[10] the secondary patency rate of 94% was reported at 4 years by using the same stent. In our series, we observed a significant difference in primary and secondary patency between stented and non-stented lesions at CIA and EIA locations. This is why we recommend the routine implantation of an endoprosthesis for any iliac occlusion. The choice of the endoprosthesis is worth debating. Any prosthesis works at the iliac location but we have seen that the choice depends on the lesion characteristics, the morphology, the approach method, and the experience of the operator. Covered stents do not give better results and need large introducers but they have specific indications for aneurysmal diseases, ulcerated plaques, may be long lesions for the new covered stents available on the market. Prospective and randomized studies are awaited. The new nitinol stents seem to give good long-term results, even for long lesions, and their implantation is possible though 7F introducers, with low risk of local complications.

Long-term results are favorable and encouraging and approach those of the surgical bypass procedure. At 8 years follow-up, we observed a PI of 73% and a PII of 86% for recanalized lesions with a small difference for PII between CIA and EIA. The same results are reported in the literature. At 4 years, Vorwerk obtained a primary patency rate of 78% and a secondary patency rate of 88%, whereas Colapinto obtained a primary and secondary patency of 76% and 80%, respectively, at 2 years. The same rates in the series of Gupta et al[28] were 76% and 81% at 4 years and in Blum et al.'s series[15] they were 76% and 87% at 3 years. The result of these different series is difficult to compare, due to the limited follow-up and because techniques differ.

Despite favorable results reported by various authors,[15–18,24–28,38,39] the interventional treatment of iliac occlusions is still a debatable issue. The Society of Cardiovascular and Interventional Radiology[40] still rates class III and IV iliac occlusions as unsuitable for PTA alone. With the advent of new techniques and prostheses, and with these published data, it is hoped that the interventional treatment will be the treatment of choice of iliac occlusions. Probably, covered stents will be improved so that real internal bypass could be performed via the percutaneous approach.

Conclusion

Long-term results of the interventional treatment for iliac occlusions have been encouraging. This therapy should be the first proposed technique. With the use of endoprostheses, the results have improved considerably, but larger randomized studies are required to clearly define the exact status of this endovascular therapy in the management of iliac occlusions and to define the prosthesis best suited for the lesion.

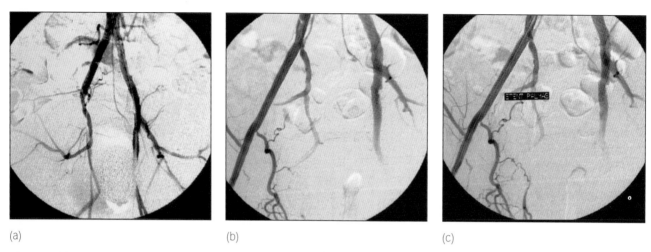

(a)   (b)   (c)

Figure 28.1

(a) Thrombosis of the external iliac artery. (b) Recanalization and placement of a long medium spiral stent. Thrombus in the lower part of the right internal iliac artery. (c) Final result after thromboaspiration.

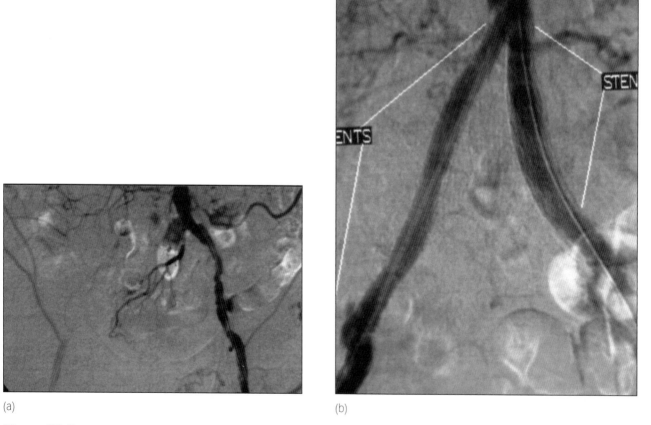

(a)   (b)

Figure 28.2

(a) Right iliac artery thrombosis. Left iliac artery polystenosis. (b) Placement of Cragg Endopro System 1/ Passager Stents.

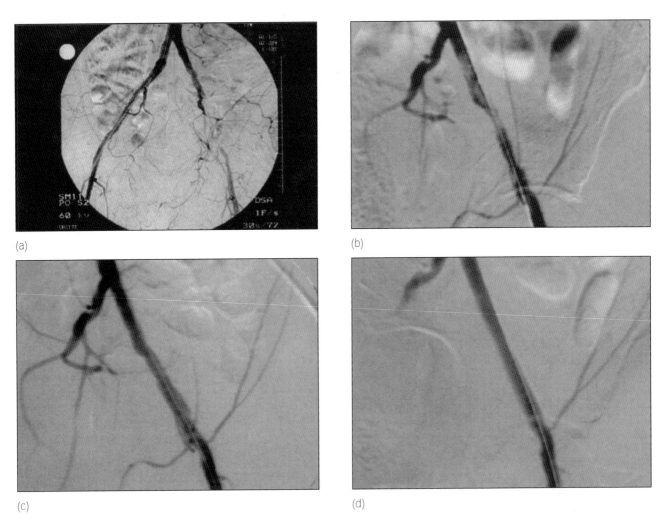

(a)

(b)

(c)

(d)

Figure 28.3
(a) Left external iliac artery occlusion. (b) Result after thrombolysis. (c) Result after balloon angioplasty. (d) Final result.

References

1 Brewster DC. Direct reconstruction for aortoiliac occlusive disease. In: Rutherford RB (ed.), *Vascular surgery*. Philadelphia: WB Saunders, 1989: 667–91.

2 De Vries SO, Hunink MG. Results of aortic bifurcation grafts for aortoiliac occlusive disease: a meta-analysis. *J Vasc Surg* 1997, **26**: 558–69.

3 Hertzer NR, Avellone JC, Farrel CJ et al. The risk of vascular surgery in a metropolitan community: with observation on surgeon experience and hospital size. *J Vasc Surg* 1984, **1**: 13–31.

4 Ansel GM, George BS, Botti CF. Percutaneous iliac arterial intervention: current indications, results, and techniques. *Intervent Cardiol* 1999; **1**: 303–9.

5 Becker GJ, Katzen BT, Dake MD. Non coronary angioplasty. *Radiology* 1989; **170**: 403–12.

6 Van Andel GJ, Van Erp WFM, Krepel M. Percutaneous transluminal dilatation of the iliac artery. Long term results. *Radiology* 1985; **156**: 321–3.

7 Tegtmeyer CJ, Hartwell GD, Selby JB et al. Results and complications of angioplasty in aortoiliac disease. *Circulation* 1991; **83**(suppl. I): 153–60.

8 Wilson SE, Wolf GL, Cross AP. Percutaneous transluminal angioplasty versus operation for peripheral atherosclerosis. *J Vasc Surg* 1989; **9**: 1–9.

9 Richter GM, Roeren TK, Noeldge G et al. Superior clinical results of iliac stent placement versus percutaneous transluminal angioplasty: four year success rate of a randomized study [Abstract]. *Radiology* 1991; **181**(suppl.): 161.

10 Henry M, Amor M, Ethevenot G et al. Palmaz stent placement in iliac and femoropopliteal arteries: primary and secondary patency in 310 patients with 2–4 year follow-up. *Radiology* 1995; **197**: 167–74.

11 Ring E, Freiman D, Mc Lean G et al. Percutaneous recanalization of common iliac artery occlusions: an unacceptable complication rate. *AJR* 1982; **139**: 587–9.

12 Graziani I. Percutaneous recanalization of total iliac and femoro-popliteal artery occlusions. *Eur J Radiol* 1987; 7.

13 Johnston KW, Rae M, Hogg-Johnston SA et al. Five-year results of a prospective study of percutaneous transluminal angioplasty. *Ann Surg* 1987; **206**: 403–13.

14 Cardon JM, Joyex A, Noblet D et al. Recanalisation endovasculaire des thromboses artérielles iliaques primitives. *J Med Vasc* 1996; **21**: 107–10.

15 Blum U, Gabelman A, Redecker M et al. Percutaneous recanalization of iliac artery occlusions: results of a prospective study. *Radiology* 1993; **189**: 536–40.

16 Vorwerk D, Günther RW. Mechanical revascularisation of occluded iliac arteries with use of self-expandable endoprostheses. *Radiology* 1990; **175**: 411–15.

17 Vorwerk D, Günther RW, Schurmmann K et al. Primary stent placement for chronic iliac artery occlusions: follow-up results in 103 cases. *Radiology* 1995; **194**: 745–9.

18 Colapinto RF, Stronell RD, Johnston WK. Transluminal angioplasty of complete iliac obstructions. *AJR* 1986; **146**: 859–62.

19 Fabregues S, Baijens K, Rieu R et al. Hemodynamics of endovascular prostheses. *J Biomech* 1998, **3**: 45–54.

20 Scheinert D, Schröder M, Balzer J et al. Stent supported reconstruction of the aortoiliac bifurcation using the kissing balloon technique. ETC Book Paris, 1999; 323–9.

21 Damaraju S, Cuasay L, Le D et al. Predictors of primary patency failure in Wallstent self expanding endovascular prostheses for iliofemoral occlusive disease. *Tex Heart Inst J* 1997, **24**: 173–8.

22 Vorwerk D, Gunther RW. Stent placement in iliac arterial lesions: three years of clinical experience with the Wallstent. *Cardiovasc Intervent Radiol* 1992, **15**: 285–90.

23 Henry M, Amor M, Henry I. First clinical experience with new nitinol self-expanding stents in peripheral arteries. *J Endovasc Surg* 1999, **6**: 92–3.

24 Rutherford RB, Becker GJ. Standards for evaluating and reporting the results of surgical and percutaneous therapy for peripheral arterial disease. *J Vasc Intervent Radiol* 1991; **2**: 169.

25 Tegtmeyer CJ, Moore TS, Chandler JG et al. Percutaneous transluminal dilatation of a complete block in the right iliac artery. *AJR* 1979; **133**: 532–5.

26 Motarjeme A, Kweifer JW, Zuska AJ. Percutaneous transluminal angioplasty of the iliac arteries: 66 experiences. *AJR* 1980; **135**: 937–44.

27 Pilla TJ, Peterson GJ, Tantana S et al. Percutaneous recanalization of iliac artery occlusions: an alternative to surgery in the high-risk patient. *AJR* 1984; **143**: 313–16.

28 Gupta AK, Ravamndalam K, Rao VRK et al. Total occlusion of iliac arteries: results of balloon angioplasty. *Cardiovasc Intervent Radiol* 1993; **16**: 165–77.

29 Biamino G, Skarabis P, Böttcher H et al. Excimer laser assisted angioplasty of peripheral vessels. In: Serruys PW, Strauss BH, King SB III (eds), *Restenosis after intervention with new mechanical devices.* Kluwer Academic Publishers, 1992: 427–73.

30 Rees CR, Palmaz JC, Garcia O et al. Angioplasty and stenting of completely occluded iliac arteries. *Radiology* 1989; **172**: 953–9.

31 Auster M, Kadir S, Mitchell SE et al. Iliac artery occlusion: management with intrathrombus streptokinase infusion and angioplasty. *Radiology* 1984; **153**: 385–8.

32 Katzen BT. Technique and results of 'low dose' thrombolytic infusion. *Cardiovasc Intervent Radiol* 1988; **11**: 41–7.

33 Haussger KA, Lammer J, Klein G et al. Perkutane Rekanalisation von Beckenarterienverschlossen: fibrinolyse, PTA, stents. *Fortschr Röntgenstr* 1991; **155**: 550–5.

34 Kichikawa K, Uchida H, Yoshioka T. Iliac artery stenosis and occlusion: preliminary results of treatment with Gianturco expandable metallic stents. *Radiology* 1990; **177**: 799–802.

35 Rominger M, Rauber K, Matthes B et al. Interventionell-radiologisches vorgehen bei längerstreckigen kompletten becken-arterienverschlossen. *Fortschr Röntgenstr* 1991; **154**: 301–14.

36 Reekers JA, Kromhout JG, Van der Waal K. Catheter for percutaneous thrombectomy: first clinical experience. *Radiology* 1993; **188**: 871–4.

37 Henry M, Amor M, Porte JM et al. The Hydrolyser catheter: clinical experience in 41 cases. *J Endovasc Surg* 1997;

38 Long AL, Page PE, Maynar AC et al. Percutaneous iliac artery stent. Angiographic long term follow-up. *Radiology* 1991; **180**: 771–8.

39 Zollikoffer CL, Antonucci F, Pfyffer M et al. Arterial stent placement with use of the Wallstent: midterm results of clinical experience. *Radiology* 1991; **179**: 449–56.

40 Standards of Practice Committee of the Society of Cardiovascular and Interventional Radiology. Guidelines for percutaneous transluminal angioplasty. *Radiology* 1990; **177**: 619–26.

29

Interventional strategies for recanalization of chronic total iliac and femoropopliteal artery occlusions

Sven Bräunlich, Dierk Scheinert and Giancarlo Biamino

Introduction

More than three decades after the first percutaneous transluminal angioplasty (PTA), chronic total occlusions (CTO) are still a technical challenge. They represent 25–30% of our catheterization laboratory activity. Considering some important pathologic features is important to improve patient selection and material choice during the procedure. The occluded part of the lumen associates two types of tissue: atheromatous plaque and old thrombus. The respective amounts of these items are largely dependent on the CTO mechanism, which may be grossly classified as two phenomena:

- late evolution of an acute occlusion (with a large quantity of old thrombus) due to a plaque rupture, usually apart from the maximal narrowing area (Figure 29.1a);
- progressive occlusion of a long-standing high-degree stenosis (with a large amount of plaque and sometimes several layers of additional thrombi) (Figure 29.1b).

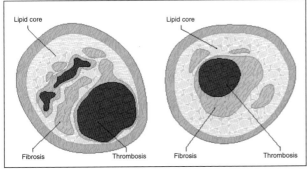

(a)   **(b)**

Figure 29.1
Two mechanisms of occlusion.

Tissue composition associates a majority of fibrous and mixed tissue and a small quantity of cholesterol, this decreases with time to be replaced by more dense collagen and calcium. Usually, the fibrous cap is located at the two edges of the occlusion. A negative remodeling of the artery is associated with the luminal process and becomes important in CTO older than 3 months. This remodeling is correlated to the fibrous replacement phenomenon within the middle of occlusion. Its importance is higher in short CTO. In long CTO, the organization of the thrombus is responsible for soft components in the middle, creating the 'piece of cake' of the lesion.[1]

Chronic iliac artery occlusions

PTA has been proved to be an effective technique for the treatment of symptomatic iliac artery stenoses and short occlusions.[2–4] When combined with the use of adjunctive stent placement, the immediate technical success rate improved significantly by up to 95%.[5–10] Patency rates of 80–90% after 5 years, reported for short iliac stenoses, are comparable to surgical results.[11–13]

Long total occlusions of iliac arteries have not yet been considered as a generally accepted indication for percutaneous treatment.[14–16] Results reported with balloon dilatations of iliac occlusions showed a technical failure rate of up to 22%[17] and a less favorable long-term outcome when compared with iliac stenoses.[17,18] Primary stenting after percutaneous recanalization of long iliac occlusions may contribute to an improvement of the long-term results.[19–21]

Because of the relatively high complication rate, due to dislodgement of thromboembolic material and distal embolization, the use of thrombolytic therapy prior to balloon angioplasty has been advocated.[15,22] Lysis therapy, however, has not been uniformly reported as being effective for chronic iliac occlusions. Alternatively, the use of percutaneous debulking techniques prior to primary stenting may improve the acute and long-term results, especially after recanalization of chronic occlusions of > 5 cm in length, which are normally not considered for percutaneous procedures. Pulsed laser systems with a short absorption depth, such as the 308 nm xenon chloride excimer laser, have been shown to permit controlled photoablation of sclerotic material.[23,24]

To evaluate the initial and long-term results of primary stent implantation after excimer-laser-assisted recanalization of chronic iliac artery occlusions, we analyzed the data of 212 consecutive patients with unilateral chronic iliac artery occlusions who were percutaneously treated in our institution.[25]

Study population

Only patients with angiographically proven iliac occlusion and stable clinical symptoms of at least 3 months duration were included. The baseline clinical characteristics of the study population are given in Table 29.1.

Table 29.1 Baseline characteristics of the study groups and pre-interventional clinical categories

Characteristic	Value	Percentage
Age (years)		
Mean ± SD	60 ± 10.6	
Range	38–89	
Sex		
Male	166	78.3
Female	46	21.7
Cardiovascular risk factors		
Smoking	186	87.7
Arterial hypertension	109	51.4
Hyperlipoproteinemia	86	40.6
Diabetes mellitus	28	13.2
Family history	47	22.2
Pre-interventional clinical categories (Rutherford classification)		
1 – Mild claudication	9	4.2
2 – Moderate claudication	51	24.0
3 – Severe claudication	126	59.4
4 – Rest pain	17	8.0
5 – Minor trophic changes	9	4.2
6 – Major trophic changes	–	–

According to the guidelines of the American Heart Association (AHA), the Rutherford categories were used for clinical classification.[15,16,26] The majority of patients presented with markedly impaired walking capacity due to claudication. Accordingly, pre-interventional standardized treadmill tests (5 minutes at 2 mph on a 12% incline) were completed by only nine of the 212 patients (4.2%). On the side of the occlusion, the mean ankle brachial index (ABI) was 0.53 ± 0.16 before and 0.41 ± 0.18 after exercise testing. On the contralateral leg, ABI values of 0.88 ± 0.21 at rest and 0.71 ± 0.22 after treadmill tests were found.

Pre-interventional angiography showed occlusions that involved the common iliac artery in 67 cases, the external iliac artery in 74 cases, and both vessel segments in 71 cases. The mean length of the occlusion was 8.9 ± 3.9 cm (range 3–19 cm). In 24 cases, a contralateral ostial stenosis of the common iliac artery was present. Based on the criteria of the Society of Cardiovascular and Interventional Radiology,[16] lesions were graded class III (occlusion length < 5 cm) in 46 cases and class IV (> 5 cm or bilateral) in 166 cases. A poor runoff with additional occlusion of the ipsilateral superficial femoral artery (SFA) was observed in 43 patients.

Recanalization procedure and stent implantation

In 193 cases (91%) the initial passage of the obstruction with the guide wire was performed by the crossover technique, whereas the retrograde approach was used in only 19 patients (9%).

In the case of unilateral iliac occlusion (Figure 29.2), after retrograde puncture and sheath placement into the contralateral common femoral artery, the occlusion was initially passed by the crossover technique with a 0.035 inch hydrophilic guide wire (length 260 cm, stiff type, angled tip, Terumo™, Tokyo, Japan) finally placed in the SFA. Using the guide wire as a marker, the ipsilateral common femoral artery was punctured under fluoroscopic control and a second 8F introducer sheath was positioned. Using an angled shaped wire loop, introduced through the ipsilateral sheath, the tip of the guide wire in the crossover position was snared and retrieved from the sheath.

Using this technique, the crossover position of the guide wire enabled the maneuvre of a 2.5 mm multifiber laser catheter through the occlusion, minimizing the risk of perforation and avoiding the possibility to track the laser catheter subintimally in the area of the aortic bifurcation.

In order to achieve an optimal debulking of the occluded vessel, several retrograde passes with the laser catheter were performed. Pulsed excimer laser systems, which work at a wavelength of 308 nm (LAIS DYMER 200+, pulse duration 200 nanoseconds, calibrated fluence 40–60 mJ/mm^2 or

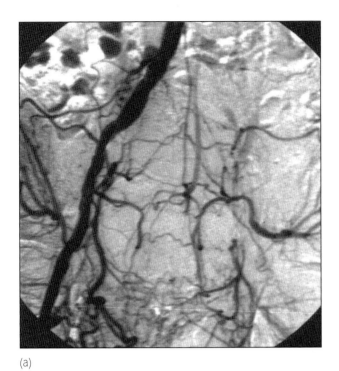

(a)

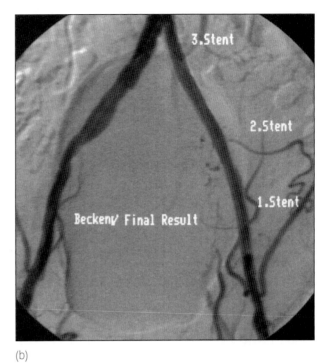

(b)

Figure 29.2
(a) Total chronic occlusion of the left common and external iliac artery. (b) Final result after excimer-laser-assisted recanalization and implantation of three Palmaz stents (length proximal to distal: 7.6, 4 and 4 cm; final balloon diameter: proximal 8 mm, distal 7 mm).

Spectranetics CVX 300, pulse duration 120 nanoseconds, fluence 45 mJ/mm^2) were used for the generation of the laser beam. In a considerable number of patients ($n = 149$; 70%) a primary laser canal with a diameter > 2 mm was achieved. Additional predilatations with an undersized balloon (mean diameter 6.3 mm, range 5–7 mm) were performed in the majority of cases ($n = 168$; 80%) prior to stent implantation.

After excimer-laser-assisted recanalization, a total number of 527 stents were implanted in 196 patients in order to stabilize the treated vessel segment. According to the morphology and location of the lesions, different types of stents were implanted (Table 29.2). Palmaz stents were used in the majority of cases (132 patients), mainly for highly calcified and ostial lesions of the common iliac arteries. Self-expanding Wallstents were placed to stabilize longer, less calcified vessel segments distal to the aortic bifurcation. In 31 patients, who showed major dissections after recanalization, Dacron-covered self-expanding nitinol stents were used to repair the vessel wall. In 53 patients, a combination of two different stents was chosen.

With the intention of stabilizing the entire target lesion, implantation of a single stent was sufficient in only 42 patients (21%). In the remaining cases, multiple stents (mean number 3.1, range 2–6) were implanted. The mean length of the stented segment was 10.2 ± 4.4 cm (range 3–22 cm). Diameters of the implanted devices ranged from 6 to 8 mm (mean 7.3 ± 0.6 mm) and were selected by comparison with

the contralateral corresponding artery or with residual patent segments in order to avoid overdilatation.

Most of the stents were delivered using a retrograde approach ($n = 421$). In patients recanalized by a single crossover approach, stents (Palmaz stent $n = 73$, Wallstent $n = 26$, Strecker stent $n = 7$) were implanted by the crossover technique. In patients with proximal lesions of the

Table 29.2   Endovascular stents used for stabilization of the recanalized vessel segment

Type of stent	No. of stents	
	Value	Percentage
Total number	527	100.0
Palmaz stent (P 394)*	346	65.7
Wallstent†	94	17.8
Strecker stent‡	38	7.2
EndoPro System 1§/Passager‖	49	9.3

* Johnson & Johnson Interventional Systems, Warren, NJ, USA.
† Schneider Europe/Boston Scientific, Bülach, Switzerland.
‡ Medi-tech/Boston Scientific, Jyllinge, Denmark.
§ Mintec, Freeport, Bahama Islands.
‖ Meadox/Boston Scientific, Natick, MA, USA.

common iliac artery, which involved the aortic bifurcation and additional ostial stenosis of the contralateral common iliac artery ($n = 24$), after initial recanalization of the occlusion the aortic bifurcation was reconstructed by bilateral simultaneous implantation of Palmaz stents by the 'kissing-balloon technique'.[10] In a further 32 patients, the 'kissing-balloon technique' was used to protect the contralateral common iliac artery during stent implantation into the proximal common iliac artery. In these cases only low-pressure balloon inflations in the non-affected common iliac artery without stent implantation were performed.

Postprocedural treatment

During intervention, all patients received 10 000 units (U) of unfractionated heparin intra-arterially, followed by intravenous heparin 1000–1200 U/hour for 24 hours (aPTT 60–80 seconds). Anticoagulation was continued with 0.3 mg subcutaneous low-molecular-weight heparin (Fraxiparin™, Sanofi Winthrop GmbH, Munich, Germany) twice daily for 2 weeks. Oral anticoagulation with phenprocoumon (INR > 2.5) was given in 78 patients, which included those with low blood-flow conditions due to impaired peripheral runoff. The remaining patients ($n = 112$) received ticlopidine (250 mg BID for 4 weeks) concomitant to ASA (100 mg OD).

Follow-up protocol

Clinical follow-up examinations, which included the standardized treadmill test and color-coded duplex sonography (Hewlett Packard, Sonos 1000 and Sonos 2000, 7.5 MHz linear transducer) were performed on hospital discharge, and then 1, 3, 6 and 12 months and every year thereafter. Mean follow-up time was 31 ± 19 months (range 3 –67 months). In 148 patients of 190 successfully recanalized patients (78%), follow-up angiographies were obtained after a mean period of 17 ± 8 months (range 3–62 months).

Definitions

Technical success was defined as patency of the vessel with an angiographic residual diameter stenosis < 30% and a residual translesion pressure gradient < 5 mmHg.

Angiographic patency at follow-up was defined as < 50% diameter restenosis. Cumulative patency rates were calculated, according to the criteria of Rutherford,[26] on the basis of clinical, sonographic or angiographic findings of the last available investigation. **Primary patency** refers to uninterrupted patency with no procedures performed on or at the margins of the treated segment. **Assisted primary patency** was defined as patency after reintervention of a restenosis (patent vessel) at the treatment site to prevent an eventual reocclusion. **Secondary patency** was defined as patency of the target vessel including reintervention of a reocclusion (non-patent vessel).

Primary technical results

Out of 212 patients the occlusion was successfully passed with a guide wire in 196 cases (92%). After excimer-laser-assisted recanalization, primary stent implantation was performed in these 196 patients. In three cases a patent vessel could not be achieved due to subintimal tracking, even after stent implantation. Furthermore, acute thrombosis immediately after recanalization and stent implantation, which could not be recanalized by local thrombolysis and PTA, occurred in two patients. In one case, an iliac vessel ruptured during stent implantation, which required emergency surgical intervention. Consequently, a primary technical success was achieved in 190 of the 212 patients (90%).

Primary clinical results

A marked clinical improvement of +3 Rutherford categories, according to the AHA guidelines, was achieved in 112 (53%) patients and an improvement of +2 in 67 cases (32%). In seven patients (3%) symptoms improved only slightly (+1 grade), and in 26 cases (12%), which includes the technical failures, no changes were observed. Nine of these 33 patients with no or minor clinical improvement had coexistent occlusions of the ipsilateral SFA, which were not considered for recanalization at the time. After successful recanalization, in all patients the mean ABI at rest increased from 0.53 ± 0.16 to 0.91 ± 0.13 ($p < 0.001$) and after exercise from 0.41 ± 0.18 to 0.84 ± 0.16 ($p < 0.001$). The average length of hospital stay was 4.8 days.

Complications

The overall rate of major procedure-related complications was 1.4% ($n = 3$). In addition to the patient with arterial rupture during stent implantation, one patient had embolic occlusion of the ipsilateral tibioperoneal trunk. Local recombinant tissue plasminogen activator (rt-PA) thrombolysis resulted in complete resolution of the thrombus. In another patient, who underwent stent implantation into the proximal common iliac artery, peripheral embolization of the contralateral leg occurred. This was due to dislodgement of thrombotic material, which occurred during balloon inflation and stent placement at the aortic bifurcation. The contralateral peripheral occlusion was recanalized by PTA and concomitant application of a weight-adjusted bolus of abciximab (ReoPro; Eli Lilly & Co, Basingstoke, Hampshire, UK) of 0.25 mg/kg, followed by a standard abciximab infusion of 0.125 g/kg/minute for 12 hours.

There were no cases of major bleeding or extensive hematoma. Minor puncture site complications occurred in 14 patients (6.6%), which included eight hematomas (3.8%) and six false aneurysms (2.8%) that were successfully treated by ultrasound-guided compression. Considering the fact that in 172 cases a bilateral percutaneous access was used, the total number of groins at risk was 384. Accordingly, the adjusted incidence of puncture site complications was 3.6%, which included hematomas in 2.1% and false aneurysms in 1.6%.

On the first or second post-interventional day an intermittent rise in body temperature (range 38.2–39.6°C) occurred in 13 of the 31 patients (42%) after implantation of the Dacron-covered nitinol stents (EndoPro1/Passager). Concomitantly, white blood cell counts were elevated up to a mean of 14.6 /nl in nine patients (29%) and C-reactive protein concentrations were increased (mean 17.8 mg/dl) in 17 cases (55%) of this subgroup. Repeated blood cultures did not show any bacterial growth. In all patients, fever resolved spontaneously after a mean of 2 days.

Follow-up results

Cumulative primary, assisted primary and secondary patency rates were calculated, which included those patients with primary interventional failure (Table 29.3). In three patients with markedly impaired peripheral runoff, thrombotic reocclusions of the target vessel occurred within the first 30 days after the intervention, which led to a 1 month primary patency rate of 88%. In two of these three cases the reoccluded segment was successfully recanalized by rt-PA thrombolysis and PTA. Thus, the secondary patency rate at 1 month was 89%.

During the long-term follow-up two patients (0.9%) died due to acute cardiac events. In only 13 patients (6.1%) was a deterioration of the initial clinical improvement, according to the classification of the AHA, observed. The mean ABI remained almost stable during the follow-up period and was 0.89 ± 0.15 before and 0.81 ± 0.16 after exercise testing at the last available follow-up (mean 31 ± 19 months, range 3–67 months).

Acute or subacute reocclusions of the stented segment were found in five patients, three of whom were successfully treated by excimer-laser-assisted angioplasty. In one case the secondary intervention failed and the patient was referred for elective bypass surgery. One patient refused further intervention.

Restenosis of the stented segment was revealed by follow-up angiography in 17 cases. However, restenosis never

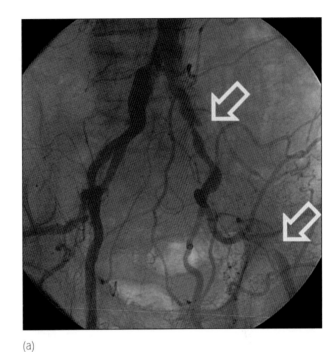

(a)

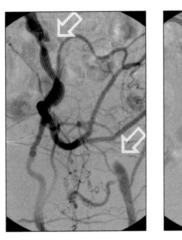

(b)

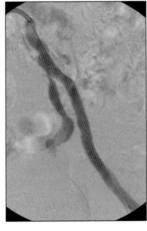

(c)

Figure 29.3
(a and b) Total chronic occlusion of the left external iliac artery. (c) Final result after implantation of a self-expanding Nitinol stent (8.0/100 mm) and postdilatation (final balloon diameter 7 mm).

involved the complete stented segment but was located in the proximal portion in nine patients and in the distal portion in two patients. In six patients with multiple stents, restenosis was located at the overlap site between the stents. In 13 of the 17 patients, restenosis was successfully treated by secondary interventions.

To identify predictors of reobstructions, univariate regression analysis of angiographic, clinical and procedural variables was performed. Variables with $p < 0.02$, including gender, hypertension, diabetes, pre-interventional clinical

Table 29.3   Cumulative patency rates (Kaplan-Meier life table method)

Follow-up (months)	No. of patients	Lost to follow-up	Local events	Patency	SD (%)
Primary cumulative patency					
0	212	0	22	89.6	2.1
6	176	16	4	87.7	2.3
12	145	21	7	83.9	2.6
24	110	34	4	81.2	2.8
36	83	19	4	77.9	3.2
48	54	28	2	75.7	3.5
60	15	35	4	66.1	5.8
Assisted primary patency					
0	212	0	22	89.6	2.1
6	176	16	4	87.7	2.3
12	149	21	3	86.1	2.4
24	113	38	2	84.7	2.5
36	83	24	1	83.8	2.7
48	54	29	1	82.4	3.0
60	15	38	1	77.5	5.5
Secondary patency					
0	212	0	22	89.6	2.1
6	178	16	2	88.7	2.2
12	153	21	1	88.2	2.2
24	114	42	1	87.5	2.3
36	83	25	1	86.5	2.5
48	54	29	1	85.1	2.8
60	15	38	1	80.0	5.6

category, occlusion length, vessel segment, stent type, number of stents, final balloon diameter and post-interventional drug treatment, were entered into a multivariate model. The only parameters that independently predicted restenosis were occlusion length (cm) (odds ratio (OR), 2.7; 95% confidence interval (CI), 1.9–3.6) and the number of stents (OR 1.7; 95% CI, 1.2–2.5).

To assess the influence of the lesion length on the long-term outcome in more detail, patients were divided into two groups according to the length of the occluded vessel segment (occlusions ≤ 10 cm in length, $n = 114$; occlusions > 10 cm in length, $n = 98$). Reocclusions and restenoses were more frequent for occlusions > 10 cm in length and resulted in primary and assisted primary patency rates that were significantly lower than the corresponding values for occlusions ≤ 10 cm in length (Figures 29.4a and b). In both groups a considerable number of reobstructions were successfully treated by PTA. As a result, there were no significant differences between either group with regard to the secondary patency rate (Figure 29.4c).

Discussion

After the first successful percutaneous recanalization procedure of a completely occluded iliac artery, reported in 1979 by Tegtmeyer et al.,[27] several small studies have been published, all of which show a high rate of failure to pass the occlusion.[14,28] Concomitantly, complication rates of up to 20% were reported, which raised the question as to whether an iliac artery occlusion is an appropriate indication for angioplasty.[14,29]

More recently, larger studies that investigated the initial and long-term success of percutaneous transluminal balloon angioplasty for the treatment of iliac occlusions have been published.[17,18,30] Johnston et al.[30] achieved a considerable primary recanalization rate of 82% (67 of 82 patients treated successfully); however, the long-term results were disappointing and showed a cumulative patency rate of 58% after a mean follow-up of 36 months.[18]

There are three major challenges in the percutaneous treatment of chronic iliac occlusions, discussed below.

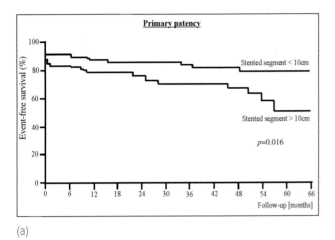

(a)

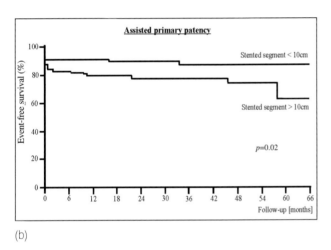

(b)

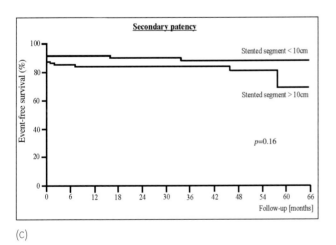

(c)

Figure 29.4

Kaplan–Meier curves comparing (a) primary, (b) assisted primary and (c) secondary patency rates for stented segments > or <10 cm in length.

Passage of the occlusion with the guide wire

Safe advancement of a guide wire through the occluded segment must be achieved. Colapinto et al.[17] described the technical problems that can occur with mechanical traversal of an occluded artery and found that the chance of successful recanalization decreases with increased length of the occluded segment. Vorwerk et al.[19] reported that subintimal passage of the occlusion with an eccentric re-entry through the aortic wall occurred in 5.8% of the cases, which may eventually cause technical failure. In contrast to the majority of authors, who prefer a primary retrograde approach, in our study the initial passage of the occlusion was performed by the crossover technique whenever possible (91%). Using this technique we were successful in initially passing the lesion with a guide wire in 92% of cases, which compares favorably with the results reported in the literature.[11,12,14,19] Furthermore, in patients with occlusions of the proximal common iliac artery, this approach may have contributed to the avoidance of major aortoiliac dissections.

Debulking of atherosclerotic and thrombotic material

A second aspect for successful recanalization of occluded iliac arteries is the fact that clot material usually extends both proximally and distally to the underlying stenotic lesion. Various techniques for removal of the occluding thrombotic material have been proposed. Several authors used local thrombolytic therapy as an adjunct to balloon angioplasty.[29,31,32] Blum et al.[22] reported an excellent primary recanalization rate of 98% by the combined use of local fibrinolysis and PTA in patients with relatively new thrombotic iliac occlusions (0.1–12 months; mean 4.2 months between onset of symptoms and recanalization). Additional stent placement was performed in 18 of 47 patients (38%). In contrast, Hausegger et al.[33] treated 42 patients for chronic iliac occlusions. They achieved instant recanalization after local thrombolysis in only 12 patients (28%) and reduction of thrombotic mass in five cases (12%). The overall complication rate in both studies was approximately 15% with a 7% rate of peripheral embolizations.

In our study, the removal of obstructing material was attempted by performing several passes with an excimer laser catheter prior to balloon dilatation and stent implantation. The excimer laser is a pulsed laser system that induces photoablation during a so-called athermic process. It is predominantly a local, very fast micro-explosion, which is provoked by an extremly high-temperature rise of the irradiated volume with energy densities of about 3–6 J/cm.^{2} As a result of the excimer laser beam's small penetration depth and the extremely short pulse duration, the thermal damage induced is minimal, even when high-energy densities are used.[23,24] In 70% of the cases, effective debulking with a primary laser canal of at least 2 mm was achieved, which facilitated subsequent balloon dilatation and stent implantation. As a result, the frequency of peripheral embolic events (0.9%) was considerably lower than in previously published studies.[19,22]

Stabilization of the recanalized vessel segment

Maintaining patency of the vessel lumen after transluminal angioplasty represents the third major challenge after achieving the initial technical success. Endoluminal stent placement in iliac artery stenoses has been proved to be efficient in eliminating residual stenoses and for providing a high long-term patency rate.[5–7,10] Patency rates reported for stent placement after recanalization of iliac artery occlusions are somewhat lower than for treatment of iliac artery stenoses.[19,20,22,29] Including interventional failures, we observed cumulative primary patency rates of 83% after 1 year, 81% after 2 years and 76% after 4 years. Vorwerk et al.[19] reported on 103 patients with chronic iliac occlusions and achieved a primary 2-year patency rate of 83% and a 4-year patency rate of 78%; however, primary interventional failures were excluded from their calculations and the mean occlusion length was only 5.1 cm.

Analyzing the influence of various clinical and procedural variables in a multivariate analysis, the only parameters that independently predicted restenosis were occlusion length and the number of stents. Comparing two clinical groups with lesion lengths of > or < 10 cm, we found a significantly higher rate of reocclusions and restenoses in the subgroup with a treated segment > 10 cm in length. However, secondary interventions within the stent were successfully performed in almost all of the patients with reobstructions, independent of the lesion length. As a result, the secondary patency rate did not show any significant differences between the two subgroups.

Chronic femoropopliteal artery occlusions

Clinical significance of femoropoliteal obstructions

Chronic atherosclerotic obstructions of the SFA are a leading cause of lifestyle limiting intermittent claudication, which occurs in about 6–10% of the population over 65 years of age.[34] PTA is normally recommended as the primary

treatment for short segment femoropopliteal stenoses and occlusions. In contrast, long chronic occlusions of the SFA are still mainly considered for vascular surgery.[15,16] Since bypass grafting is associated with a considerable procedure-related morbidity and mortality, surgical intervention is usually reserved for patients with ischemic rest pain or advanced claudication.[35] Consequently, many patients with long chronic SFA occlusions remain untreated, systematically underestimating the subjective discomfort induced by the disease for the single patient.

As percutaneous revascularization techniques permit a lower threshold of intervention than has been traditionally practiced for surgical procedures, improvement of endovascular recanalization techniques for treatment of total occlusions is particularly desirable. Adjunctive techniques may have the potential to improve the acute and long-term results. The pulsed excimer laser has been extensively evaluated in debulking atherosclerotic material in vitro and in vivo, demonstrating that the photoablative effect of laser light can be used to recanalize even lesions not amenable to conventional PTA.[36–40]

Study population

The objective of this study was to assess the acute and follow-up results of excimer-laser-assisted recanalization of long chronic SFA occlusions. We analyzed the data of 318 consecutive patients with occlusions of the SFA that were percutaneously treated by excimer-laser-assisted angioplasty in our institution during a 1-year period.[41]

The baseline clinical characteristics of the study population are listed in Table 29.5. On average, there were 2.7 cardiovascular risk factors per individual, with smoking, arterial hypertension and hyperlipoproteinemia the most frequent predisposing factors. According to the guidelines of the AHA, the Rutherford categories were used for clinical classification. The majority of patients presented with markedly impaired walking capacity due to claudication. Pre-intervention standardized treadmill testing (5 minutes at 2 mph on a 12% incline) was successfully completed by only 21 of 318 patients (6.6%). Critical lower limb ischemia with rest pain or minor tissue loss was present in six and 15 patients, respectively. The mean ABI determined in the index leg before and after exercise was 0.62 ± 0.15 and 0.40 ± 0.18, respectively.

In 93 patients a bilateral SFA occlusion was present so that, in total, 411 occluded vessels were treated in 318 patients (Table 29.6). The mean occlusion length was 19.4 cm. The medial and distal segment of the SFA down to the level of the adductor canal was the most common site of occlusion. The mean length of the patent proximal stump was 4.6 cm; however, in 53 cases the artery stump was shorter than 1 cm.

Table 29.4 Comparison of our data with interventional and surgical data from the literature

Author: (ref. no.)	No. patients	Technical success rate (%)	Rate of major complications* (%)	Rate of minor complications† (%)	Rate of primary patency (%)	Follow-up time (months)
Iliac stent studies						
Scheinert et al.[25]	212	89.6	1.4	6.6	77.9	36
Vorwerk et al.[19]	103	79.5	10.6	2	81‡	36
Reyes et al.[20]	59	92	8.5	5.1	73	24
Iliac PTA studies						
Johnston[18]	82	81.7	8.4	6	66	36
Colapinto et al.[17]	64	78	3.1	0	78	6-48
Gupta et al.[79]	50	78.6	8.9	14.3	76	36

	No. patients	Operative mortality (%)	Systemic morbidity (%)	Local morbidity (%)	Rate of primary patency (%)	Follow-up time (months)
Aortoiliac bypass studies						
Szilagyi et al.[80]	1748	5.0	18.9	6.0	85.3	60
Nevelsteen et al[81]	912	5.5	8.6	9.0	88.9	60
Van den Akker et al.[82]	518	3.3	NA	NA	86.5	60

* Such as acute ischemia, distal embolisms, dissections, vessel rupture and mortality.
† Puncture site complications including haematomas, false aneurysms, arterio-venous fistulas.
‡Technical failures excluded.
NA, Not available.

Technique of excimer laser angioplasty

One main limitation of conventional recanalization techniques remains the inability to cross total occlusions of lengths > 5 cm, in up to 50% of cases. This relevant disadvantage of the technique is magnified by the Achilles' heel of balloon angioplasty: the high degree of restenosis or reocclusions in approximately 50% in peripheral arteries.[42,43]

Analyzing this data, the idea was born that with debulking of obstructive material it may be possible to transform an occlusion in a stenosis, so that the final balloon dilatation, which remains necessary in the majority of the cases, may provoke limited damage of the arterial wall and, consequently, may reduce the stimuli activating the mechanisms of restenosis. Subsequently, a variety of new techniques designed to remove obstructive vessel material have been developed.[44]

In the early 1980s the innovative idea that laser energy can be used to vaporize sclerotic material[45–47] convinced several groups to rapidly introduce laser angioplasty as a clinical modality.[48–54] Overly enthusiastic, maybe success-dictated, reports presaged the science fiction fantasy that by aiming a laser beam through an optical fiber at the obstructive material,

blood flow might be restored without spasm, embolism, dissection or perforation. The clinical debacle of the first systems using continous-wave laser irradiation was the consequence of an uncritical use of such a powerful, inadequate energy source for debulking sclerotic vessel material. Furthermore, the partial use of the acronym laser without regard to the specific-tissue related properties of different laser sources led to many simplifications and misunderstandings and may explain the actual scepticism towards laser angioplasty by a large number of interventionalists.

Laser physics – basic considerations

During recent years, it has been demonstrated that the majority of laser wavelengths of the electromagnetic spectrum can debulk vessel material.[23,51,54–57] Two main parameters must be considered for laser–tissue interaction effects: the interaction time (between laser beam and tissue) and the tissue-specific absorption or effective energy density.[58]

Table 29.5   Study population – baseline data

	n	Percentage
Number of patients		
Male	207	65.1
Female	111	34.9
Total	318	100.0
Mean age (years)	64.2±10.7 (range 33–91)	
Cardiovascular risk factors		
Smoking	240	75.5
Arterial hypertension	222	69.8
Hyperlipoproteinemia	168	52.8
Diabetes mellitus	99	31.1
Family history	89	27.9
Cerebrovascular disease	36	11.3
Clinical category (Rutherford classification)		
1 – Mild claudication	21	6.6
2 – Moderate claudication	24	7.5
3 – Severe claudication	252	79.2
4 – Rest pain	6	1.9
5 – Minor trophic changes	15	4.7
6 – Major trophic changes	–	–
Walking capacity		
Relative (m)	102±92.5	
Absolute (m)	142±90.0	
ABI		
At rest	0.62±0.15	
After exercise	0.40±0.18	

ABI, Ankle–brachial index.

Table 29.6   Lesion characteristics

	n	Percentage
Number of lesions		
Right	199	48.4
Left	212	51.6
Total	411	100.0
Bilateral lesions (no. patients)	93	29.2
Involvement of vessel segment		
Proximal SFA	255	62.0
Medial SFA	381	92.7
Distal SFA	369	89.8
Length of occlusion (cm)	19.4±6.0 (range 10–31)	
Length of proximal SFA stump (cm)	4.6±5.5 (range 0–20. median 2)	
Runoff		
one vessel	97	23.6
two or three vessels	314	76.4

SFA, Superficial femoral artery.

At lower energy densities and longer interaction times, tissue ablation is a consequence of local heating with resulting dessication and subsequent vaporization.[59] Examples of these thermal effects are the continous wave Nd:YAG or argon laser systems. Although the laser light of the continous-wave laser sources has been transmitted via bare fibers or with metal tips,[60,61] quartz windows[62] or sapphire probes[63,64] at the distal end of the optical fiber, heat can be regarded as the main cause of tissue vaporization of all systems. Particularly when the recanalization speed is slower than 1.5 mm/second, considerable transversal temperature rises are observed,[59] and thermal damage of adjacent tissue structures can hardly be avoided. The increase of the vessel-surrounding temperature to 60–80°C may be deleterious with regard to the long-term results of those interventions. Furthermore, because heavily calcified material is refractory to the ablation mechanism of thermal systems,[65] a recanalization stop due to a calcified obstacle will cause an unacceptably high risk of perforation.[56]

In contrast to the vaporization caused by the continous-wave lasers, the excimer laser is a pulsed system that induces photoablation during a so-called athermic process.[66,67] This photoablation phenomenon was first described in 1982 by Srinivasan and co-workers.[68,69] Electrical fields large enough to break chemical bonds can only be produced at very high energy densities with extremly short interaction times. This effect, called optical breakdown or photoablation, can be obtained with the pulsed excimer laser with high-energy densities.[53,66,70] The medical systems introduced for angioplasty use a xenon chloride 308 nm excimer laser as the source of energy. At this wavelength the ablation of the irradiated tissue is no longer a consequence of a photochemical disruption of molecular chains. It is predominately a local, very fast micro-explosion provoked by an extremly high temperature rise of the irradiated volume with energy densities of about 3–6 J/cm.[2] As a result of the excimer laser beam`s small penetration depth and the extremely short pulse duration in comparison with the pulse repetition rate used, the thermal damage induced by the excimer laser is minimal, even when high-energy densities are used.[23]

Excimer-laser-assisted recanalization technique

The contralateral access with subsequent crossover recanalization of the occlusion can be considered the standard approach for recanalization of long SFA occlusions. After retrograde femoral puncture and introduction of a 7–8F hemostatic sheath, a hydrophilic guide wire (Terumo 0.035 inch, stiff type, angled tip; Terumo Inc., Tokyo, Japan) is navigated in crossover position with the help of suitably shaped diagnostic catheters (Cobra or Hook shape, 5F). After obtaining the pre-interventional selective angiography of the target leg (a 20–30° lateral view may be helpful to identify the origin of the totally occluded SFA) (Figure 29.5a and b), the guide wire is advanced into the origin of the occlusion. Then, the multifiber excimer laser catheter (7 or 8F) is placed at the origin of the occlusion and the activated catheter is advanced the first few millimeters into the occlusion without wire guidance. For further recanalization of the occluded vessel segment the activated laser catheter is advanced stepwise for a short (< 5 mm) distance without wire guidance, followed by further crossing with the guide wire ('step-by-step technique'). The advancement of the activated laser catheter has to be performed very slowly, not exceeding 1 mm/second. To enter the patent distal segment of the artery it is recommended to cross the last 2 cm of the occlusion with the guide wire alone (angled or straight tip) before lasering. Particular attention should be paid to the avoidance of vessel wall dissections distal to the original occlusion.

Fluoroscopic 'road mapping' is used throughout to verify the alignment of guide wires and catheters to the vessel lumen. Particular attention is given to thoroughly flushing the vessel with saline before lasering to remove remaining contrast medium, as the interaction of laser energy with the contrast medium can produce shock waves which may result in disruption of the vessel wall. After initial laser passage, the 0.035 inch hydrophilic guide wire is changed to a 0.018 inch guide wire to allow distal saline flushing during a second or third passage of the obstructed area. Angiographic controls of the target vessel and the distal runoff are performed to verify the effect of the laser debulking procedure (Figure 29.5c and d). Finally, the recanalization procedure is completed by complementary balloon dilatations. The dimensions of the balloon, as well as dilatation pressure and dilatation time, adheres to the standards described above (Figure 29.5e and f).

Postprocedural treatment

During intervention all patients receive 5000–10 000 U heparin intra-arterially. Anticoagulation may be continued for 24 hours (1000–1200 U/hour intravenous heparin) with an activated partial thromboplastin time of 60-80 seconds. ASA (100 mg/day) is given to all patients.

Primary technical results

Table 29.7 details the technical results of the initial recanalization procedures. In 342 of 411 cases (83.2%) the primary approach to cross the occlusion was successful. In 44 of the 69 initially failed procedures (63.8%) a secondary procedure was performed, mainly utilizing the transpopliteal technique. Of these secondary recanalization procedures, 68.2% were completed successfully. Thus, the total primary recanalization success rate was 90.5%.

Table 29.7 Interventional data

	n	Percentage
Primary approach		
Crossover	369	89.7
Antegrade	27	6.6
Popliteal	15	3.6
Successful	342	83.2
Failed	69	16.8
Secondary approach		
Attempted	44	63.8*
Crossover	2	
Antegrade	3	
Popliteal	39	
Successful	30	68.2†
Crossover	1	
Antegrade	2	
Popliteal	27	
No secondary approach	25	36.2
Success of excimer-laser-assisted angioplasty (total)	372	90.5
Size of laser catheter (mm)		
2.0	117	28.5
2.2	234	56.9
2.5	60	14.6
Final balloon diameter (mm)		
5	78	21.0‡
6	288	77.4
7	6	1.6
Implantation of stents		
Number of cases	30	7.3
Number of stents	87	
Wallstents	5	
Palmaz stents	81	
Length of stented segment (cm)	11.3	(range 4–24)

* Percentage of primarily failed cases (n = 69).
† Percentage of secondary attempts.
‡ PTA performed in 372 cases after successful laser passage.

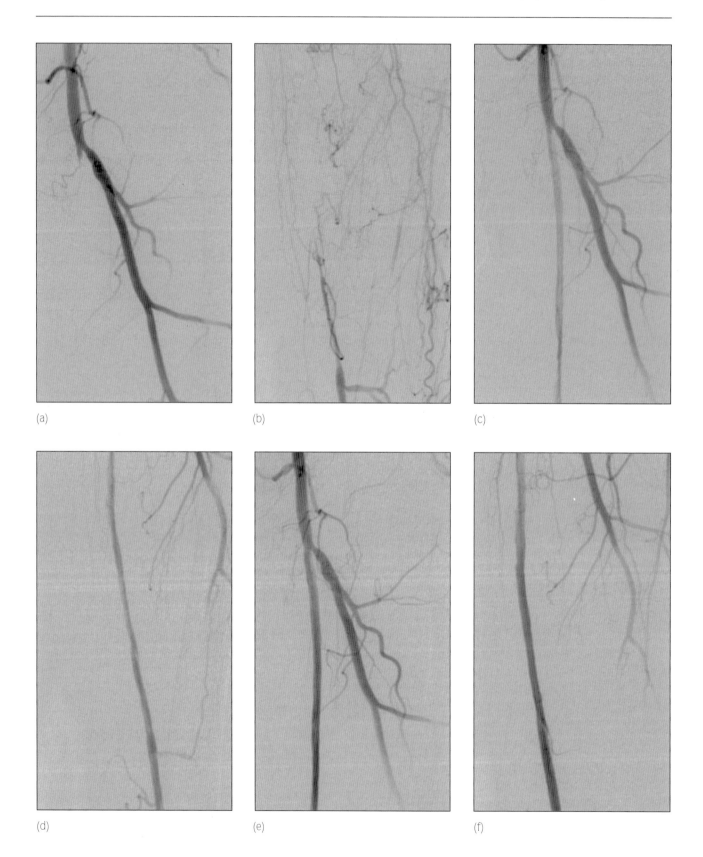

(a)

(b)

(c)

(d)

(e)

(f)

Figure 29.5

(a and b) Chronic occlusion of the left superficial femoral artery. (c and d) angiographic image after successful recanalization with a 2.5 mm multifiber laser catheter (two passes) and (e and f) final result after balloon dilatation (diameter 5 mm, length 80 mm, dilatation pressure 10 atm).

The average diameter of the multifiber laser catheter used for recanalization was 2.18 ± 0.16 mm. Balloon dilatations were performed in all 372 cases after successful initial laser passage. The mean balloon diameter was 5.8 ± 0.43 mm. Implantation of endovascular stents into the SFA was performed in 30 cases (7.3%) with threatened reocclusion due to extensive dissection or significant recoil (mean percentage diameter stenosis, $76 \pm 15\%$) after excimer-laser-assisted angioplasty. A total of 87 stents were implanted with a mean length of the stented segment of 11.3 ± 3.3 cm.

Complications

In this considerably large group of patients with complex femoral obstructions, there were no procedure-related major adverse events such as death, amputation or acute surgical intervention (Table 29.8). Relevant complications involving the target lesion or the distal runoff vessels were encountered in 29 cases (7.1%). Distal embolization or peri-interventional thrombosis of the infragenouidal arteries occurred in 16 cases (3.9%). Using adjunctive interventional techniques, including mechanical recanalization of the occlusion and catheter-based local thrombolysis with rt-PA (10 mg bolus, followed by continuous infusion of 1 mg/hour for 24 hours), complete resolution of the thrombus was achieved in 11 cases. In the remaining five patients, patency of only one runoff vessel could be achieved. None of these patients suffered any adverse sequellae as a result. Minor puncture site complications occurred in 27 patients (6.5%), including 12 hematomas (2.9%) and 15 false aneurysms (3.6%), all of which could be successfully treated by ultrasound-guided compression. In no case was surgical intervention required.

Table 29.8 Interventional complications and serious adverse events

	n	Percentage
Death	0	
Amputation	0	
Acute surgical intervention	0	
At target lesion		
acute reocclusion	4	1.0
perforation	9	2.2
embolization/distal thrombosis	16	3.9
At puncture site		
false aneurysm	15	3.6
hematoma (reduced Hb > 3 mg/dl)	12	2.9

Primary clinical results

A marked clinical improvement of +2 or more according to the limb-status grading scale was observed in 247 patients. Minor clinical improvement (+1) occurred in 26 cases and in 45 patients no changes in clinical status were observed. The group of patients with no or minor improvement included those with primary interventional failures ($n = 33$ including six cases with bilateral failure), as well as patients with limitations in walking capacity due to contralateral ($n = 28$) iliac or femoral obstructions. The remaining 10 patients were limited by diffuse disease in the ipsilateral infragenouidal arteries which, despite treatment ($n = 6$), remained symptomatic. Postinterventional treadmill testing was completed by 272 patients (85.4%) without the development of any claudication symptoms. As compared to the pre-interventional reference value, the ABI showed a significant increase from 0.62 ± 0.15 to 0.95 ± 0.15 (at rest) and 0.40 ± 0.18 to 0.87 ± 0.17 (after exercise).

Follow-up

Follow-up was continued over a 1-year period using clinical examination, standardized treadmill testing and transcutaneous color-coded duplex ultrasound. Cumulative primary, assisted primary and secondary patency rates were calculated, including those patients with primary interventional failures (Table 29.9). During 1 year, 257 cases of restenosis or reocclusion were observed, with the majority of events occurring between 6 and 12 months. Because of close monitoring intervals during follow-up, a considerable number of restenotic lesions could be detected opportunistically. Thus, the majority of restenotic vessels ($n = 158$) could be successfully retreated before reocclusion occurred, resulting in an assisted primary patency rate of 64.6% after 1 year. Furthermore, in 40 cases with partial or complete reocclusion of the originally treated vessel segment, successful reintervention could be performed. The secondary patency rate after 1 year was 75.1%.

The treatment of patients in the case of interventional failure or failure during follow-up was based on the clinical situation of the patient. In 41 cases with severe claudication, patients were referred for bypass surgery. In the remaining cases conservative treatment was applied.

Discussion

Two decades after the clinical introduction of PTA as a de-occluding technique in the femoropopliteal segment, a number of factors affecting the primary and long-term success of the procedure have been identified. Short lesion length,

Table 29.9 Interventional complications and serious adverse events

Follow-up (months)	Lesions at risk	Events	Event-free survival	SD
Primary patency				
0	411	39	0.905	0.014
3	370	34	0.822	0.019
6	318	66	0.651	0.024
9	232	109	0.345	0.025
12	115	48	0.201	0.021
Assisted primary patency				
0	411	39	0.905	0.014
3	370	31	0.829	0.018
6	321	36	0.736	0.022
9	263	28	0.658	0.024
12	223	4	0.646	0.024
Secondary patency				
0	411	39	0.905	0.014
3	370	19	0.859	0.017
6	333	20	0.807	0.020
9	291	16	0.763	0.021
12	263	4	0.751	0.022

minimal vascular disease elsewhere, with good peripheral runoff, symptoms of claudication as opposed to limb-threatening ischemia, stenosis rather than occlusion and absence of diabetes all correlate with improved primary success and long-term patency.[30,71] Unlike other vascular beds, occlusions predominate by a factor of at least 3 in the femoropopliteal arteries. Furthermore, most femoropopliteal occlusions are long and there is often coexistent multilevel atherosclerotic disease. As a consequence, patients with long chronic occlusions of the SFA are generally not considered 'good candidates' for percutaneous recanalization. Surgical bypass is often considered the treatment of choice.

According to a meta-analysis by Dalman and Taylor,[35] 4-year primary patency rates of surgical above-knee revascularization vary from 60 to 70%, for below-knee procedures, the 4-year secondary patency ranges from 70% for venous grafts to 40% for PTFE grafts. Despite these satisfactory long-term results, even at the infrainguinal level, vascular surgery is associated with substantial procedure-related morbidity and mortality. Accordingly, it is common practice to reserve femoropopliteal bypass surgery for patients with at least category 3 chronic limb ischemia.[15,16] As percutaneous procedures are generally associated with a significantly lower rate of general and local complications, effective transluminal recanalization techniques would offer a treatment option for many patients with long SFA occlusions and life-style limiting claudication.

Initial recanalization procedure

The first major challenge in percutaneous treatment of chronic SFA occlusions is to achieve a safe initial passage of the occlusion. Using conventional recanalization techniques, with a guiding-catheter-supported navigation of a guide wire through the occlusion followed by PTA, initial technical failure rates of 18–26% have been reported for chronic SFA occlusions.[30,71] After the first clinical feasibility study of PTA of peripheral arteries using a continuous-wave laser was reported in 1984,[72] many different laser sources and catheter delivery systems have been developed. A number of randomized trials were performed in the early 1990s comparing these different laser sources and application systems with conventional PTA. Although none of the studies could demonstrate a statistically significant superiority of laser recanalization alone as compared to PTA, the combined treatment with guide wire and laser resulted in technical success rates of up to 91%.[73,74]

In our series with excimer-laser-assisted angioplasty, a total recanalization rate of 90.5% could be achieved. Despite our treatment of very long occlusions, with a mean occlusion length of 19.4 versus 7.8 cm in the report by Lammer et al.,[73] our technical success rate compares favorably with their results, and is substantially higher than in previously published studies without laser assistance.[30,71] The technical modifications discussed below may have contributed to the high success rate.

In most of the cases, the **step-by-step technique** (which has been described in detail in the methods section) was applied to initially cross the occluded vessel segment. This technique was developed to safely navigate the guide wire through the occlusion using the guidance and ablative force of the laser catheter. This technique was particularly beneficial to enter flush occlusions without a visible proximal stump or to pass a segment resistant to guide wire crossing. Furthermore, the routine use of this technique may have contributed to the low rate of occlusive arterial wall dissections with a resultant stent frequency of only 7.3%.

In most of the cases (89.7%) the **crossover technique** was used as the primary approach to cross the occlusion. Using this technique, peri- and post-interventional blood-flow reduction at the treated vessel segment due to obstruction of the ipsilateral common femoral artery by the introducer sheath or post-interventional compression could be prevented. As a result, early reocclusions of the recanalized vessel, which have been reported in the literature with a frequency up to 41%,[42] were extremely rare in our study (1.0%). Furthermore, this approach allows the recanalization of occlusions extending to the origin of the SFA, which would not be accessible using the antegrade technique.

Whereas the **primary interventional approach** was successful in 83.2% of the cases, the application of **alternative secondary approaches** contributed to an increment of the overall technical success rate by 7.3%. The popliteal approach was highly effective to recanalize occlusions that could not be successfully crossed from the antegrade direction. Puncture of the popliteal artery under fluoroscopic guidance using the road-map technique was safe, with only minor puncture site complications in four cases (10.2%). However, a popliteal approach should only be attempted if the distal SFA and popliteal artery are free of stenoses and there is sufficient distal runoff. The size of the introducer sheath should be chosen according to the size of the popliteal artery.

Finally, it should be mentioned that the **technical improvements** of the multifiber laser catheters, which currently consist of up to 120 single fibers, led to a significant reduction in the dead space between the fibers, allowing a higher fluence and subsequently increasing the ablation efficacy of the devices.

In the current study, excimer-laser-assisted angioplasty of long chronic SFA occlusions has been shown to be a safe technique. There were no major adverse events. All minor procedure-related complications, including hematomas and false aneurysms, could be treated without surgical intervention. In almost all cases, a successful recanalization was associated with a marked improvement of the clinical symptoms. Post-interventionally, 85.4% of all patients referred for percutaneous recanalization of long SFA occlusions were able to complete a 5 minute standardized treadmill test without claudication, which is equivalent to a pain-free walking distance of almost 300 m. In 68.8% of patients, complete relief of symptoms with an unlimited walking capacity could be achieved.

Long-term results

Maintaining long-term patency of the recanalized vessel is the ultimate goal following successful recanalization of long chronic SFA occlusions. The use of a debulking device such as the excimer laser offers the theoretical benefit of removing as much occluding atherosclerotic and thrombotic material as possible, facilitating subsequent balloon dilatation and reducing the risk of thromboembolic events. Furthermore, it is conceivable that this approach will limit the arterial wall stress during balloon inflation, which may subsequently lead to a reduction of the restenosis rate. In the current study, debulking of obstructing material was attempted by performing several passes with the excimer laser catheter prior to balloon dilatation. The debulking process of the excimer laser is predominantly a local, very fast micro-explosion provoked by an extremely high-temperature rise of the irradiated volume with energy densities of about 3–6 J/cm^2. As a result of the small penetration depth of the collimated excimer laser beam ($10 \mu m$) in connection with the extremely short pulse duration (120–200 nanoseconds) and in relation to the used repetition rate of 25 Hz, the thermal damage to the vessel wall induced by the excimer laser is minimal even when high-energy densities are used.[23,75] In the randomized comparison of excimer-laser-assisted angioplasty, continuous-wave Nd:YAG laser angioplasty and conventional PTA, published by Lammer et al.,[73] the 12-month angiographic patency rate after recanalization of long SFA occlusions (> 8 cm in length) was best in the excimer laser group (42 versus 24% for Nd:YAG and 42 versus 12% for PTA).

Since the calculation of patency rates based on recurrence of clinical symptoms tends to overestimate patency rates, in our study long-term results were evaluated using standardized treadmill testing with calculation of the Doppler indices at rest and after exercise. Duplex-derived peak systolic velocity ratios have been shown to accurately reflect the anatomic status of the arterial tree.[76,77] Accordingly, serial color-flow duplex scanning was used for long-term surveillance after recanalization and angioplasty. In cases of suspected restenosis, angiography was performed to confirm the reobstruction. Based on a standard life table survival analysis, including primary interventional failures, the primary patency rate after 1 year was 20.1%. Due to the fact that a considerable number of patients without clinical symptoms did not attend the follow-up examinations, the calculated primary patency rate may have been biased towards less favorable results. However, recurrent narrowing after femoropopliteal angioplasty is a relevant problem and restenosis seems to be even more frequent after recanalization of very long chronic SFA occlusions. With an aggressive surveillance program, including functional clinical testing as well as color-coded duplex ultrasound, restenosis can be detected opportunistically. Reintervention on the target lesion can be performed in the majority of cases on an outpatient basis. As a result, eventual reocclusion can be prevented in most patients. With this strategy we were able to achieve an assisted primary patency rate of 64.6% after 1 year. The performance of repeat recanalization procedures on reoccluded arteries contributed to a further 10.5% improvement in vessel patency, resulting in 75.1% of patients being free of symptoms after 1 year.

Summary

Total iliac artery occlusions

In conclusion, patients with chronic unilateral iliac artery occlusions can be effectively treated by the percutaneous approach. Technical modifications, which include mechanical passage of the occlusion with a hydrophilic guide wire that uses a primary crossover approach and the use of debulking techniques prior to balloon dilatation and stenting, may improve the safety of the procedure. The results with primary stenting after excimer-laser-assisted recanalization of chronic iliac occlusions are better than those that have routinely been reported for balloon angioplasty alone (Table 29.4).[48,49] However, the presented data were obtained from a non-randomized, non-controlled registry and therefore are not finally conclusive with regard to the value of excimer laser debulking and the use of primary stenting. A prospective randomized trial will be needed to investigate the value of primary stent implantation as compared to angioplasty alone. Finally, although the morbidity and mortality of interventional procedures is substantially lower than that previously reported for surgical treatment, long-term patency rates of bypass surgery remain superior to interventional treatment. Extended follow-up data on the durability and long-term patency, obtained from a randomized comparison of surgical and interventional treatment, will be needed before the endovascular approach can be considered as a first-line treatment for chronic iliac artery occlusions.

Chronic total femoropopliteal occlusions

The combination of excimer laser technology with current interventional devices and advanced recanalization techniques allows recanalization of long chronic SFA occlusions in > 90% of cases. This successful revascularization is associated with excellent immediate clinical results. A complete relief of symptoms, or at least a significant improvement in functional capacity, could be achieved in almost all patients. The high frequency of restenosis remains the major limitation of this interventional technique. An aggressive surveillance program with standardized treadmill testing and color-coded duplex sonography is essential to detect restenosis. Reintervention should be performed early to prevent reocclusion of the vessel and to maintain the achieved clinical benefit.

PTA and stenting yields higher patency rates than PTA alone. With the new Nitinolstents, stenting in the femoropopliteal arteries markedly lowers the restenosis rate. In the future it has to be proved whether primary stenting, with or without drug-eluting stents should be considered for long diffuse lesions.

Future perspectives

More favorable long-term results after successful recanalization of long SFA occlusions were achieved with stent implantation. We retrospectively compared 1-year patency rates after implantation of Nitinolstent (SMART™) versus Wallstent in 269 long SFA lesions. There were no significant differences in patient baseline characteristics. For the SMART™ stent and the Wallstent the target lesion lengths were 17.8 ± 11 and 19.7 ± 10.1 mm, respectively. Total occlusion occured in 77 and 79% of cases, with an occlusion length of 15.3 ± 9.8 and 15.8 ± 9.5 mm, respectively. The number of implanted stents were 1.8 ± 1.0 and 1.8 ± 1.0

with a stent length of 120 ± 78 and 143 ± 98 mm, respectively. Laser debulking before stent implantation was performed in 43 and 33% of cases. The primary patency rate after a 12-month follow-up was $61 \pm 5\%$ for the SMART™ stent and $30 \pm 5\%$ for the Wallstent ($p < 0.001$). Twelve-month assisted primary patency was 75 ± 4 and $53 \pm 5\%$ ($p < 0.001$). The secondary patency after 12 months was 79 ± 4 and $64 \pm 5\%$ ($p = 0.007$). With the new Nitinolstents, stenting in the femoropopliteal arteries markedly lowers the restenosis rate compared to PTA alone and compared to the first self-expanding stent, the Wallstent.

In the future, drug-eluting stents represent one of the most promising fields in interventional therapy. As recently shown by Duda et al,[78] sirolimus-eluting self-expanding stents (SMART™) are feasible in long SFA occlusions. After successful recanalization of 36 SFA lesions (mean length 85 ± 57 mm, total occlusions 57%) the patients were randomly assigned to receive either sirolimus-eluting or uncoated SMART™ stents. The occlusion rate at 6 months follow-up were 0% in the sirolimus group and 5.9% in the uncoated stent group. The in-lesion restenosis rate was 0 and 23.5%, respectively ($p = 0.10$).

This encouraging data strengthen our resolve to treat patients with long SFA occlusions. The goals are to improve vascular patency and limb perfusion, as well as to maximize quality of life while minimizing the costs of care by making interventional therapies a valid alternative to surgical procedures.

References

1 Chevalier B, Royer T, Guyon P et al. *Chronic Total Occlusion. The PCR Course Book 2002*. (Groupe Composer-Toulouse: France, 2002).

2 Tegtmeyer CJ, Hartwell GD, Selby JB et al. Results and complications of angioplasty in aortoiliac disease. *Circulation* 1991; **83** (Suppl.I):I-53–I-60.

3 Kadir S, White RI, Kaufman SL et al. Long-term results of aortoiliac angioplasty. *Surgery* 1983; **94**:10–14.

4 Becker GJ, Katzen BT, Dake MD. Noncoronary angioplasty. *Radiology* 1989; **170**: 921–40.

5 Murphy KD, Encarnacion CE, Le VA, Palmaz JC. Iliac artery stent placement with the Palmaz stent: follow-up study. *J Vasc Intervent Radiol* 1995; **6**:321–9.

6 Hausegger KA, Lammer J, Hagen B et al. Iliac artery stenting: clinical experience with Palmaz stent, Wallstent, and Strecker stent. *Acta Radiol* 1992; **33**:292–6.

7 Henry M, Amor M, Ethevenot G et al. Palmaz stent placement in iliac and femoropopliteal arteries: primary and secondary patency in 310 patients with 2–4 year follow-up. *Radiology* 1995; **197**:167–74.

8 Sullivan TM, Childs MB, Bacharach JM et al. Percutaneous transluminal angioplasty and primary stenting of the iliac arteries in 288 patients. *J Vasc Surg* 1997; **25**:829–38.

9   Laborde JC, Palmaz JC, Rivera FJ et al. Influence of anatomic distribution of atherosclerosis on the outcome of revascularization with iliac stent placement. *J Vasc Intervent Radiol* 1995; **6**:513–21.

10   Scheinert D, Schröder M, Balzer JO et al. Stent-supported reconstruction of the aorto-iliac bifurcation using the kissing balloon technique. *Circulation* 1999; **100** (Suppl II):II-295–II-300.

11   Brothers TE, Greefield LJ. Long-term results of aortoiliac reconstruction. *J Vasc Intervent Radiol* 1990; **1**:49–55.

12   Kwasnik EM, Siouffi SY, Jay ME, Khuri SF. Comparative results of angioplasty and aortofemoral bypass in patients with symptomatic iliac disease. *Arch Surg* 1987; **122**:288–91.

13   deVries SO, Hunink MG. Results of aortic bifurcation grafts for aortoiliac occlusive disease: a meta-analysis. *J Vasc Surg* 1997; **26**:558–69.

14   Ring EJ, Freimann DB, McLean GK, Schwarz W. Percutaneous recanalization of common iliac artery occlusions: an unacceptable complication rate? *Am J Roentgenol* 1982; **139**:587–9.

15   Pentecost MJ, Criqui MH, Dorros G et al. Guidelines for peripheral percutaneous transluminal angioplasty of the abdominal aorta and lower extremity vessels. *Circulation* 1994; **89**:511–31.

16   Standards of Practice Committee of the Society of Cardiovascular and Interventional Radiology. Guidelines for percutaneous transluminal angioplasty. *Radiology* 1990; **177**:619–26.

17   Colapinto RF, Stronell RD, Johnston WK. Transluminal angioplasty of complete iliac obstructions. *Am J Roentgenol* 1986; **146**:859–62.

18   Johnston KW. Iliac arteries: reanalysis of results of balloon angioplasty. *Radiology* 1993; **186**:207–12.

19   Vorwerk D, Guenther RW, Schürmann K et al. Primary stent placement for chronic iliac artery occlusions: follow-up results in 103 patients. *Radiology* 1995; **194**:745–9.

20   Reyes R, Maynar M, Lopera J et al. Treatment of chronic iliac artery occlusions with guide wire recanalization and primary stent placement. *J Vasc Interv Radiol* 1997; **8**:1049–55.

21   Dyet JF, Gaines PA, Nicholson AA et al. Treatment of chronic iliac occlusions by means of percutaneous endovascular stent placement. *J Vasc Interv Radiol* 1997; **8**:349–53.

22   Blum U, Gabelmann A, Redecker M et al. Percutaneous recanalization of iliac artery occlusions: results of a prospective study. *Radiology* 1993; **189**:536–40.

23   Biamino G, Dörschel K, Harnoss BM et al. Experience in excimer laser photoablation of atherosclerotic plaques. In: Biamino G, Müller GJ, (eds) *Advances in Laser Medicine, First German Symposium on Laser Angioplasty*. Ecomed Verlagsgesellschaft: Berlin, 1988: 147–56.

24   Cumberland DC, Sanborn TA, Tayler DI et al. Percutaneous laser thermal angioplasty: initial clinical results with a laser probe in total peripheral artery occlusions. *Lancet* 1986; **1**:1457–9.

25   Scheinert D, Schroder M, Ludwig J et al. Stent-supported recanalization of chronic iliac artery occlusions. *Am J Med* 2001; **110**:708–15.

26   Rutherford RB. Standards for evaluating results of interventional therapy for peripheral vascular disease. *Circulation* 1991; **83** (Suppl. I):I-6–I-11.

27   Tegtmeyer CJ, Moore TS, Chandler JG et al. Percutaneous transluminal dilatation of a complete block in the right iliac artery. *Am J Roentgenol* 1979; **133**: 532–5.

28   Motarjeme A, Kweifer JW, Zuska AJ. Percutaneous transluminal angioplasty of the iliac arteries: 66 experiences. *Am J Roentgenol* 1980; **135**:937–44.

29   Rees CR, Palmaz JC, Garcia O et al. Angioplasty and stenting of completely occluded iliac arteries. *Radiology* 1989; **172**:953–9.

30   Johnston KW, Rae M, Hogg-Johnston SA et al. Five year results of a prospective study of percutaneous transluminal angioplasty. *Ann Surg* 287; **206**:403–12.

31   Auster M, Kadir S, Mitchell SE et al. Iliac artery occlusions: management with intrathrombus streptokinase infusion and angioplasty. *Radiology* 1984; **153**:385–8.

32   Kichikawa K, Uchida H, Yoshioka T. Iliac artery stenosis and occlusion: preliminary results of treatment with Gianturco expandable metallic stents. *Radiology* 1990; **177**:799–802.

33   Hausegger KA, Lammer J, Klein G et al. Perkutane Rekanalisation von Beckenarterienverschlüssen: Fibrinolyse, PTA, Stents. *Fortschr Roentgenstr* 1991; **155**:550–5.

34   Kannel WB, McGee DL. Update on some epidemiologic features of intermittent claudication: the Framingham study. *J Am Geriatr Soc* 1985; **33**:13.

35   Dalman RL, Taylor LM. Basic data related to infrainguinal revascularization procedures. *Ann Vasc Surg* 1990; **4**:309–12.

36   Abela GS. Laser arterial recanalization: a current perspective. *J Am Coll Cardiol* 1988; **12**:103–5.

37   Deckelbaum LI, Isner JM, Donaldson R et al. Reduction of laser-induced pathologic tissue injury using pulsed energy delivery. *Am J Cardiol* 1985; **56**:662–7.

38   Grundfest WS, Litvack IF, Goldenberg T et al. Pulsed ultraviolet lasers and the potential for safe laser angioplasty. *Am J Surg* 1985; **150**:220–6.

39   Grundfest WS, Litvack F, Forrester JS et al. Laser ablation of human atherosclerotic plaque without adjacent tissue injury. *J Am Coll Cardiol* 1985; **5**:929–33.

40   Isner JM, Donaldson RF, Decklebaum LI et al. The excimer laser: gross, light microscopic and ultrastructural analysis of potential use in laser therapy of cardiovascular disease. *J Am Coll Cardiol* 1985; **6**:1102–9.

41   Scheinert D, Laird JR, Schroder M, Steinkamp H, Balzer JO, Biamino G. Excimer laser-assisted recanalization of long, chronic superficial femoral artery occlusions. *J Endovasc Ther* 2001; **8**:156–66.

42   Colapinto RF, Harries-Jones EP, Johnston KW. Percutaneous transluminal angioplasty of peripheral vascular disease: a two year experience. *Cardiovasc Intervent Radiol* 1980; **3**:213–18.

43   Hewes RC, White RI, Murray RR et al. Long-term results of superficial femoral artery angioplasty. *Am J Roentgenol* 1986; **146**:1025–9.

44   Waller BF. Crackers, breakers, stretchers, drillers, scrapers, shavers, burners, welders and melters. The future treatment of atherosclerotic coronary artery disease? A clinical–morphologic assessment. *J Am Coll Cardiol* 1989; **13**:969–87.

45   Choy DSJ. History of lasers in medicine. *Thorac Cardiovasc Surg* 1988; **36**:114–17.

46   Choy DSJ, Stertzer SH, Myler RK, Marco J, Fournial G. Human coronary laser recanalization. *Clin Cardiol* 1984; **7**:377–81.

47   Forrester JS, Litvack F, Grundfest WS. Laser angioplasty and cardiovascular disease. *Am J Cardiol* 1986; **57**:990–2.

48 Crea F, Davies G, Mckenna W, Pashazade M, Tayler K, Maseri A. Percutaneous laser recanalization of coronary arteries. *Lancet* 1986; **2**:214–15.

49 Ginsburg R. Percutaneous laser angioplasty in the treatment of peripheral vascular disease. *Thorac Cardiovasc Surg* 1988; **36** (Suppl 2):142–5.

50 Ginsburg R, Wexler L, Mitchell RS, Profitt D. Percutaneous transluminal laser angioplasty for treatment of peripheral vascular disease: clinical experience with 16 patients. *Radiology* 1985; **156**:619–24.

51 Nordstrom LA, Castaneda-Zuniga WR, Lindeke CC, Rasmussen TM, Burnside DK. Laser angioplasty: controlled delivery of argon laser energy. *Radiology* 1988; **167**:463–5.

52 Sanborn TA, Cumberland DC, Greenfield AJ, Welsh CL, Guben JK. Percutaneous laser thermal angioplasty: initial results and 1-year follow-up in 129 femoropopliteal lesions. *Radiology* 1988; **168**:121–5.

53 Srinivasan R, Braren B, Dreyfus RW, Hadel L, Seeger DE. Mechanism of the ultraviolet laser ablation of polymethyl methacrylate at 193 and 248 nm: laser-induced fluorescence analysis, chemical analysis, and doping studies. *J Opt Soc Am* 1986; **3**:785–91.

54 Welch AJ, Bradley AB, Torres JH et al. Laser probe ablation of normal and atherosclerotic human aorta in vitro: a first thermographic and histologic analysis. *Circulation* 1987; **76**:1353–63.

55 Abela GS, Normann S, Feldman RL, Geiser EA, Cohen D, Conti CR. Effects of carbon dioxide, Nd:YAG and argon laser radiation on coronary atheromatous plaques. *Am J Cardiol* 1982; **50**:1199–205.

56 Geschwind HJ, Boussignac G, Teisseire B, Benhaiem N, Bittoun R, Laurent D. Conditions for effective Nd:YAG laser angiolplasty. *Br Heart J* 1984; **52**:484–9.

57 Sanborn TA, Faxon DP, Haudenschild CC, Ryan TJ. Experimental angioplasty circumferential distribution of laser thermal injury with a laser probe. *J Am Coll Cardiol* 1985; **5**:934–8.

58 Berlien HP, Müller GJ. Laser in Medicine. In: Biamino G, Müller GJ, (eds) *Advances in Laser Medicine I. First German Symposium on Laser Angioplasty*. Ecomed Verlagsgesellschaft: Berlin, 45–55.

59 Dörschel K, Biamino G, Brodzinski T, Axel T, Müller G. Comparison of the feasibility of laser angioplasty using heater probes, sapphire tips, and bare fibers. *Eur Heart J* 1988; **9**:331.

60 Abela GS, Fenech A, Crea F, Conti CR. Hot tip: another method of laser recanalization. *Lasers Surg Med* 1985; **5**:327–35.

61 Hussein H. A novel fiberoptic laser probe for treatment of occlusive vessel disease. *Opt Laser Technol Med* 1986; **6**:59–66.

62 Cothren RM, Hayes GB, Kramer JR, Sacks B, Kitrell C, Feld MS. A multifiber catheter with an optical shield for angiosurgery. *Laser Life Sci* 1986; **1**:1–12.

63 Fourrier JL, Brunetaud JM, Prat A, Marache P, Lablanche JM, Bertrand ME. Percutaneus angioplasty with a sapphire tip. *Lancet* 1987; **1**: 105.

64 Geschwind HJ, Blair JD, Mongolsmai D et al. Development and experimental application of contact probe catheter for laser angioplasty. *J Am Coll Cardiol* 1987; **9**:101–7.

65 Biamino G, Kar H, Harnoss BM, Dörschel K, Müller G. Feasibility of Nd:YAG laser angioplasty. In: Biamino G, Müller GJ, (eds) *Advances in Laser Medicine I. First German Symposium on Laser Angioplasty*. Ecomed Veralgsgesellschaft: Berlin, 134–40.

66 Biamino G. Coronary and peripheral laser angioplasty. In: Hogrefe, Huber, (eds) *Interventional Cardiology*. Göttingen: 243–60.

67 Pacala TJ, McDermid IS, Laudenslager JB. Ultranarrow linewidth, magnetically switched, ion pulse, xenon chloride laser. *Appl Phys Lett* 1984; **44**:658–60.

68 Srinivasan R, Leigh W. Ablative photodecompensation: action of far ultraviolet (193 nm) laser radiation on poly films. *J Am Chem Soc* 1982; **104**:6784–5.

69 Srinivasan R, Mayne-Bauton. Self-developing photoetching of poly films by far ultraviolet excimer laser radiation. *Appl Phys Lett* 1982; **4**:576–8.

70 Linsker R, Srinivasan R, Wynne JJ, Alonso DR. Far ultraviolet laser ablation of atherosclerotic lesions. *Lasers Surg Med* 1984; **4**:201–6.

71 Capek P, McLean GK, Berkowitz HD. Femoropopliteal angioplasty: factors influencing long-term success. *Circulation* 1991; **83** (Suppl I):I-70–I-80.

72 Geschwind J, Boussignac G, Teisseire B. Percutaneous transluminal laser angioplasty in man. *Lancet* 1984; **1**:844 (letter).

73 Lammer J, Pilger E, Decrinis M et al. Pulsed excimer laser versus continuous-wave Nd:YAG laser versus conventional angioplasty of peripheral arterial occlusions: prospective, controlled randomized trial. *Lancet* 1992; **340**:1183–8.

74 Belli AM, Cumberland DC, Procter AE et al. Total peripheral artery occlusions: conventional versus laser thermal recanalization with a hybrid probe in percutaneous angioplasty: results of a randomized trial. *Radiology* 1991; **181**:57–60.

75 Cumberland DC, Tayler DI, Welsh CL et al. Percutaneous laser thermal angioplasty: initial clinical results with a laser probe in total peripheral arterial occlusions. *Lancet* 1986; **1**:1457–9.

76 Köhler TR, Nance DR, Cramer MM et al. Duplex scanning for diagnosis of aortoiliac and femoropopliteal disease: a prospective study. *Circulation* 1987; **76**:1074–80.

77 Vroegindeweij D, Tielbeek AV, Buth J et al. Patterns of recurrent disease after recanalization of femoropopliteal artery occlusions. *Cardiovasc Intervent Radiol* 1997; **20**:257–62.

78 Duda SH, Pusich B, Richter G et al. Sirolimus-eluting stents for the treatment of obstructive superficial femoral artery disease. *Circulation* 2002; **106**:1505–9.

79 Gupta AK, Ravimandalam K, Rao VRK et al. Total occlusion of iliac arteries: results of balloon angioplasty. *Cardiovasc Intervent Radiol* 1993; **16**:165–77.

80 Szilagyi DE, Elliott JP Jr, Smith RF et al. A thirty-year survey of the reconstructive surgical treatment of aortoiliac occlusive disease. *J Vasc Surg* 1986; **3**:421–36.

81 Nevelsteen A, Wouters L, Suy R. Long-term patency of the aortofemoral dacron graft: a graft limb related study over a 25-year period. *J Cardiovasc Surg (Torino)* 1991; **32**:174–80.

82 Van den Akker PJ, Van Schilfgaarde R, Brand R et al. Long-term results of prosthetic reconstruction for obstructive aortoiliac disease. *Eur J Vasc Surg* 1992; **6**:53–61.

83 Jorgensen B, Meisner S, Holstein P et al. Early rethrombosis in femoropopliteal occlusions treated with percutaneous transluminal angioplasty. *Eur J Vasc Surg* 1990; **4**:149–52.

30

Procedures for the hypogastric artery

Jacob Cynamon and Priya Prabhaker

For a long time the hypogastric artery was a neglected vessel, with few procedures being performed by interventional radiologists except for a limited number of angioplasties done for significant claudication or erectile dysfunction. Recently, this vessel has become of prime importance to various procedures. Fibroids are currently treated by embolizing the uterine artery as it stems from the anterior division of the hypogastric artery. Pudendal arteriography and iliac angioplasty are being performed for evaluation and management of impotency. Rarely, buttock claudication, which can be due to significant hypogastric artery stenosis, can be treated by angioplasty. The most frequent intervention of the hypogastric artery performed at our institution is preoperative hypogastric artery coil embolization for stent–graft or operative repair of abdominal aortic and iliac artery aneurysms to prevent collateral endoleaks. This chapter will review these indications and techniques that have now become commonplace in the angiography suite.

Claudication

Since angioplasty for claudication has been around for many years, we will begin with this topic. Isolated hypogastric artery stenosis causing significant claudication occurs rarely (Figure 30.1).[1] Occasionally, an external iliac artery occlusion occurs with a proximal hypogastric artery stenosis. In this situation, where the common femoral artery and the distal vessels are supplied by the hypogastric artery, a focal stenosis of the hypogastric artery may lead to severe thigh or calf claudication and thus may warrant treatment via angioplasty. An alternative to angioplasty would be recanalization of the external iliac artery, which is significantly more invasive than a focal hypogastric artery angioplasty. Unfortunately, there are no large series reporting the initial and long-term results of hypogastric artery angioplasties for the treatment of claudication.

Erectile dysfunction

The evaluation and possible treatment of impotency is another procedure that involves the hypogastric artery. Although there are many methods of evaluation of the cause of impotency, such as duplex ultrasonography, magnetic resonance imaging, and radionuclide imaging, pudendal arteriography remains the gold standard for penile arterial assessment. Pudendal arteriography allows for an anatomic study of the causes of impotence, which is necessary when considering penile arterial reconstructive surgery. The distal aorta, common iliac artery, proximal hypogastric artery, and the pudendal arteries must be evaluated. Pudendal arteriography is best performed by bilaterally catheterizing the hypogastric arteries and using the image intensifier to visualize in the ipsilateral anterior oblique projection, with the penis positioned across the contralateral thigh so that the dorsal and cavernosal arteries become visible (Figure 30.2). The angiogram is performed after injecting 60 mg of papaverine directly into the cavernosum using a 25 or 27 gauge needle.[2] This causes a partial or complete erection in most patients, which improves flow and helps visualize the dorsal penile artery. The classic penile anatomy is the dorsal penile, cavernosal, and bulbar arteries stemming from each pudendal artery.[3,4] A great deal of variation exists, with only 18% of cases in one study having the classic pudendal anatomy.[5] To avoid misinterpretation of normal variants, such as the dorsal penile artery branching from the iliac or common femoral artery, these variants should be searched for if a dorsal penile artery is not seen with hypogastric artery injection (Figure 30.3). If a stenosis is identified in one of the inflow vessels such as the common iliac or proximal hypogastric arteries, the patient may benefit from transluminal angioplasty. In addition, a focal lesion in the pudendal artery can be dilated with a small vessel balloon.[6] However, many patients with arterial erectile dysfunction do not have a focal lesion amenable to angioplasty. These patients can benefit from a surgical bypass to the dorsal penile artery.

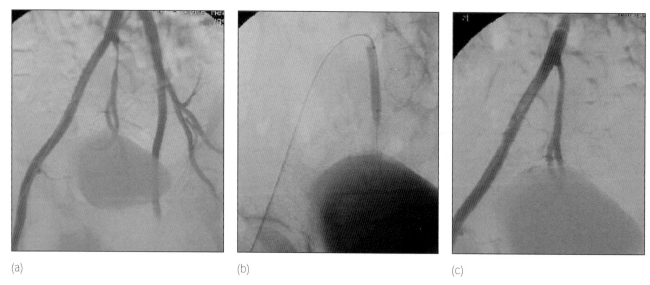

(a)   (b)   (c)

Figure 30.1
(a) A 62-year-old man with three block buttock claudication with a focal stenosis of the proximal hypogastric artery. (b) Percutaneous transluminal angioplasty (PTA) with a 6 x 4 balloon performed via an ipsilateral common femoral artery puncture. (c) Post-PTA angiogram demonstrating a good result. The patient no longer suffered from buttock claudication.

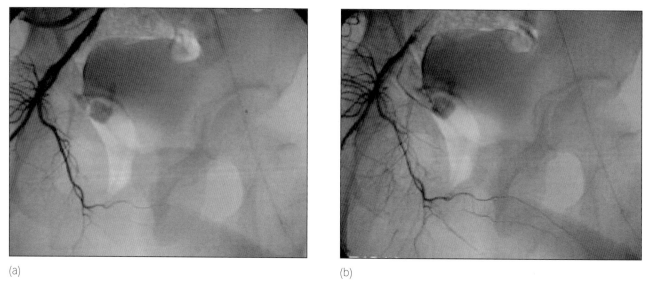

(a)   (b)

Figure 30.2
Right anterior oblique view of a selective right hypogastric artery (a) before (b) after injection of 60 mg papaverine. The pudendal artery is visualized and is seen as it enters the dorsum of the penis and becomes the dorsal penile artery. The cavernosal and bulbar arteries are also seen. Note this elongated view of the dorsal penile artery can only be obtained in the anterior oblique projection with the penis draped across the contralateral thigh.

Uterine artery embolization

Transcatheter uterine artery embolization was once an uncommon procedure performed for emergency control of hemorrhage related to pelvic trauma, postpartum and postcesarean bleeding, placental abnormalities, ectopic pregnancy, hemorrhage from gestational trophoblastic disease, intraoperative bleeding, and pelvic arteriovenous malformations.[7] Recent use of uterine artery embolization for the treatment and management of symptomatic uterine leiomyomas has further stretched the application of this procedure. Uterine leiomyomas produce significant morbidity by causing uterine enlargement, abnormal bleeding, anemia, pelvic pain, and infertility. Prior therapeutic

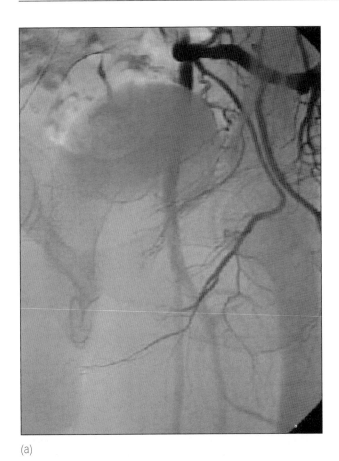

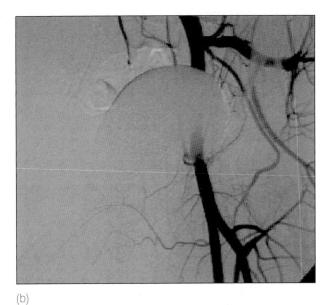

(a)   (b)

Figure 30.3

(a) The left dorsal penile artery is not seen on the selective hypogastric artery injection. (b) An external iliac artery injection demonstrates the dorsal penile artery to be a branch off the superficial femoral artery, which is an unusual variant.

techniques, such as treatment with gonadotrophin-releasing hormone (GnRH) analogs, myomectomy, or hysterectomy, have proved to be either inadequate or associated with significant morbidity, mortality, and potential infertility. Thus, the utilization of uterine artery embolization to shrink leiomyomas by obstructing their blood supply appears to be a better and less-invasive approach to the treatment of symptomatic fibroids.[8,9]

Uterine artery embolization is performed via selective catheterization of the hypogastric and uterine arteries. Bilateral embolization is required for treatment of symptomatic leiomyomas since bilateral arterial anastomoses provide the blood supply to fibroids. The most common agents used include Gelfoam sponges and polyvinyl alcohol particles (Figure 30.4).[10] Other agents such as Biospheres and Onyx are being evaluated. Complications have been infrequent, with the most common complication being groin hematomas and arterial perforations. Post-embolization pain resulting from leiomyoma ischemia is also fairly common and is controlled with appropriate narcotics. Other observed but very rare complications include endometritis and ischemia to pelvic organs seen with emergency embolization done for

hemostasis. Studies have shown a high rate of success, with decreased symptomatology and reduction in leiomyoma volume of between 20 and 80%. Limited follow-up of patients undergoing uterine artery embolization has prevented knowledge of the exact frequency of embolization failure and of the consequences on post-embolization fertility. However, successful pregnancies have been reported after the procedure, which offers hope that uterine artery embolization may one day be the main modality of treatment for symptomatic uterine fibroids. Randomized clinical trials should be performed to further elucidate the applications of and indications for uterine artery embolization.[7,11,12,13]

Hypogastric artery embolization

Stent–grafts have become an alternative to standard surgical repair in the management of aortoiliac aneurysms. Two grafts are currently FDA (Food and Drug Administration) approved and others are in clinical trials. If an endoleak occurs, which is

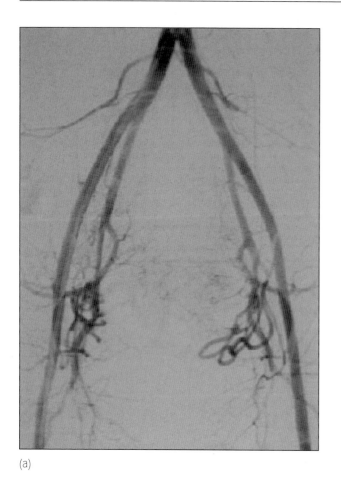

(a)

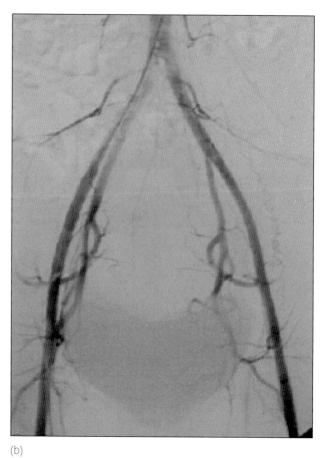

(b)

Figure 30.4
(a) A 44-year-old patient with a large fibroid and severe pelvic pain related to menstruation. Pelvic angiogram demonstrates hypertrophied uterine arteries. Bilateral uterine artery embolization performed with polyvinyl alcohol (250–400 μm particles). (b) The hypertrophied uterine arteries are no longer seen. The patient's symptoms have dramatically improved.

the leakage of blood into a treated aneurysm, the procedure is considered a failure. Endoleaks may occur as a result of an incomplete seal around the proximal or distal attachment of a stent–graft (type I) or due to retrograde flow from collateral arterial branches (type II). Midgraft tears or modular disconnections are called type III endoleaks, and type IV endoleaks are due to graft porosity. When a stent–graft crosses the origin of one of the hypogastric arteries, cross-pelvic collaterals may allow retrograde flow through the hypogastric artery and into the treated aneurysm, resulting in a type II endoleak. To prevent this occurrence, coils can be placed in the hypogastric artery prior to placing the endovascular graft across its origin. Stent–grafts will cross the origin of the hypogastric artery in the following circumstances:

1. abdominal aortic aneurysms (AAAs) with short common iliac arteries (CIAs), making stent anchorage in one of the common iliac arteries difficult
2. CIA aneurysms extending near the CIA bifurcation

3. an AAA with an aorto-unifemoral stent–graft, a cross-femoral bypass, and a contralateral CIA occlusion device, such as the type placed frequently at our institution [The Montefiore Endovascular Graft System (MEGS)] (Figure 30.5).

Hypogastric artery coil embolization can decrease the incidence of these endoleaks. It will prevent retrograde flow via the hypogastric artery into the aneurysm. The hypogastric artery branches can still continue to be perfused via cross-pelvic collaterals. Unfortunately, many patients treated in this manner will develop buttock claudication. This occurred in 41% of all patients in a study conducted at our institution.[14]

The location at which the hypogastric artery is coil embolized is important in reducing the incidence of buttock claudication. A more proximal embolization may have a lower incidence of buttock claudication. In our study, 10% of patients with proximal hypogastric artery coil embolizations developed buttock claudication vs 55% of those with distal embolizations. Coils, as opposed to other embolic agents, permit proximal placement while also preventing backflow, but still preserve distal vessel patency, thus minimizing possible resultant ischemia. Proximal occlusion of the hypogastric artery at its origin, before its anterior–posterior bifurcation, sufficiently impedes retrograde filling of the aneurysm and the development of endoleaks. In addition, proximal occlusion still allows collaterals to contribute to the anterior and posterior divisions of the hypogastric artery and permits continued communication between the anterior and posterior divisions. The vessels distal to the embolization site continue to fill via collaterals and can thus help prevent ischemia-induced claudication (Figure 30.6).[14,15]

To ensure more accurate proximal placement of embolization coils and maintain communication between the branches of the hypogastric artery, nonfibered GDC coils can be used in conjunction with Gianturco coils. GDC coils may be used in cases where Gianturco coils are likely to embolize to the hypogastric bifurcation or beyond, which can occur in patients with difficult anatomy, such as a hypogastric artery

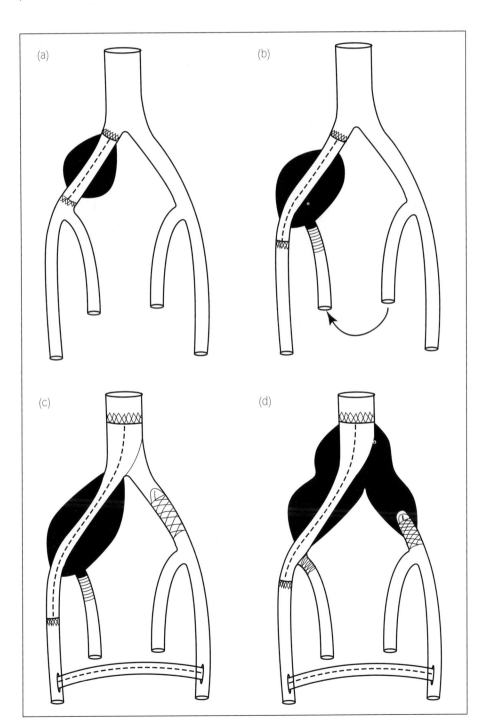

Figure 30.5
(a) Common iliac artery with enough normal distal common iliac artery to anchor the distal stent–graft above the hypogastric artery. Therefore, embolization of the hypogastric artery is not needed. (b, c, d) Iliac and aortoiliac aneurysms with insufficient normal common iliac artery requiring extension of the stent–graft into the external iliac artery. Coil embolization of the hypogastric artery is thus indicated.

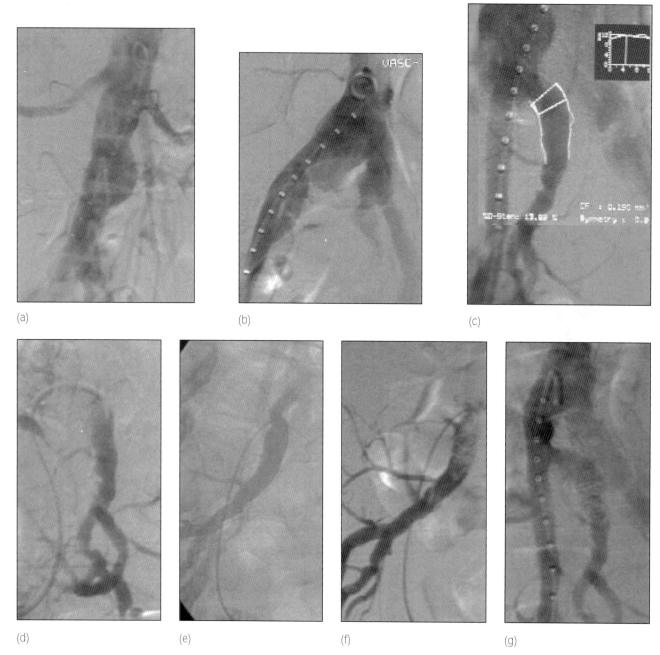

(a)   (b)   (c)

(d)   (e)   (f)   (g)

Figure 30.6

(a, b) Aortic and right common iliac artery aneurysms. Coil embolization of the right hypogastric artery was performed via an ipsilateral common femoral artery approach. (c) Measurement of the hypogastric artery helps us choose the coil size required to limit the incidence of coil migration. (d) Selective catheterization with a Cobra catheter is performed in the posterior oblique projection. (e) The anterior and posterior divisions are best seen in the anterior oblique projection. (f, g) Adequate coil placement in the hypogastric artery proximal to the bifurcation and the iliolumbar artery.

that does not taper as one moves distally towards its bifurcation. A nonfibered GDC coil will prevent microcoils and Gianturco coils from embolizing into the branches of the hypogastric artery while still allowing communication between the anterior and posterior divisions of the hypogastric artery even if it is lodged at the hypogastric bifurcation. In addition, GDC coils can be useful in difficult

ipsilateral hypogastric artery catherterizations where a reversed curve catheter may be necessary to adequately seal the proximal hypogastric artery. Gianturco coils cannot always easily advance through a reverse curve catheter. Instead, a nonfibered GDC coil can be first placed to prevent distal embolization and then followed by Tornado or Vortex coils placed through a Tracker catheter (Figures 30.7 and 30.8).[16]

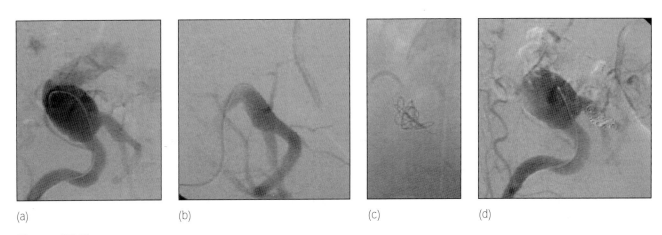

(a)   (b)   (c)   (d)

Figure 30.7

(a) A common iliac artery aneurysm. (b) Reverse taper of the hypogastric artery. Note that any coil placed in the proximal hypogastric artery is likely to embolize as the artery is enlarging as it nears the bifurcation. (c) A GDC coil is being placed in the hypogastric artery. (d) Post-GDC coil and proximal Gianturco coil embolization.

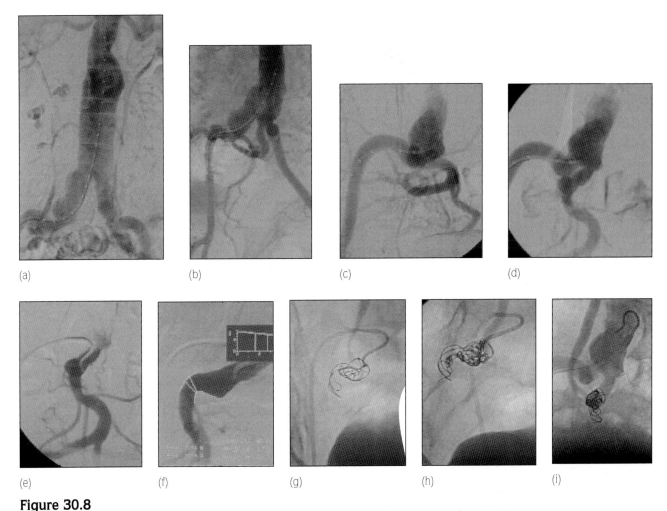

(a)   (b)   (c)   (d)

(e)   (f)   (g)   (h)   (i)

Figure 30.8

((a) Aorto–right common iliac artery aneurysm. (b, c) The origin of the hypogastric artery is not easily identified on either oblique view. (d, e) Craniocaudal angulation demonstrates the origin of the hypogastric artery, allowing its catheterization with an SOS Omni catheter. (f) Measuring the diameter of the hypogastric artery. (g) GDC coil placed via a Tracker catheter. (h) Post-microcoil embolization. The microcoils were not able to travel beyond the GDC coil. (i) Post-embolization completion angiogram demonstrates well-positioned coils above the hypogastric artery bifurcation and cessation of prograde flow in the hypogastric artery.

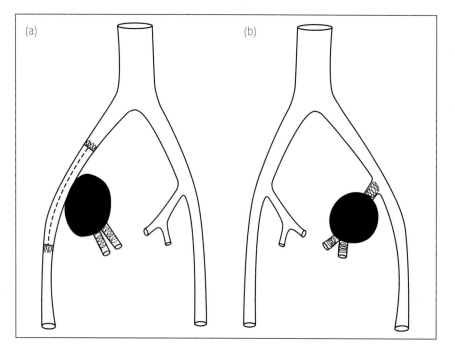

(a) (b)

Figure 30.9
Hypogastric artery aneurysms are managed by coil embolizing its branches and occluding the proximal hypogastric artery by either (a) using a stent–graft from the common iliac artery to the external iliac artery or (b), if an adequate proximal neck exists, an occluder can be placed in the proximal hypogastric artery.

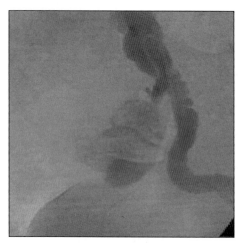

(a)

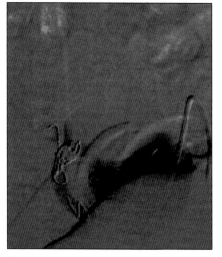

(b)

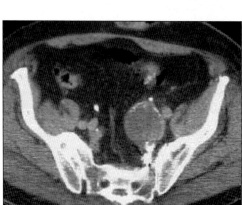

(c)

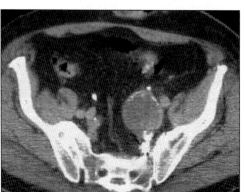

(d)

Figure 30.10
(a) A patient with a hypogastric artery aneurysm. (b) Branches of the hypogastric artery are coil embolized. (c) An occluder is placed in the proximal hypogastric artery. (d) The hypogastric aneurysm is isolated and thrombosed.

When treating a hypogastric artery aneurysm, one must occlude the distal and proximal end of the hypogastric artery. If the anterior and posterior divisions arise from the body of the aneurysm, as they often do in a hypogastric aneurysm, proximal embolization would not be possible. Coil embolization of its branches and a common iliac artery to external iliac artery endoluminal graft would isolate or occlude the aneurysm. If there is enough space in the proximal hypogastric artery, an occluder can be placed in this vessel instead of the common iliac to external iliac stent–graft (Figures 30.9 and 30.10).[17]

Common iliac aneurysms or arteriovenous fistulas involving the common iliac arteries provide another challenge. The usual hypogastric artery embolization may not prevent endoleaks into the aneurysm or flow through the fistula even after the proximal common iliac artery to external iliac artery stent–graft is placed. This occurs because of a communication between the iliolumbar and lumbar arteries that allows flow into the common iliac artery and through the fistula. In these cases, coils should extend above the iliolumbar artery or be placed into the iliolumbar artery to prevent a persistent lumbar to iliolumbar collateral (Figure 30.11).[14]

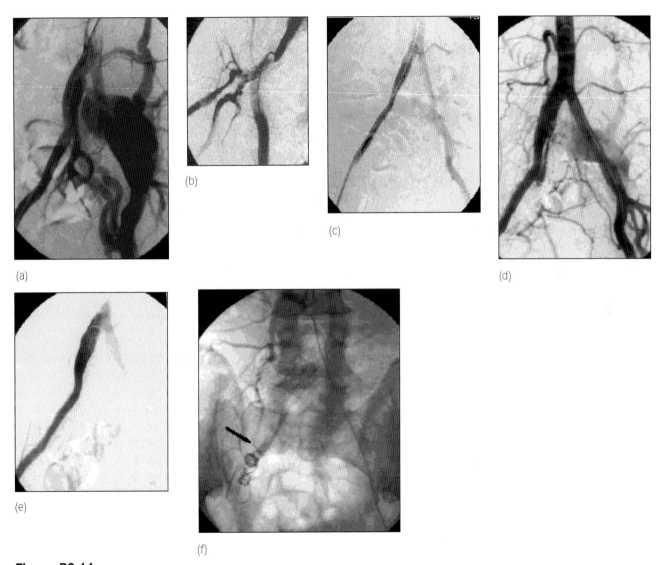

Figure 30.11

(a) A 49-year-old man s/p back surgery developed a right common iliac artery to vein fistula. (b, c) The planned procedure was a common iliac artery to external iliac artery stent–graft to prevent retrograde flow in the hypogastric artery from leaking into the common iliac artery behind the stent–graft and having a persistent fistula, and thus the hypogastric artery was embolized. (d) Follow-up 3 months later shows a persistent small fistula. (e) There was no proximal or distal endoleak. (f) The leak turned out to be a lumbar to iliolumbar collateral. In retrospect, the most proximal coil was just beyond the iliolumbar artery. This allowed a persistent lumbar to iliolumbar collateral with retrograde flow in the proximal hypogastric artery and in the common iliac artery behind the stent–graft and through the fistula.

Hypogastric artery embolization prior to the surgical repair of aortoiliac or iliac aneurysms may also prove advantageous. Cases where hypogastric artery embolization would be most useful include those in which the proposed surgical procedure would require either a surgical anastomosis at the common iliac artery bifurcation or ligation of the hypogastric artery. This can be difficult with a common iliac artery aneurysm, especially on the left side because of the need to mobilize the sigmoid mesocolon. A study performed at our institution revealed that in all cases after hypogastric artery embolization, the actual surgical procedure was modified to

an external iliac artery or common femoral artery bypass with ligation of the proximal artery, thereby excluding the common iliac artery aneurysm. This technique avoids the need to operate in the region of the iliac aneurysm, thus significantly simplifying the operation. Our study demonstrated simplification of the open aneurysm repair with a low occurrence of complications, which suggests that hypogastric artery embolization should be considered for patients with iliac aneurysms prior to open aortoiliac or iliac aneurysm repair (Figure 30.12).

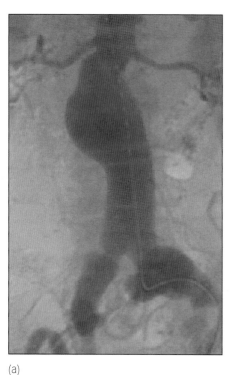

(a)

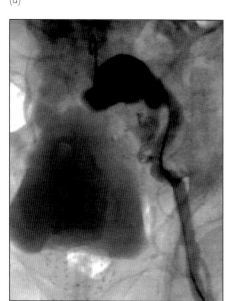

(c)

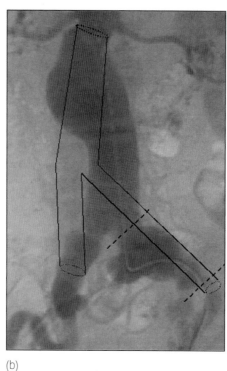

(b)

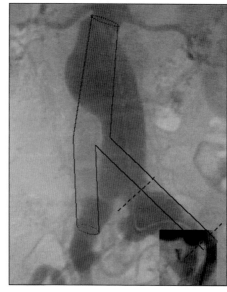

(d)

Figure 30.12

(a) A patient with an aortoiliac aneurysm. Surgical options include a bifurcated graft to the right common iliac artery and to the distal left common iliac artery. This can be a difficult operation. A less optimal alternative is (b) a bifurcated graft to the right common iliac artery and ligation of the proximal left common iliac artery and its external iliac artery, with the left limb of the bifurcated graft inserting into the left external iliac artery below the ligation. This procedure does not address preventing retrograde left hypogastric artery flow and maintains a pressurized left common iliac artery. If the left hypogastric artery is coil embolized (c) prior to open repair, the latter procedure can be performed (d) and there is no concern regarding retrograde flow so the common iliac artery aneurysm will also occlude.

So far, our discussion has focused on unilateral hypogastric artery. Bilateral hypogastric artery embolization is usually avoided for fear of causing significant morbidity in the form of perineal necrosis, severe lower extremity neurological deficits, ischemic colitis, impotency, and buttock claudication.[18] Bilateral occlusion is more likely required in aortic aneurysm cases that also affect the iliac arteries. This occurs in about 20% of aortic aneurysms, which often involve the distal common iliac artery.[19] Interruption of one or both hypogastric arteries may be necessary in these cases along with aortoiliac or aortofemoral bypass in order to completely exclude the aneurysm. A study performed by vascular surgeons at our institution reveals that the incidence of severe morbidity might actually be quite low for bilateral hypogastric artery interruption.[20] No patients in this study suffered perineal necrosis, ischemic colitis, or death. In addition, only a small percentage experienced impotency, neurological deficits, or persistent buttock claudication after occlusion of the hypogastric artery unilaterally or bilaterally. These results suggest that unilateral or bilateral hypogastric artery occlusion is most probably not a dangerous procedure and thus can be performed to completely exclude aneurysms that involve the iliac bifurcation or hypogastric arteries. It is proposed that the complications seen in other series are more likely due to other intraoperative events such as hypotension and severing of important collaterals that stem from the distal external iliac, common femoral, and profunda femoral arteries.

In conclusion, the hypogastric artery has become a very important vessel in interventional radiology. More knowledge and research is needed to prevent unanticipated complications that may occur when treating claudication, impotency, uterine leiomyomas, and most importantly, aortoiliac aneurysms.

References

1   Smith G, Train J, Mitty H, Jacobson J. Hip pain caused by buttock claudication. *Clin Orthop Rel Res* 1992; **284**: 176–80.
2   Wahl S, Rubin M, Bakal C. Radiologic evaluation of penile arterial anatomy in arteriogenic impotence. *Int J Impot Res* 1997; **6**: 93–7.
3   Ferner H, Strubesand J (eds). *Sobotta atlas of human anatomy*, Vol. 2, 10th edn. Baltimore: Urban & Schwartzberg. 1983: 200–1.
4   Kadir S. *Atlas of normal and variant angiographic anatomy*. Philadelphia: WB Saunders, 1991: 227–93.
5   Bookstein JJ, Lang EV. Penile magnification pharmaco-arteriography: details of intrapenile arterial anatomy. *Am J Radiol* 1987; **146**: 883–8.
6   Valji K, Bookstein J. Transluminal angioplasty in the treatment of arteriogenic impotence. *CVIR* 1988; **11**: 245–52.
7   Abulafia O, Sherer D. Transcatheter uterine artery embolization for the management of symptomatic uterine leiomyomas. *Obst Gynecol Sur* 1999; **54**(12): 746.
8   Wallach E. Myomectomy. In: Thompson J, Rock J (eds), *Te Lindes's operative gynecology*, 7th edn. Philadelphia: Lippincott, 1992: 647–62.
9   Dubuisson J, Lecuru F, Foulot H. Laparoscopic myomectomy. In: Sutton C, Diamond M (eds), *Endoscopic surgery for gynaecologists*. London: WB Saunders, 1993: 71–6.
10   Markoff G, Quagliarello J, Rosen R, Bechman E. Uterine arteriovenous embolization successfully embolized with a liquid polymer isobutyl 2-cyanoacrylate. *Am J Obst Gynecol* 1987; **156**: 1179–80.
11   McLucas B, Goodwin S, Vedantham S. Embolic therapy for myomata. *Minimally Invas Ther Allied Technol* 1996; **5**: 336–8.
12   Braf Z, Knootz W. Gangrene of bladder: complications of hypogastric artery embolization. *Urology* 1977; **9**: 670–1.
13   Stancato-Pasik A, Mitty H, Richard H, Eshkar N. Obstetric embolotherapy: effects on menses and pregnancy. *Radiology* 1996; **201**: 179.
14   Cynamon J, Lerer D, Veith F et al. Hypogastric artery coil embolization prior to endoluminal repair of aneurysms and fistulas: buttock claudication, a recognized but possibly preventable complication. *J Vasc Intervent Radiology* 2000; **11**(5): 573–7.
15   Lee, C, Kaufman J, Fan C et al. Clinical outcome of internal iliac artery occlusions during endovascular treatment of aortoiliac aneurysmal diseases. *J Vasc Intervent Radiology* 2000; **11**(5): 567–71.
16   Cloft H, Joseph G, Tong et al. Use of three-dimensional Guglielmi detachable coils in the treatment of wide-necked cerebral aneurysms. *Am J Neuroradiol* 2000; **21**(7): 1312–4.
17   Cynamon J, Marin M, Veith F et al. Endovascular repair of an internal iliac artery aneurysm with use of a stented graft and embolization coils. *J Vasc Intervent Radiology* 1995; **6**: 509–12.
18   Andriole G, Sugarbaker P. Perineal and bladder necrosis following bilateral internal iliac artery ligation. Report of a case. *Dis Colon Rectum* 1985; **28**(3): 183–4.
19   Armon M, Wenham P, Witake S et al. Common iliac artery aneurysms in patients with abdominal aortic aneurysms. *Eur J Vasc Endovas Surg* 1998; **15**(3): 255–7.
20   Mehta M, Veith F, Ohki T et al. Unilateral and bilateral hypogastric artery interruption during aortoiliac aneurysm repair in 154 patients: a relatively innocuous procedure. Presented at the 54th Annual Meeting of the Society of Vascular Surgery, June 10–14, 2000.

31

Percutaneous endovascular treatment of femoropopliteal occlusive diseases

Michel Henry, Isabelle Henry, Christos Klonaris and Michèle Hugel

Introduction

The number of patients who have peripheral artery occlusive diseases is steadily increasing worldwide, primarily as a result of the aging of the population. It is estimated that 10–20% of individuals more than 70 years of age sustain some degree of chronic, lower-extremity ischemia. This percentage is greater in some subgroups of patients, such as those having diabetes or end-stage renal failure. Femoropopliteal arterial occlusive diseases are found alone or more often in combination with other lesions at the aortoiliac and/or infrapopliteal level. The extent, severity, and combination of the atherosclerotic lesions determine the severity of the disease and the type of treatment.

Types of peripheral vascular diseases are generally classified as claudication or critical limb-threatening ischemia. The distinction is made because the natural history and progression of the two types are different. The prognoses are different as well: better for patients with claudication and worse for those with more advanced stages of ischemia. In addition, this claudication serves as a guide for decisions that must be made concerning the best treatment option. Patients with disease limited to the superficial femoral artery (SFA) usually present with variable levels of claudication. However, popliteal artery involvement often leads to more significant functional limitation, whereas multilevel vascular involvement often leads to critical limb ischemia. Patients who have severe, lifestyle-limiting claudication, rest pain, or tissue necrosis should be offered relatively aggressive therapy. Invasive therapy is indicated for these patients.

During the past 40 years, bypass surgery has been the mainstay of treatment at this level. Results of revascularization are satisfactory but not ideal. The patency rates vary according to several factors: the vessel inflow and outflow status, clinical status (claudication vs ischemia), type of graft selected (vein vs synthetic), the quality of graft when vein is used, the site of distal anastomosis (above or below the knee), the patient comorbidity, and the experience of the vascular center and surgeons in performing these demanding procedures. Veith et al.,[1] published the results from a 6-year prospective muticenter trial, in which saphenous vein and polytetrafluoroethylene (PTFE) grafts in 845 infrainguinal arterial reconstructions were randomly compared. Total 4-year patency rates were 68 ± 8% for veins and 47 ± 9% for synthetic grafts. When the distal anastomosis was infrapopliteal, patency rates were even lower – 49 ± 10% for vein and only 12 ± 7% for synthetic grafts.

Endovascular therapy, inspired by the work of Dotter and Judkins[2] in the United States in the mid-1970s and Grüntzig and Hopff[3] in Europe in the mid-1980s, is, however, a relatively new field of vascular medicine. Only within the last decade has this new concept of treatment become widely recognized and accepted. During that time, the applications of endovascular therapy have been broadened dramatically in all vessels, including those at the aortoiliac and femoropopliteal levels. Currently, interventional procedures are the first treatments to be proposed for most patients who have peripheral artery diseases. Balloon angioplasty alone may offer good immediate and long-term results; however, the addition of stents has been proposed in order to increase the procedural success of angioplasty and extend its application to more types of lesions. Nevertheless, stenting is controversial. Although it is well accepted at the aortoiliac level, it is less so at the femoropopliteal level.[4–26] Moreover, the rapid development of endovascular stents for peripheral applications, the different designs, the unique properties, and even name changes as a result of corporate mergers have made stent selection a confusing issue in everyday clinical practice. Therefore, an overview of currently available stents and their characteristics is necessary before the indications and proper stent selection in different clinical settings can be considered.

Indications for invasive therapy – patient selection

The cornerstone of therapy for the claudicant is aggressive risk factor reduction and regular aerobic activity.[27] Any treatment should take into account the risk of limb loss (usually low) versus the risk of death (significantly elevated.[28,29] A supervised walking program has been shown to improve ambulation more significantly than a home walking program.[30,31] Recent advances in medical therapy such as cilostazol may also improve ambulation.[32,33]

Invasive therapy is indicated for chronic critical leg ischemia and acute leg ischemia (stages III and IV of Fontaine's classification).

In intermittent claudication, indications for invasive therapy have been summarized in Recommendation 21 of the Trans Atlantic Inter Society Consensus (TASC) working Group.[34] Before offering a patient the option of any invasive therapy endovascular or surgical, the following consideration must be taken into account:

- a predicted or observed lack of adequate response to exercise therapy and risk factor modification
- the patient must have a severe disability, either being unable to perform normal work or having very serious impairment of other activities important to the patient
- absence of other disease that would limit exercise even if the claudication was improved (e.g. angina or chronic respiratory disease)
- the individual's anticipated natural history and prognosis
- the morphology of the lesion must be such that the appropriate intervention would have low risk and high probability of initial and long-term success.

Indications for invasive therapy have also to take into account that patients with isolated aortoiliac disease tend to be younger and have a low likelihood of coronary heart disease comorbidity, whereas those with femoropopliteal diseases tend to have the highest likelihood of coronary heart disease comorbidity.[28,29,35,39] Preservation of the saphenous veins for coronary bypass grafting is a potential advantage in such patients. A percutaneous transluminal angioplasty (PTA) should be the first choice for these patients.

Femoropopliteal lesions have been categorized in morphological terms with preferred therapeutic options as follows (Recommendation 34 of TASC):

TASC type A lesions:
1. single stenosis < 3 cm.

TASC type B lesions:
2. single stenosis 3–10 cm in length, not involving the distal popliteal artery (CIRSE – single stenosis or *occlusion* 3–10 cm long)
3. heavily calcified stenoses up to 3 cm in length

4. multiple lesions, each less than 3 cm (stenoses or occlusions)
5. single or multiple lesions in the absence of continuous tibial run off to improve inflow for distal surgical bypass.

TASC type C lesions:
6. single stenosis or occlusion longer than 5 cm (CIRSE – single stenosis or occlusion > 10 cm long)
7. multiple stenoses or occlusions, each 3–5 cm, with or without heavy calcification.

TASC type D lesions:
8. complete common femoral artery or superficial femoral artery occlusions or complete popliteal and proximal trifurcation occlusions.

According to recommendation 35 of the TASC, endovascular procedure is the treatment of choice for type A lesions and surgery the procedure of choice for type D lesions. For type B and C lesions we have the choice between endovascular procedure and surgery. However, developments of new catheters and wires, new techniques (e.g. recanalization devices, atherectomy devices) the use of fibrinolysis, thromboaspiration, mechanical thrombectomy devices, and the large number of stents available on the market have improved the technical success rate and seem also to improve the long-term patency rate. For these reasons, the tendency is to enlarge the indications for interventional procedure and to reserve surgery in case of endovascular procedure failures or complications. PTA is preferred in high-risk patients, elderly patients, diabetics and in patients with multivascular diseases. The low complication rates, the less invasive nature of these procedures, and the preservation of the surgical option have made them increasingly popular. The repeatability of these procedures is an important feature to consider. The patency rates of percutaneous procedures do not necessarily need to be equivalent with surgical methods to allow them to be the procedures of choice.[33] Maintaining ambulation and limb viability, together with the lowest procedural morbidity and mortality, should be the goal of these procedures; coupled with the use of improving vascular closure devices that allow for short-term outpatient care, endovascular procedures appear poised to revolutionize the treatment of arterial occlusive diseases.[33]

Technical considerations
Preprocedural evaluation of the lesion

During preprocedural evaluation of the lesion, the segment of the vessel to be treated and the total vasculature of the lower extremities must be evaluated thoroughly. Preprocedural arteriography is indispensable for analyzing the lesion (exact location, percentage and length of the stenosis, diameter of the artery), for collecting information about the nature of the lesion (eccentric, ulcerated, or calcified), the inflow vessels, the runoff, and the collateral circulation, and for choosing the best approach. Duplex ultrasonography is also performed before the procedure to characterize the lesion and to provide a baseline study. In cases of arterial occlusions, a computed tomographic (CT) scan is performed to exclude the presence of aneurysms. Angioscopy and intravascular ultrasound also provide valuable information for making decisions about the appropriate treatment; however, they are not part of our routine diagnostic workup, mainly because the cost is prohibitive.

The access sites

For the treatment of femoropopliteal lesions, one can choose one of four different access sites depending on:

- the location of the lesion
- the status of the artery above and below the segment to be treated
- the type of endoprostheses available
- the operator's experience.

The antegrade ipsilateral access site

This is the most commonly used access site since one can use large introducers (9F) which allow for the introduction either of a simple balloon catheter or a stent–balloon combination. This is the access site of choice for lesions located in the lower two-thirds of the superficial femoral artery.

The contralateral access site

This access site allows us to treat lesions of the common femoral, deep femoral and the upper part of the superficial artery. It is not advisable to use this access site in the event of tortuous iliac lesions; otherwise, failure of stent implantation may result because of stent length, rigidity, or the deployment system. One can use large introducers (9F) at this site, and long curved introducers could facilitate stent placement. This approach allows for the combined treatment of lesions at the iliac and femoral level. It has the advantage of not blocking blood flow in the superficial femoral artery and avoids compression of the ipsilateral femoral artery after withdrawal of the introducer.

The brachial access site

We use the brachial access site in case of failure or when other sites are impossible to access. This access point requires the use of long introducers, long guide wires, and balloons with long sheaths, consequently limiting indications. The choice of this site is also limited by the size and length of the required introducers (≤ 7F). In the case of bilateral lesions, the two femoral arteries may be treated at the same time through a single access site.

The popliteal access site

The popliteal access site may be the access site of choice for the treatment of proximal lesions of the superficial or common femoral artery when the contralateral approach is not possible. It is also used after access failure via the antegrade site, which is essential in long recanalizations. Furthermore, any angioplasty technique can be used with any available stent.

Technical aspects

Femoropopliteal stenoses

Whatever the access site, the stenoses are crossed either by peripheral guide wires (hydrophilic wires for tight stenoses impossible to cross with other wires) or by coronary wires in case of very tight stenoses. Some lesions (e.g. calcified, long lesions) may be treated before dilatation by debulking devices such as Rotablator or Rotarex. Then a balloon angioplasty is performed. If a 'stent like result' is obtained, PTA alone is sufficient. With no 'stent like result', stenting has to be considered. Some lesions may be treated by direct stenting without predilatation (see later).

Femoropopliteal occlusions

Acute occlusions. These occlusions may be treated by several techniques, fibrinolysis (urokinase, rt-PA) thromboaspiration, mechanical thrombectomy, or combined techniques. After reopening the artery, the underlying lesion should be treated as previously.

Chronic occlusions. These occlusions are treated in most cases by hydrophilic wires. The subintimal recanalization technique seems promising: 90% of chronic occlusion can be recanalized, even long occlusions. In the case of failure, the laser technique or some other technique with new recanalization devices can be used.

Femoropopliteal aneurysms

These lesions can now be treated by interventional procedures with covered stents with promising results (see Chapter 47).

Treatment and follow-up

Adjunctive medical therapy includes preprocedural aspirin (160–300 mg/day), starting at least 1 day before the procedure and intraprocedural heparin (5000 units intravenously).

All patients received aspirin (100 mg/day) continuously after the procedure and ticlopidine (250–500 mg/day) or clopidogrel (75 mg/day) for 1 month if a stent is placed.

Low molecular weight heparin is sometimes given for 2–8 days in some specific cases, such as lesions with a high risk of thrombosis.

The follow-up is similar to the one used after any angioplasty: a Doppler echocardiography examination is performed at 24 hours, 3 months, 6 months, and annually, including, if possible, an angiography at 6 months.

Results of femoropopliteal PTA

Several important studies of femoropopliteal PTA with long-term results have been published and recently summarized.[34]

A technical success is obtained in 82–96 % of the cases[5,40–46] greater than 90% in stenoses, 80–85% in occlusions.

The long-term patency rates are listed in the Table 31.1.

The weighted average for the primary patency rate is 61% at 1 year, 51% at 2 years, and 48% at 5 years.

Becker et al.[48] also found a 4–5 year patency rate of 67%, Vogelzang[49] recorded a patency rate of 49% at 5 years and 35% at 10 years.

Several factors may affect the outcome of angioplasty:[40–46,50–55]

- Morphologic features:
    eccentric vs concentric plaques
    heavy vs no calcification
    postangioplasty residual stenosis
    extensive dissection.
- Identified risk factors:
    critical limb ischemia vs claudication
    long lesions vs short lesions
    occlusion vs stenosis
    poor runoff
    diabetes
    smoker.

Table 31.2 summarizes the dependence of the primary patency rate (PI) on lesion length and run off.

In the older literature long-term results are better for stenoses than for occlusions. For Johnston,[41] the 5-year cumulative clinical success rate was 53% for stenoses with good run off, 31% for stenoses with poor run off, 36% for occlusions with good run off, and 16% for occlusions with poor run off.

The apparently lower long-term clinical success of PTA for femoropopliteal occlusion compared with stenoses was attributable in large part to lower technical success (lesion crossing) and a resultant lower starting point or an otherwise identical life table curve (lower, but parallel).[34]

Once an occlusion is crossed with a guide wire and successfully dilated, it generally exhibits the same expected patency as that of a stenosis of equivalent length if all other factors are equal.[40–42,45–57] This means that occlusion is a confounding variable that lowers the critical technical success but that has no other established impact on long-term patency.

Alback[58] recently reported a 2-year patency rate of 61% in claudicants and 38% in critical ischemia.

Golledge[59] reported a 1-year restenosis rate of 24% when the post-procedural ankle brachial index (ABI) is ≥ 0.9 and 64% when the ABI is < 0.9.

Results of femoropopliteal stenting

Although arterial stenting is well accepted at some locations – iliac, renal, carotid and coronary arteries – it is controversial at the femoropopliteal level. Accepted indications are elastic recoil, extensive dissection, poor cosmetic results, significant post-angioplasty residual stenosis and restenosis. In general, the immediate and early results have been excellent and many cases of angioplasty failures have been converted to early successes. However, restenosis caused by intimal hyperplasia in the stented segment is frequent and may limit stent implantation and stent indications. The first published results with a variety of stents were less than promising because of the high restenosis rate[13,17–19,60–68] and the risk of compression of balloon expandable stents, caused by external trauma or muscle compression within the adductors canal.[65] Can we improve the stent results with the new generation of stents – nitinol self-expandable stents, covered stents?

It seems that the stent design greatly influences the outcome of femoropopliteal stenting and to choose a stent we have to take into account that:

- flexing and elongation of the artery occurs constantly in association with the movements of the leg
- the popliteal artery crosses a joint
- we have a risk of stent fatigue and fracture.

Table 31.1   Results of femoropopliteal PTA

Authors	Number of limbs	Claudicants (%)	Primary patency rate PI (%)		
			1 year	3 years	5 years
Gallino et al.[44] 1984	329	61	62	60	58
Krepel et al.[45] 1985	164	90	68	57	57
Jeans et al.[47] 1990	190	51	50	45	41
Capek et al.[40] 1991	217	74	71	51	48
Johnston et al.[41] 1992	254	80	63	51	38
Huninck et al.[46] 1993	131	58	57	45	45
Matsi et al.[42] 1994	140	100	47	42	–
Murray et al.[43] 1995	44	89	86	53	–

Table 31.2   Primary patency rate (PI) dependence on lesion length and runoff

Authors	Lesion length/ run off	PI (%)	
Depending on the lesion length			
Currie et al.[56] 1994	< 5 cm	59	6 months
	> 5 cm	4	6 months
Murray et al.[43] 1995	< 7 cm	81	6 months
	> 7 cm	23	6 months
Krepel et al.[45] 1985	< 2 cm	77	5 years
	> 2 cm	54	5 years
Jeans et al.[47] 1990	< 1 cm	76	5 years
	> 1 cm	50	5 years
Depending on the runoff			
Gallino et al.[44] 1984	Good run off	71	2 years
	Bad run off	37	2 years
Hunink et al.[54] 1994	Stenosis and good run off	62	5 years
	Occlusion and good run off	48	5 years
	Stenosis and bad run off	43	5 years
	Occlusion and bad run off	27	5 years

Stent types

The properties of an ideal intravascular stent are as follows:

- high radiopacity for clear visualization, which facilitates accurate placement
- high hoop strength to resist arterial recoil
- minimal or no foreshortening in deployment, for precise placement
- simple and easy-to-use delivery system
- longitudinal flexibility to cross tortuous vessels and aortic bifurcation with the contralateral approach
- radial elasticity to resist external compression without permanent deformation, especially at flexion sites
- it should bend in concert with the artery (joint flexion)
- it should respond to flexion and elongation

- it should reduce the risk of stent fatigue and fracture (absence of joints or bonding points)
- high expansion ratio and low profile for passage through small introducers or guiding catheters or through tight stenoses
- retrievability in case of faulty deployment
- side branch accessibility
- minimal induction of intimal hyperplasia
- resistance to thrombosis and corrosion
- durability
- low price.

Unfortunately, no currently available endoprosthesis combines all of the above properties. However, many of these properties can be found in the various stent designs, which can be divided into three main categories:

1   balloon-expandable
2   self-expandable
3   covered.

A brief description of the stents currently available for clinical use is presented.

Balloon-expandable stents

The Strecker stent (Boston Scientific Corp,; Natick, MA). The Strecker stent is made of a tubular wire mesh knitted from a single electropolished tantalum filament. It has a premounted balloon and good radiopacity. The flexibility of this stent is a valuable feature. It is available in diameters from 4 to 12 mm, with lengths of 20, 40, 60, and 80 mm.

The Palmaz stents (Cordis Corporation, a Johnson & Johnson company: Warren, NJ). The classic Palmaz stents are made of rigid stainless steel and can be dilated to various diameters, depending on the size of the balloon chosen for deployment. These stents range from 4 to 9 mm in diameter and from 10 to 39 mm in length. They can be implanted precisely because of their minimal foreshortening and good radiopacity. These characteristics are of particular value for treating lesions situated at or near a bifurcation. The large Palmaz stents have diameters from 8 to 12 mm and lengths up to 30 mm, and they are available for iliac and transhepatic use. In addition, extra-large stents are available for aortic applications.

The newer Palmaz stents (Cordis). The Palmaz-Schatz Long Medium Stent is articulated and is thus more flexible and can be easily implanted using the contralateral approach. Diameters range from 6 to 10 mm and lengths from 41.8 to 77.8 mm. The new Palmaz Corinthian Stent also has improved flexibility. Its short length (12–18 mm) is useful for focal tight lesions in the iliac and femoral arteries. Diameters range from 5 to 8 mm.

The Perflex stent (Cordis). The flexibility of the Perflex stent is important. The diameters vary between 6 and 10 mm and the lengths between 22 and 88 mm.

The Medtronic AVE stents (Medtronic AVE: Santa Rosa, CA). The Medtronic AVE stents comprise both rigid and flexible types, ranging from 5 to 10 mm in diameter and from 20 to 60 mm in length. They combine the minimal foreshortening and good radiopacity of the Palmaz stent and the flexibility of the new nitinol stents, even though they are made of stainless steel.

The MegaLink stent (Guidant France S.A.; Rueil Malmaison, France). The MegaLink stents are stainless steel, flexible stents with satisfactory radial strength and minimum recoil. They are available in diameters of 6–10 mm and in lengths of 18–38 mm.

Other stents are available on the market and are similar to MegaLink or AVE stents.

Self-expandable stents

The Wallstent Endoprosthesis (Boston Scientific). The Wallstent is made of a stainless steel alloy mesh and is soft and flexible along its longitudinal axis. Its radial strength enables a progressive dilation of the artery. The radiopacity of this stent is rather poor. The main disadvantage of this stent is shortening, which makes precise placement difficult. With the new Easy Wallstent, repositioning of the stent is possible even after partial deployment.

Nitinol Stents. Nitinol alloys are known as shape-memory alloys. Nitinol prostheses recover their predetermined diameters at body temperature. They are resistant to arterial wall radial strength; however, most of them are not well suited for use with hard, calcified plaques. The nitinol stents can be divided into different types:

- laser-cut stents (Symphony Nitinol Stent with Radiopaque Markers, Boston Scientific; Optimed Sinustent, Optimed Medizinische Instrumente GmbH, Ettlingen, Germany; Optimed Sinus Flex [formerly Amadeus], Optimed; SMART™ Stent, Cordis; Memotherm™ Nitinol Stent, Bard Peripheral Technologies, Covington, GA; Jomed stent, IntraTherapeutics stent)
- braided stents (Expander™, Bolton Medical)
- coil stents (IntraCoil™, IntraTherapeutics, St. Paul, MN)
- ZA Stent (Cook)

All nitinol stents are not equivalent. Some are very flexible (e.g. IntraCoil, Sinus Flex, Expander, SMART Stent, and ZA Stent) and can be implanted at locations where there is an angulation. Others, such as the Symphony, are more rigid. Some stents may even break when they are bent or placed in a flexion site (e.g. Sinustent and Memotherm).

Covered stents

The Cragg Endopro System 1 and the Passager™ Stent Graft (Boston Scientific). The Cragg/ Passager stent was the first covered stent. Made of nitinol, it is self-expandable, and is covered with an ultrathin 0.1-mm woven polyester fabric (Dacron). The rigidity of the stent and of the delivery system makes contralateral implantation difficult.

The Corvita Endoluminal Graft (Boston Scientific). The two principal characteristics of the Corvita stent are its self-expandable cylindrical wire structure and its highly porous coating of polycarbonate polyurethane. It can be cut with scissors by the user to adapt its length to the length of the lesion.

The Hemobahn™ Endoprosthesis* (W. L. Gore Associates, Inc.; Flagstaff, AZ). The Hemobahn stent is a self-expandable endovascular stent graft. The inner wall surface is composed of ultrathin PTFE graft material; on the exterior is a self-expanding nitinol stent. It is well suited to the contralateral approach.

The Wallgraft™ Endoprosthesis* (Boston Scientific). The Wallgraft stent is a flexible, self-expanding, covered stent made of cobalt and titanium and covered with PET graft material.

The Jostent Coronary Stent Graft (Jomed France SARL, Voisins le Bretonneux, France). The Jostent graft is the only balloon-expandable, covered-tube stent with radial strength. It is composed of stainless steel and ultrathin PTFE graft material.

All these stents are not equivalent: their characteristics are summarized in Tables 31.3 and 31.4.

Stent implantation

The medical literature reveals some inconsistencies in the use of the term 'primary stenting'. The first usage refers to stent placement before predilation of the lesion with balloon angioplasty.[8,69] We prefer the term 'direct stenting' to refer to this procedure. Other authors[25,26,63] use 'primary stenting' to describe procedures in which stents are predetermined to be inserted after balloon predilation, regardless of angioplasty results. We agree with this usage and will apply it accordingly. A third usage[25,26,63] pertains to procedures in which selective stent deployment is performed only after suboptimal angioplasty results. We will refer to this as 'selective stent placement'.

Advantages of direct stenting.

Direct stenting has the advantage of shortening the duration of both the procedure and the radiation exposure. Moreover, direct stenting may decrease the restenosis rate due to diminution of arterial wall damage. It is as yet unknown whether this procedure will be cost-effective in the long term. Some authors[8] have advocated the use of this technique to prevent peripheral embolism when treating occlusions. (In our series of patients with iliac occlusions,[14] however, we did not see an increased rate of peripheral embolism when stents were placed after lesion predilation.) Covered stents can be implanted directly in cases of aneurysm, arterial trauma or rupture, and arteriovenous fistulas.

Advantages of primary stenting.

Generally, stents are implanted after predilation. Primary stenting can be considered for use in some lesions that have a high risk of restenosis (such as eccentric, ulcerated, diffuse, and long lesions), in occlusions, in cases of restenosis, or in specific locations (such as the external iliac artery). This approach facilitates proper stent selection because predilation provides important information about the lesion (soft, fibrous, or calcified plaques), its length, the correct pressure to use for balloon inflation, and the exact diameter of the artery.

Table 31.3 Stent characteristics					
Characteristic	Palmaz BE stents	Wallstent	IntraCoil	Z Stent	Optimed Memotherm™
Flexibility	±	+++	+++	+++	+
Precise placement	+++	−	−	+	++
Radial force	+++	+	+	+	+++
Lengthening	−	−	+++	++	−
Contralateral approach	+	+++	+++	+++	+++

BE = Balloon expandable.

Table 31.4 Stent characteristics				
Characteristic	Expander™	Smart™	Symphony	Covered stents
Flexibility	+++	+++	+	+
Precise placement	++	++	++	++
Radial force	++	++	+++	++
Lengthening	−	−	−	−
Contralateral approach	+++	+++	+	++

Technical notes.

With the direct, primary, or selective technique, the stent should cover the entire lesion. The diameter of the stent must precisely match the size of the vessel. When occlusion makes the exact diameter of the artery difficult to measure, it is helpful to refer to the contralateral site. In cases of direct stenting, the use of a long introducer enables crossing of the lesion; therefore, the stent is placed at the appropriate level while protected by the introducer. After progressive withdrawal of the introducer, the stent is deployed. This avoids problems of stent and balloon progression over the wire in the presence of very tight or severely calcified lesions. Moreover, if they are unprotected, balloon-expandable stents can slide over the balloon, leading to incorrect placement.

In addition to appropriate sizing of the stent, we emphasize gradual and gentle dilation during deployment in order to avoid complications such as adjacent dissection, perforation, or rupture of the arterial wall. Self-expandable nitinol stents take several hours or even days after their deployment to expand fully. By that time, acute in-stent thrombosis may have occurred. For this reason, these stents should be dilated immediately after placement rather than waiting for the stent to expand on its own. Distal embolism and vessel occlusion might be eliminated by continuous blood flow and saline perfusion through the introducer and by appropriate antiplatelet therapy. If this protocol is followed, the procedure may have to be delayed until the full antiplatelet effect is achieved. The guide wire should be placed in the largest distal artery: thus, if the target vessel should become occluded, it would be easier to treat the distal artery.

Results

Classical non-covered stents

Published data. Several studies have been published in the literature on the first stents available and are summarized in the TASC consensus document[34] and in Table 31.5. All these data show large differences in terms of primary patency 22–79% at 1 year). It is difficult to compare all these non-randomized studies. Indications for stenting, lesion length stented, lesion characteristics are different. No conclusion can be drawn from these studies.

Recently, three randomized studies were published showing that femoropopliteal stenting does not improve long-term success compared with PTA alone.

Cejna et al.[71] performed a multicenter randomized trial in which PTA was compared to Palmaz stent implantation in femoropopliteal artery obstruction in 142 patients (154 lesions). Cumulative primary angiographic patency rates for PTA were 79%, 64%, and 53% at 6, 12, and 24 months, respectively. Primary patency rates for stent placement were 86%, 63%, and 58% at 6, 12, and 24 months ,respectively. Thus, despite better short-term and mid-term results, long-term success rates are not better after stenting.

Vroegindeweij et al.[26] studied 51 claudicants with short lesions and good run off. PTA alone (27 lesions) was compared to Palmaz stenting (24 lesions): 1-year patency was 74% vs 62% (NS).

Zdanowski et al.[72] compared 17 PTA vs 15 PTA + Strecker stenting in 32 patients with total occlusion (median lesion length 7 cm): 1-year reocclusion 75% vs 33% and 1-year restenosis 25% vs 50%.

Table 31.5 Classical non-covered stents

Authors	Stent type	Number of limbs	Primary/secondary patency (%)		Follow-up
Rousseau et al.[18] 1989	Wallstent	40	76		1 year
Zollikoper et al.[62] 1991	Wallstent	15	55		1 year
			18		3 years
Do et al.[63] 1992	Wallstent	26	59		1 year
Sapoval et al.[17] 1992	Wallstent	22	49	67	1 year
			49	67	2 years
Liermann et al.[19] 1992	Strecker	48	71		1 year
Martin et al.[61] 1995	Wallstent	96	61	84	1 year
			49	72	2 years
White et al.[66] 1995	Wallstent	32	75		1 year
Bray et al.[67] 1995	Wallstent	57	79		1 year
Bergeron et al.[20] 1995	Palmaz	42	77	89	2 years
Chatelard and Guibourt[70] 1996	Palmaz	35	75.7	83.3	32 months
Strecker et al.[64] 1997	Strecker	80	76		1 year
			48		3 years
Gray et al.[22] 1997	Wallstent	58	22	46	1 year
Damaraju et al.[21] 1997	Wallstent		41		2 years

These three randomized studies do not support femoropopliteal stenting as a primary approach and, along with Recommendation 36 of the TASC Consensus document,[34] stents may have a limited role in salvage of acute PTA failures or complications.

Our experience. The stenting procedure is considered technically successful if the residual stenosis is lower than 30% of the reference diameter at follow-up angiography, and if the mean residual pressure gradient is lower than 5 mmHg without the addition of vasodilators.

The Classical Palmaz Stent[13] (Figures 31.1 and 31.2). A total of 126 patients received 188 stents at the femoropopliteal level. 85 presented with a stenosis and 41 with an occlusion. The mean length of the lesions was 3.8 cm (1–15 cm). Technical success was achieved in 125 patients (99.2%) and with 187 out of 188 stents. One stent did not deploy correctly in a severely calcified lesion of the common femoral artery. This patient required bypass surgery. During the same period, 184 patients received 230 stents in the iliac arteries, with a technical success rate of 100%.

The restenosis rate in the femoropopliteal arteries is given in Table 31.6, and is compared to the restenosis rate obtained for the iliac arteries. This rate increased as we descended to the femoral level. It depended on the lesion type and length, the diameter of the artery, and the number of stents placed.

Primary and secondary patencies at 4 year follow-up were as follows: primary patency at the femoral level was 81% ± 3.5% at 1 year, 73 ± 4.4% at 2 years, 72 ± 5.2% at 3 years, and 65 ± 7.5% at 4 years. At the popliteal level, primary patency was 50 ± 11.2% at 1 year, 50 ± 15.8% at 2 years, 50 ± 17.7% at 3 years, and 50 ± 17.7% at 4 years. In comparison, at the iliac level, it was 94 ± 1.8% at 1 year, 91 ± 2.3% at 2 years, 86 ± 3.3% at 3 years, and 86 ± 4.1% at 4 years. Secondary patency at the femoral level was 96 ± 1.8% at 1 year, 95 ± 2.2% at 2 years, 95 ± 2.6% at 3

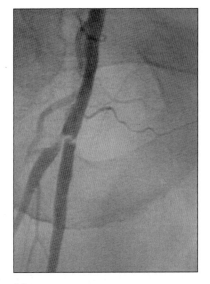

(a)

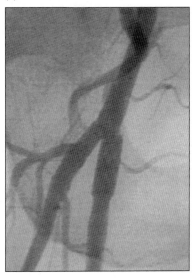

(b)

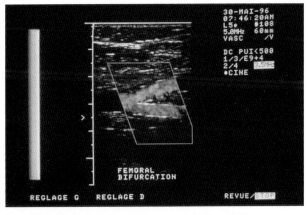

(c)

Figure 31.1

(a) Femoral bifurcation stenoses. (b) Results after placement of Palmaz stents. (c) Duplex scan results.

Table 31.6 Six-month restenosis rates.

Lesion	Percent restenosis	
Location of lesion		
Iliac	0.6	(p < 0.01)
Femoropopliteal	13	(p < 0.01)
Femoral	12	
Upper one-third SFA	4.4	
Mid one-third SFA	9.8	
Lower one-third SFA	18.5	
Popliteal	20	
Type of lesion		
Iliac stenosis	0.6	

SFA = superficial femoral artery.

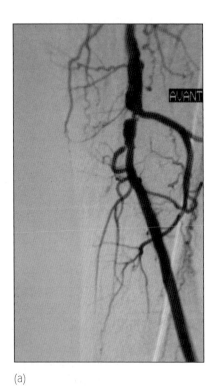
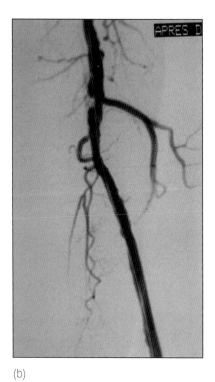
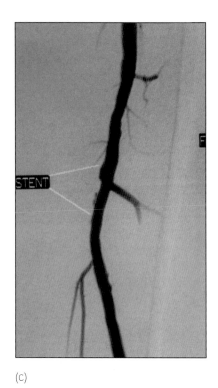

(a)   (b)   (c)

Figure 31.2
(a) Calcified superficial femoral artery stenosis. (b) Results after balloon dilatation. (c) Results after Palmaz stent

Table 31.7 Primary and secondary patencies following the nature and the length of the lesion and the number of stents placed

Type	Primary patency	Secondary patency
Stenoses	80	94
Occlusions	39	86
Lesions < 3 cm	82	94
Lesions > 3 cm	69	87
1 stent	82	93
> 1 stent	70	91

years, and 95 ± 3.5% at 4 years. At the popliteal level, secondary patency was 90 ± 9.5% at 1 year, 80 ± 13.4% at 2 years, 80 ± 13.4% at 3 years, and 69 ± 16% at 4 years. At the iliac level it was 98 ± 1% at 1 year, 96 ± 1.5% at 2 years, 94 ± 2.1% at 3 years, and 94 ± 2.8% at 4 years.

We note that the primary patencies were different for the iliac and femoral arteries (86% vs 65%), whereas the secondary patencies were relatively similar (94% vs 95%).

Table 31.7 indicates primary (PI) and secondary (PII) patencies for the femoropopliteal arteries, depending on the nature of the lesion (stenosis or occlusion), lesion length, and the number of stents placed.

A Palmaz stent also seems a good prosthesis to treat short lesions at the femoral bifurcation and at the ostium of the

profunda. We have treated 26 femoral bifurcations by the contralateral approach with coronary techniques with a 3-year primary patency of 86% and a secondary patency of 94%.

The Long Medium Spiral Stent. In our series, 145 stents were placed in 135 patients for:

- 84 stenoses (iliac, 45; femoropopliteal, 39)
- 51 occlusions (iliac, 22; femoropopliteal, 29).

The secondary patency obtained with the long medium spiral stent is encouraging and similar to that obtained with the other Palmaz stents (Table 31.8).

Table 31.8 Primary and secondary patencies

	At 6 months (%)	At 30 months (%)
Primary patency:		
Global	91.8	87.3
Iliac	98.3	98.3
Femoropopliteal	85.1	77.5
Secondary patency		
Global	96.7	94.5
Iliac	100	100
Femoropopliteal	93.6	90.1

Nitinol stents

Our experience. We have been using nitinol self-expandable stents for several years, but all the stents are not equivalent (see Tables 31.3 and 31.4). We would like to report our experience with two types of nitinol stents.

Sinus Optimed stent[73–76] Figure 31.3a–d: This is a tubular laser-cut stent without welding, with good flexibility, high radial force, no shortening: it is available in diameters from 4 to 12 mm and in lengths 3–8 cm. These stents are implanted through 7F introducers over 0.035-inch guide wire.

A total of 231 lesions were stented, 204 at femoral level (131 stenoses and 73 occlusions, with mean lesion length of 66.2 ± 51.5 mm), 27 at the popliteal level (19 stenoses, and 8 occlusions, with mean lesion length 44.3 ± 27.2 mm). A technical success was obtained in all cases. Three-year primary patency (PI) and secondary patency (PII) rates are as shown in Table 31.9.

With this stent we have obtained a good global long-term patency rate, but better for stenoses than for occlusions. The patency rate depends on the length of the lesions. It is low for occlusions longer than 8 cm. In these cases surgery seems better than the endovascular procedure.

The long-term results at the common femoral artery level (CFA) are excellent: similar to those obtained at the iliac level.

We have observed some fractures of the stent, at Hunter canal level, so it is better to avoid implantation of this stent at this location and, maybe, at all joint locations.

Intracoil Stent[75–78] (Figure 31.4a–c, 31.5a–c)
The IntraCoil Stent is a self-expandable coil stent, a combination of nitinol and coil design, which provides:

- excellent flexibility in all planes
- longitudinal flexibility – elongation without migration
- exceptional conformability
- strong compression resistance

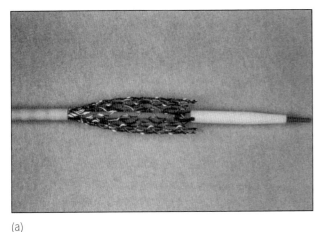

(a)

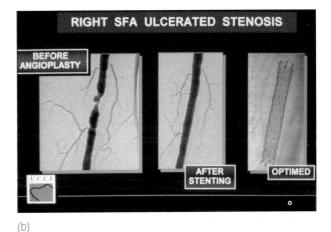

(b)

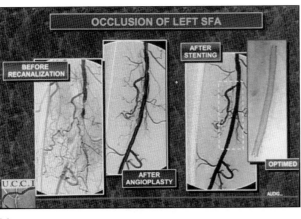

(c)

(d)

Figure 31.3

(a) Optimed Sinus Stent. (b) Treatment of a right (SFA) ulcerated stenosis. (c)Treatment of a left SFA occlusion. (d) Treatment of a calcified common femoral artery stenosis.

Table 31.9   Three-year primary patency (PI) and secondary patency (PII) rates

Femoral	Number of lesions	PI (%)		PII (%)	
All lesions	204	62.1		72.4	
Stenoses	131	69.6	p < 0.004	79.8	p < 0.002
Occlusions	73	49		60.4	
CFA	24	87.9	NS	93.3	NS
Upper one-third	45	48.4	NS	60.9	NS
Mid one-third	81	59.9	p < 0.02	72.7	p < 0.01
Lower one-third	54	65.5	p < 0.02	74.1	p < 0.001
Lesions ≤ 4 cm	94	79.9		86.1	
Stenoses	79	84.4	p < 0.07	94.5	p < 0.06
Occlusions	15	59.2	p < 0.07	55.4	p < 0.06
Lesions ≤ 8 cm	172	66.4	NS	76.9	NS
Stenoses	127	69.8		80.6	
Occlusions	45	55.7		67.2	
Lesions >8 cm	32	36.4	NS	48	NS
Stenoses	4	66.7		66.7	
Occlusions	28	31		45.8	
Popliteal					
All lesions	27	66.1		78.6	
Stenoses	19	67.3		78.4	
Occlusions	8	62.5		81.8	

CFA = common femoral artery.

This stent is ideal for tortuous vessels – vessels susceptible to external compression – and must respond to flexing and elongation. It bends in concert with the artery and reduces the risk of stent fatigue and fractures (absence of joints or bending points).

A total of 140 lesions were treated with this stent: 75 at the femoral level (61 stenoses and 14 occlusions, with mean lesion length of 51.3 ± 29.7 mm), 65 at popliteal and tibioperoneal trunk level (38 stenoses and 27 occlusions, with mean lesion length of 45.1 ± 20.9 mm).

The 5-year primary (PI) and secondary (PII) patency rates are given in Table 31.10.

These long-term patencies are excellent and much better than the patencies published with other stents. The stent design is probably one of the reasons for these very good results. We have also used other nitinol stents at the femoropopliteal level: the SMART stent, the Expander stent, the Symphony, and the new ZA Cook stent. All these stents are not equivalent and we will try to define their specific indications later.

Table 31.0   Five-year primary (PI) and secondary (PII) patency rates

	PI (%)	PII (%)
Femoral	78.4	85.2
Popliteal + tibioperoneal trunk	86.8	95

Other published data. With the IntraCoil stent, good results were recently published by Rosenfield[79] who observed a 9-month freedom-free target lesion revascularization of 85.9% and by Jahnke et al.[80] after treatment of 29 lesions with 40 stents and who has reported a 1-year PI of 81.3% and a PII of 100%.

Starke[81] published a 30-month primary patency of 71% without stent and a 16-month primary patency of 83% with nitinol stent. He also related a large number of mechanical instability deformations and fractures with the Memotherm stent (77%) and with the Optimed Stent (15%).

Covered stents[5,6,82] Figures 31.6, 31.7a and b, 31.8a and b)

Covered stents have also been used at the femoropopliteal level. In 50 femoral artery occlusive lesions, Dake's group[15] used the Hemobahn device and reported a 6-month PI of 83% and a PII of 87%. Diethrich,[83] using a customized PTFE-coated Palmaz device, reported a 9-month PI of 72% and a PII of 84%.

We evaluated the Cragg Endopro/Passager grafts in 92 lesions (29 stenoses, 50 occlusions, and 13 aneurysms). The mean lesion length was 10.2 ± 7.7 cm. The respective PIs and PIIs at 5 years were 65% and 73% at the femoral level, 40% and 50% at the popliteal level, 82% and 93% for lesions less than 10 cm, 51% and 59% for lesions 10 cm or

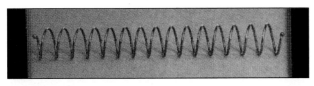

(a)

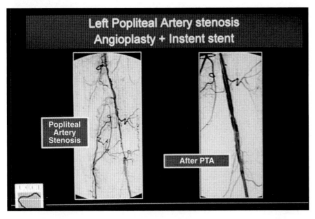

(b)

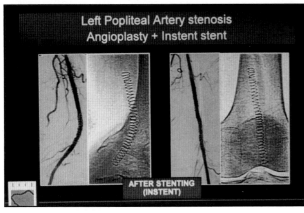

(c)

Figure 31.4
(a) IntraCoil Stent. (b and c) Treatment of a left popliteal artery stenosis.

longer, 63% and 73% for stenoses, and 61% and 72% for occlusions. Although the results are satisfactory in femoral lesions shorter than 10 cm, they are less favorable in longer lesions, particularly in the popliteal artery.

We also treated 25 femoropopliteal lesions with the Corvita covered stent (8 stenoses, 12 occlusions, and 5 aneurysms). The respective PIs and PIIs at 3 years were 55% and 72% overall, 54% and 82% for lesions less than 10 cm, 55% and 64% for longer lesions, 78% and 78% for stenoses, and 31% and 64% for occlusions.

We have started implanting Wallgraft and Jomed stents, but longer series are awaited to analyze the results.

In our experience, covered stents do not yield better results than those achieved with noncovered stents in the treatment of arterial occlusive diseases.

We expected a lower restenosis rate with these stents, but a restenosis can appear not only at the extremities of the stents but also inside the stents; therefore, we suggest that it is preferable, in general, to reserve their use for aneurysms, arterial rupture, and arteriovenous fistulae, as in the iliac vessels. Ideally, covered stents developed in the future will enable the performance of a true endoluminal arterial bypass (as an alternative to surgery) to treat long lesions.

Treatment of bypass stenosis

About 20–30% of bypass vein grafts and synthetic grafts develop graft-threatening stenosis, especially during the first 12 months after surgery.[84–86] If untreated, the stenosis will lead to graft failure. The therapeutics options are percutaneous procedures and reoperation for surgical reconstruction. Several series[87–90] have shown that short focal lesions respond well to angioplasty or to angioplasty and stenting in combination. When angioplasty is insufficient, stents with good radial force may be the best opinion: either balloon-expandable stents (such as Palmaz and Medtronic AVE) or some of the nitinol stents (e.g., Optimed stents and Symphony).

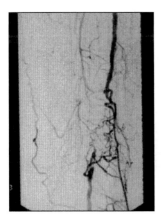

(a)

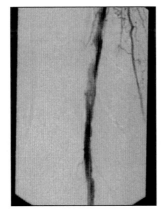

(b)

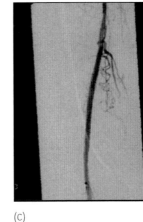

(c)

Figure 31.5
(a) Superficial femoral artery (SFA) occlusion. (b) Result after recanalization and balloon dilatation. (c) Result after IntraCoil Stent.

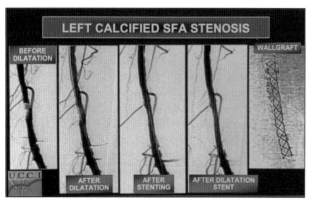

Figure 31.6
Treatment of a left calcified ulcerated superficial femoral artery
(SFA) stenosis with a Wallgraft covered stent.

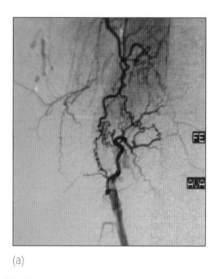

(a)

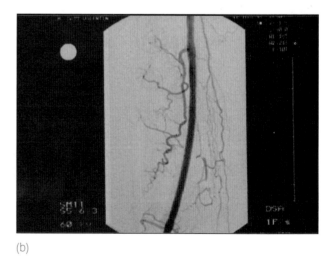

(b)

Figure 31.7
(a) Left superficial femoral artery (SFA) occlusion. (b) Results after recanalization and covered stent (Passager).

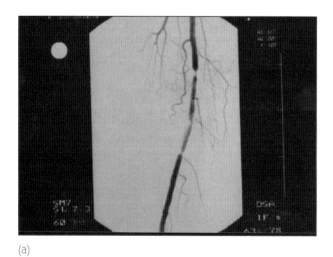

(a)   (b)

Figure 31.8
(a) Superficial femoral artery (SFA) instent restenosis (Palmaz stent). (b) Results after placement of a covered stent (Passager).

Recently, Bandyk[91] summarized the indications for PTA/stenting in cases of vein graft stenosis > 70%:

- time from primary grafting procedure: > 3 months
- vein diameter: > 3.5 mm
- stenosis length: < 2 cm.

The 2-year patency rate was 63% (same as surgery).

Indications for Stenting[75]

The goals of all stents used are the same:

- prevent immediate recoil
- eliminate residual stenoses and post-angioplasty pressure gradient
- give a smooth, regular parietal surface, in order to reduce the restenosis rate and improve long-term patency.

Earlier studies show that following PTA, the risk of restenosis is significantly higher when there is a persistent residual stenosis associated with a pressure gradient.[92,93] Long-term patency is 75% when the arterial lumen is smooth, 66% when it is irregular, 80% in the case of short lesions, and 55% in the case of long lesions.[45,93] Complex lesions (long, irregular, or ulcerated) have poorer results.

As compared with the results of balloon angioplasty, our results show that we can hope to improve long-term patency for patients treated with stents. However all stents are not equivalent: each stent has specific indications. It is important to have access to various stents in a catheterization laboratory in order to implant the one which is the best adapted for specific lesions and locations. Generally speaking, the indications for femoropopliteal stenting do not differ from indications for other localizations. Some of these indications are well accepted:

- post-angioplasty residual stenosis (stenosis greater than 30% at angiography or IVUS or pressure gradient > 5 mmHg)
- undilatable stenosis (elastic or rigid)
- post-angioplasty dissection, resulting in occlusion or serious flow reduction
- restenoses
- poor cosmetic results.

Other indications may be discussed, but the implantation of a stent as a first intention can be considered in the event a lesion is at risk for restenosis or bad outcome (e.g. occlusion, complex lesion, ulcerated lesion, eccentric lesion, etc).

All endoprostheses are not equivalent, and indication for stent implantation also depends on the location of the lesion, its nature, and its morphology. The stent should therefore be chosen depending on the nature of the lesion.

Stent indications

The indications of the main stents used are summarized in Tables 31.11–31.14.

Balloon-expandable stents such as Palmaz and Medtronic AVE stents keep the same specific indications because of their radial force and their very accurate placement. Ostial lesions, short lesions, and fibrous and calcified lesions may be treated with these stents with good results. We have observed compression of balloon-expandable stents in the lower part of the SFA and in the popliteal artery, so we recommend avoiding implantation of the stents at these levels.

We currently tend to prefer nitinol stents, which are flexible, self-expandable, and cannot be compressed: therefore, they may be implanted in any artery. Their radial force seems sufficient at least for some of them to treat fibrous or calcified lesions. But all nitinol stents are not equivalent: e.g. the Sinustent has better radial force than the

Table 31.11 Stent indications

	Palmaz BE stents	Wallstent	IntraCoil	Z stent	Optimed Memotherm
Iliac	+++	+++	+	++	+++
CFA	+	++	++	+++	++
DFA	++	+	+	+	++
SFA					
Ostium	+++	−	−	+	++
one-third >	++	++	+++	+++	+++
mid one-third	+	++	+++	+++	+++
one-third <	−	+	+++	+++	+++
Popliteal	−	+	+++	++	+
Bifurcation	+++	−	+	+	++
Distal leg	+	+	+	−	−
Bypass	+++	++	+	+	+++

BE = Balloon-expandable stents. CFA = common femoral artery. DFA = distal femoral artery. SFA = superficial femoral artery.

Table 31.12   Stent indications

	Expander	SMART	Symphony	Covered stents
Iliac	+++	+++	++	+++
CFA	+++	+++	+	+
DFA	+	++	−	−
SFA				
Ostium	++	++	++	+
one-third >	+++	+++	+++	+++
Mid one-third	+++	+++	+++	+++
one-third <	+++	+++	++	++
Popliteal	++	++	−	+
Bifurcation	++	++	+	−
Distal leg	−	−	−	−
Bypass	+++	+++	+++	++

CFA = common femoral artery, DFA = distal femoral artery, SFA = superficial femoral artery.

Table 31.13   Stent indications

	Palmaz BE stents	Wallstent	IntraCoil	Z Stent	Optimed Memotherm
Tortuous arteries	±	+++	+++	+++	+
Calcifications	+++	+	−	+	+++
Joint	−	+	+++	+++	+
Length > 8 cm	−	+	−	++	+++
Ostium	+++	−	−	+	++
Branches	+	+	+++	+	+

BE = balloon-expandable stents.

Table 31.14   Stent indications

	Expander	SMART	Symphony	Covered stents
Tortuous arteries	++	+++	−	++
Calcifications	++	+	+++	++
Joint	++	++	−	+
Length > 8 cm	+++	+++	+++	+++
Ostium	++	++	++	+
Branches	+	+	++	−

IntraCoil and seems more suitable for use in fibrous or calcified lesions. The Symphony stent also has a good radial force but is more rigid, so is difficult to implant at joint location. The IntraCoil is the most flexible stent, with a lengthening characteristic, and may be the best choice for popliteal use.

We have observed breaking of the Sinustent in the lower part of the SFA and in the popliteal artery. All laser cut stents may have the same problem, so we suggest avoiding these stents at these locations and prefer coil stents or stents that have a good flexibility and a lengthening characteristic.

Thanks to the use of covered stents, true internal bypasses may be performed; they may be an alternative to surgery for the treatment of aneurysms, arteriovenous fistulas, arterial traumas, and ruptures. However treatment of long lesions with these prostheses is still debatable. For the time being, long-term results do not seem superior to those obtained with non-covered stents, particularly the nitinol stent. Restenosis and thrombosis rates are still high. Technical improvements are expected. Their indications in the femoral artery are well accepted, but they are more debatable in the popliteal artery.

Complications of endovascular procedures

Complications of the interventional procedure include the risks of all therapeutic modalities employed: lysis, PTA, stent, anticoagulation, and antiaggregation.

Complications can be classified as major, or minor. Becker et al.[48] reviewed 4662 published PTA procedures. Major complications were observed in 5.6%. In 2.5% surgery was required; limb loss was observed in 0.2% and death in 0.26%. Minor complications were observed in 4.6%. Matsi and Manninen[94] published a complication rate of 10.5%, of which 2% required surgery. Complications are more frequent in limb salvage patients than in claudicators, with a 30-day mortality rate of 10% vs 0.5%.[94] Cardiac and renal comorbidities are frequently found in this group and favored by obesity and diabetes.

For Gardiner et al.[95] the rate of major complications was lower: 3%.

The majority of these complications can now be treated by interventional procedures, with a success rate of 75%.[94]

Thromboembolic vessel occlusions and puncture site injury are the most common complications. Less commonly, complications occur at the PTA site itself, including thrombosis, dissection, perforation, and occlusion.

The use of thrombolytic drugs, mechanical thrombectomy devices, stents, and covered stents for perforation decrease morbidity for these procedures and avoid the need for surgery in most cases.

The risk of puncture site complications (e.g. hematomas, bleeding, pseudoaneurysms) is decreasing with the use of puncture site closure devices.

With stenting procedures, the thrombosis rate was high in the first published data;[17–19] with antiaggregant drugs (ticlopidine, clopidogrel) this risk seems low.

The future

Restenosis remains a major problem after PTA, with or without stent implantation at the femoropopliteal level. Several therapies or techniques have been proposed to improve the results:

- platelet receptor antagonists
- antithrombotic agents
- lipid-lowering therapy
- gene therapy
- photodynamic therapy
- smooth muscle cell inhibitors
- sonotherapy.

Two further techniques are now discussed.

Brachytherapy

Minar,[96] in a randomized study of 113 patients with long–segment femoropopliteal lesions (> 15 cm) treated either by PTA alone or by PTA + brachytherapy (the gamma-ray emitter iridium-192 or ^{192}Ir), published a 6-month restenosis rate of 28.3% after brachytherapy and 53.7% after placebo ($p < 0.005$) and a 12-month patency of 63.6% after brachytherapy and 35.3% after placebo ($p < 0.005$).

Pötter[97] published a 6-month restenosis rate of 30% after brachytherapy; after PTA + stenting, the expected restenosis rate being 70%.

Waskman et al.,[98] after treatment of 35 patients presenting with femoropopliteal lesions (mean lesion length 9.8 ± 3 cm) with an ^{192}Ir source, noticed an angiographic 6-month restenosis rate of 17.2% and a clinical 12-month restenosis rate of 13.3%.

Brachytherapy seems promising and may be a way, in the future, to limit intimal proliferation, but there may be an unfavorable interaction between radiation and freshly implanted stents. Stent endothelialization is inhibited with a risk of late thrombosis, which necessitates prolonged antiplatelet therapy (> 6 months): Terstein.[99]

Coated stents

The aim of coated stents is to reduce intimal hyperplasia and prevent thrombus formation. Heparin, hirudine, and iloprost have been proposed but paclitaxel and rapamycin seem the most efficient drugs and have shown excellent results at the coronary level.

Conclusions

Femoropopliteal diseases are often not life threatening, but claudication can be life altering. Conservative treatment and surgery have to be reconsidered.

PTA is a simple procedure that is safe and effective, with low risks even in elderly patients, and should be proposed as a first treatment.

Restenosis remains the main problem. Stents may improve long-term patency but all stents are not equivalent and we have specific stent indications depending on location and lesion characteristics, for example.

The stent chosen must have significant flexibility and resistance to external compression, longitudinal lengthening/shortening, as well as torsion/flexion forces. It must also be resistant to thrombosis and neointimal proliferation.

The treatment of biological and mechanical components of the restenosis has to be considered. Brachytherapy and drug-eluting stents will probably play a role in the near future to improve long-term patency, so that these techniques could be in competition with surgery, even for long and complex lesions.

References

1 Veith FJ, Gupta SK, Ascer E et al. Six year prospective multicenter randomized comparison of autologous saphenous vein and expanded PTFE grafts in infrainguinal arterial reconstructions. *J Vasc Surg* 1986; **3**: 104–14.

2 Dotter CT, Judkins MP. Transluminal treatment of arteriosclerotic obstruction. Description of a new technique and a preliminary report of its application. *Circulation* 1964; **30**: 654–70.

3 Grüntzig A, Hopff H. Percutaneous recanalization after chronic arterial occlusion with a new dilator–catheter [in German]. *Dtsch Med Wochenschr* 1974; **99**: 2502–11.

4 Beyar R, Henry M, Shofti R et al. Self-expandable Nitinol stent for cardiovascular applications: canine and human experience. *Cathet Cardiovasc Diagn* 1994; **32**: 162–70.

5 Henry M, Amor M, Cragg A et al. Occlusive and aneurysmal peripheral arterial disease: assessment of a stent–graft system. *Radiology* 1996; **201**: 717–24.

6 Henry M, Amor M, Henry I et al. Application of a new covered endoprothesis in the treatment of occlusive and aneurysmal peripheral arterial disease: [in French]. *Arch Mal Cœur Vaiss* 1997; **90**: 953–60.

7 Strecker EP, Hagen B, Liermann D et al. Iliac and femoropopliteal vascular occlusive disease treated with flexible tantalum stents. *Cardiovasc Intervent Radiol* 1993; **16**: 158–64.

8 Vorwerk D, Guenther RW, Schurmann K et al. Primary stent placement for chronic iliac artery occlusions: follow-up results in 103 patients. *Radiology* 1995; **194**: 745–9.

9 Bosch JL, Hunink MG. Meta-analysis of the results of percutaneous transluminal angioplasty and stent placement for aortoiliac occlusive disease. *Radiology* 1997; **204**: 87-96.

10 Tetteroo E, Van der Graaf Y, Bosch JL et al. Randomized comparison of primary stent placement versus primary angioplasty followed by selective stent placement in patients with iliac artery occlusive disease. Dutch Iliac Stent Trial Study Group. *Lancet* 1998; **351**: 1153–9.

11 Vorwerk D, Guenther RW, Schurmann K et al. Aortic and iliac stenoses: follow-up results of stent placement after insufficient balloon angioplasty in 118 cases. *Radiology* 1996; **198**: 45–8.

12 Palmaz JC, Laborde JC, Rivera FJ et al. Stenting of the iliac arteries with the Palmaz stent: experience from a multicenter trial. *Cardiovasc Intervent Radiol* 1992; **15**: 291–7.

13 Henry M, Amor M, Ethevenot G et al. Palmaz stent placement in iliac and femoropopliteal arteries: primary and secondary patency in 310 patients with 2–4 year follow-up. *Radiology* 1995; **197**: 167-74.

14 Henry M, Amor M, Ethevenot G et al. Percutaneous endoluminal treatment of iliac occlusions: long-term follow-up in 105 patients. *J Endovasc Surg* 1998; **5**: 228–35.

15 Dake MD, Semba CP, Kee ST et al. Early results of Hemobahn for the treatment of peripheral arterial disease. In: *Ninth International Course Book of Peripheral Vascular Intervention. Endovascular Therapy Course* May 5–8, 1998; Paris, France. Toulouse: Europa Organisation, 1998: 259–60.

16 Ohki T, Veith FJ. Endovascular grafts for the treatment of arterial lesions. In: *Ninth International Course Book of Peripheral Vascular Intervention. Endovascular Therapy Course* May 5–8, 1998; Paris, France. Toulouse: Europa Organisation, 1998: 269–82.

17 Sapoval MR, Long AL, Raynaud AC et al. Femoropopliteal stent placement: long-term results. *Radiology* 1992; **184**: 833–9.

18 Rousseau HP, Raillat CR, Joffre FG et al. Treatment of femoropopliteal stenoses by means of self-expandable endoprostheses: midterm results. *Radiology* 1989; **172**(3 Pt 2): 961–4.

19 Liermann D, Strecker EP, Peters J. The Strecker stent: indications and results in iliac and femoropopliteal arteries. *Cardiovasc Intervent Radiol* 1992; **15**: 298–305.

20 Bergeron P, Pinot JJ, Poyen V et al. Long-term results with the Palmaz stent in the superficial femoral artery. *J Endovasc Surg* 1995; **2**: 161–7.

21 Damaraju S, Cuasay L, Le D et al. Predictors of primary patency failure in Wallstent self-expanding endovascular prostheses for iliofemoral occlusive disease. *Tex Heart Inst J* 1997; **24**: 173–8.

22 Gray BH, Sullivan TM, Childs MB et al. High incidence of restenosis/reocclusion of stents in the percutaneous treatment of long-segment superficial femoral artery disease after suboptimal angioplasty. *J Vasc Surg* 1997; **25**: 74–83.

23 Cikrit DF, Dalsing MC. Lower-extremity arterial endovascular stenting. *Surg Clin North Am* 1998; **78**: 617-29.

24 Criado FJ. Endovascular treatment of occlusive lesions in the femoropopliteal territory. In: Criado FJ, (ed.), *Endovascular intervention: basic concepts and techniques*. Armonk, NY: Futura Publishing Company, 1999: 105–14.

25 Cejna M, Schoder M, Lammer J. PTA vs. stent in femoropopliteal obstruction [in German]. *Radiologe* 1999; **39**: 144–50.

26 Vroegindeweij D, Vos LD, Tielbeek AV et al. Balloon angioplasty combined with primary stenting versus balloon angioplasty alone in femoropopliteal obstructions: a comparative randomized study. *Cardiovasc Intervent Radiol* 1997; **20**: 420–5.

27 Weitz JL, Byrne J, Clagett GP et al. Diagnosis and treatment of chronic arterial insufficiency of the lower extremities: a critical review. *Circulation* 1996; **94**: 3026–49.

28 Smith GD, Shipley MJ, Rose G. Intermittent claudication, heart disease risk factors, and mortality: The Whitehall study. *Circulation* 1990; **82**: 1925–31.

29 Newman AB, Siscovick DS, Manolio TA et al. Ankle/arm index as a marker of atherosclerosis in the cardiovascular health study. *Circulation* 1993; **88**: 837–45.

30 Ernst E, Fialka V. A review of the clinical effectiveness of exercise therapy for intermittent claudication: indications, methods and results. *Surgery* 1978; **84**: 640–3.

31 Ekroth R, Dahllof AG, Gundevall B et al. Value of a supervised exercise program for the therapy of arterial claudication. *J Vasc Surg* 1997; **25**: 312–19.

32 Dawson DL, Cutler BS, Meissner MH et al. Cilostazol has beneficial effects in treatment of intermittent claudication. *Circulation* 1998; **98**: 678–86.

33 Ansel GM. Endovascular treatment of superficial femoral and popliteal arterial occlusive disease. *J Invas Cardiol* 2000; **12**: 382–8.

34 TASC. Management of peripheral arterial disease. Trans Atlantic Inter Society Consensus. *Int Angiol* 2000; **19**(Suppl 1): 1–304.

35 Criqui MH, Langer RD, Fronek A et al . Mortality over a period of 10 years in patients with peripheral arterial disease. *N Engl J Med* 1992; **326**: 381–6.

36 Criqui MH, Fronek A, Klauber MR et al. The sensitivity, specificity, and predictive value of traditional clinical evaluation of peripheral arterial disease: results from non-invasive testing in a defined population. *Circulation* 1985; **71**: 516–22.

37 Vogt MT, Cauley JA, Newman AB et al. Decreased ankle/arm blood pressure index and mortality in elderly women. *JAMA* 1993; **270**: 465–9.

38 Newman AB, Sutton-Tyrrell K, Vogt MT et al. Morbidity and mortality in hypertensive adults with a low ankle/arm blood pressure index. *JAMA* 1993; **270**: 487–9.

39 Applegate WB. Ankle/arm blood pressure index: a useful test for clinical practice? *JAMA* 1993; **270**; 497–8.

40 Capek P, McLean GK, Berkowitz HD. Femoropopliteal angioplasty. Factors influencing long-term success. *Circulation* 1991; **83**: I-70–I-80.

41 Johnston KW. Femoral and poplital arteries: reanalysis of results of balloon angioplasty. *Radiology* 1992; **183**: 767–71.

42 Matsi PJ, Manninen HI, Vanninen RL et al. Femoropopliteal angioplasty in patients with claudication: primary and secondary patency in 140 limbs with 1–3 year follow-up. *Radiology* 1994; **191**: 727–33.

43 Murray JG, Apthorp LA, Wilkins RA. Long segment (> 10 cm) femoropopliteal angioplasty: improved technical success and long-term patency. *Radiology* 1995; **195**: 158–62.

44 Gallino A, Mahler F, Probst P et al. Percutaneous transluminal angioplasty of the arteries of the lower limbs: a 5 year follow-up. *Circulation* 1984; **70**(4): 619–23.

45 Krepel VM, Van Andel GJ, Van Erp WF et al. Percutaneous transluminal angioplasty of the femoropopliteal artery: initial and long term results. *Radiology* 1985; **156** (2): 325–8.

46 Hunink MG, Donaldson MC, Meyerovitz MF et al. Risks and benefits of femoropopliteal percutaneous balloon angioplasty. *J Vasc Surg* 1993; **17**(1): 183–92.

47 Jeans WD, Armstrong S, Cole SE et al. Fate of patients undergoing transluminal angioplasty for lower limbs ischemia. *Radiology* 1990; **177**: 559–64.

48 Becker GJ, Katzen BT, Dake MD. Noncoronary angioplasty. *Radiology* 1989; **170**: 921–40.

49 Vogelzang RL. Long term results of angioplasty. *J Vasc Interv Radiol* 1996; **7**(Suppl):179.

50 Adar R, Critchfield GC, Eddy DM. A confidence profile analysis of the results of fempop percutaneous transluminal angioplasty in the treatment of lower extremity ischemia. *J Vasc Surg* 1989; **10**: 57–67.

51 Yucel EK. Femoropopliteal angioplasty: Can we predict success with duplex sonography? *ARJ* 1994; **162**: 184–6.

52 Mewissen MW, Kinney EV, Bandyk DF et al. The role of duplex scanning versus angiography in predicting outcome after balloon angioplasty in the femoropopliteal artery. *J Vasc Surg* 1992; **15**: 860–6.

53 Sacks D, Robinson ML, Summers TA et al. The value of duplex sonography after peripheral artery angioplasty in predicting subacute restenosis. *ARJ* 1994; **162**: 179–83.

54 Hunink MG, Wong JB, Donaldson MC et al. Patency results of percutaneous and surgical revascularizations for femoro-popliteal arterial disease. *Med Decis Making* 1994; **14**: 71–81.

55 Jeans WD, Cole SF, Horrocks M et al. Angioplasty gives good results in critical lower limb ischemia: a 5 year follow-up in patients with known ankle pressure and diabetic status having femoropopliteal dilatations. *Br J Radiol* 1994; **67**: 123–8.

56 Currie IC, Wakeley CJ, Cole SE et al. Femoropopliteal angioplasty for severe limb ischemia. *Br J Surg* 1994; **81**: 191–3.

57 Wilson SE, Wolf GL, Cross AP et al. Percutaneous transluminal angioplasty versus operation for peripheral arteriosclerosis: report of a prospective randomized trial in a selected group of patients. *J Vasc Surg* 1989; **9**: 1–9.

58 Alback A. Hemodynamic results of femoropopliteal percutaneous transluminal angioplasty. *Eur J Vasc Endovasc Surg* 1998; **16**: 7–12.

59 Golledge J. Outcome of femoropopliteal angioplasty. *Ann Surg* 1999; **229**: 146–53.

60 Henry M, Amor M, Henry I et al. Femoropopliteal stenting results, indications: choice of the stent. *Radiology* 1999; **213**: 50.

61 Martin EC, Katzen BT, Benenati JF et al. Multicenter trial of the Wallstent in iliac and femoral arteries. *JVIR* 1995; **6**: 843–9.

62 Zollikofer CL, Antonucci F, Pfyffer M et al. Arterial stent placement with use of the Wallstent: midterm results of clinical experience. *Radiology* 1991; **179**: 449–56.

63 Do-dai-Do, Triller J, Walpoth BH et al. A comparison study of self-expendable stents vs balloon angioplasty alone in femoropopliteal artery occlusions. *Cardiovasc Intervent Radiol* 1992; **15**: 306–12.

64 Strecker EP, Boos IB, Gottmann D. Femoropopliteal artery stent placement: evaluation of long-term success. *Radiology* 1997; **205**(2): 375–83.

65 Rosenfield K, Schainfeld R, Pieczek A et al. Restenosis of endovascular stents from stent compression. *J Am Coll Cardiol* 1997; **29**: 328–38.

66 White GH, Liew SC, Waugh RC et al. Early outcome and intermediate follow-up of vascular stents in femoral and popliteal arteries without long-term angiocoagulation. *J Vasc Surg* 1995; **21**(2): 270–9.

67 Bray AE, Liu WG, Lewis WA et al. Strecker Stents in the femoropopliteal arteries: value of duplex ultrasonography in restenosis assessment. *J Endovasc Surg* 1995; **2**(2): 150–60.

68 Gray BH, Olin JW. Limitations of percutaneous transluminal angioplasty with stenting for femoropopliteal arterial occlusive disease. *Semin Vasc Surg* 1997; **10**(1): 8–16.

69 Doros G, Jaff M, Jain A et al. Follow-up of primary Palmaz–Schatz stent placement for atherosclerotic renal artery stenosis. *Am J Cardiol* 1995; **75**: 1051–5.

70 Chatelard P, Guibourt C. Long-term results with a Palmaz stent in the femoropopliteal arteries. *J Cardiovasc Surg* 1996; **37**: 67–72.

71 Cejna M, Thurnher S, Illiasch H et al. PTA versus Palmaz Stent placement in femoropopliteal artery obstructions: a multicenter prospective randomized study. *J Vasc Interv Radiol* 2001; **12**: 23–31.

72 Zdanowsky Z, Albrechtsson U, Lundin A et al. Percutaneous transluminal angioplasty with or without stenting for femorpopliteal occlusions? A randomized controlled study. *Int Angiol* 1999; **18**: 251–5.

73 Henry M, Henry I, Tzvetanov K et al. Angioplasty and stenting with the optimal sinius stent in peripheral arterial occlusion diseases: long-term follow-up. *Am J Cardiol* 2000; TCT 190–76Ii.

74 Henry I, Henry M, Tzvetanov K et al. Influence of lesion characteristics in long-term results after peripheral artery stenting. *Am J Cardiol* 2000; TCT 74,31i.

75 Henry M, Klonaris C, Amor M et al. Which stent for which lesion in peripheral interventions? *Tesc Heart Invest J* 2000; **27**: 119–26.

76 Henry M, Amor M, Berger R et al. Clinical experience with a new Nitinol self-expanding stent in peripheral arteries. *J Endovasc Surg* 1996; **3**: 369–79.

77 Beyar R, Henry M, Schofti R et al. Self expandable nitinol stent for cardiovascular applications: canine and human experience. *Cath Cardiovasc Diagn* 1994; **32**: 162–70.

78 Henry M, Amor M, Beyar R et al. Clinical experience with the instent nitinol self-expanding stent. In: Henry M, Amor M (eds), *Tenth International Course Book of Peripheral Vascular Intervention* Toulouse: Europa Edition, 1999: 193–204.

79 Rossenfield K, Intra Coil trial, current results. ISET Meeting, Miami, January 21–25, 2001.

80 Jahnke T, Brossmann J, Voshage G et al. Endovascular placement of a new self-expanding Nitinol Coil stent (Intra coil™) for the treatment of femoropopliteal occlusive disease [Abstract]. *JVIR* 2001; **12**(Suppl S1–S195): S50.

81 Stark E. Femoropopliteal occlusive diseases. *J Interv Cardiol* 1999; **12**: 505–12.

82 Henry M, Amor M, Henry I et al. Role of covered stents in peripheral arterial diseases. *Tenth International Course Book of Peripheral Vascular Intervention. Endovascular Therapy Course,* May 18–21, 1999, Paris, France. Toulouse: Europa Organisation, 1999: 229–46.

83 Diethrich EB. Endoluminal graft delivery system for femoropopliteal arterial occlusive disease. In: *Ninth International Course Book of Peripheral Vascular Intervention. Endovascular Therapy Course,* May 5–8, 1998, Paris, France. Toulouse: Europa Organisation, 1998: 283–94.

84 Mills JL, Fujitani RM, Taylor SM. The characteristics and anatomic distribution of lesions that cause reversed vein graft failure: a five-year prospective study. *J Vasc Surg* 1993; **17**: 195–206.

85 Grigg MJ, Nicolaides AN, Wolfe JH. Detection and grading of femorodistal vein graft stenoses: duplex velocity measurements compared with angiography. *J Vasc Surg* 1988; **8**: 661–6.

86 Berkowitz HD, Hobbs CL, Roberts B et al. Value of routine vascular laboratory studies to identify vein graft stenosis. *Surgery* 1981; **90**: 971–9.

87 Tonnesen KH, Holstein P, Rordam L et al. Early results of percutaneous transluminal angioplasty (PTA) of failing below-knee bypass grafts. *Eur J Vasc Endovasc Surg* 1998; **15**: 51–6.

88 Avino AJ, Bandyk DF, Gonsalves AJ et al. Surgical and endovascular intervention for infrainguinal vein graft stenosis. *J Vasc Surg* 1999; **29**: 60–71.

89 Sanchez LA, Suggs WD, Marin MI et al. Is percutaneous balloon angioplasty appropriate in the treatment of graft and anastomotic lesions responsible for failing vein bypasses? *Am J Surg* 1994; **168**: 97–101.

90 Houghton AD, Todd C, Pardy B et al. Percutaneous angioplasty for infrainguinal graft-related stenoses. *Eur J Vasc Endovasc Surg* 1997; **14**: 380–5.

91 Bandyk DF. Treatment of vein graft stenoses. ISET Meeting, Miami, January 21–25, 2001.

92 Colapinto AF. Long term results of iliac and femoropopliteal angioplasty. In: Dotter CT, Grundig A, School W, Zeitler E (eds), *Percutaneous transluminal angioplasty.* Berlin: Springer-Verlag, 1983: 202–6.

93 Van Andel GJ, VanErp WFM, Krepel VM et al. Percutaneous transluminal dilatation of the iliac artery: long term results. *Radiology* 1985; **156**: 321–3.

94 Matsi PJ, Manninen HI. Complications of lower-limb percutaneous transluminal angioplasty: a prospective analysis of 410 procedures on 295 consecutive patients. *Cardiovasc Int Radiol* 1998; **21**: 361–6.

95 Gardiner GA Jr, Meyerovitz MF, Stokes KR et al. Complications of transluminal angioplasty. *Radiology* 1986; **159**: 201–208

96 Minar E, Pokrajac B, Maca T et al. Endovascular brachytherapy for prophylaxis of restenosis after femoropopliteal angioplasty. *Circulation* 2000; **102**: 2694–9.

97 Pötter R. SFA Brachytherapy. The Vienna Experience [abstract] Radiation Therapy V Syllabus, Washington, 5–7 February, Washington, 2001.

98 Waksmann R, Laird JR, Jurkovitz CT. Intravascular radiation therapy following balloon angioplasty of narrowed femoral. Popliteal arteries to prevent restenosis: results of the PARIS feasibility clinical trial [abstract]. Radiation therapy V Syllabus, 5–7 February, Washington, 2001.

99 Terstein P. Fullfilling the promise of percutaneous angioplasty. *Circulation* 2000; **102**: 2674–6.

32

Infragenicular percutaneous transluminal angioplasty

Emilio Calabrese

Introduction

The efficacy of dorsalis pedis, tibialis posterior and even plantar artery bypass in limb salvage, has been repeatedly demonstrated by Lo Gerfo, Veith, Gupta and several other surgeons, showing a high long-term patency rate and a significant improvement in the clinical status of the limb.[1,2] While they are certainly the standard of care for long infragenicular arterial obstructions, distal bypasses are long and technically demanding procedures which require the availability of a suitable long vein and a reasonable minimal distance between the surgical field of the distal anastomosis and the gangrenous or infected area.

Patients with severe cardiac disease and deteriorated general conditions may sometimes be poor candidates for lengthy surgery, even if performed with sophisticated anesthesia and attentive monitoring. Several diabetic patients have extensively infected feet, which do not respond to local and antibiotic treatment unless a proper blood supply is provided. This subset of patients with no suitable veins available, with extensive infection in proximity of a planned distal anastomosis and with expected poor tolerance for long surgery, is an ideal candidate group for alternative minimally invasive procedures, provided that a reasonable limb salvage rate is attainable with these techniques (Table 32.1).

In the early 1990s, a few centers around the world started performing infragenicular percutaneous transluminal angioplasty (PTA) with some encouraging results. The crudeness of the earlier available tools had limited the reach and efficacy of the technique, and during the 1980s, infrapopliteal PTA was performed with boogies and tapered catheters.[3] It is assumed that unreported failures must have been widespread: the procedure did not gain favor for several years, until the application of delicate coronary PTA instrumentation to the lower limbs rendered distal PTA a less traumatic procedure.

Table 32.1 Indications for infragenicular PTA
• No suitable vein available for bypass • Severe infection near the sites of planned anastomosis • Poor general conditions and high surgical risk • Short lesions • Patient's refusal of surgery • Previously failed bypass • Unavailability of highly skilled surgeon

Sivananthan et al, from Leeds in England, reported a technical success rate of 96% when performing tibial artery angioplasty and a clinical improvement rate of 58%. They observed the improvement of ankle-brachial index in 52% of the treated limbs and improvement in the isotope flow studies in 43% of the limbs. Angiograms were not used to assess patency, except in those few cases where PTA failed. The authors correctly pointed out the need to relieve the arterial spasm that occurs during below the knee angioplasty.[4]

Treiman et al, from Los Angeles, in a joint study performed by surgeons and radiologists, observed early recurrence of previously dilated stenosis as the main cause for early failure, and deemed the clinical results from the procedures unsatisfactory.[5] Their angiographic observation of locally recurrent stenosis formed the foundation for later studies at the National Center for Limb Salvage, based on the insertion of tiny stents in the treatment of short occlusions and difficult stenosis.

Appropriate medical treatment was also an issue and, while Treiman could not observe any benefit from the use of dipiridamole + aspirin, Bull et al[6] emphasized the use of sodium warfarin: the drug was not to be recommended (neither in more recent studies nor in our experience). Bull also noticed a very poor success rate in angioplasty of completely occluded tibial segments.[6] Lofberg et al,[7] reported a Swedish study from Uppsala on 94 infragenicular procedures performed on 82 patients, 90% of whom were in Fontaine IV, between 1989 and 1993. In this series, 196 PTAs were performed, involving either the infragenicular vessels only or both the infragenicular and femoral vessels. Seventy-one of the procedures were performed for complete occlusion (none longer than 5 cm below the knee and none longer than 10 cm above the knee). Patients were followed up at 6, 12, 24 and 36 months post PTA: the primary clinical success rate was 55%, 51%, 36% and 36%, respectively. The cumulative secondary clinical success rate was 44%, while limb salvage was 72% at 36 months. Clinical success was defined as a subjective improvement of symptoms and possibly an associated increase of ankle-brachial index of 0.10, based on the old reporting standards of the Society of Vascular Surgery – International Society of Cardiovascular Surgery (SVS-ISCVS), published in 1986. The presence of diabetes, preop ankle brachial pressure index (ABPI) <0.2 and the type of lesion (occlusion versus stenosis) did not affect long-term results.

Performance of a surgical bypass, major amputation or death were considered endpoints in this study. Of the 82 patients, one patient had immediate bypass for acute ischemia post PTA; 13 patients had elective bypass because of PTA occlusion at a mean 7.2 months post PTA; 20 patients underwent amputation at a mean 4.7 months after reocclusion of PTA. Of the remaining patients, 15 died during the follow-up (mean 10.8 months – range 1–40 months). The remaining 34 patients were followed for mean 16.2 months (range 1–60 months). Eventually, 34 out of the 82 patients (41%) were alive and had retained their limbs at a mean 16.2 months follow-up. The data from the Lofberg study pointed out both the efficacy of infragenicular procedures for limb salvage and the high mortality associated with severe peripheral vascular disease.[7]

ABPI, Doppler analysis and clinical observation may be inaccurate in determining patency rates for the procedure, and the only certain determining factor of clinical success is having been able to save a limb in a patient who is still alive.

Brown et al, while reporting enthusiastic results on infragenicular PTA, observed dismal failure rates when PTA was associated with surgical bypass.[8] In our series, when distal angioplasty was performed after bypass, results were excellent whenever stenting was used to support PTA of distal anastomoses or to warrant long-term patency of stenosed runoff arteries.

Veith et al supported the use of distal PTA in combination with bypass and confirmed the higher mortality of bypass (3.3% in their series) when compared with PTA.[9]

Fraser et al, in 1996, and Bakal et al reviewed the literature on infragenicular PTA, observing how accurate selection of patients for PTA improved results. They also noticed that clinical results and limb salvage after PTA were higher than the patency rate, while in surgical bypasses patency always exceeded limb salvage rate. Bakal specifically emphasized the need for the achievement of a so called 'straight-line flow' to the foot to achieve a good outcome. We were unable to reproduce Bakal's findings in our studies and, in fact, we observed that straight-line flow to the foot is not a requirement to achieve long-term patency and limb salvage, especially when stenting is utilized. We did notice that the status of distal runoff vessels is much less critical after infragenicular PTA than after surgical bypass in maintaining long-term patency. Fraser observed that diabetic patients fared slightly worse than non-diabetic ones. Establishing limb salvage as a main goal instead of hemodynamic patency gave a significant push to the popularity infragenicular PTA, because it was repeatedly noticed that healed ischemic lesions do not often recur even if the dilated vessel restenoses with time.[11]

Boyer et al from France, carried out a retrospective study on 49 patients who underwent 71 infrapopliteal PTAs. Immediate technical success was achieved in 91%, but two of the four failures required major amputation. Operative mortality was 2% and morbidity 16%. They reported an exceptional three-year limb salvage of 87% and a primary patency rate of 81% determined by duplex ultrasound.[12]

Söder et al, from Finland, had a realistic 48% primary patency, 56% secondary patency and 80% cumulative limb salvage at 18 months. Lack of angiographic improvement at the site of ischemia, as well as renal insufficiency, were determined as major factors in poor long-term outcome, a finding that we, too, observed in our series.[13]

In 2001, Dorros and Jaff published a five-year follow-up of 284 ischemic limbs in *Circulation*. They had an immediate technical success in 95% of cases, and, in addition to the infragenicular vessel angioplasty, they had to perform a proximal PTA in 59% of limbs. At follow-up, bypass surgery was performed on 8% of the studied limbs, major amputation in 9% and 91% of them were eventually salvaged. Their Fontaine IV patients had a 5-year survival of 33%, compared to the 58% of Fontaine III and 56% of the whole series (most cases were in Fontaine class III). Their results point out the efficacy of infragenicular PTA, but also the need of attentive follow-up and general medical work-up to improve a dismal survival rate. Careful aggressive studies and treatment of associated coronary disease, renal artery and cerebrovascular disease may significantly improve survival, when performed as indicated.[14]

Graziani and his collaborators in Italy, have performed a large number of infragenicular PTAs with success, and having cooperated with internists, diabetes specialists and surgeons, achieved encouraging rates of limb salvage at a 14-month follow-up.[15]

Nasr et al observed how, in their series, PTA had progressively replaced surgery, obtaining a limb salvage rate of 85% at 5 years, but still observing a high patient mortality of 55% in the same time period.[16]

At the National Center for Limb Salvage in Novara, while simple PTA provided a high limb salvage rate in the short term, long-term angiographic patency remained low, and gangrenous lesions reoccurred in the long term. Recurrency of ischemic lesions greatly improved with the use of stents in those patients who had complete occlusions. In a prospective study of 43 consecutive patients with infrapopliteal stenting, 55% were alive, with patent stented vessels and with markedly improved limb status, after a mean follow-up of 24 months.

Techniques

Four different yet interlacing techniques are available for below the knee PTA:

Transluminal simple PTA

The patient is properly prepared with ticlopidine 250 mg bid starting at least 3 days prior to the procedure, plus coated aspirin 160 mg qd. A complete selective diagnostic angiogram is performed. Under road-mapping, the omolateral common femoral artery or the superficial femoral artery is punctured in-current, and a 4F introducer is inserted. Heparin (5000 IU) is given. Accurate magnified diagnostic angiograms are repeated in-current through this access. Stenosis are crossed with a 0014 coronary straight high support guide (SciMed's Choice Pt grafix), and are dilated with either short coronary balloons or longer, low profile peripheral balloons (Invatec's Submarine, Abbott/Jomed's Opera, BS' Bijoux, Cordis' Savvy, Guidant's Viatrak). Overstretching and excessive balloon diameters are avoided. The balloons are inflated at 6–14 atm. When using coronary balloons, dilatation up to 24 atm may help win resistant calcific lesions, and the most recalcitrant stenosis may require a low-pressure cutting balloon. Long occlusions can sometimes be reopened, thus obtaining direct flow to the foot.

It is our policy to generally open only one out of three infragenicular vessels to avoid the risk of generalized thrombosis should complications occur: a leeway for emergency distal bypass should always be left open just in case things go very wrong.

To advance a Choice Pt grafix through a long occlusion, the guide should never be pushed alone because it would coil and become useless. The guide is kept inside a rapid exchange coronary balloon, usually 2 mm in diameter, and must be pushed just a few millimeters ahead of the tip of the balloon, which must be advanced progressively. Coronary balloons have the lowest profile, and are the most useful in crossing difficult lesions. Longer low profile peripheral balloons may later smoothen the inner wall of the vessel with a more homogeneous pressure over a long stretch.

Balloons as long as 12 cm are used to obtain a smooth surface and to reduce the operator's exposure to X rays, because they require a smaller number of sequential inflations.

Upon completion of the procedure, the introducers are immediately removed and protamine 50 mg is given to reverse the effects of heparin. Antiplatelet drugs are given for a long time: ticlopidine for the first 6 months at a dose of 250 mg qd and aspirin indefinitely. In no case is post-op heparin given either intraveneously or subcutaneously (unless needed for other reasons: implanted heart mechanical valve, previous embolism, etc).

In terms of limb salvage, early clinical results with this technique are quite good, with prompt healing of the lesions and time to develop new collaterals and more resilient granulation tissue before the vessel reoccludes. Reocclusion is a problem, but doesn't necessarily produce recurrence of symptoms. Published studies are generally unreliable when they consider a vessel as open by means of direct doppler signal or improved distal ABPI: such data are not very reliable when evaluating post PTA infragenicular vessels. Angiograms are the golden standard, and the reocclusion rate of simple, non-stented infragenicular PTA is very high in the treatment of completely occluded vessels, especially when the obstructed segment is long.

Subintimal angioplasty

Dr Bolia, in Leicester, accidentally developed, and then perfected a technique for subintimal angioplasty of the femoral artery, which he later applied to infragenicular vessels yielding positive clinical success. In a paper from 1994, he reported excellent early results in the recanalization of long occluded segments of tibioperoneal vessels using his technique.

While the transluminal PTA requires a straight 0.014 guide which the operator attempts to maintain centered in the vessel, in subintimal PTA a loop technique is used, and after exiting the inner lumen of the vessel above the obstruction, it is re-entered below it when feasible. In good hands, and with proper training and experience, this technique will reopen even the longest occlusions: long-term patency is still to be studied by means of arteriograms in order to demonstrate flux with certainty; limb salvage rates, however, are very encouraging.[17,18]

PTA and spot stenting

While effective in the presence of stenosis, simple PTAs show good clinical results but poorer anatomical ones in long-term follow-up of complete occlusions of tibioperoneal vessels.

Spot stenting of complete occlusions seems to provide better results both in terms of patency and of limb salvage. There is the need for low French size stents, which must be self expandable because external compression is always possible in the calf and ankle.

Nitinol stents, such as the 4F Abbott/Jomed XPERT and more distally the 3F SciMed RADIUS, are quite suitable for this

purpose (Figure 32.1). When necessary, even the dorsalis pedis can be reached by positioning a 3F/3mm RADIUS stent.

Stents should probably be inserted when cutting balloons are used, because when practiced alone this technique is generally followed by complete reocclusion of the vessel. A further possibility is to insert stents in a Y fashion at the tibioperoneal bifurcation (Figure 32.2).

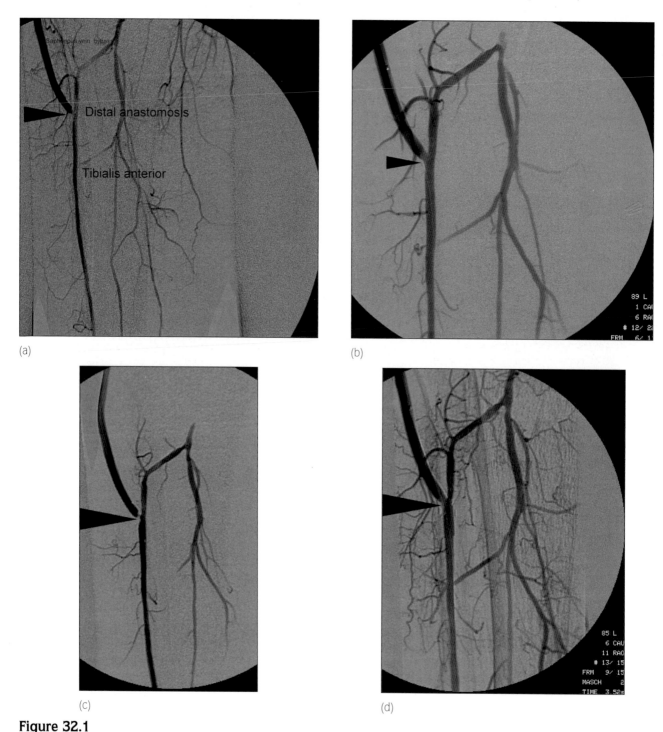

(a) (b) (c) (d)

Figure 32.1

(a) Stenosis at the distal anastomosis of a femoral to tibialis anterior saphenous vein bypass. (b) Simple PTA of the anastomosis yields excellent immediate result. (c) Recurrent severe stenosis 4 months later. (d) Repeated PTA and insertion of an Abbott/Jomed Xpert stent.

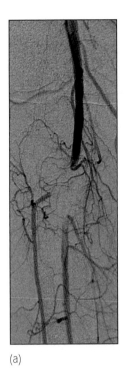

(a)

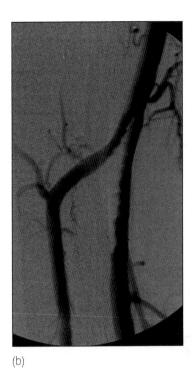

(b)

Figure 32.2
(a) Complete thrombosis of stenotic lesions in the infrapopliteal trifurcation (b) Thrombolysis, PTA and Y stenting.

PTA and long segment retro and infragenicular stenting

This is an extreme limb salvage technique, to be performed when surgery is not feasible and when dealing with long calcified occlusions, after a failed unstented PTA, or when dealing with dissected arteries and multiple resistant stenosis. Indications should be kept strict and the procedure should be performed by well trained operators. In such cases, long flexible stents are required. Nitinol appears to be the best material currently available, provided that stents with three interlinks are used, such as the Abbott/Jomed SELFX, or better yet, the Abbott/Jomed XPERT. The Cordis SMART, while being an outstanding stent in rectilinear structures, bends unnaturally under flexion, due to its six-interlinks system, which makes it very rigid and prone to early fracture under transversal flexion stress. Besides, six-interlinks systems significantly reduce flow during knee flexion. When multiple stents are used, they should be slightly overlapped and, upon completion of the procedure, a flexion angiogram should be performed to assure proper positioning and absence of kinks.

Long-term results of over 2 years have angiographically demonstrated that primary patency is highest in non-diabetic patients, and lowest in diabetic women. Unlike surgical bypass, it appears that poor distal runoff does not produce early closure of sequential stenting, making this procedure a reasonable alternative when the most distal vessels are severely diseased.

Conclusion

Infragenicular PTA is progressively replacing surgical bypass for limb salvage in selected patients, and, granted the application of strict criteria, results are very encouraging. Proper antiplatelet treatment, impeccable atraumatic coronary-type techniques, strict patient follow-up and additional medical (control of diabetes, microbiologic work-up and treatment) and wound treatment (debridement, minor amputations, skin transplants), result in excellent limb salvage.

The insertion of properly placed self-expanding nitinol stents promises to significantly improve patency in complete occlusions and may win a significant place in the treatment of recurrent stenotic lesions.

Aggressive invasive studies of coronary, renal and cerebro-vascular circulation, along with the treatment of severe even if asymptomatic arterial lesions, seem to promise an improvement of the current long-term dismal survival of patients with severe foot ischemia. In terms of survival, patency and limb salvage, patients with chronic terminal renal failure provide the least encouraging results with the use of below the knee PTA.

References

1   Sanchez LA, Schwartz ML, Veith MJ. Bypass surgery into plantar vessels: an effective extension of limb salvage surgical techniques. *Perspect Vasc Surg* 1994; **7**: 47–55.

2   Friedman SG, Safa TK. Pedal branch arterial bypass for limb salvage. *Am Surg* 2002; **68**(5): 446–8.

3   Brown K, Schoenberg N, Moore E. Saddekni A. Percutaneous transluminal angioplasty of infrapopliteal vessels: preliminary results and technical considerations. *Radiology* 1988; **169**(1): 75–8.

4   Sivananthan U, Browne T, Thorley P, Rees M. Percutaneous transluminal angioplasty of the tibial arteries. *Br J Surg* 1994; **81**(9): 1282–5.

5   Treiman G, Treiman R, Ichikawa L, Van Allan R. Should percutaneous transluminal angioplasty be recommended for treatment of infrageniculate popliteal artery or tibioperoneal trunk stenosis? *J Vasc Surg* 1995; **22**(4): 457–65.

6   Bull PG, Mendel H, Hold M, Denck H. Distal popliteal and tibioperoneal transluminal angioplasty: long term follow-up. *J Vasc Interv Radiol* 1992; **3**(1): 45–53.

7   Löfberg AM, Lörelius LE, Karacagil S, Westman B, Almgren B, Berqgvuist D. The use of below-knee percutaneous transluminal angioplasty in arterial occlusive disease causing chronic critical limb ischemia. *Cardiovasc Interv Radiol* 1996; **19**(5): 317–22.

8   Brown KT, Moore ED, Getrajdman GI, Saddekni S. Infrapopliteal angioplasty: long-term follow-up. *J Vasc Interv Radiol* **4**(1): 139–44.

9   Veith F, Gupta SK, Wengerter KR. Changing arteriosclerotic disease patterns and management strategies in lower-limb-threatening ischaemia. *Ann Surg* 1009; **212**: 402–12.

10   Fraser S, Al-Kutoubi A, Wolfe J. Percutaneous transluminal angioplasty of the infrapopliteal vessels: the evidence. *Radiology* 1996; **200**(1): 33–6.

11   Bakal CW, Cynaman J, Sprayregen S. Infrapopliteal percutaneous transluminal angioplasty: what we know. *Radiology* 1996; **200**(1): 36–43.

12   Boyer L, Therre T, Garcier JM et al. Infrapopliteal percutaneous transluminal angioplasty for limb salvage. *Acta Radiol* 2000; **41**(1):73–7.

13   Söder H, Manninen H, Jaakkola P et al. Prospective trial of infrapopliteal artery balloon angioplasty for critical limb ischemia: angiographic and clinical results. *J Vasc Interv Radiol* 2000; **11**(8): 1021–31.

14   Dorros G, Jaff MR, Dorros AM, Mathiak LM, He T. Tibioperoneal (outflow lesion) angioplasty can be used as primary treatment in 235 patients with critical limb ischemia – five-year follow-up: *Circulation* **2001**; 2057–62.

15   Faglia E, Mantero M, Caminiti M et al. Extensive use of peripheral angioplasty, particularly infrapopliteal, in the treatment of ischameic diabetic foot ulcers: clinical results of a multicentric study of 221 consecutive diabetic subjects. *J Int Med* 2002; **252**: 225–32.

16   Nasr MK, McCarthy RJ, Hardman J, Chalmers A, Horrocks M. The increasing role of percutaneous transluminal angioplasty in the primary management of critical limb ischaemia. *Eur J Vasc Endovasc Sugery* 2002; **23**(5): 298–403.

17   Bolia A, Sayers RD, Thompson MM, Bell PR. Subintimal and intraluminal recanalization of occluded crural arteries by percutaneous balloon angioplasty. *Eur J Vasc Surg* 1994; **8**(2): 214–9.

18   Varty K, Bolia A, Naylor A, Bell P, London N. Infrapopliteal percutaneous transluminal angioplasty : a safe and successful procedure. *Eur J Vasc Endovasc Surgery* 1995; **9**(3): 341–5.

33

Endovascular treatment for lower extremity bypass failure

Zvonimir Krajcer and Michael Levy

Introduction

The goals of lower extremity bypass grafting are to maximize long-term patency and prevent the return of ischemic symptoms. In order to achieve these goals, efforts have focused on preventing grafts from failing, and salvaging failed grafts. This chapter summarizes the various treatment options for failing and failed grafts, focusing particularly on endovascular treatment.

Defining failing versus failed grafts

The term 'failing graft' was first used and defined by Veith et al.[1] in 1984. They described a lower extremity graft which was patent, but was encountering reduced flow, which presented as worsening hemodynamic changes (ischemic symptoms, poor distal pulses, reduced ankle–brachial index and abnormal Duplex scanning).

The failing graft may present with stenosis in the inflow or outflow tracts, at the proximal and distal anastomoses, or in the body of the graft itself.[2] This is in contrast to a graft that has 'failed', in which there is thrombosis, or total occlusion in the aforementioned areas, as well as severe claudication, or acute ischemia (rest pain, ulceration, gangrene).[3]

Once a failing graft has been diagnosed, it is considered standard to begin immediate treatment.[1,4] When a graft has failed, its treatment is more difficult, often resulting in lower patency and limb salvage rates.[5]

Natural history of lower extremity bypass conduits

Several authors[3,6] have speculated as to why a bypass conduit fails. Reasons for failure differ, depending on the length of time since the bypass operation. Failure during the earliest stage (<30 days) is thought to be due to either technical errors (residual thrombus, intimal flaps) or judgement errors (poor vein quality, inadequate inflow or run-off). In rare cases graft thrombogenicity or hypercoagulable states are thought to play a role. Futjitana[4] reports that early failure is observed in 3–10% of cases, and is most commonly seen within the first 72 h postoperatively. Graft failure at 30 days to 18 months is attributed to intimal hyperplasia. Failure after 18 months is attributed to progression of atherosclerosis.

The existing literature on patency rates for bypass conduits divides them roughly into two categories: suprainguinal grafts (originating above the inguinal ligament), and infrainguinal grafts (originating below the inguinal ligament). Although there is more literature concerning infrainguinal grafting, reports on suprainguinal (aortoiliac/aortofemoral) grafting maintain that they are the most durable of all arterial reconstructive procedures.[7] Previous studies have revealed that the 5-year primary patency rate of suprainguinal grafts ranges from 77%[8] to 88%.[9]

However, 5-year primary patency rates for infrainguinal grafts range from 47%[10] to 80%.[11] Taylor and Porter[10] reported that their 5-year cumulative patency was 79%, although, when a good-quality autogenous saphenous vein was used, the patency rate improved to 85%. Furthermore, they noted that patients undergoing redo bypass surgery after their primary failure showed a 5-year patency rate of 57%.

Success of reoperation in the setting of lower extremity bypass failure

Reoperation in the setting of bypass failure has historically met with poor results. Whittemore et al,[12] presented a landmark study examining reconstruction following failure of femoropopliteal grafts. This study included 72 limbs that were treated with reoperation for acute, subacute and chronic bypass failure. They reported a cumulative 5-year patency of 50%. However, it is noted that the majority of their reoperative procedures yielded 5-year patency rates of less than 37%: vein patch after thrombectomy (n = 18) 19%, saphenous vein bypass (n = 32) 37%, arm vein bypass (n = 16) 34%, prosthetic bypass (n = 19) 0%, and bypass to or from original vein graft (n = 18) 36%. The only category showing good 5-year patency rates was the smallest group (n = 8), vein patch without thrombectomy, 86%.

The grafts with the worst reoperative outcome are infrainguinal grafts that experience early failure: Robinson et al,[13] report a 10-year experience with 112 infrainguinal bypass grafts which underwent early graft failure (<30 days). Reoperation of these early failed grafts met with poor results: limb salvage rates were 74% after 1 month, 54% at 1 year, and 31% at 5 years. Patency rates after reoperation were 70% at 1 month, 37% at 1 year, and 23% at 5 years. Furthermore, results suggest that reoperation in the setting of acute limb ischemia for early graft failure met with a worse prognosis than reoperation for claudication.

Fewer reports have dealt with reoperation for suprainguinal graft failure; however, the results are generally better. Erodes et al,[14] report their experience with 46 patients undergoing secondary revascularization for aortofemoral graft occlusion (rest pain/severe ischemia presented in 85% of patients). Five-year cumulative patency for all procedures was 68%, with limb salvage achieved in 85%. Nevelsteen et al,[15] reported similar results for reoperation on 930 aortobifemoral Dacron grafts. Five-year cumulative primary patency was 59%, and 8-year limb salvage was 79%.

Endovascular treatment for lower extremity bypass occlusion

Endovascular interventions for failing and failed lower extremity bypass grafts have garnered significant enthusiasm owing to the generally poor results yielded by reoperative and medical[16] interventions. Catheter-directed thrombolysis, percutaneous transluminal angioplasty (PTA), stenting and rheolytic thrombectomy are some of the major treatments currently under investigation for use in the setting of graft failure.

Thrombolysis for lower extremity bypass failure

A discussion regarding indications for thrombolysis in peripheral vascular disease cannot begin without mention of the three major landmark trials that gave legitimacy to this intervention: The Rochester Trial, the STILE trial, and the TOPAS trial. It is noted that none of these trials specifically addressed lytic treatment for lower limb bypass failure.

The Rochester trial[17] was a prospective, randomized, controlled trial involving 114 patients with lower extremity arterial occlusion presenting to a single institution. This was the first trial to randomize patients to thrombolytic therapy (urokinase) or a surgical intervention. Only patients with severe ischemia (<7 days) were included. Limb salvage rates at 1 year were similar in both groups (82%). The trial showed that the magnitude of intervention, and cardiopulmonary complications, were higher in the surgical group (49% surgery versus 16% lysis), whereas major bleeding complications were higher in the thrombolytic group (11% lysis versus 2% surgery). Cost was slightly higher in the lysis group. Cumulative survival was increased in the thrombolysis group (84% lysis versus 58% surgery at 1 year); however, two out of three of the thrombolysis group required adjuvant treatment including angioplasty and elective surgery.

The STILE Trial (Surgery versus Thrombolysis for Ischemia of the Lower Extremity)[13] was a multicenter trial involving 31 centers in the USA and Canada. Patients were selected based on lower extremity ischemia <6 months in duration. Patients were randomized to thrombolysis with recombinant tissue plasminogen activator (r-tPA), urokinase, or surgery. Although target enrollment was 1000 for this study, an interim analysis performed on 393 patients caused the study to be terminated. The analysis revealed a highly significant increase in recurrent/ongoing ischemia in the thrombolysis patients (45.4% in the lysis group compared to 23.6% in the surgical group, p = 0.001). Despite termination due to poor results in the thrombolysis group, several points are noted:

1. No difference was observed between the surgical or thrombolysis groups when looking at rate of major amputation or death.
2. Patients with acute bypass graft occlusions did better with lysis than surgery.
3. Of thrombolysis patients, 55.8% had a reduction in the magnitude of surgery.
4. Patients with acute ischemia (<14 days) had improved amputation-free survival, and shorter hospital stays, with thrombolysis.

The TOPAS trial (Thrombolysis Or Peripheral Artery Surgery)[19] involved 79 centers in North America and Europe. The trial took place in two phases.

Phase 1 involved 213 patients with ischemic symptoms of <14 days' duration. Patients were randomized to one of three dosing regimens of recombinant urokinase, or surgical revascularization. The magnitude of surgical procedures was reduced by 49.7% in lysis patients compared to 13.8% in surgical patients ($p < 0.001$). Amputation rates were comparable in all groups, and no significant difference was found in overall survival.

Phase II of the trial involved 544 patients randomized to lytic treatment or primary operation. This trial showed no major differences between groups for death or major amputation rates. One-year amputation-free survival was 65% in the lysis group and 69.9% in the surgery group. The investigators concluded that urokinase reduced the magnitude of open procedures without a significant increase in risk of amputation or death.

These trials facilitated the increase in the use of intra-arterial thrombolysis as first-line treatment in lower limb ischemia. Further studies have examined the use of catheter-directed thrombolysis specifically for lower extremity bypass failure:

Bhatnagar et al[20] reported the results of 55 patients undergoing 81 thrombolytic treatments for both suprainguinal and infrainguinal graft failure. The results showed that 1-year primary patency rates were highest for cases undergoing lysis alone ($n = 11$), at 56% (3-year limb salvage 82%). Those who underwent successful lysis, but later required arterial reconstruction or PTA ($n = 37$), yielded a 47% 1-year primary patency rate (3-year limb salvage 76%). Cases in which lysis failed, resulting in arterial reconstruction or amputation ($n = 33$), yielded a 24% 1-year primary patency rate (3-year limb salvage 37%). In total, 25 amputations in 55 patients were observed during a total of 4.5 years of follow-up.

Wholey et al[21] reported the results of a retrospective multicenter study that compared thrombolysis of lower extremity occlusions classified as acute, subacute, and chronic. Both suprainguinal and infrainguinal grafts were included. Two hundred and thirty-five patients were treated with urokinase infusion. Results suggest that thrombolysis is most effective for acute occlusion. Primary patency at 1 year was 87% for acute, 85% for subacute and 75% for chronic occlusions.

Nackman et al[22] described the results of a 10-year surveillance examining thrombolysis of occluded infrainguinal vein grafts. Forty-four patients underwent 44 infusions of urokinase. Cumulative primary patency at 1 year was 25%. These results suggest that vein graft replacement is better than vein graft thrombolysis. Univariate analysis of data suggested that, at presentation, diabetes, infrapopliteal grafting and graft age of less than 12 months were associated with worse patency rates. However, post-lysis, factors affecting primary patency were graft age less than 12 months, diabetes, and ankle–brachial index at discharge.

In summary, thrombolysis has been shown to be a good treatment method, both as an alternative to and in combination with surgery for lower extremity bypass occlusion. Several authors have commented that its best use is as a diagnostic tool allowing for better visualization of inflow and outflow lesions to assist in planning further interventions.[20–23] It is best used in cases where identifiable lesions are present. It is also considered good treatment for limbs with poor collateral flow, allowing for collateral lesions to be opened before further treatment.[22] Thrombolysis has also been shown to reduce the magnitude of surgical intervention from urgent to elective.[20]

Further benefits of lysis may include the conservation of autogenous veins for future bypass, as well as less risk of intimal damage than surgical balloon thrombectomy.[23] Thrombolysis should not be used on failed grafts < 1 month old due to poor long-term patency rates, and increased risk of bleeding.[22]

PTA for lower extremity bypass failure

Since the 1964 landmark article in which Dotter and Judkins[24] reported using arterial dilators to alleviate obstructions producing lower extremity ischemia, techniques of peripheral angioplasty have undergone many changes. At the present time much controversy surrounds the indications of PTA for failed or failing grafts. There have been few published reports. Often, PTA of occluded grafts is grouped in with procedures performed on native vessels for limb salvage.

Several authors have reported severe limitations of the use of PTA for vein graft stenosis and failure. Whittemore et al[25] described a study of 30 patients undergoing PTA at a mean of 17.8 months after infrainguinal bypass with autogenous vein grafts. Five-year cumulative primary patency was 18%. Brown et al[26] reported a 78% clinical failure rate in patients for 14 failed and 9 failing grafts at an average follow-up of 25.8 months.

Sanchez et al[2] reported their experience over 10 years of treating failing lower extremity grafts. one hundred and fifty grafts with 285 lesions were reported. Lesions were divided into two types: simple and complex. Simple lesions were defined as: < 1.5 cm long, in a vein graft $\geq$ 3 mm in diameter. Complex lesions were defined as: > 1.5 cm long, in grafts < 3 mm in diameter, often multiple lesions. Results showed that PTA was superior for simple lesions, yielding a 2-year extended patency rate of 93%, in contrast to 54% when complex lesions were treated. Five-year secondary patency rates for PTA were 58% versus 71% for surgery; however, this difference did not achieve statistical significance ($p = 0.25$). The final recommendations of this study suggest PTA for small stenotic lesions, and surgery for all other cases.

Gonsalves et al,[27] undertook a study to determine criteria which correlated with successful outcomes for PTA of vein graft stenosis. This was a 5-year single-institution study which examined 76 failing grafts with 87 stenoses. Twenty-eight grafts (32%) were ultimately treated with PTA (over a mean interval of 11 months). Three factors were found to correlate with PTA success for vein graft stenosis: (1) vein diameter ≥ 3.5 mm; (2) lesion length <2 cm; (3) appearance of failing graft >3 months post-bypass surgery. Repeat surgery was indicated for grafts without these features. PTA for grafts with these characteristics yielded a 1-year cumulative primary patency rate of 88%. Furthermore, grafts with these characteristics underwent significantly less intervention than grafts that did not meet these characteristics.

Avino et al[28] reported a study in which stenosis-free patency of open surgical repair of infrainguinal graft stenosis was compared to PTA. A stenosis was detected by duplex scanning in 144 vein grafts, of which 77 were treated with open repair and 67 were treated with angioplasty. Stenosis-free patency was identical at 2 years (63% for surgery and 63% for PTA). The rate of reintervention was reported to be higher after PTA (22%) than surgery (14%). However, fewer graft failures occurred in the PTA group (2 versus 8). Twenty-six patients underwent simultaneous duplex scanning during their angioplasty procedure. Duplex scanning was very useful in assessing the hemodynamic impact after angioplasty, and in 9 of the 26 (34%) cases the duplex findings led to the use of a larger balloon, or a longer inflation time. The overall result was a 1-year stenosis-free patency of 89%, in contrast to 61% for the non-duplex scanned PTAs.

In summary, although some studies show limitations in using PTA for lower extremity graft occlusion, others report acceptable success rates. Balloon angioplasty appears to work best in small isolated lesions in large vessels, for grafts that have failed later than 3 months. Furthermore, PTA achieves comparable rates to surgery in terms of patency and overall morbidity, and remains a viable alternative to surgery in patients who have a higher operative risk, or no available vein conduit.

Stenting for lower extremity bypass failure

It is argued that stents were developed primarily as a device to deal with the major limitations of PTA: intimal dissection and elastic recoil. In fact, in 1969, Dotter[29] proposed a supportive endoskeleton, or scaffolding device, to deal with these limitations. Acute dissection and residual stenosis have been reported to occur in up to 15% of patients undergoing PTA.[30]

There are numerous reports on the efficacy of PTA and stenting in native peripheral arteries, but there is a distinct absence of reports concerning the use of stenting in the setting of lower limb graft failure. Schneider et al[31] suggested several theoretical advantages that can be applied to stenting in the setting of graft occlusion: (1) access via remote site; (2) reduced morbidity to patients at high operative risk; (3)

decreased use of general anesthesia; and (4) decreased blood loss during the procedure. However, there are disadvantages of stenting, and these include: (1) variability in technical expertise; (2) expense of the procedure; (3) risk of vascular injury (including dissection); and (4) the risk of hemorrhage with the concurrent use of thrombolysis.

Few randomized trials have examined the efficacy of stenting for the treatment of lower limb ischemia. Vroegindeweiji et al[32] reported a randomized, controlled trial comparing PTA and stenting versus angioplasty alone for the treatment of femoropopliteal occlusions. Of the 51 patients enrolled in the study, none experienced rest pain. Follow-up results were determined by duplex ultrasound and ankle–brachial index and showed no advantage of stenting over angioplasty alone. Clinical and hemodynamic success at 1 year was 74% for PTA and stenting, versus 85% for angioplasty alone. Cumulative primary patency at 1 year was 74% for PTA and 62% for stenting, with no statistically significant differences noted.

Stenting, much like PTA, in the suprainguinal area has met with good results: Nawaz et al[33] reported the results of 140 patients or 163 limbs undergoing iliac stenting over a 3-year period. Results demonstrated primary clinical success of 90% at 1 year, and 84% at 3 years. Primary assisted cumulative patency was 95% at 1 year and 91% at 3 years. Palmaz et al[34] reported similar results with iliac artery stenting with a Palmaz stent in 486 patients.

Results of infrainguinal stenting proved to be inferior. Gray and Olin[35] looked at 55 patients at a single institution over 3 years who underwent PTA and stenting of 57 superficial femoral arteries. Multiple stents were used in long segments in 81% of the cases. Of the 57 segment-stented, 40 (70%) developed restenosis and 21 (52.5%) of those had reintervention. Primary patency at 1 year was 22% and secondary patency was 46%.

Henry et al[36] reported the results of 126 patients with 188 infrainguinal stents. Results showed 4-year primary patency rates of 65% for femoral stents and 50% for popliteal stents. They also noted that the more stents used in a single limb, the worse the long-term outcome.

Martin et al[37] reported the results of a multicenter trial of Wallstents in iliac and femoral arteries. For iliac stenting, primary clinical patency was 81% at 1 year and 71% at 2 years. For femoral stenting, primary clinical patency was 61% at 1 year and 49% at 2 years.

It must be noted that the best results appear to occur in conjunction with surgical interventions. Schneider et al[31] reported on the results of staged and simultaneous procedures involving both open repair and PTA with stenting for lower extremity ischemia. They examined 274 patients undergoing lower extremity revascularization. Of those, 38 underwent both surgical and endovascular procedures (21 simultaneous and 17 staged). The decision to undertake combined procedures was reflected by the severe degree of ischemia in this subpopulation: 19 presented with gangrene

(50%), 12 had rest pain (31.6%), and seven had severe claudication (18.4%). Cumulative primary patency at 1 year was 82% in the staged group, and 83% in the simultaneous group. Both surgical patency (82% in staged group, 86% in simultaneous) and endovascular patency (90% in staged group, 92% in simultaneous group) were high.

Some of the biggest problems encountered with stents in the long term are thrombosis and restenosis due to intimal hyperplasia and progressive atherosclerosis.[35] Cikrit and Dalsing[38] report that with failure to cover arteriosclerotic lesions proximal and distal to the stent, these lesions will grow at a rate of 5% per year.

In summary, although good patency rates have been reported for stenting in native vessels, it is important to see more studies dedicated to stenting for limb salvage, and lower limb bypass occlusion. This is a useful intervention that provides a good alternative to patients with dissection and recoil after PTA.

Rheolytic thrombectomy for lower limb bypass occlusion

Rheolytic thrombectomy is gaining popularity for use in patients with acute lower extremity ischemia associated with heavy thrombus burden, and where an alternative to surgical thrombectomy is sought. Rheolytic thrombectomy involves a catheter that utilizes high-speed saline jets to create a low-pressure zone (creating a Bernoulli effect) in the lumen of the vessel to pull thrombus off the wall. Another set of jets within the catheter creates a Venturi effect to pull the thrombus material into the catheter.

Wagner et al[39] reported the results of a multicenter trial using a rheolytic thrombectomy device for acute occlusive disease of the lower extremity. Of the 50 patients included in the study, 39 had native arterial occlusion and 11 had thrombosis of a bypass graft. Thrombus material was successfully removed in 45 (90%) cases, although technical success was only 52%. Adjunctive procedures, including thrombolysis, PTA, or aspiration thrombectomy, were performed in the 45 (90%) cases. Primary patency at 1 year (after adjunctive procedures) was 69%.

Silva et al[40] treated 21 patients (22 limbs) for lower extremity ischemia due to acute occlusion using rheolytic thrombectomy. Technical success was achieved in 20 of the 22 (91%) limbs. Four patients died during follow-up (three during hospitalization), all due to causes unrelated to treatment. A 6-month limb salvage rate of 89% (16 of 18) was observed in those who survived.

In summary, rheolytic thrombectomy is a promising intervention that achieves good patency rates in conjunction with other interventions. Further study will be required to better assess its efficacy.

Our experience with endovascular intervention for lower extremity bypass failure

From July 1994 to June 2000, 33 patients underwent endovascular treatment for stenosis or occlusion of 42 lower extremity bypass grafts at our institution. Patient characteristics are listed in Table 33.1. The majority of the patients were male (mean age 61±15 years). Evaluation of their presenting symptoms revealed that 23 patients (70%) presented with acute ischemic changes, 4 (12%) had non-healing ulcers, and 2 (6%) had gangrene. Most (88%) patients had multiple comorbidities, including 4 patients (12%) who were non-surgical candidates. In total, 49 interventions were performed in 42 grafts (33 primary, 13 secondary, 3 tertiary).

Table 33.1 Patient characteristics.

Characteristics and Demographics	
Total number of patients	33
Males	25 (76%)
Females	8 (24%)
Mean Age (years)	61±15
History of:	
Hypertension	26 (79%)
Diabetes	11 (33%)
Smoking	11 (33%)
Three-vessel coronary artery disease	18 (55%)
Congestive heart failure	3 (9%)
Chronic renal insufficiency	6 (18%)
Stroke	3 (9%)

Table 33.2 Procedural features.

Mean age of grafts	38 months
Range	1–125 months
Total number of grafts	42
Graft Types:	
Aortoiliac	1 (2.4%)
Aortofemoral	4 ((9.5%)
Aortopopliteal	1 (2.4%)
Iliofemoral	1 (2.4%)
Femoropopliteal	26 (62%)
Femorotibial	5 (12%)
Popliteal–tibial	1 (2.4%)
Popliteal–peroneal	1 (2.4%)
Superficial femoral stent graft	1 (2.4%)
Aortic stent graft	1 (2.4%)

Procedural features and graft characteristics are listed in Table 33.2. In total, 22 patients received various thrombolytic regimens (3 had retavase, 14 received urokinase, 4 had tPA and 1 had streptokinase), with 2 of those receiving adjunctive abciximab and 14 undergoing stent implantation utilizing 22 stents (Figures 33.1–33.3).

Results

Results are summarized in Table 33.3. Acute technical success was achieved in 31 (94%) patients, while in 2 patients the bypasses could not be recanalized. Complications were experienced by 13 patients (39%) 1 had bleeding at the groin

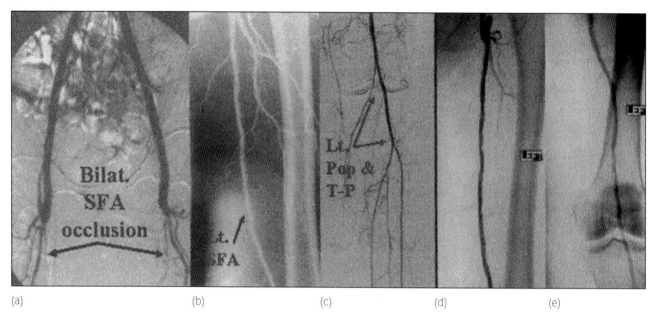

(a)   (b)   (c)   (d)   (e)

Figure 33.1
Recannalization of a chronic superficial femoral artery total occlusion in a 78-year old woman who had a history of previous aorto-bifemoral and bilateral femoro-popliteal bypass surgery and a 2-year old femoro-popliteal bypass graft occlusion. (a) Pre intervention. (b) After thrombolysis and balloon angioplasty shows the left popliteal, tibial and peroneal arteries are patent. (c) Distal runoff after thrombolysis and balloon angioplasty shows the left popliteal, tibial and peroneal arteries are patent. (d) Four months later follow-up angiography demonstrates patent left superficial femoral and (e) popliteal arteries remain patent.

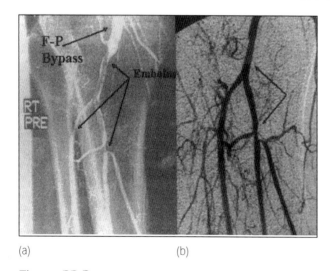

(a)   (b)

Figure 33.2
Pre-intervention in a 56-year old man post femoro-popliteal bypass shows an extensive thrombo-embolism to the trifurcation vessels. (b) Post rheolytic thrombectomy (Angiojet®) angiography revealed resolution of thrombus and good trifurcation run-off.

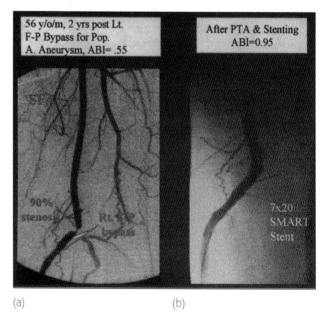

(a)   (b)

Figure 33.3
Proximal anastomosis (inflow lesions).

Table 33.3 Results and complications

Technical success	31 of 33 patients (94%)
Thrombolytic therapy alone	5 patients
Thrombolytic + rheolytic thrombectomy	3 patients
Thrombolytic + PTA	8 patients
Thrombolytic + PTA + Stenting	4 patients
Thrombolytic + PTA + Stenting + IIbIIIa therapy	2 patients
PTA only	3 patients
PTA + stenting	8 patients
Failure to recanalize	2 patients (6%)
Complications	
Minor	9 patients (27%)
Hematoma	7 patients
Access site pseudoaneurysm	2 patients
Major	4 patients (12%)
Access site bleeding requiring transfusion	2 patients
Gastrointestinal bleeding requiring transfusion	1 patient
Myocardial infarction	1 patient

site and 1 had gastrointestinal bleeding; 6 had hematomas at the puncture site; 2 developed pseudoaneurysms at the arterial access site; and 1 patient suffered a myocardial infarction.

The long-term follow-up (mean 21±8 months) revealed that 16 patients required re-intervention (7 due to thrombosis and 9 due to significant restenosis). Limb amputation was necessary in 3 patients, and 4 patients died of unrelated causes. Using the Kaplan–Meier estimates of survival method, primary patency at 1 year was 41% and secondary patency 85%.

Patency rates for different treatment modalities were as follows: lysis alone, 29%; PTA alone, 67%; PTA and lysis 70%, PTA and stent, 38%; and PTA, lysis and stent, 34%. Limb salvage rates at 1 year were calculated to be 67%.

These results are consistent with the results of others for the various interventions, as reported in this chapter. Our periprocedural and chronic complication rates appear to be higher than those reported in the literature; however, this may be accounted for by variance in definitions of complications. Furthermore, although our experience has demonstrated promising results, longer follow-up with larger numbers of patients will be crucial to better determine the outcomes of these interventions.

Conclusion

Previous studies and our data indicate that endovascular interventions in the setting of lower extremity bypass failure offer good options for patients with multiple comorbidities and severe peripheral vascular disease. Previous studies have demonstrated that combined surgical and endovascular treatments in the setting of acute lower limb ischemia offer better results in a great majority of patients than either modality alone.[41] It will be important that more studies be undertaken with newer endovascular treatments to determine the best treatment options for these patients.

References

1   Veith FJ, Weiser RK, Gupta SK et al. Diagnosis and management of failing lower extremity arterial reconstructions prior to graft occlusion. *J Cardiovasc Surg* 1984; **25**: 381–4.

2   Sanchez LA, Gupta SK, Veith FJ et al. A ten-year experience with one hundred fifty failing or threatened vein and polytetrafluoroethylene arterial bypass grafts. *J Vasc Surg* 1991; **14**: 729–38.

3   Belkin M, Whittemore AD. Reoperative approaches for failed infrainguinal vein grafts. *Semin Vasc Surg.* 1994; **7**: 158–64.

4   Fujitani RM. Revision of the failing vein graft: outcome of secondary operations. *Semin Vasc Surg* 1993; **6**: 118–29.

5   Welch HJ, O'Donnell TF. Role of thrombolytic, antiplatelet, antithrombotic, and other drugs in the management of failed arterial grafts. *Semin Vascu Surg* 1994; **7**: 201–9.

6   Fowl RJ, Kempczinski RF. Success rates and failure rates, and causes of failure for common arterial reconstructive procedures. *Semin Vasc Surg* 1994; **7**: 132–8.

7   Szilagyi DE, Elliott JP Jr, Smith RF et al. A thirty year survey of the reconstructive surgical treatment of aortoiliac occlusive disease. *J Vasc Surg* 1986; **3**: 421–36.

8   Martinez BD, Hertzer NR, Beven EG. Influence of distal arterial occlusive disease on prognosis following aortobifemoral bypass. *Surgery* 1980; **88**: 642–53.

9   Berkowitz HD, Greenstein SM. Improved patency in reversed femoral–infrapopliteal autologous vein grafts by early detection and treatment of the failing grafts. *J Vasc Surg* 1987; **5**: 755–61.

10 Taylor LM Jr, Porter JM. Present status of reversed vein bypass grafting: five year results of a modern series. *J Vasc Surg* 1990; **11**: 193–206.

11 Taylor LM Jr, Porter JM. Clinical and anatomical considerations for surgery in femoropopliteal disease and the results of surgery. *Circulation* 1991; **83**(suppl I): I-63–I-69.

12 Whittemore AD, Clowes AW, Couch NP, Mannick JA. Secondary femoropopliteal reconstruction. *Ann Surg* 1981; **193**: 35–42.

13 Robinson KD, Sato DT, Gregory RT et al. Long-term outcome after early infrainguinal graft failure. *J Vasc Surg* 1997; **26**: 425–38.

14 Erodes LS, Bernhard VM, Berman SS. Aortofemoral graft occlusion: strategy and timing of reoperation. *Cardiovasc Surg* 1995; **3**: 277–83.

15 Nevelsteen A, Suy R. Graft occlusion following aortofemoral Dacron bypass. *Ann Vasc Surg* 1991; **5**: 32–7.

16 Taylor LM, Moneta GL, Porter JM. Nonoperative management of femoropopliteal occlusive disease. In: Yao JST, Pearce WH, eds. *Practical Vascular Surgery*, 1st edn. McGraw-Hill, St Louis, MO, 1999: 24.

17 Ouriel K, Shortell CK, De Weese JA et al. A comparison of thrombolytic therapy with operative revascularization in the initial treatment of acute peripheral arterial ischemia. *J Vasc Surg* 1994; **19**: 1021–30.

18 The STILE Investigators. Results of a prospective randomized trial evaluating surgery versus thrombolysis for ischemia of the lower extremity. *Ann Surg* 1994; **220**: 251–68.

19 Ouriel K, Veith FJ Sasahara AA et al. A comparison of recombinant urokinase with vascular surgery as initial treatment for acute arterial occlusion of the legs. *N Engl J Med* 1998; **338**: 1105–11.

20 Bhatnagar PK, Ierardi RP, Ikeda Y et al. The impact of thrombolytic therapy on arterial and graft occlusions: a critical analysis. *J Cardiovasc Surg* 1996; **37**: 105–12.

21 Wholey MH, Maynar MA, Wholey MH et al. Comparison of thrombolytic therapy of lower-extremity acute, subacute, and chronic arterial occlusions. *Catheter Cardiovasc Diagn* 1998; **44**: 159–69.

22 Nackman GB, Walsh DB, Fillinger MF et al. Thrombolysis of occluded infrainguinal vein grafts: predictors of outcome. *J Vasc Surg* 1997; **25**: 1023–32.

23 Chalmers RTA, Hoballah TF, Kresowik TF et al. Late results of a prospective study of direct intra-arterial urokinase infusion for peripheral arterial and bypass graft occlusions. *Cardiovasc Surg* 1995; **3**: 293–7.

24 Dotter CT, Judkins MP. Transluminal treatment of arterial obstruction: description of a new technique and a preliminary report of its application. *Circulation* 1964; **30**: 654.

25 Whittemore AD, Donaldson MC, Polak JF et al. Limitations of balloon angioplasty for vein graft stenosis. *J Vasc Surg* 1991; **14**: 340.

26 Brown KT, Moore ED, Getrajdman GI, Saddekni S. Infrapopliteal angioplasty: long-term follow-up. *J Vasc Intervent Radiol* 1993; **4**: 139–44.

27 Gonsalves C, Bandyk DF, Avino AJ, Johnson BL. Duplex Features of vein graft stenosis and the success of percutaneous transluminal angioplasty. *J Endovasc Surg* 1999; **6**: 66–72.

28 Avino AJ, Bandyk DF, Gonsalves AJ et al. Surgical and endovascular intervention for infrainguinal vein graft stenosis. *J Vasc Surg* 1999; **29**: 60–71.

29 Dotter CT. Transluminally placed coil spring endarterial tube grafts – long term patency in canine popliteal artery. *Investi Radiol* 1969; **4**: 329.

30 Johnston KW, Rae M, Hogg-Johnson SA et al. Five-year results of a prospective study of percutaneous transluminal angioplasty. *Ann Surg* 1987; **206**: 403–13.

31 Schneider PA, Abcarian PW, Ogawa RVT et al. Should balloon angioplasty and stents have any role in operative intervention for lower extremity ischemia? *Ann Vasc Surg* 1997; **11**: 574–80.

32 Vroegindeweiji D, Vos LD, Tielbeek AV et al. Balloon angioplasty combined with primary stenting versus balloon angioplasty alone in femoropopliteal artery occlusions. *Cardiovasc Intervent Radiol* 1997; **20**: 420–5.

33 Nawaz S, Cleveland T, Gaines P et al. Aortoiliac stenting, determinants of clinical outcome. *Eur J Vasc Endovasc Surg* 1999; **17**: 351–59.

34 Palmaz JC, Laborde JC, Rivera FJ et al. Stenting of the iliac arteries with the Palmaz stent: experience from a multicenter trial. *Cardiovasc Intervent Radiol* 1992; **15**: 291–7.

35 Gray BH, Olin JW. Limitations of percutaneous transluminal angioplasty with stenting for femoropopliteal arterial occlusive disease. *Semin Vasc Surg* 1997; **10**: 8–16.

36 Henry M, Amor M, Ethevenot G et al. Palmaz stent placement in iliac and femoropopliteal arteries: primary and secondary patency in 310 patients with 2–4 year follow-up. *Radiology* 1995; **197**: 167–74.

37 Martin EC, Katzen BT, Benenati JF et al. Multicenter trial of the wallstent in the iliac and femoral arteries. *J Vasc Intervent Radiol* 1995; **6**: 843–9.

38 Cikrit DF, Dalsing MC. Lower-extremity arterial endovascular stenting. *Surg Clin North Am* 1998; **78**: 617–29.

39 Wagner HJ, Muller-Hulsbeck S, Pitton MB et al. Rapid thrombectomy with a hydrodynamic catheter: results from a prospective, multicenter trial. *Radiology* 1997; **205**: 675–81.

40 Silva JA, Ramee SR, Collins TJ et al. Rheolytic thrombectomy in the treatment of acute limb-threatening ischemia. *Catheter Cardiovasc Diagn* 1998; **45**: 386–93.

41 Rutherford RB, Baker JD, Ernst C. et al: Recommended standards for reports dealing with lower extremity ischemia: Revised version. *J Vasc Surg* 1997; **26**: 517.

34

Renal artery stenosis: when and how to treat it

Christopher J White

Introduction

Renovascular hypertension occurs in response to a significant hemodynamic obstruction to renal bloodflow. The resultant stimulation of renin and angiotensin production causes systemic hypertension and fluid retention. Atherosclerotic renal artery stenosis, the most common cause of secondary hypertension, affects fewer than 5% of the general hypertensive population.[1] There are, however, several clinical 'high-risk' subsets of patients in which atherosclerotic renal artery stenosis is much more common, such as poorly controlled hypertensives with renal insufficiency,[2] and patients with severe hypertension-associated coronary or peripheral vascular disease (Table 34.1).[3–6]

In patients undergoing coronary angiography for suspected coronary artery disease, the incidence of renal artery stenosis ranges from 15% to 18%.[3–6] In patients with known aneurysmal or occlusive peripheral vascular disease, associated renal artery stenosis is found in 28%.[7] In patients with renal insufficiency, the incidence of unsuspected renal artery stenosis is as high as 24%.[8]

The natural history of renal artery stenosis is to progress over time. The incidence of progression in angiographic studies ranges from 39% to 49%.[9–12] Many of these lesions progress to complete occlusion with loss of renal function.[11] In a prospective study of patients with renal artery stenosis treated medically, progression occurred in 42% (11% progressed to occlusion) of the patients over a 2-year period.[13] Of particular importance is the realization that progression of renal artery stenosis and loss of renal function are *independent* of the ability to medically control blood pressure.[14] Renal artery stent placement can significantly slow the progression of renal failure in these patients.[15]

A consensus is now developing that patients with significant renal artery stenosis ($\geq 50\%$ diameter stenosis and/or $\geq 15\,mmHg$ pressure gradient) in the setting of uncontrolled hypertension or renal insufficiency are appropriate candidates for percutaneous revascularization. Other indications for renal artery revascularization include patients with congestive heart failure (flash pulmonary edema) and unstable angina. Patients on hemodialysis whose parenchyma is supplied by stenotic renal arteries may also be considered candidates for endovascular stent placement.[16–22]

Patient selection and indications for treatment

History and physical examination

Patients with early (<20 years) or late (>55 years) onset of hypertension are more likely to have renal artery stenosis than the general hypertensive population (Table 34.1). Other groups at increased risk for renovascular hypertension are those with refractory hypertension on multiple medications,

---

Table 34.1 Hypertensive patients at increased risk of renal artery stenosis.

- Abdominal bruit (systolic and diastolic)
- Onset of hypertension <20 years or >55 years
- Malignant hypertension
- Refractory or difficult-to-control hypertension
- Azotemia with ACE inhibitors
- Atrophic kidney
- Hypertension and associated atherosclerotic disease
- Elderly with renal insufficiency

those with malignant hypertension, patients with flash pulmonary edema and those who develop renal insufficiency when treated with angiotensin-converting enzyme inhibitors (ACEIs). Patients with known atherosclerotic disease of the coronary or peripheral vasculature should be suspected of atherosclerotic renal artery stenosis if they are hypertensive or develop renal insufficiency. On physical examination, patients with a diastolic and systolic abdominal or flank bruit should be suspected of having renal artery stenosis.

Laboratory tests

Screening tests for renal artery stenosis and associated renovascular hypertension are designed to either image the anatomic obstruction to bloodflow in the renal arteries or to assess the physiologic significance of the obstruction. Screening tests designed to detect differences between the kidneys suffer from decreased sensitivity due to the high incidence (approximately 30%) of bilateral atherosclerotic renal artery stenosis.

Historically, screening tests for renal artery stenosis and renovascular hypertension consisted of intravenous urography and random or stimulated measurements of plasma renin activity. While a normal plasma renin level in an untreated patient is useful to rule out the presence of renovascular hypertension, the sensitivity and specificity of an elevated plasma renin level are too low to be useful as a screening test.[23]

Captopril renal scintigraphy is based upon the renal response to a dose of the ACEI, causing a reduction in the glomerular filtration rate of the stenotic kidney, resulting in a delayed clearance of the radioisotope which is compared to the function of the contralateral kidney.[24] Initial studies reported sensitivities and specificities as high as 90% for this test in a highly selected population of patients; however, more recent investigations have demonstrated a wide variation in the test's accuracy. The high incidence of bilateral atherosclerotic lesions (approximately 30%) and the difficulty in interpreting this test in patients with renal insufficiency are problematic. This, combined with the high cost and the duration of the examination (imaging is performed over 2 days in some centers), makes this test unattractive for routine patient screening.

Selective renal vein renin measurements have been shown to correlate with reduction in hypertension following revascularization of a stenotic renal artery.[25] However, the requirement to perform these tests under controlled circumstances, withdrawing confounding medications, and its insensitivity in the presence of bilateral renal artery disease makes it unattractive for routine screening.

Spiral computerized tomography provides three-dimensional reconstructions of the aorta and renal arteries.[26,27] While it may be useful in detecting renal artery stenosis, it requires that a high volume of radiographic contrast be given to the patient. It has not gained acceptance as a standard screen-

ing test, but may be useful in selected patients such as those with suspected aneurysmal disease of the abdominal aorta.

Magnetic resonance angiography (MRA) is a promising technique for imaging the abdominal aorta and renal arteries without the use of radiographic contrast.[28–30] Artifactual drop-out of images at sites of increased turbulence (ostia of the renal arteries) and its relatively high cost continue to be problems in its general application as a screening tool.

Renal duplex ultrasound imaging has become the noninvasive diagnostic test of choice over the past several years.[31] It does not require the patient to receive a contrast agent, and is relatively inexpensive and easy to perform. Several investigators have demonstrated sensitivities and specificities in excess of 90% for this test. The major drawback to this test is that it requires a skilled technician to perform the examination, and in some patients their body habitus makes imaging very difficult.

Renal arteriography remains the gold standard for diagnosing renal artery stenosis. This test can be performed in an outpatient setting, and in skilled hands has very low risk. In our center, patients suspected of renal artery stenosis undergo diagnostic angiography with intervention at the same time, which is both cost-effective and efficient for the management of these patients.

Indications and contraindications

Clinical indications

A presumptive diagnosis of renovascular hypertension may be made in a patient with hypertension and an angiographically demonstrated diameter stenosis of ≥ 50%. Jean et al[4] published their experience in 196 patients undergoing cardiac catheterization for suspicion of coronary artery disease. Some degree of renal artery stenosis was demonstrated in one-third of the patients and was significant (>50% diameter stenosis) in 18%. Of those patients with coronary atherosclerosis (n = 152), 22% were found to have significant renal artery stenosis. Univariate analysis revealed that the presence of coronary disease and renal insufficiency correlated with the presence of significant renal artery stenosis.[4] In our cardiology practice, screening renal angiography is routinely performed in hypertensive (≥ 150/90 mmHg) patients, on two or more antihypertensive medications, undergoing cardiac catheterization for suspicion of atherosclerotic coronary artery disease.

The clinical indications for percutaneous renal artery revascularization are similar to those for surgical revascularization. Patients with ≥ 50% diameter stenosis of the renal artery and poorly controlled hypertension are candidates for percutaneous intervention. For aorto-ostial lesions, restenosis lesions, or following a suboptimal balloon angioplasty (≥ 30%

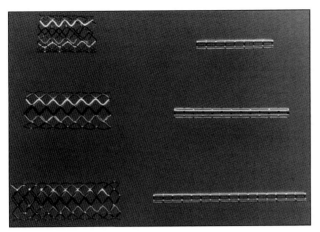

Figure 34.1
Palmaz stents, undeployed (left) and deployed (right) in sizes
from 104, 154, and 204.

residual diameter stenosis or dissection), the use of endovascular stents is preferred (Figure 34.1).[32] For patients with fibromuscular dysplasia or renal branch artery lesions, we prefer balloon angioplasty with provisional stenting for unsatisfactory results.[33,34]

Patients with renal failure and associated renal artery stenosis may benefit from percutaneous revascularization, although this has not been demonstrated in any systematic study. Traditional teaching requires that both renal arteries be compromised to cause renal failure, but in the setting of patients with hypertensive renal insufficiency, a unilateral stenosis may serve to protect the affected kidney from hypertensive damage. This kidney might be expected to respond with improved function if the offending stenotic lesion is treated.[16,17]

Finally, treatment of isolated renal artery stenotic lesions which do not cause uncontrolled hypertension or renal insufficiency has been debated as a means to preserve renal function. The natural history of atherosclerotic renal artery stenosis is to progress with time.[9–13] Timely intervention and correction of these lesions may prevent progressive narrowing of the vessel and loss of renal function. Patients on hemodialysis whose parenchyma is supplied by stenotic renal arteries, and those with renal artery stenosis and refractory congestive heart failure or unstable angina should also be considered candidates for angioplasty or stenting.[18,19]

Contraindications

Contraindications to renal angioplasty and stenting are relative and not absolute. The risk versus benefit of the procedure must be weighed. Patients with atheroembolic disease or a 'shaggy' aorta are at increased risk of cholesterol emboli with catheter manipulation in the aorta. Patients with renal artery aneurysms are at risk of rupture, and surgical correction should be considered.

Renovascular hypertension

A randomized trial comparing balloon angioplasty to medical therapy in 106 patients with uncontrolled hypertension and renal artery stenosis (≥ 50% diameter stenosis) demonstrated failure of medical therapy in 44% (n = 22/50 patients) at 3 months, requiring crossover to angioplasty therapy.[35] At 3 months, there was evidence of improved blood pressure control, a requirement for fewer medications, and improved renal function in the angioplasty group. At 1-year follow-up, 16% (n = 8) of the medically treated patients experienced occlusion of the stenotic renal artery versus none in the angioplasty group.

There have been many reports of successful percutaneous therapy for renovascular hypertension.[20,22,36–41] Dorros et al[40] demonstrated that renal artery stent placement was more effective than balloon angioplasty alone in improving or abolishing pressure gradients across renal artery lesions treated. In 76 patients (92 renal arteries) undergoing primary renal artery stent placement, the technical success rate was 100% and the angiographic restenosis rate at 6 months was 25%. Clinical follow-up demonstrated that 78% of their patients had stable or improved renal function, with a significant decrease in blood pressure and number of antihypertensive medications for the entire group.[41]

A randomized trial comparing balloon angioplasty versus stent placement in 85 patients with atherosclerotic renal artery stenosis and hypertension demonstrated a higher success rate and superior long-term patency rate with stent placement compared to balloon angioplasty.[42] At 6 months the angiographic restenosis rate for the balloon angioplasty group was 48% compared to only 14% (P < 0.01) for the stent group.

We have reported our experience in 100 consecutive patients with renovascular hypertension and lesions difficult to treat with balloon angioplasty alone.[32] Our patient population consisted predominantly of females (58%) with an overall mean age of 67 ± 10 years. All of the patients had poorly controlled hypertension (systolic ≥ 150 mmHg and/or diastolic > 90 mmHg) while taking at least two antihypertensive drugs. The average number of antihypertensive medications they were taking before renal stent placement was 2.6 ± 1.0. Renal artery stenosis (> 50% diameter stenosis) was bilateral in one-third (33%) and unilateral in one-third (67%), with five patients having a solitary kidney with renal artery stenosis.

The indications for stent placement in our series are shown in Figure 34.2 and include aorto-ostial lesions, failed angioplasty, and recurrent stenosis after prior balloon dilation. In total, 149 stents were placed in 133 arteries of 100 consecutive patients. Angiographic success (<30% residual diameter stenosis) was obtained in 99% (132/139) of arteries attempted (Figure 34.3). Clinical success, defined as normalization of the blood pressure on the same or fewer medications, occurred in 76% of the patients at the 6-month clinic visit. We were unable to withdraw medications in many

of the patients because of the concomitant presence of ischemic heart disease which required antianginal therapy.

One major complication, stent thrombosis 3 days following placement, occurred in this series. The patient was immediately taken to the catheterization laboratory and the occlusion reopened with balloon dilation. The renal artery remained patent at the 6-month follow-up angiogram. Several minor complications occurred. There were no renal artery perforations or need for emergency surgery in any patient. Two patients experienced transient contrast nephropathy which resolved without the need for dialysis. There were seven access site complications, including groin hematomas in five patients, one femoral pseudoaneurysm which resolved with ultrasound-guided compression, and one brachial artery occlusion which occurred following sheath removal and was resolved with a percutaneous balloon dilation from a femoral access site. One patient suffered a sudden cardiac death several days following stent implantation which was unrelated to the stent procedure.

At the 6-month follow-up, there continued to be a statistically significant improvement in blood pressure control (Figure 34.4), the average number of antihypertensive medications per patient was reduced from 2.6 ± 1.0 to 2.0 ± 0.9 ($P < 0.001$), and the angiographic restenosis rate (>50% diameter stenosis) was 18.8% (15/80) in the 67 patients undergoing follow-up angiography. Quantitative angiographic analysis of the restenosis lesions demonstrated that the only procedural variable associated with angiographic restenosis was the immediate post-stent minimal lumen

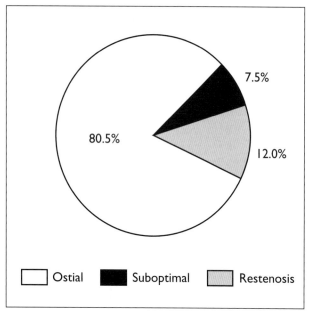

Figure 34.2
Pie chart showing the indication for stent placement (n=133).

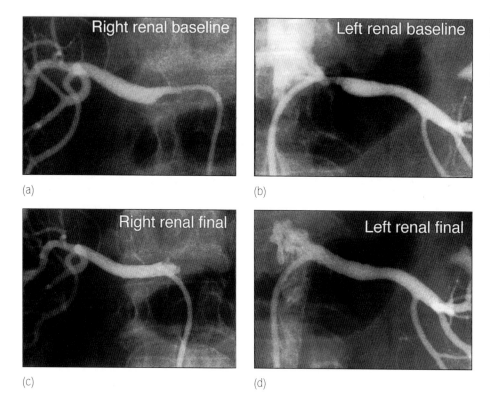

(a)　　　　　(b)

(c)　　　　　(d)

Figure 34.3
Baseline angiogram showing significant lesions in proximal right (a) and left (b) renal arteries. (c, d) following stent placement.

diameter (MLD). We found that the post-stent MLD following stent placement was significantly higher in the patients with continued patency (4.9 ± 0.9 mm) than in those with angiographic restenosis (4.3 ± 0.7 mm, $P = 0.025$). We identified a non-significant trend for higher systolic blood pressure in those patients with angiographic restenosis, but there was no difference in diastolic blood pressures.

Unstable angina and congestive heart failure

We have analyzed the results of renal artery stent placement in another group of 48 patients with unstable angina ($n = 23$) or congestive heart failure ($n = 25$) who had hypertension

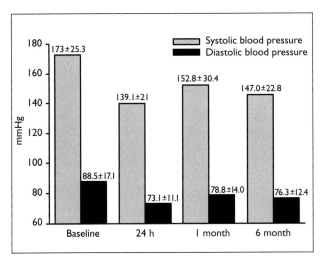

Figure 34.4
Blood pressure results at baseline, post-stent, and 6 months.

refractory to medical therapy and ≥ 70% stenosis of one ($n = 30$) or both ($n = 18$) renal arteries.[21] Results of renal artery stenting for each subgroup are shown in Table 34.2. For the entire cohort of patients, hypertension control was achieved within 24 h in 87% and a sustained benefit was seen in 74% at 6 months.

Preservation of renal function

In our series of 100 consecutive patients receiving renal stents for refractory hypertension, there were 44 patients with renal insufficiency (serum creatinine > 1.5 m/dL), with a mean serum creatinine of 2.4 ± 1.6 mg/dl.[32] There was no significant change in renal function following stent placement for the entire group. However, nine (22.5%) of the patients with renal failure did normalize their serum creatinine values (1.8 ± 0.1 to 1.4 ± 0.1 mg/dL) following successful stent placement.

A recent series showed that renal artery stent placement slowed the progression of renal artery stenosis in a group of patients with impaired renal function and atherosclerotic renal artery stenosis.[15] A group of 23 patients had their renal function analyzed by plotting the slopes of the reciprocal serum creatinine values before and after successful stent placement. The authors found that the progression of renal failure was significantly slowed after stent placement.

Conclusion

In patients with atherosclerotic cardiovascular disease and poorly controlled hypertension, the incidence of renal artery stenosis is higher than previously suspected and should be looked for in patients at increased risk (Table 34.1). A preponderance of the evidence suggests

Table 34.2	Outcome results for renal stents in hypertensive patients with unstable angina and congestive heart failure.					
	Unstable angina (n=23)			Heart failure (n=25)		
	Pre-stent	24 h	6 months	Pre-stent	24 h	6 months
Survival	–	100%	96%	–	100%	88%
Event-free	–	100%	96%	–	100%	84%
Sx improved	–	91%	82%	–	76%	75%
Functional class	3.1±0.7	1.5±0.8*	1.5±1.3*	3.2±0.8	1.8±0.9*	1.4±1.4*
SBP (mmHg)	176±24	133±20*	151±24*	163±31	128±19*	146±28*
DBP (mmHg)	90±13	70±11*	81±11	83±17	71±7*	75±15*
Serum Cr (mg%)	1.5±0.4	1.6±0.8	1.7±0.8	1.8±0.4	1.8±0.3	2.0±0.6

SBP, systolic blood pressure; DBP, diastolic blood pressure;
*, p < 0.05 at 24 h or 6 months versus pre-stent value.

that, in patients with renovascular hypertension that is poorly controlled with medical therapy, revascularization is the appropriate strategy. The current standard of practice, supported by randomized trials, suggests that in selected patients stent placement is superior to balloon angioplasty.[42] The advantage of endovascular stents over balloon angioplasty alone is their ability to scaffold the lumen of the renal artery to defeat the elastic recoil of the dilated lesion. This is particularly important for the aorto-ostial lesions, in which elastic recoil is difficult for balloons to overcome.[43]

Percutaneous revascularization of renal arterial obstructive disease has been dramatically enhanced by the addition of vascular stents to the interventionalist's armamentarium. Stent placement enhances both the safety and long-term efficacy of percutaneous revascularization compared to balloon angioplasty alone, but requires a higher level of operator skill to achieve optimal results.

Surgical revascularization of atherosclerotic renal artery stenosis is an effective treatment for renovascular hypertension.[22] However, renovascular surgery is associated with the morbidity and hospital stay of a major operation as well as complications including bypass graft thrombosis and nephrectomy in up to 4% and operative mortality rates of up to 3%.[44,45]

We successfully placed stents in lesions which are difficult to treat successfully and durably with balloon angioplasty alone.[32] Our patients were not randomized, so we cannot directly compare our results to balloon angioplasty alone; however, given the historically poor results in this group of lesions, we did not believe we could ethically randomize our patients to balloon angioplasty versus stent placement.

Our experience with renal stenting in patients with renovascular hypertension and refractory unstable angina or congestive heart failure is also very encouraging.[21] These patients were unmanageable with medical therapy alone. The placement of renal stents successfully reduced their afterload and allowed these patients to be managed medically.

Improvement or stabilization of renal function appears to be possible with intervention in patients with atherosclerotic renal artery stenosis. The goals of therapy include reversing the relentless regression of the renal artery stenosis and preservation of renal function. In our series of patients with renovascular hypertension, the initial benefit in blood pressure reduction was sustained in the majority of patients, with a reduction in the number of antihypertensive medications required to control blood pressure. The 6-month restenosis rate was <20%, which is a marked improvement over the reported restenosis rates for balloon angioplasty in atherosclerotic lesions. In conclusion, when considering the treatment strategies for renal artery stenosis causing medically refractory hypertension, the percutaneous placement of renal artery stents is the treatment of choice in selected patients.

Acknowledgement

I would like to express my appreciation to Mr Mario Vaz for assistance in the preparation of the manuscript and to Mr James O'Meara for design and preparation of the graphics.

References

1   Simon N, Franklin SS, Bleifer KH et al. Clinical characteristics of renovascular hypertension. *JAMA* 1972; **220**: 1209–18.

2   Jacobsen HR. Ischemic renal disease: an overlooked clinical entity? *Kidney Int* 1988; **34**: 729–43.

3   Eyler WR, Clark GJ, Rian RL et al. Angiography of the renal areas including a comparative study of renal arterial stenosis with and without hypertension. *Radiology* 1962; **78**: 879–92.

4   Jean WJ, Al-Bittar I, Xwicke DL et al. High incidence of renal artery stenosis in patients with coronary artery disease. *Cathet Cardiovasc Diagn* 1994; **32**: 8–10.

5   Olin JW, Melia M, Young JR et al. Prevalence of atherosclerosis renal artery stenosis in patients with atherosclerosis elsewhere. *Am J Med* 1990; **88**: 46N–51N.

6   Harding MB, Smith LR, Himmelstein SI et al. Renal artery stenosis: prevalence and associated risk factors in patients undergoing routine cardiac catheterization. *J Am Soc Nephrol* 1992; **2**: 1608–16.

7   Valentine RJ, Clagett GP, Miller GL et al. The coronary risk of unsuspected renal artery stenosis. *J Vasc Surg* 1993; **18**: 433–40.

8   O'Neil EA, Hansen KJ, Canzanello VJ et al. Prevalence of ischemic nephropathy in patients with renal insufficiency. *Am Surg* 1992; **58**: 485–90.

9   Meany TF, Dustan HP, Novick AC. Natural history of renal arterial disease. *Radiology* 1968; **9**: 877–87.

10 Greco BA, Breyer JA. The natural history of renal artery stenosis: who should be evaluated for suspected ischemic nephropathy? *Semin Neph* 1996; **16**: 2–11.

11 Schreiber MJ, Pohl MA, Novick AC. The natural history of atherosclerotic and fibrous renal artery disease. *Urol Clin North Am* 1984; **11**: 383–92.

12 Wollenweber J, Sheps SG, Davis GD. Clinical course of atherosclerotic renovascular disease. *Am J Cardiol* 1968; **21**: 60–71.

13 Zierler RE, Bergelin ROP, Isaacson JA et al. Natural history of atherosclerotic renal artery stenosis: a prospective study with duplex ultrasonography. *J Vasc Surg* 1994; **19**: 250–8.

14 Dean RH, Kieffer RW, Smith BM et al. Renovascular hypertension: anatomic and renal function changes during drug therapy. *Arch Surg* 1981; **116**: 1408–15.

15 Harden PN, MacLeod MJ, Rodger RSC et al. Effect of renal artery stenting on progression of renovascular renal failure. *Lancet* 1997; **349**: 1133–6.

16 Novick AC, Pohl MA, Schreiber M et al. Revascularization for preservation of renal function in patients with atherosclerotic renovascular disease. *J Urol* 1983; **129**: 907–12.

17 Kaylor WM, Novick AC, Ziegelbaum M et al. Reversal of end stage renal failure with surgical revascularization in patients with atherosclerotic renal artery occlusion. *J Urol* 1989; **141**: 486–8.

18   Pickering TG, Devereux RB, James GD et al. Recurrent pulmonary edema in hypertension due to bilateral renal artery stenosis: treatment by angioplasty or surgical revascularisation. *Lancet* 1988; **2**: 551–2.

19   Messina LM, Zelenock GB, Yao KA et al. Renal revascularizatiron for recurrent pulmonary edema in patients with poorly controlled hypertension and renal insufficiency: a distinct subgroup of patients with arteriosclerotic renal artery occlusive disease. *J Vasc Surg* 1992; **15**: 73–82.

20   Tami LF, McElderry MW, al-Adli NM et al. Renal artery stenosis presenting as crescendo angina pectoris. *Cath Cardiovasc Diagn* 1995; **35**: 252–6.

21   Khosla S, White CJ, Collins TJ et al. Effects of renal artery stent implantation in patients with renovascular hypertension presenting with unstable angina or congestive heart failure. *Am J Cardiol* 1997; **80**: 363–6.

22   Scoble JE. Is the 'wait-and-see' approach justified in atherosclerotic renal artery stenosis? *Nephrol Dial Trans* 1995; **4**: 588–9.

23   Pickering TG. Diagnosis and evaluation of renovascular hypertension. *Circulation* 1991; **83**(suppl 1): I-147–I-154).

24   Fommei E, Ghione S, Palla L et al. Renal scintigraphic captopril test in the diagnosis of renovascular hypertension. *Hypertension* 1987; **10**: 212–20.

25   Vaughan ED Jr, Buhler FR, Laragh JH et al. Renovascular hypertension; renin measurements to indicate hypersecretion and contralateral suppression, estimate renal plasma flow, and score for surgical curability. *Am J Med* 1973; **55**: 402–14.

26   Olbricht CJ, Paul K, Prokop M et al. Minimally invasive diagnosis of renal artery stenosis by spiral computed tomography angiography. *Kidney Int* 1995; **48**: 1332–7.

27   Rubin GD. Spiral (helical) CT of the renal vasculature. *Semin Ultrasound CT MR* 1996; **17**: 374–97.

28   Kim D, Edelman RR, Kent KC et al. Abdominal aorta and renal artery stenosis: evaluation with MR angiography. *Radiology* 1990; **174**: 727–31.

29   Bakker J, Beek FJ, Beutler JJ et al. Renal artery stenosis and accessory renal arteries: accuracy of detection and visualization with gadolinium-enhanced breath-hold MR angiography. *Radiology* 1998; **207**: 497–504.

30   De Cobelli F, Vanzulli A, Sironi S et al. Renal artery stenosis: evaluation with breath-hold, three-dimensional, dynamic, gadolinium-enhanced versus three-dimensional, phase-contrast MR angiography. *Radiology* 1997; **207**: 689–95.

31   Olin JW, Piedmonte MR, Young JR et al. The utility of duplex ultrasound scanning of the renal arteries for diagnosing significant renal artery stenosis. *Ann Intern Med* 1995; **122**: 833–8.

32   White CJ, Ramee SR, Collins TJ et al. Renal artery stent placement: utility in difficult lesions for balloon angioplasty. *J Am Coll Cardiol* 1997; **30**: 1445–50.

33   Archibald GR, Beckmann CF, Libertino JA. Focal renal artery stenosis caused by fibromuscular dysplasia: treatment by percutaneous transluminal angioplasty. *Am J Radiol* 1988; **151**: 593–6.

34   Cluzel P, Raynaud A, Beyssen B et al. Stenosis of renal branch arteries in fibromuscular dysplasia: results of percutaneous transluminal angioplasty. *Radiology* 1994; **193**: 227–32.

35   van Jaarsveld BC, Krijnen P, Pieterman H et al. The effect of balloon angioplasty on hypertension in atherosclerotic renal artery stenosis. *N Engl J Med* 2000; **342**: 1007–14.

36   Losinno F, Zuccala A, Busato F et al. Renal artery angioplasty for renovascular hypertension and preservation of renal function: long-term angiographic and clinical follow-up. *Am J Radiol* 1994; **162**: 853–7.

37   Weibull H, Bergqvist D, Bergentz SE et al. Percutaneous transluminal angioplasty versus reconstruction of atherosclerotic renal artery stenosis: prospective randomized study. *J Vasc Surg* 1993; **18**: 841–52.

38   Martin LG, Cork RD, Kaufman SL. Long-term results of angioplasty in 110 patients with renal artery stenosis. *J Vasc Intervent Radiol* 1992; **3**: 619–26.

39   Weibull H, Bregqvist D, Jonsson K et al. Long term results after percutaneous transluminal angioplasty of atherosclerotic renal artery stenosis: the importance of intensive follow up. *Eur J Vasc Surg* 1991; **5**: 291–301.

40   Dorros G, Prince C, Mathiak L. Stenting of a renal artery stenosis achieves better relief of the obstructive lesion than balloon angioplasty. *Cathet Cardiovasc Diagn* 1993; **29**: 191–8.

41   Dorros G, Jaff M, Jain A et al. Follow-up of primary Palmaz–Schatz stent placement for atherosclerotic renal artery stenosis. *Am J Cardiol* 1995; **75**: 1051–5.

42   van de Ven PJ, Kaatee R, Beutler JJ et al. Arterial stenting and balloon angioplasty in ostial atherosclerotic renovascular disease: a randomised trial. *Lancet* 1999; **353**: 282–6.

43   Rensing BJ, Hermans WRM, Beatt KH et al. Quantitative angiographic assessment of elastic recoil after percutaneous transluminal coronary angioplasty. *Am J Cardiol* 1990; **66** 1039–44.

44   Hansen KJ, Starr SM, Sands E et al. Contemporary surgical management of renovascular disease. *J Vasc Surg* 1992; **16**: 319–31.

45   Novick AC, Ziegelbaum M, Vidt DG et al. Trends in surgical revascularization for renal artery disease: ten years experience. *JAMA* 1987; **257**: 498–501.

35

Protected renal angioplasty and stenting with the PercuSurge device

Michel Henry, Isabelle Henry, Christos Klonaris and Michèle Hugel

Introduction

Endovascular treatment of atherosclerotic renal artery stenosis is now a well-accepted alternative for renal artery revascularization.[1,2] This method has been proposed as a standard of care for non-ostial renal artery lesions and, although initial studies concerning the treatment of ostial lesions yield varying results,[3,4] recent series suggest that their management with vascular endoprostheses is highly effective.[5-9] However, a post-procedural deterioration in renal function in a subset of patients represents an important complication associated with this technique.[10-12] Atheroembolism during the steps of the procedure has been implicated as a precipitating factor for this complication.[13-15] In order to eliminate the risk of atheroembolic material being flushed into the renal parenchyma, we applied a novel technique consisting of balloon angioplasty and stenting with distal balloon protection followed by debris aspiration, a concept currently being utilized in aorto-coronary saphenous vein graft restenosis and carotid artery angioplasty.[16]

Materials and methods

From January 1999 to June 2000, 32 renal artery atherosclerotic stenoses in 28 patients were treated with percutaneous transluminal angioplasty and stenting under balloon protection using the PercuSurge Guardwire™ system (PercuSurge Inc., Sunnyvale, CA). All patients had hypertension and/or renal insufficiency. All had a diagnostic renal duplex scan and digital subtraction arteriography performed prior to the intervention. Due to the current available dimensions of the protection balloon, patients with a renal artery diameter larger than 6 mm were excluded from this study. Patient demographics, risk factors, associated coronary, carotid or other peripheral arterial disease, the existence of diffuse atherosclerotic aortic disease, blood pressure, and serum creatinine values were recorded. Written informed consent was obtained from all patients.

Description of the protection device

The PercuSurge Guardwire™ system consists of three main components (Figures 35.1 and 35.2):

1. The Guardwire temporary occlusion catheter is a 0.014-inch or 0.018-inch hollow tube angioplasty wire constructed of nitinol. Incorporated into its distal segment is an inflatable compliant elastomeric balloon capable of occluding vessel outflow. A marker shows the location of the balloon. The diameter of the balloon (5 or 6 mm) is chosen depending on the diameter of the artery. The distal 3.5 cm of the wire is floppy and shapable. The wire

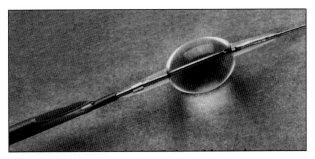

Figure 35.1
Export™ aspiration catheter mounted on GuardWire™ temporary occlusion catheter.

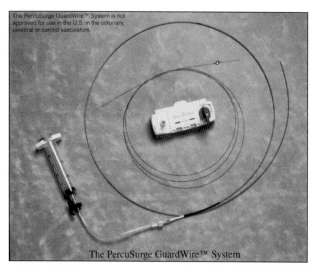

Figure 35.2
The PercuSurge GuardWire™ system.

is available in lengths of 190 cm and 300 cm, allowing 'monorail' or 'over the wire' techniques for angioplasty and stenting.

2. The proximal end of the hypotube wire incorporates a Microseal™, which allows inflation and deflation of the distal occlusion balloon. The device keeps the elastomeric balloon inflated to protect the kidney from atheroembolism during the maneuvers of the procedure and at same time allows catheter exchange at the proximal end, similar to commonly used guide wires.

3. The Export™ aspiration catheter is placed over the shaft of the Guardwire to aspirate the debris generated by the procedure prior to distal balloon deflation. Its external diameter is 5.2F and aspiration occurs through a 1 mm side-hole. This catheter is tapered to the Guidewire to avoid the risk of debris generation or stent dislodgment during its advancement into the renal artery.

Angioplasty and stenting technique (Figure 35.3)

Using the femoral approach, an 8F guiding catheter was initially placed at the ostium of the renal artery. In cases of subocclusive tight lesions or in cases with an acute angle between the aorta and the renal artery, a coaxial technique with a 5F Simmons-type selective catheter placed inside the guiding catheter was used to catheterize the renal artery. The lesion was then crossed with a coronary 0.014-inch wire and the guiding catheter was slowly advanced at the renal ostium, over the Simmons catheter. Then, the coronary wire and the Simmons catheter were both removed. The Guardwire was

then carefully advanced across the lesion and the marker of the protection balloon placed 2 or 3 cm beyond it. The Microseal™ adapter was attached and the occlusion balloon inflated to occlude the renal artery. On detaching the adapter, the occlusion balloon remained inflated. Balloon angioplasty was then performed for the non ostial lesions ($n = 3$) and predilatation with a 4–5 mm angioplasty balloon in 15 ostial lesions. In these 18 cases, subsequent stenting was performed after the guiding catheter had been advanced into the renal artery, sliding over the shaft of the angioplasty balloon, in order to facilitate safe stent placement and avoid dislodgment of debris. In the remaining 14 ostial lesions, direct stenting without predilation was chosen because the guiding catheter could easily slide over a selective Simmons-type catheter and the stent could safely be placed in the right position. For ostial lesions, care was given to the position of the stent, which should slightly protrude approximately 1–2 mm into the aortic lumen. The proximal part of the stent was afterwards redilated with a balloon of 1 mm larger diameter. After stent deployment, the aspiration catheter was advanced over the wire to the level of the lesion and close to the protection balloon, and any debris generated was sucked out using a 20 ml syringe connected to the proximal end of this catheter.

The aspirated blood was subsequently sent to the laboratory for analysis. The aspiration catheter was then removed. The Microseal adapter was reattached to the Guardwire™ and the occlusion balloon was deflated, allowing normal vessel flow. If the angiographic result was satisfactory, the device was removed.

Definitions

Ostial lesions were defined as stenoses greater than 50% of the diameter of the renal artery within 5 mm of the aortic lumen, as assessed by arteriography.[9] Immediate technical success was defined as residual stenosis less than 30% of the reference diameter, as measured by quantitative angiographic analysis without significant periprocedural complications. Inability to successfully place the PercuSurge Guardwire at the right position to protect the kidney throughout the procedure was considered failure of the device. Duplex criteria for restenosis were a loss of the early systolic notch and a systolic velocity > 1.5 m/s. The angiographic criterion for restenosis was the development of luminal narrowing > 50% of the reference diameter. Reversal of hypertension was defined as diastolic blood pressure ≤ 90 mmHg and no need for any medication. Improvement corresponded to a diastolic pressure of 91–109 mmHg with at least a 15% decrease from the preprocedural level or a diastolic pressure of 91–109 mmHg, a decline of at least 10% from the preprocedural level, and withdrawal of at least one drug from the treatment regimen.[17] Baseline serum creatinine values between 1.5 mg/dl and 1.9 mg/dl and ≥ 2.0 mg/dl represented moderate and severe

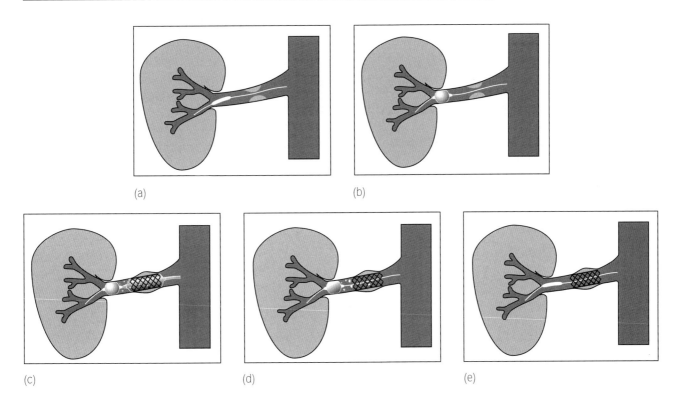

(a)   (b)

(c)   (d)   (e)

Figure 35.3
(a) The Guardwire temporary occlusion balloon-on-a-wire catheter has crossed the lesion. (b) The distal protection balloon is inflated, occluding arterial flow, to protect the renal parenchyma from atheroembolism during the procedure. (c) During balloon angioplasty or stent deployment, generated debris is collected proximal to the balloon. (d) The Export catheter is advanced over the Guardwire to aspirate the debris. (e) The balloon is deflated and withdrawn. Angiographic control follows.

renal insufficiency respectively.[9,18] A decrease of more than 0.2 mg/dl from preprocedural creatinine values represented an improvement, whereas values within ± 0.2 mg/dl of baseline were considered unchanged, and an increase of > 0.2 mg/dl was considered as a deterioration in renal function.[18] Determination of vessel diameter was made by sizing the guiding catheter against the normal vessel distal to the lesion using quantitative analysis.

Continuous data are presented as mean ± SD and categorical data as percentages. Statistical differences between groups were determined by the Student's t-test. Statistical significance was taken at $p < 0.05$. All calculations were performed with the SPSS Program (SPSS version 7.5, Chicago, IL).

Periprocedural management and follow-up

All procedures were performed under local anesthesia and intravenous sedation. An intravenous bolus of 5000 units of unfractionated heparin and 3 mg of cefamandole nitrate were routinely administered at the beginning of the procedure.

Postprocedural drug regimen included aspirin (100 mg/day) indefinitely and ticlopidine (250–500 mg/day) or clopidogrel (75 mg/day) for 1 month. Patients remained in the hospital for 48 hours to monitor serum creatinine levels and adjust blood pressure medications. A renal duplex scan was scheduled at 6 and 12 months and then annually and angiography at 6 months or when restenosis was suspected on the basis of positive clinical and duplex scan findings. Serum creatinine values were measured before and after the procedure at day 1, 30, at 6 months, and thereafter every 6 months.

Results

Immediate results

Thirty-two renal artery angioplasties and stenting were performed under balloon protection (15 right, 17 left) using the PercuSurge system in 28 patients (18 males, 10 females, mean age 71.3 ± 8.6 years, range 49–87 years). Bilateral lesions were treated as a part of the same procedure. All patients were hypertensive. Sixteen patients had normal renal function (serum creatinine ≤ 1.4 mg/dl), 10 had moderate renal insufficiency, and 2 had severe renal dysfunction. Renal artery stenosis was located at the ostium in 29 cases (91%); the mean percentage diameter stenosis was 81.6 ± 8.5%, range 70–95%. Mean lesion length was 12.1 ± 3.9 mm, range 10–29 mm. The diameter of the artery was estimated at 6 mm in 21 cases and 5 mm in 11 cases. Nineteen patients (68%) had diffuse, severe atherosclerosis of the abdominal aorta. Five patients (18%) had diabetes mellitus, 20 (71%) were current smokers, and 14 (50%) had hyperlipidemia. Associated coronary artery disease was found in 16 (57%), cerebrovascular disease in 8 (29%) and peripheral arterial disease in 14 (50%) patients.

All procedures were performed by a femoral approach according to the technique described above. All stenoses were easily crossed with the Guardwire. All ostial lesions were treated with stent placement. In the 3 non-ostial lesions, stent placement was necessary because of unsatisfactory angioplasty results (significant residual stenosis). In these cases, we had to reinflate the protection balloon and to perform a new aspiration after stent deployment. For ostial lesions, predilatation was performed in 15 cases and direct stent deployment in the remaining 14 lesions. In all cases, stents were advanced and placed at the deployment site while protected with the guiding catheter. Thirty-six balloon-expandable stents of different types were implanted: 14 AVE, 6 Palmaz, 12 Herculink, and 4 Corinthian stents. We were familiar with each of these stent types used; no specific selection criteria were applied. Four patients received 2 stents in the same artery to treat a long lesion. Technical success was obtained for all arteries with good stent deployment, no significant residual stenosis, and complete covering of the lesion (Figure 35.4). Mean time of renal artery occlusion was 6.58 ± 2.52 min (2.29–13.17 min). When stents were deployed primarily, mean occlusion time was 5.02 ± 1.53 min. In cases of predilatation and subsequent stenting, mean occlusion time was 7.57 ± 2.48 min ($p = 0.015$).

After angioplasty and stenting procedures, aspiration was routinely performed, allowing removal of visible particles in all patients (Figure 35.5). The aspirated blood samples were analyzed and studied by optic and electron microscopic techniques (Figure 35.6). Different particles were isolated and identified. Their number varied from 13 to 208 per procedure (mean: 98.1 ± 60) and diameter varied from 38 to 6206 μm (mean: 201.25 ± 76.2 μm). Excluding the 6.2 mm fragment, which may skew the mean value, the mean diameter was 188 ± 49.8 μm. In cases of direct stenting, the mean number of extracted particles per procedure was 112 ± 73.5. When predilatation of the lesion was performed, the mean number was 86 ± 47 ($p = 0.36$). Also, we did not notice a significant statistical difference between the mean diameters of the particles according to the use of a direct approach of stenting or after predilatation (190 ± 44.5 μm vs 210 ± 96 μm, respectively, $p = 0.56$). For the 3 non-ostial lesions, aspiration was performed both after angioplasty and after stenting, and more particles were collected with the second aspiration (64 vs 79.5). The particles were atheromatous plaques, cholesterol crystals, necrotic cores, fibrin, thrombi, platelets, and macrophage foam cells.

One patient developed an arterial spasm at the site of the protection balloon which immediately responded to local vasodilation therapy. Additionally, a puncture-site hematoma was seen with no further consequences.

Follow-up

The mean follow-up period was 6.7 ± 2.9 months (range 2–17 months); in all cases, follow-up was beyond the period required for the development of clinical manifestations of atheroembolism. No deterioration of renal function in any

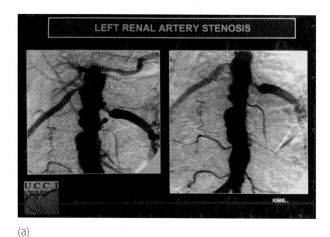

(a)

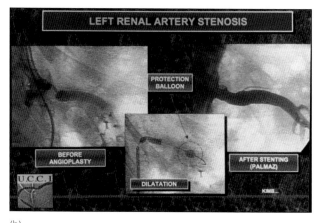

(b)

Figure 35.4

(a) Bilateral ostial renal artery stenosis in a patient with hypertension and renal insufficiency. (b) Left renal artery angioplasty and stenting (Palmaz stent) under protection with the PercuSurge device.

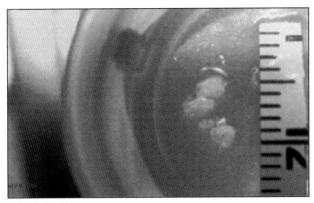

Figure 35.5
(a) Visible debris removed with CL Aspiration catheter.

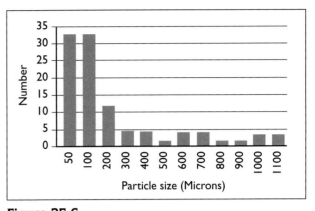

Figure 35.6
(b) Distribution of the aspirated particles in one patient after electron microscopic analysis.

patient was observed. The mean creatinine value was 1.34 ± 0.35 mg/dl preprocedurally ($n = 28$), 1.22 ± 0.36 mg/dl at 24 hours ($n = 28$), 1.35 ± 0.43 mg/dl at 1 month ($n = 28$), and 1.24 ± 0.30 mg/dl at 6 months ($n = 20$). Five patients with baseline renal insufficiency had improvement at 6 months after the procedure. Concerning the effects of the procedure on hypertension, 4 patients were cured (14.3%), 15 improved (53.6%) and 9 remained unchanged (32.1%). Systolic blood pressure dropped from 167 ± 15.2 mmHg to 154.7 ± 12.3 mmHg after the procedure in this group of patients. The mean reduction in systolic blood pressure was 12.3 ± 9.5 mmHg, range $7.4–17.3$ mmHg ($p = 0.001$). Diastolic blood pressure dropped from 103 ± 12 mmHg to 93.2 ± 6.8 mmHg after the procedure; mean reduction in diastolic blood pressure was 10.3 ± 8.6 mmHg, range $5.9–14.7$ mmHg ($p = 0.001$). The number of medications in this group also dropped from 2.17 ± 0.8 to 1.17 ± 0.7 per patient; mean reduction was 1 ± 0.7 per patient. One patient died 3 days after the procedure from myocardial infarction. This patient underwent coronary angioplasties of the circumflex and left anterior descending arteries 3 days before.

One patient developed a bilateral restenosis at 6 months, treated by new percutaneous transluminal angioplasty (PTA) with success.

Discussion

In recent years, PTA techniques have become the cornerstone of therapeutic strategy for renal artery stenosis. The goals of endovascular management are the improvement in the control or, ideally, normalization of blood pressure and stabilization or improvement of renal function.

Summarized results of recent publications[8–11,18–21] regarding the effects of angioplasty or stenting on renal function show that a large percentage of patients seem to benefit from the procedure. However, in many of these series, even after successful initial technical results, a decline in renal function was noted in a subset of patients. In a prospective study, Dorros et al.[10] reported the results of primary stent placement for atherosclerotic renal artery stenosis in 76 patients with 6-months follow-up. Serum creatinine values improved in 30%, remained unchanged in 48%, and deteriorated in 22% of the patients. In a later study[18] including 141 patients with 6-months follow-up, they reported that renal function had stabilized or improved in two-thirds of unilateral stenosis patients, whereas one-third of patients had an increase in their creatinine of > 2.0 mg/dl above baseline. Lack of complete angiographic follow-up limited their understanding of the worsening of renal function in patients with normal baseline creatinine after successful revascularization. Recently, Isles et al.[11] published a review of 10 studies, including 416 stent placement procedures in 379 patients treated for renal artery stenosis. Although technical success was high in all studies (96–100%), renal function improved in 26%, stabilized in 48%, and deteriorated in 26% of the patients.

Many factors may account for this deterioration: contrast media-induced nephrotoxicity, progression of concomitant nephrosclerosis, restenosis of the renal artery, and atheroembolism during the procedure.[10] It should be appreciated that the majority of the above factors are iatrogenic in origin.[22] Consequently, proper patient selection, application of strict indications for intervention, meticulous techniques, and adequate follow-up are of paramount importance. Although many efforts have been made towards more effective and safer endovascular procedures for renal artery stenosis, little attention has been given to the detrimental effects of atheroembolism on renal function. This entity is caused by the release of microscopic plaque fragments and cholesterol crystals from the renal artery lesion or the atherosclerotic aorta into parenchymal renal vasculature during the procedure.[22–25] Instrument manipulation in the aorta and renal arteries can result in detachment and embolism of atheromatous debris from ulcerated plaques. The large size of the devices used, an increased length, or specific difficulties of the procedure may be promoting factors. There is also evidence that both oral and intravenous use of anticoagulants and thrombolytic drugs can induce atheroembolism.[26,27]

The true incidence of atheroembolism is uncertain because many patients can have a silent course due to the large functional kidney reserve, which allows for normal serum creatinine values despite a significant decline of total glomerular filtration. Therefore, only the most severe cases, especially patients with preprocedural renal dysfunction and limited functional reserve, may be detected. Clinical manifestations of the disease are nonspecific as well. Thadhani et al.[28] retrospectively evaluated 52 patients with both renal failure and histologically proven atheroembolism after angiography or cardiovascular surgery over a 10-year period. Within 30 days of their procedure, 50% of patients had cutaneous signs of atheroembolism and 14% had documented blood eosinophilia. Most patients reach a peak serum creatinine level over 3–8 weeks,[29] but onset is usually sooner.[12] Although proteinuria and nephrotic syndrome are uncommon, Haggie et al.[29] reported 4 patients with documented histopathological atheroembolism who developed nephrotic-range proteinuria and suggested that atheroembolism should be considered in the differential diagnosis of nephrotic syndrome in elderly patients with serious vascular disease. Similar conclusions were made by Greenberg et al.,[30] after reviewing the clinical features and histological findings of 24 patients found to have cholesterol atheroembolism at renal biopsy. 19 of these patients had recently undergone an invasive vascular procedure.

Even in cases of clinical suspicion, the diagnosis of this complication is difficult to establish using routine laboratory tests. Renal biopsy is the only definite diagnostic tool, valuable to exclude other potentially treatable disease processes, but its routine application for confirmation of a disease amenable to supportive treatment only is problematic. For these reasons, it is not surprising that atheroembolism after renal artery interventions is often misdiagnosed as drug-induced nephrotoxicity or is attributed to the progression of nephrosclerosis.

Few studies have addressed the problem of atheroembolism after renal artery interventions. Interestingly, in all of them, this was the predominant complication. Boisclair et al.[12] published their results of stent placement in 33 patients either for immediate angioplasty failure or recurrent stenosis. They reported immediate technical success in all cases. However, 7 patients developed complications, including 4 renal artery emboli. In another study, Van de Ven et al.[13] reported that after successful immediate revascularization with stents in 24 patients with an atherosclerotic ostial renal artery stenosis, 2 patients

developed renal insufficiency due to cholesterol embolism. Also, Wilms et al.[15] reported 2 cases of renal deterioration in a group of 11 patients after stent-supported renal angioplasty, including a case of massive cholesterol embolism.

Renal atheroembolism definitely poses a risk of renal function deterioration and decreased survival in patients undergoing endovascular procedures for renal artery stenosis. Due to the increasing number of such patients being treated, the cost of renal function deterioration and subsequent end-stage renal disease with need for dialysis represents a significant long-term problem. Its importance is clearly demonstrated in a recent work by Krishnamurthi et al.[31] who evaluated its impact on survival in 44 patients who had surgery for atherosclerotic renal artery stenosis and concomitant intraoperative renal biopsy for detection of atheroemboli. Atheroembolic disease was identified in the biopsy specimens in 16 patients (36%) and correlated significantly with decreased survival. The 5-year survival in this group was 54% versus 85% in patients without atheroembolism ($p = 0.011$).

In order to avoid the occurrence of atheroembolic events during renal interventions, one should emphasize that the procedure should be as atraumatic as possible, with utilization of small devices and adaptation of coronary angioplasty techniques. Recently, Feldman et al.,[32] recognizing the risk of atheroembolism, reported their 'no-touch' technique consisting of placing a second 0.035-inch J wire within the guiding catheter during cannulation of the renal artery to prevent the tip of the catheter from rubbing the aortic wall in an effort to minimize its contact with atherosclerotic plaques and reduce the potential for embolization. Beyond these technical considerations, in our efforts to eliminate this complication, we applied the concept of protected renal angioplasty and stenting. Our results show stabilization or improvement of renal function with no case of deterioration. This may well be attributed to the utilization of the protection system during the intervention. It is very important that visible atherosclerotic debris were extracted in all cases. In one case, we removed a fragment measuring 6.2 mm at its maximum diameter, a size large enough to produce a macroembolism or even a renal artery occlusion.

In our study, protected renal angioplasty and stenting seems to have the same effect on hypertension as that of renal angioplasty and stenting without protection:[33] significant decreases in systolic and diastolic blood pressure, easier blood pressure control, and reduction in the number of antihypertensive medications. Larger randomized studies are needed to confirm these observations.

The absence of renal deterioration after protected renal angioplasty and stenting could influence the long-term prognosis of hypertension. Further studies and long-term follow-up studies are needed to appreciate the impact of the maintenance of renal function on hypertension.

Although in this small series of patients no device-related complications occurred, adding another device to the procedure, trying to prevent complications, could potentially create new problems. The potential of renal artery thrombosis during protection balloon inflation and flow occlusion is negligible, since the patients are under heparin and antiplatelet therapy and the duration of the occlusion is usually short – less than the time required to perform the distal anastomosis of a conventional aorto-renal bypass. One could also state that there is a potential increased risk for distal atheroembolism by the application of this technique, since the generated debris could be directed into the lower extremities. To reduce the risk of this complication, debris was removed by aspiration alone and flushing of the treated area not performed. The predetermined volume capacity of the balloon in order to reach its final diameter of 5–6 mm and its compliant nature eliminate the risk of renal artery dissection. Inability to deflate the protection balloon after stenting is a possible but rare scenario; however, it could be easily managed by cutting the Guardwire distally to the Microseal adapter segment. We have faced this complication once, during our ongoing study on protected carotid interventions with the same device.

To facilitate balloon withdrawal and prevent it from getting caught on the stent, the guiding catheter was routinely advanced into the stent to its distal extremity. One should also remember that this technique does not protect the kidney from atheroembolism during attempts to initially catheterize the renal artery and cross the lesion. Finally, the additional cost of the protection device must be balanced with its potential benefit.

The rationale for protected renal artery angioplasty and stenting is similar to that of brain protection during angioplasty of the carotid arteries. This technique, based on the pioneering work of Theron et al.,[34] is being applied by multiple groups to prevent stroke. Our concept was that the same technique could be suitable in the management of renal artery stenosis, mitigating the risk of atheroembolism. To our knowledge, this is the first study that presents the results of protected angioplasty for renal artery interventions.

This study raises a number of questions that remain unanswered. Is this technique indicated for all patients undergoing endovascular treatment for renal artery stenosis or should it be limited to those with pronounced aortic atherosclerosis or with ostial renal artery lesions? Is there any role for intravascular ultrasound in this arena? Should its applicability be restricted to patients with baseline renal insufficiency? In this study the feasibility and safety of balloon-protected renal angioplasty and stenting in the prevention of renal atheroembolism have been demonstrated in a small cohort. Larger randomized trials are needed to definitively address the utility of this approach and to better document its beneficial effect on renal function, and, maybe, on hypertension and its long-term prognosis.

References

1 Novick AC. Options for therapy of ischemic nephropathy: role of angioplasty and surgery. *Semin Nephrol* 1996; **16**: 53–60.

2 Zuccala A, Zucchelli P. Ischemic nephoropathy: diagnosis and treatment. *J Nephrol* 1998; **11**: 318–24.

3 Klinge J, Mali WP, Puijlaert CB et al. Percutaneous transluminal renal angioplasty: initial and long-term results. *Radiology* 1989; **171**: 501–6.

4 Canzanello VJ, Millan VG, Spiegel JE et al. Percutaneous transluminal renal angioplasty in management of atherosclerotic renovascular hypertension: results in 100 patients. *Hypertension* 1989; **13**: 163–72.

5 Sos TA, Pickering TG, Sniderman K et al. Percutaneous transluminal renal angioplasty in renovascular hypertension due to atheroma or fibromuscular hyperplasia. *N Engl J Med* 1983; **309**: 274–9.

6 Van de Ven PJ, Kaatee R, Beutler JJ et al. Arterial stenting and balloon angioplasty in ostial atherosclerotic renovascular disease: a randomized trial. *Lancet* 1999; **353**: 282–6.

7 Henry M, Amor M, Henry I et al. Stents in the treatment of renal artery stenosis: long-term follow-up. *J Endovasc Surg* 1999; **6**: 42–51.

8 Henry M, Amor M, Henry I et al. Stent placement in the renal artery: three-year experience with the Palmaz stent. *J Vasc Interv Radiol* 1996; **7**: 343–50.

9 Blum U, Krumme B, Flugel P et al. Treatment of ostial renal artery stenoses with vascular endoprostheses after unsuccessful balloon angioplasty. *N Engl J Med* 1997; **336**: 459–65.

10 Dorros G, Jaff M, Jain A et al. Follow-up of primary Palmaz–Schatz stent placement for atherosclerotic renal artery stenosis. *Am J Cardiol* 1995; **75**: 1051–5.

11 Isles CG, Robertson S, Hill D. Management of renovascular disease: a review of renal artery stenting in ten studies. *QJM* 1999; **92**: 159–67.

12 Boisclair C, Therasse E, Oliva VL et al. Treatment of renal angioplasty failure by percutaneous renal artery stenting with Palmaz stents: midterm technical and clinical results. *Am J Roentgenol* 1997; **168**: 245–51.

13 Van de Ven PJ, Beutler JJ, Kaatee R et al. Transluminal vascular stent for ostial atherosclerotic renal artery stenosis. *Lancet* 1995; **346**: 672–4.

14 Wilms G, Staessen J, Baert AL et al. Percutaneous transluminal renal angioplasty and renal function. *Radiology* 1989; **29**: 195–200.

15 Wilms GE, Peene PT, Baert AL et al. Renal artery stent placement with use of the Wallstent endoprosthesis. *Radiology* 1991; **179**: 457–62.

16 Henry M, Amor M, Henry I et al. Carotid stenting with cerebral protection. First clinical experience using the PercuSurge Guardwire system. *J Endov Surg* 1999; **6**: 321–31.

17 Standards of Practice Committee of the Society of Cardiovascular and Interventional Radiology. Guidelines for percutaneous transluminal angioplasty. *Radiology* 1990; **177**: 619–26.

18 Dorros G, Jaff M, Mathiak L et al. Four-year follow-up of Palmaz–Schatz stent revascularization as treatment for atherosclerotic renal artery stenosis. *Circulation* 1998; **98**: 642–7.

19 Taylor A, Sheppard D, Macleod MJ et al. Renal artery stent placement in renal artery stenosis: technical and early clinical results. *Clin Radiol* 1997; **52**: 451–7.

20 Paulsen D, Klow NE, Rogstad B et al. Preservation of renal function by percutaneous transluminal angioplasty in ischaemic renal disease. *Nephrol Dial Transplant* 1999; **14**: 1454–61.

21 Rodriguez-Lopez JA, Werner A, Ray LI et al. Renal artery stenosis treated with stent deployment: indications, technique and outcome for 108 patients. *J Vasc Surg* 1999; **29**: 617–24.

22 Scolari F, Bracchi M, Valzorio B et al. Cholesterol atheromatous embolism: an increasingly recognized cause of acute renal failure. *Nephrol Dial Transplant* 1996; **11**: 1607–12.

23 Meyrier A. Renal vascular lesions in the elderly: nephrosclerosis or atheromatous renal disease? *Nephrol Dial Transplant* 1996; **11**(Suppl 9): 45–52.

24 Saleem S, Lakkis FG, Martinez-Maldonado M. Atheroembolic renal disease. *Semin Nephrol* 1996; **16**: 309–18.

25 Mayo RR, Swartz RD. Redefining the incidence of clinically detectable atheroembolism. *Am J Med* 1996; **100**: 524–9.

26 Rauh G, Spengel FA. Blue toe syndrome after initiation of low-dose oral anticoagulation. *Eur J Med Res* 1998; **3**: 278–80.

27 Belenfant X, d'Auzac C, Bariety J et al. Cholesterol crystal embolism during treatment with low-molecular-weight heparin. *Presse Med* 1997; **26**: 1236–7.

28 Thadhani RI, Camargo CA Jr, Xavier RJ et al. Atheroembolic renal failure after invasive procedures. Natural history based on 52 histologically proven cases. *Medicine (Baltimore)* 1995; **74**: 350–8.

29 Haggie SS, Urizar RE, Singh J. Nephrotic-range proteinuria in renal atheroembolic disease: report of four cases. *Am J Kidney Dis* 1996; **28**: 493–501.

30 Greenberg A, Bastacky SI, Iqbal A et al. Focal segmental glomerulosclerosis associated with nephrotic syndrome in cholesterol atheroembolism: clinicopathological correlations. *Am J Kidney Dis* 1997; **29**: 334–44.

31 Krishnamurthi V, Novick AC, Myles JL. Atheroembolic renal disease: effect on morbidity and survival after revascularization for atherosclerotic renal artery stenosis. *J Urol* 1999; **161**: 1093–6.

32 Feldman RL, Wargovich TJ, Bittl JA. No-touch technique for reducing aortic wall trauma during renal artery stenting. *Cathet Cardiovasc Intervent* 1999; **46**: 245–8.

33 Henry M, Amor M, Henry I et al. Stents in the treatment of renal artery stenosis: long-term follow-up. *J Endovasc Surg* 1999; **6**: 42–51.

34 Theron JG, Payelle GG, Coskun O et al. Carotid artery stenosis: treatment with protected balloon angioplasty and stent placement. *Radiology* 1996; **201**: 627–36.

36

Renal angioplasty and stenting: techniques, indications and results

Emilio Calabrese and Luigi Inglese

Introduction

Atherosclerosis and fibromuscular dysplasia are the two main causes of renovascular disease. Atheromas are characterized by cholesterol plaque, thickening of the intima and often calcium deposits, which frequently involve the ostium of the renal artery.

Fibromuscular dysplasia affects young individuals, more commonly women, producing hyperplasia and fibrosis of the intima, the media or the adventitia: dysplasia of the media accounts for over two thirds of cases and produces the typical 'string of beads' appearance of the renal artery.

Renal artery stenosis (RAS) can be associated with hypertension, renal failure and, less frequently, with non-cardiac precordial pain, 'apparent' heart failure and 'flash' pulmonary edema (FPE).

Surgical repair of a renal aneurysm and bypass, or patch reconstruction, have been utilized with significant success when dealing with renal artery disease. While initial experience with percutaneous transluminal renal angioplasty (PTRA) showed inferior results when compared with surgery, subsequent refinements in techniques, along with the introduction of primary stenting, have greatly improved the efficacy of interventional techniques. Geroulakos et al.[1] observed how percutaneous procedures have almost completely supplanted surgery in RAS, but they were still not convinced about the absolute indications of stenting and its superiority over simple PTA.

A subsequent editorial by Dietrich,[2] observed that renal stenting, particularly in the ostium region, is to be recommended. Rees et al.[3] also reported good results when inserting stents in patients who had poor results and restenosis after non-stented conventional angioplasty. Primary stenting is now the procedure of choice in most cases of atherosclerotic renal artery disease.

Clinical aspects of renal artery stenosis (RAS)

Five to 10% of cases of hypertension in adults may be directly related to or caused by RAS. Lawson[4] showed that renal artery disease was a very common cause of hypertension in children. Improvement of hypertension after resolution of RAS may be expected if appropriate studies on the renin–angiotensin system are conducted to confirm a reasonable cause–effect relationship between RAS and hypertension.

Simultaneous, double catheter sampling of renin levels in both renal veins, allowing measurement of the renal vein: systemic renin activity ratio, is especially useful in assessing unilateral renal stenosis and its relationship to systemic hypertension.[5,6]

RAS, especially bilateral, is responsible for 20% of cases of renal failure in patients with other manifestations of peripheral vascular disease.[7] Recently, worsening renal function with evidence of severe RAS has been shown to respond to PTRA.

RAS has been incidentally observed in 50% of patients studied angiographically for peripheral vascular disease and it has been observed that RAS progresses to complete occlusion.[8]

In one study, untreated RAS of > 60% was shown to progress to complete occlusion within 2 years, thus justifying PTRA as an organ–salvage procedure. Further studies are needed to clarify this matter, especially when dealing with patients with multisite arterial stenoses where RAS is incidentally found by means of arteriography.

Bilateral RAS, due to the possibility of progression to complete bilateral occlusion and severe renal failure, and in consequence of the increasing awareness of its association with episodes of FPE, provides a strong indication for PTRA or surgery.

Some endovascular therapists advocate the use of PTA in the presence of asymptomatic renal stenosis with no increase in creatinine as a means of organ preservation, to delay aggravation of the stenosis and the possible manifestation of renal insufficiency.[9]

A study performed in the UK, on 85 patients who had had incidental diagnosis of RAS, showed that > 30% of patients with concomitant renal artery and peripheral artery disease died within 2 years, mostly due to cardiovascular causes. (At the time of this study, FPE and nephrogenic apparent heart failure had not been associated with RAS). All patients who required dialysis died within 1 year. All unilateral renal stenoses in this group were treated medically, while 35% of bilateral stenosis were treated with angioplasty. The type of treatment did not change the survival outcome in this small group.

Renal Artery Stenosis (RAS): Diagnosis

Relevant data pointing toward the presence of RAS include the presence of diastolic hypertension, elevated creatinine levels, recent onset of renal failure, presence of multiple peripheral vessel disease, unexplained precordial pain and recurrent pulmonary edema (PE) in hypertensive patients without evidence of primary heart disease.

Testing includes: 24-hour Holter pressure monitoring, measurement of renin levels (either systemic or, better, with selective renal vein catheterization), renal scan and radionephrogram (before and after administration of 50 mg captopril).

B-mode Doppler ultrasound, both plain and contrast enhanced, will detect many RAS,[10] but unsuitable patients, limitations of the technique itself and lower sensitivity, when compared to helical computerized tomography (CT) (0.75 versus 0.94), would suggest integration with a CT scan.[11,12] Contrast-enhanced B-mode scans can be most useful in follow-up studies of renal stents whose presence produce artefacts that interfere with both CT scan and magnetic resonance imaging (MRI) accuracy.[13]

MRI with gadolinium is an effective diagnostic tool when multiplanar reformatting (MPR) or 3D volume rendering is applied, instead of the less accurate maximum intensity projection (MIP) protocol.[14] (Figure 36.1).

Multislice, contrast-enhanced, spiral CT scans provide reliable data on the status of the renal arteries, provided that there has been no previous stenting. The presence of a stent in the renal artery may produce artefacts and errors in the evaluation of residual and in-stent stenosis. Contrast media toxicity in CT scans is no more than that reported for arterial angiograms performed with iodinated media.[15]

Absence of detectable renal function on iodinated contrast studies and a silent technetium renal scan should not

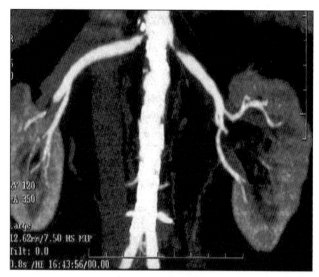

(a)

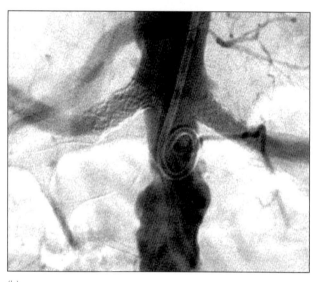

(b)

Figure 36.1
(a) Magnetic resonance imaging of bilateral renal artery stenosis.
(b) Bilateral PTA and stenting for treatment of renal failure.

discourage revascularization procedures when dealing with complete chronic renal artery occlusion (CCRAO). Core-needle biopsy is an essential tool when evaluating the possible benefits of recanalizing CCRAO. Experience accumulated in surgical procedures has shown that preoperative (and intraoperative) biopsies, showing that < 50% of glomeruli are hyalinized, predicted clinical success with effective renal function after restoring perfusion. The status of the tubuli is not determinant in predicting results of recanalization and kidneys with severe tubular necrosis can still do well after restoring the blood flow. Collaterals from the lumbar arteries may have provided enough blood flow for the kidney to survive, but not to thrive and function. Kidneys that failed to grow beyond 6 cm in maximal diameter are poor candidates for revascularization and smaller kidneys may be prone to rupture after restoration of blood flow.

Technique

Through a 4F introducer, a Cordis Universal Flush or a piggy-tail catheter is inserted in the abdominal aorta. Three-dimensional rotational arteriograms or multiple-angle angiograms should be performed in AP, LAO and RAO to identify the ostium of both renal arteries very clearly. Aortograms will identify polar renal arteries; selective angiograms carried out with a 4F Cobra 1 or Cobra 2 catheter will be needed to clarify details. When renal failure is present, or when investigating renal transplants, CO_2 injection will avoid complications related to allergic reactions and contrast toxicity. No evidence of renal damage produced by CO_2 has been reported, provided that injecting the contrast with the patient in the lateral decubitus position be avoided (Figure 36.2).

The diagnostic catheter is then removed and the 4F introducer replaced with a 6F one, and 5000 U heparin (intravenously) is given. The patient should already have been given ticlopidine or aspirin for at least 2–3 days, otherwise, rapid antiplatelet drug protocols should be enacted immediately (Eptifibade [Schering's Integrilin®], Tirofiban [MSD's Aggrastat®] or Abciximab [Reopro®]).

The angling of the renal artery in respect to the aorta is essential in deciding the most appropriate approach. Steep downward angling should prompt the use of a transbrachial or transradial approach because negotiating a steep angle from the femoral artery could be troublesome. Transbrachial access is safe and feasible for steep aortorenal angles and when iliac arteries cannot be crossed. Galli et al.[16] demonstrated the feasibility of a transradial approach to renal artery stenting with a 6F introducer and guiding catheter (6F Zuma 2: Medtronic).

A 6F introducer and a 6F multipurpose guiding catheter is generally the best support from the upper limbs. When the procedure is carried out from the lower limb, a Shepherd hook, a standard J renal guiding catheter or an arrow renal short introducer will support a femoral approach in an appropriate manner. The guiding systems should be completed by a Y connector to allow for dye injection during positioning of the stent. The catheter should be initially mounted on a 0.035 inch high support guide to avoid damage of the vessel wall and the guide should be removed when the catheter is in the abdominal aorta in proximity of the renal ostium.

When the positioning of the guiding catheter appears difficult, a coaxial internal 4F diagnostic catheter will reach the target more easily and directly without trauma. This will permit the insertion of a 0.014 inch guide into the renal artery, thus stabilizing the position of the guiding catheter. Inserting a guide through a diagnostic catheter, removing it and then inserting a hard guiding catheter along the guide is usually traumatic and difficult to accomplish with a thin 0.014 inch guide.

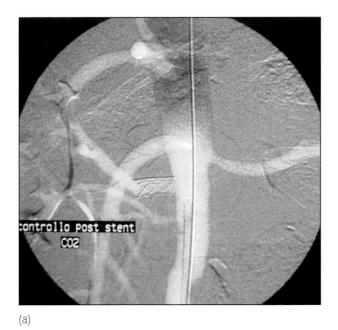

(a)

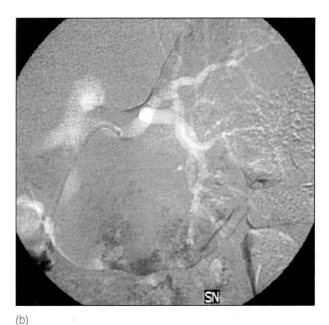

(b)

Figure 36.2
(a) Carbon dioxide arteriogram to assess renal artery and stent (b) Carbon dioxide selective arteriogram of left renal artery.

The lesion should be crossed with a 0.014 inch high support coronary guide, which should be positioned in a distal branch, possibly of the inferior tree. Hydrophilic nitinol guides, such as Terumo or Choice PT grafix, should be absolutely avoided because they may perforate the parenchyma and produce significant hematoma. Guides of 0.035 inch are rarely used, and 0.020 inch Schneider and 0.018 inch guides, popular up until some time ago, are now being abandoned because thinner balloons cannot accommodate them. A stent with a very low profile, such as an AACHEN® renal stent should be positioned on a rapid-exchange coronary balloon. Rapid-exchange low-profile balloons significantly reduce difficulties and trauma to the vessel during complex procedures.

Ostial lesions require perfect positioning and the stent should cover the plaque completely up to the aortic wall. It is not necessary to have the stent protrude 1–2 mm into the aortic lumen, but it is essential that it lines up with the margin of the intima of the aorta. Inglese and JoMed teamed up to produce a stent specifically designed for ostial lesions with a reinforced proximal structure to exert maximal force against the aortic wall and the ostium itself: this design is intended to limit the occurrence of recoil (see Figure 36.3).

Proper angling of the angio-tube is essential to position the proximal part of the stent.

Kim et al.[17] studied the angle of origin of the renal arteries as compared to the long axis of the L1 spinous process (L1SP) in 160 CT scans. The right renal artery arises ventrally at an angle of 30° (SD±15) from a plane orthogonal to the long axis of L1SP. The left renal artery arises dorsally at an angle of 7° (SD±13). Therefore the optimal initial angle for visualization of the ostium is: LAO 30° (relative to L1SP) for the right renal artery and LAO 7° for the left renal artery.

Pre-dilatation should be avoided whenever possible except in fibrodysplasia, to limit the chances of embolization, and direct primary stenting should be the preferred procedure with a low-profile stent. If pre-dilatation becomes unavoidable, then a 3 mm coronary balloon should provide the maximum acceptable pre-dilatation diameter. The stent should be shorter than the balloon on top of which it has been pre-mounted, in such a way that, when the balloon is inflated, it will assume a donut shape and reduce distal embolization during initial delivery of the stent.

When choosing the balloon for initial delivery of the stent, one should avoid insisting on large balloons, to avoid dissection and damage to the renal artery distal to the stent. When the balloon inflates, it expands freely for a few millimeters beyond the stent and even a minimal oversizing may damage the vessel. In the presence of calcified ostial stenosis, the balloon must be exposed to high pressures in order to open the stent: this may overinflate the distal portion of the balloon beyond the stent and damage the artery, especially when dealing with compliant balloons. To refine the initial stent dilatation, it is always possible to use a second, shorter and larger balloon. Proximal renal arteries will usually require a 6 mm dilatation,

ranging from 5 mm in females to 7 mm in larger arteries. Polar or multiple renal arteries will accommodate 3–4 mm stents and should never be overdilated.

Since several studies have shown a high incidence of restenosis in the presence of insufficient dilatations,[3] residual stenosis should not exceed 15%. Weibull et al.[18] suggest that the initial stenosis must be totally eliminated in order for the procedure to be deemed a complete success.

When dealing with stenosis at the bifurcation, one should have guides inserted in both branches, and simple dilatation should be performed (Figure 36.4). If there is significant recoil, then the guide from the minor branch, previously dilated, should be removed, and the major branch should be stented. The stent mesh should then be crossed by a guide wire to reach the minor branch, the ostium of which should be redilated (see Figures 36.5 and 36.6). When significant recoil of the minor branch is observed, or when both branches appear to be of significant diameter, then one may consider inserting a second stent through the mesh of the first one to cover both ostia.

Results of percutaneous transluminal renal angioplasty (PTRA)

Rodriguez-Lopez et al.[19] reported data on 108 patients with renal stenting under blood pressure control, but observed no significant improvement in renal function. They also reported a 3.2% operative mortality. They reported restenosis in six patients (5.5%), in three instances due to initial misplacement of the stent beyond the ostium. In any case, it is possible that the incidence of restenosis be higher because only 76% of the patients had a follow-up duplex scan or angiography.

Dorros et al.[20] reported a group of > 1000 patients who were treated with renal artery stenting to improve control of hypertension (85%), to preserve renal function (59% with elevated creatinine levels) and because of congestive heart failure (15%): 64% had unilateral stenosis and 36% had bilateral stenosis. A 4-year follow-up showed improved control of both systolic and diastolic blood pressure, and a significant decrease in creatinine levels. The improvement in renal function was more evident in patients treated for bilateral stenosis. At the 4-year follow-up no patients with bilateral stenosis and only 6% with unilateral stenosis had worsening of renal functions. This shows that stenting has a positive impact on renal function when performed on patients with elevated creatinine levels. The results were persistent over time, while adverse effects on renal function are extremely rare. Survival in this group was severely affected by initial creatinine levels, with 85% of patients with creatinine < 1.5 mg/ml alive after 4 years and only 36% of those with creatine ≥ 2 mg/ml alive after 4 years.

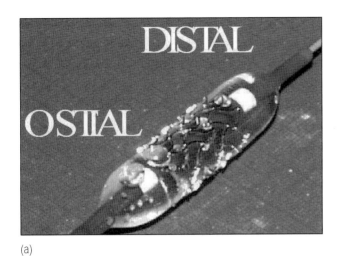

(a)

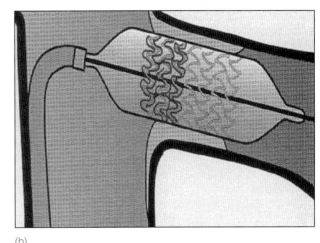

(b)

(c)

Figure 36.3

(a) Wave stent by Abbott/Jomed mounted on a balloon. (b) Scheme of Wave stent being positioned. Proximal structure appears thicker for increased radial strength. (c) Wave Stent by Abbott/Jomed inserted in renal ostium: the stent is designed to have a harder structure in its proximal part to produce higher radial force within the ostium.

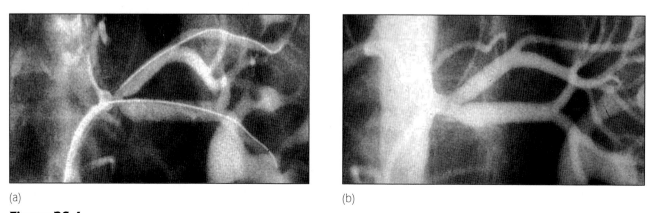

(a)   (b)

Figure 36.4
(a) Early bifurcation with stenosis of both branches. (b) Bilateral simple PTA. Small confined area of dissection with good distal flow.

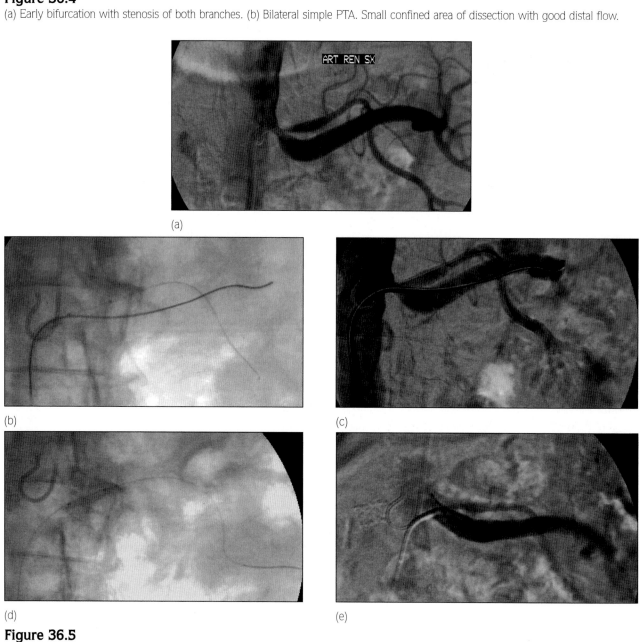

(a)

(b)   (c)

(d)   (e)

Figure 36.5
(a) Ostial stenosis with early origin of small stenotic upper branch. (b) 0.035 guide in main branch and 0.014 with coronary balloon in minor branch. (c) Stenting of major branch. (d) Coronary balloon passed through stent to re-dilate the minor branch. (e) Procedure complete.

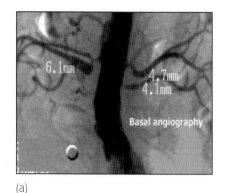

(a)

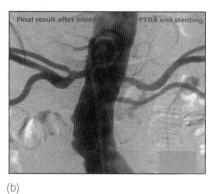

(b)

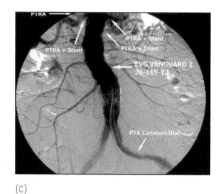

(c)

Figure 36.6

(a) Aneursysm of the abdominal aorta wih complex bilateral renal artery stenoses. (b) Bilateral PTA and stenting of renal arteries. (c) Insertion of Vanguard endoprosthesis to exclude the aortic aneurysm.

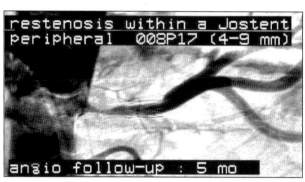

(a)

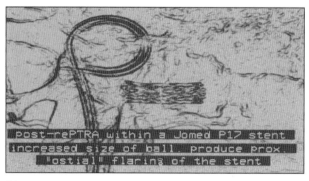

(b)

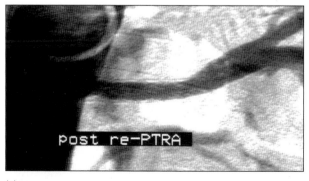

(c)

Figure 36.7

(a) In-stent re-stenosis. (b) Ostial flaring of the stent with larger balloon. (c) Final result post Re-PTA.

Bloch et al.[21] studied the effect of renal ostium PTA end stenting in patients of over 75 years of age, and observed that 74% had improved control of hypertension and the conditions of only 5% showed worsening. Over a 2-year follow-up, 79% of patients presented with either improved or stable renal function.

Schillinger et al.[22] analyzed potential risk factors predictive of post-PTRA renal failure and found that preoperative impaired renal function and contrast dosage were independent predictors of acute renal failure. Hypertension and congestive heart failure were associated factors. They came to the conclusion that while transient renal dysfunction occurs in 10% of patients post-PTRA within 24 hours, persistent renal failure is rare.

Long-term patency of the stents remains a problem, influenced by various factors and either watchful observation of recurrent stenosis, repeated dilation, or bypass surgery are indicated (Figure 36.7). Residual stenosis at the original dilatation, as low as 15%, noticeably increases the incidence of restenosis. Incorrect positioning of the proximal part of the stent within ostial stenosis, when one does not cover the diseased vessel at the aorta, is another problem. Data accumulated in women undergoing iliac angioplasty and taking estrogen replacement therapy has shown that while at 1 year the patency rate is similar in both users and non-users, non-users have a patency rate of 74% at 5 years and users a rate of 49%.[23]

In a randomized group of 58 non-diabetic patients Weinbull et al.[24] compared PTA to surgery. Primary patency at 2 years was 75% in the PTA study group and 96% in the surgical group. Secondary patency was 90% in the PTA group and 98% in the surgical group. Concerning the effect of blood pressure control and renal function protection, the efficacy of the two systems proved to be similar.

When dealing with RAS, the issue of concomitant diseases related to cerebrovascular circulation should also be considered. In a study by Missouris et al.,[25] only 55% of patients in a group of 38 who underwent PTRA had normal carotid arteries, 26% of which presented moderate stenosis and 18% of which were severe. Nine out of 38 patients had previously suffered a stroke and one had had a transient ischemic attack (TIA). In conclusion, four out of every 10 patients undergoing PTRA presented carotid stenosis that might have required either medical or interventional and/or surgical treatment. Accurate carotid evaluation is thus paramount in renal artery disease.

Apparent heart failure is another fundamental issue when dealing with RSA.[26] Hypertension, increased fluid retention and decreased glomerular filtration rate all contribute to the development of signs resembling heart failure with effort dyspnea, paroxysmal nocturnal dyspnea or edema. Sometimes, patients experience precordial pain without significant coronary disease. Resolution of RAS by PTRA produced a rapid fall of plasma atrial natriuretic factor and creatinine levels, and a reduction in mean blood pressure and weight. Symptoms of congestive heart failure subsided, especially in patients with a single functioning kidney and RAS.

FPE is a lethal complication that is being recognized with increasing frequency as usually being associated with bilateral renal stenosis or with stenosis in an isolated functioning kidney. Patients with FPE present with severe hypertension, fluid retention and acute or subacute renal failure, severe respiratory distress, and fluid overload in the lungs. They do not respond to conventional treatment even when dialysis and automatic ventilation are supplied.

Weatherford et al.[27] reported successful treatment in five consecutive patients with surgical renal revascularization. Basaria and Fred[28] also observed the association of FPE with RAS. Harker et al.[29] reported FPE as an acute and rare complication of PTRA.

Bloch et al.[30] studied the incidence of PE in RAS. They observed that in a series of patients, 41% of those with bilateral RAS had episodes of PE. Of those treated with PTRA and stenting, 77% suffered no further episodes. The only cases of recurrent PE were reported in patients with thrombosis or restenosis of the PTRA. Results were less evident in patients with unilateral RAS.

Reports of congestive heart failure and/or precordial pain in the absence of coronary heart disease and the occurrence of an episode of refractory FPE, should draw attention to the need for an attentive evaluation of the renal arteries. Some of the so-called 'cardiac deaths' in multivessel peripheral atherosclerotic disease, previously attributed to heart disease, might possibly be caused by underestimation of the effects of severe RAS. Patients who have peripheral artery disease and concomitant severe RAS, especially when involving both kidneys or a single solitary functioning kidney, may require treatment both for the preservation of renal function and for the prevention of FPE and refractory congestive heart failure.

Complications

Incidence of arterial perforation and rupture is < 1%,[1] but delayed rupture can appear up to 24 hours after the procedure. Some early reports of arterial rupture describe a technique of simple balloon inflation to obtain sealing, but insertion of a covered stent is certainly a superior and safer technique when feasible (see Figure 36.8). Delayed formation of hyatrogenic pseudoaneurysms have been reported, and have also been successfully treated with covered stents (Figure 36.9). McWilliams et al.[31] reported a pseudoaneurysm of the distal renal artery following PTA for ostial stenosis, which was treated with bench surgery and autotransplantation.

Distal embolism during PTRA is a problem, which has been addressed by using gentle techniques, avoiding crossing the lesion with the guiding catheter, utilizing primary stenting and donut balloons.

Some operators have attempted to use distal protection systems such as PercuSurge®,[32] Cordis' Angioguard® or similar systems. Unfortunately, there is often limited space to position a protection system distal to the site of stenosis because early bifurcations are common. Besides, complications related to the protection device may arise, such as dissection, and they can be extremely difficult to repair in the distal renal artery.

Hematoma of the kidney may be produced by placing the guide in a position too distal, or by using thick, rigid 0.035 inch guides or slippery Terumo ones, which may easily penetrate

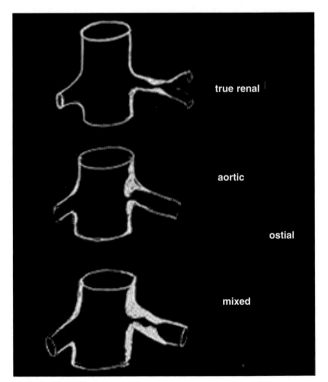

Figure 36.8
Definition of anatomy renal artery stenosis

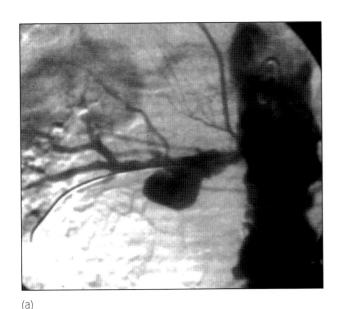

(a)

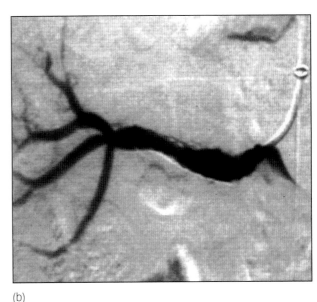

(b)

Figure 36.9
(a) Pseudoaneurysm of the right renal artery. (b) Pseudoaneurysm excluded by means of a covered Jomed stent.

the parenchyma. An asymptomatic hematoma needs strict surveillance with several postprocedural echoes or CT scans, and it usually stabilizes after reversal of heparin. A symptomatic, painful hematoma needs stricter surveillance in the intensive care unit, and may occasionally require surgery and even nephrectomy. Rupture of the kidney is rarely observed, and mostly in hypoplastic kidneys after PTRA for severe stenosis and in patients suffering from other systemic diseases. Emergency nephrectomy is the choice treatment unless complex organ-salvage procedures are attempted in patients who have only a single functioning kidney.

Dissections distal to the stent should be fixed with a second stent: only when this is impractical should it be left alone, with no treatment or with simple ballooning. Thrombosis of the artery may be associated with lack of appropriate preoperative antiplatelet preparation or by insufficient anticoagulation during the procedure. Excessive guide manipulation, the use of a distal protective device or a large bore guide may all induce thrombosis, but dissection is the most common cause of arterial occlusion during PTRA and it should be properly addressed.

Segmental infarction of the kidney may be due to distal vessel thrombosis, following guide manipulation, or to distal embolization: it rarely requires treatment unless it is very extensive, but it may dispel the advantages on blood pressure control and renal function that one would have expected from the PTRA.

Mann and Sos[33] reported a single case of successful treatment of distal atheroembolism in the renal artery with corticosteroids, producing sustained improvement of renal function. Further studies and experience are needed to confirm the efficacy of this approach.

Renal failure due to excess contrast injection has been reported and the use of diluted, limited amounts of contrast

help limit this complication. CO_2-assisted PTRA, which utilizes CO_2 as a contrast medium in borderline renal failure, almost completely resolves the contrast toxicity issue[34] (Figure 36.2a).

Fibrodysplasia, aneurysms and trauma

Fibromuscular hyperplasia (Figure 36.10) was generally treated by simple dilatation without stenting, but a few recent reports suggest better results with stenting.

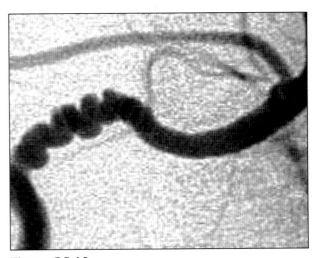

Figure 36.10
Fibrodysplasia.

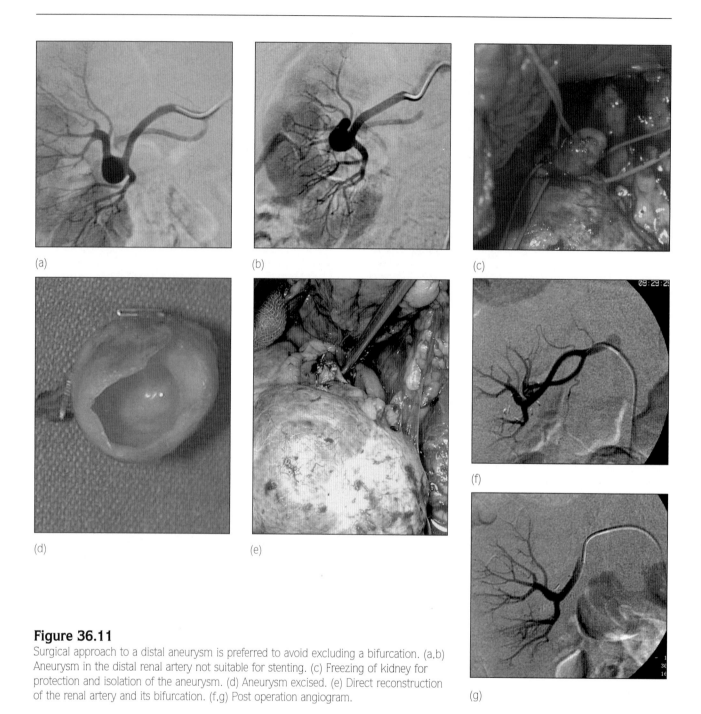

Figure 36.11

Surgical approach to a distal aneurysm is preferred to avoid excluding a bifurcation. (a,b) Aneurysm in the distal renal artery not suitable for stenting. (c) Freezing of kidney for protection and isolation of the aneurysm. (d) Aneurysm excised. (e) Direct reconstruction of the renal artery and its bifurcation. (f,g) Post operation angiogram.

However, primary stenting should always be avoided in fibromuscular dysplasia and the lesion should be predilated, occasionally even with cutting balloons. Failure to predilate, may induce unfavourable hourglass shaping of the stent. In seven of 31 patients treated with PTRA for fibromuscular dysplasia, a restenosis developed within 12 months. Primary patency at 12 months was 77%. A persistent moderate residual stenosis (30–59%) after PTRA was a strong predictor of late restenosis. In 93% of cases, successful PTRA was followed by a drop in blood pressure. Renal function either improved or stabilized in all cases. Only in one of the 31 patients was a Palmaz stent inserted.

Tshomba et al.[35] successfully excluded a distal renal artery aneurysm by inserting multiple coils. The aneuryms had a small neck and contained a thrombus. The patient presented an abnormal captopril scintigram, elevated blood pressure under treatment and moderately elevated BUN and creatinine. The patient showed improved BUN and creatinine levels after the procedure and became normotensive. Complex renal aneurysms involving a bifurcation require surgery, under local cooling, or with ex-vivo 'bench' techniques (Figure 36.11).

Aneurysm in the kidney may produce arterial hypertension that normalizes after excision of the aneurysm.[36,37] Even a large-neck aneurysm can be thrombosed with a balloon-assisted coil embolization.[38] Aneurysms can be excluded with PTFE-covered stents or even with stents covered with autologous saphenous vein. In renal trauma, the endovascular approach can prove very useful.[39]

Conclusions

PTRA is one of the most technically demanding procedures in the interventional field, and inaccurate techniques lead to severe complications and to early recurrence of stenosis.

Improvements in technical results have led the operator to perform PTRA as an incidental procedure, even when moderate arterial stenosis is found, in the course of a routine aortogram, thus pushing the indications for the procedure.

Early success in PTRA depends on selective indications, complete diagnostic procedures, accurate techniques and a 'traumatic' stenting, technical prowess, and strict follow-up.

Incidence of restenosis remains an important problem, which could be further reduced by aggressive-lipid lowering therapy,[40] the use of drug-eluting stents (currently undergoing clinical evaluation) and by new developments in antiplatelet treatments. Through the use of properly performed PTRA, it is possible to obtain control of hypertension, protect organ functions and possibly improve survival in selected cases with nephrogenic congestive failure and FPE.

References

1. Geroulakos G, Missouris C, Mitchell A, Greenhalgh RM. Endovascular treatment of renal artery stenosis. *J Endovasc Ther* 2001; **8**: 177–85.

2. Dietrich EB. Treating renal artery stenosis: one point of view. *J Endovasc Ther* 2001; **8**:186–7 (commentary)

3. Rees CR, Palmaz JC, Becker GJ et al. Palmaz stent in atherosclerotic stenoses involving the ostia of the renal arteries: preliminary report of a multicenter study. *Radiology* 1991; **181**: 507–14.

4. Lawson JD, Boerth RK, Foster JH et al. Diagnosis and management of renovascular hypertension in children. *Arch Surg* 1977; **112**: 1307.

5. Vaughn ED, Buhler FR, Larach JH. Renovascular hypertension: measurements to indicate hypersecretion and contralateral suppression, estimate renal plasma flow and score for surgical curability. *Am J Med* 1973; **55**: 402.

6. Stanley JC, Gewertz BL, Fry WJ. Renal: systemic renin indices and renal vein renin ratios as prognastic indicators in remedial renovascular hypertension. *J Surg Res* 1976; **20**: 149–55.

7. Hansen KJ. Prevalence of ischemic nephropathy in the atherosclerotic population. *Am J Kidney Dis* 1994; **24**: 615–21.

8. Caps MT, Perissinotto C, Zierler RE et al. Prospective study of atherosclerotic disease progression in the renal artery. *Circulation* 1998; **8**: 2866–72

9. Hood DB, Hodgson KJ. Renovascular disease. In: (Moore, Ahn, eds) *Endovascular Surgery*, 3rd edn. (Saunders: 2001): 342.

10. Missouris CG, Allen CM et al. Non-invasive screening for renal artery stenosis with ultrasound contrast enhancement. *J Hypertension* 1996; **14**: 519–24

11. Elkhonen M, Artaud D et al. Evaluation of spiral computed tomography of the renal arteries alone or combined with Doppler ultrasonography in the detection of renal artery stenosis. Prospective study of 114 renal arteries. *Arch Mal Coeur et Vaiss* 1995; **88**: 1159–64.

12. Equine O, Gautier C, Desmoucelles F et al. Importance of the echo-Doppler and helical angioscanner of the renal arteries in the management of renovascular diseases. Results of a retrospective study in 113 patients. *Arch Mal Coeur et Vaiss* 1999; **92**: 1043–5.

13. House MK, Dowling RJ, King P et al. Doppler ultrasound (pre- and post-contrast enhancement) for detection of recurrent stenosis in stented renal arteries: preliminary results. *Australas Radiol* 2000; **44**: 36-40.

14. Baskaran V, Pereles FS, Nemcek AA et al. Gadolinium-enhanced 3D MR angiography of renal artery stenosis: a pilot comparison of maximum intensity projection, multiplanar reformatting, and 3D volume-rendering post-processing algorithms. *Acad Radiol* 2002; **9**: 50–9

15. Lufft V, Hoogestraat-Lufft L, Fels LM et al. Contrast media nephropathy: intravenous CT-angiography in renal artery stenosis: a prospective randomized trial. *Am J Kidney Dis* 2002; **40**: 236-42.

16. Galli M, Tarantino F, Mameli S et al. Transradial approach for renal percutaneous transluminal angioplasty and stenting: a feasibility pilot study. *J Invas Cardiol* 2002; **14**: 386–90.

17. Kim PA, Khilnani NM, Trost DW, Sos TA, Lee L. Fluoroscopic landmarks for optimal visualization of the proximal renal arteries. *J Vasc Intervent Radiol* 1999; **10**: 37–9.

18. Weibull H, Berqvist D, Jonsson K et al. Long-term results after percutaneous transluminal angioplasty of atherosclerotic renal artery stenosis. The importance of intensive follow-up. *Eur J Vasc Surg* 1991; **5**: 291–301.

19. Rodriguez-Lopez JA, Werner A, Lance I et al. Renal artery stenosis treated with stent deployment: indications, technique and outcome for 108 patients. *J Vasc Surg* 1999; **29**: 617–24.

20. Dorros G, Jaff M, Mathiak L et al. Multicenter Palmaz stent renal artery stenosis revascularization registry report: four-year follow-up of 1,058 successful patients. *Cath Cardiovasc Intervent* 2002; **55**: 182–8.

21. Bloch MJ, Trost DA, Whitmer J, Pickering TG, Sos TA, August P. Ostial renal artery stent placement in patients 75 years of age or older. *Am J Hyperten* 2001; **14**: 983–8.

22. Schillinger M, Haumer M, Mlekusch W, Schlerka G, Ahmadi R, Minar E. Predicting renal failure after balloon angioplasty in high-risk patients. *J Endovasc Ther* 2001; **8**: 609–14.

23 Timaran CH, Stevens SL, Grandas OH, Freeman MB, Goldman MH. Influence of hormone replacement therapy on the outcome of iliac angioplasty and stenting. *J Vasc Surgery* 2001; **33** (Suppl 2): S85–S92.

24 Weibull H, Berqvist D, Bergentz SE et al. Percutaneous transluminal renal angioplasty versus surgical reconstruction of atherosclerotic renal artery stenosis: a prospective randomized study. *J Vasc Surg* 1993; **18** 841–52.

25 Missouris CG, Papavassiliou MB, Khaw K, Belli AM, Buckenham T, McGregor GA. High prevalence of carotid artery disease in patients with atheromatous renal artery stenosis. *Nephrol Dial Transplant* 1998; **13**: 945–8.

26 Missouris CG, Belli AM, McGregor GA. 'Apparent' heart failure: a syndrome caused by renal artery stenoses. *Heart* 2000; **83**: 152–5.

27 Weatherford DA, Freeman MB et al. Surgical management of flash pulmonary edema secondary to renovascular hypertension. *Am J Surg* 1997; **174**: 160–3.

28 Basaria S, Fred HL. Images in cardiovascular medicine. Flash pulmonary edema heralding renal artery stenosis. *Circulation* 2002; **105**: 899

29 Harker CP, Steed M, Althaus SJ, Coldwell D. Flash pulmonary edema: an acute and unusual complication of renal angioplasty. *J Vasc Intervent Radiol* 2000; **6**: 130–2.

30 Bloch MJ, Trost DW, Pickering TG, Sos TA, August P. Prevention of recurrent pulmonary edema in patients with bilateral renovascular disease through renal artery stent placement. *Am J Hypertension* 1999; **12**: 1–7.

31 McWilliams RG, Godfrey H, Bakran A, Schultze LJ, van Bockel JH, van Oostayen JA. Delayed pseudoaneurysm after renal artery angioplasty. *J Endovasc Therapy* 2002; **9**: 48–53.

32 Henry M, Klonaris K, Henry I et al. Protected renal stenting with the PercuSurge® GuardWire device: a pilot study. *J Endovasc Therapy* 2001; **8**: 227–37

33 Mann SJ, Sos TA. Treatment of atheroembolization with corticosteroids. *Am J Hypertension* 2001; **14**: 831–4.

34 Calabrese E, Garaffo S, Quattrone C. Angiography and PTA with CO_2. Rome: MET, 2000.

35 Tshomba Y, Deleo G, Ferrari S, Marina R, Biasi G. Renal artery aneurysm: improved renal function after coil embolization. *J Endovasc Ther* 2002; **9**: 54–8

36 Martin RS, Meacham PW et al. Renal artery aneurysm: selective treatment for hypertension and prevention of rupture. *J Vasc Surg* 1989; **9**: 26–34.

37 Lebel M, Laroche GP. Renal artery aneurysms and hypertension. *J Hum Hyperten* 1998; **12**: 765–6.

38 Mounayer C, Aymaud A, Saint-Maurice JP et al. Balloon-assisted coil embolization for large-necked renal artery aneurysms. *Cardiovasc Intervent Radiol* 2000; **23**: 228–30

39 Dinkel HP, Danuser H, Triller J. Blunt renal trauma: minimally invasive management with microcatheter embolization – Experience in nine patients. *Radiology* 2002; **223**: 723–30.

40 Khong TK, Missouris CG, Belli AM, McGregor GA. Regression of atherosclerotic renal artery stenosis with aggressive lipid lowering therapy. *J Hum Hypertension* 2001; **15**: 431–3.

41 Pillay WR, Kan YM, Crinnion JN et al. Prospective multicentre study of the natural history of atherosclerotic renal artery stenosis in patients with peripheral vascular disease. *Bri J Surg* 2002; **89**: 737–40.

42 Sos TA, Pickering TG, Sniderman K et al. Percutaneous transluminal renal angioplasty in renovascular hypertension due to atheroma of fibromyuscular dysplasia. *N Eng J Med* 1983; **309**: 274–9.

43 Birrer M, Do DD, Mahler F, Triller J, Baumgartner I. Treatment of renal artery fibromuscular dysplasia with balloon angioplasty: a prospective follow-up study. *Eur J Vasc Endovasc Surg* 2002; **23**: 146–52.

44 Kaukanen ET, Manninen HI, Matsi PJ, Soider HK. Brachial artery access for percutaneous renal artery intervention. *Cardiovasc Intervent Radiol* 1997; **20**: 353–8.

45 Zeller T, Frank U et al. Color duplex ultrasound imaging of renal arteries and detection of hemodynamically relevant renal artery stenoses. *Ultraschall Med* 2001; **22**: 116–21.

37

Mesenteric and celiac angioplasty and stenting

Dieter Liermann and Johannes Kirchner

Introduction

Chronic mesenteric ischemia is a rare, but serious, cause of abdominal pain. It commonly presents with weight loss and abdominal angina (Orthner's disease).[1–3] The entity has been known, described and studied for a long time,[4] with experimental work dating back to 1875.[5] As simple as the pathophysiological model may appear to be at first, its correct assessment and the evaluation of the symptoms are difficult owing to diagnostic differentiation from non-vascular causes of abdominal complaints.[2,3] Most often, atheromatous occlusive disease is the primary cause of abdominal angina,[8] although anatomical studies on asymptomatic patients with a relatively high rate of atherosclerotic changes in the visceral arteries often do not result in any symptoms.[7,8] An explanation for this phenomenon is the very slow progression of the disease in some patients, with the development of collaterals over time. Other causes (non-occlusive mesenteric ischemia, systemic vasculitis, external compression, retractile mesenteritis, Shneddon's syndrome) for the mesenteric ischemia have been described less frequently. Women appear to be affected by the disease more often than men.[3]

The lethality of an acute arterial occlusion of the superior mesenteric artery ranges from 70% to 90%,[9] and the postoperative mortality rate from 3% to 20%. An emergency operation in these patients is connected with a considerable increase of both the operative risk and perioperative mortality. This restricts the indications for surgery, and makes it necessary to search for alternative treatment methods. Percutaneous transluminal angioplasty (PTA) was recommended for the treatment also of the abdominal angina.[10] However, compared to iliac or peripheral vessels, it is obvious that PTA is usually more difficult in the mesenteric arteries, which are curved and show an acute angle to the abdominal aorta. This holds true in particular if the superior mesenteric artery shows considerable atherosclerotic change

or is partially ectatic. Nevertheless, today PTA has been well described in the treatment of mesenteric artery stenoses. Thus, several studies were undertaken to determine the safety and efficacy of PTA of the superior mesenteric artery.[11–17] These studies demonstrated that the initial success rate was excellent, with the majority of patients showing complete improvement of the symptoms and continued relief of symptoms at follow-up.[11] Thus, a primary success rate of 90%, with a recurrence rate necessitating redilation of 50%, is achieved.[15]

PTA seems to be better than surgery in cases of stenotic or short occlusive lesions in patients with chronical mesenteric ischemia, and surgery only may be preferred in patients with long occlusions and low operative risk.[14] Also, local thrombolytic therapy can be useful in the treatment of complete occlusion of the superior mesenteric artery,[18] and PTA of the inferior mesenteric artery was reported to be highly effective in abolishing symptoms of mesenteric ischemia.[19] Thus, today, PTA of a recognizable stenosis or occlusion of the superior mesenteric artery seems to be the first measure, even under acute conditions. PTA is worth trying because of the low risk involved.[20–24] This does not hold true for cases of intestinal necrosis.

Indication for stenting

Although stent implantation in cases of insufficient result after PTA or restenosis following PTA has become a common and widespread interventional procedure, stent implantation in occlusive vascular disease of the abdominal vessels is only indicated when PTA fails. Successful PTA with signs of restenosis alone does not justify the use of stents.[25,26] Also, the use of stents in abdominal vessels is impossible if there is a contraindication for long-term anticoagulation treatment.

If the clinical signs are decisive, there are no age- or sex-specific restrictions. Increased operative risk or inoperability with severe abdominal angina is a clear indication. A necessary condition is sufficient transbrachial or femoral access. As a rule, the transbrachial path should be selected for interventions in the area of the abdominal vessels, because of better leverage. If stents with a larger diameter are applied, either the brachial artery must be exposed transbrachially in order to avoid complications, or the transfemoral path must be selected.

Method

Stent selection

The appropriate stent selection is somewhat controversial. We assumed only highly flexible stents to be suitable for stenting the superior mesenteric artery, because they can be removed in the case of detachment difficulties or misplacement.[25–29] We showed that only the tantalum stent was sufficiently flexible and removable with a flexible three- or four-armed forceps.[25,28] Nevertheless, other authors also reported the use of the Palmaz stent in this locality[30,31] or in ostial celiac artery stenosis.[30]

Highly flexible tantalum stents with diameters between 5 and 7 mm and lengths of 4–8 cm are suitable for implantation. If a diameter of up to 6 mm at the end is sufficient, transbrachial exposure can usually be done without surgery and the 8F sheath can be inserted percutaneously to the incision.

Anticoagulation

An essential condition for successful mesenteric and celiac angioplasty and stenting is a strict peri-interventional anticoagulation protocol. In cases of transbrachial approach, no relevant complications have been observed to date in our own patients when initially 5000 IU heparin and an antispasmodic agent were given. In the following heparinization of 100–150 IU/kg body weight should be attempted. A 72-h anticoagulation with heparin 1000 IU/h through a perfusor follows stent implantation. Phenoprocumon (Marcumar® Roche, Germany) therapy for 6 months, or for an unlimited period in difficult cases, is recommended. In the other cases, long-term therapy with aspirin should follow the 6-month phenprocoumon treatment.

Procedure

At first, diagnostic digital subtraction angiography (DSA) with special focus on the upper abdominal vessels (selective celiac and mesenterial angiography) has to be performed, demonstrating the status quo (stenoses, occlusions, collateral vessels)

in total. The vessel origin of the celiac artery or the superior mesenteric artery is probed after an angiography catheter is positioned through a Terumo wire, the tip of which should be either slightly bent or straight, depending on the degree of stenosis. After the catheter has been advanced beyond the stenosis, a more stable wire should be substituted. The dilation catheter, and, in cases of insufficient result, the stent catheter, can be positioned through this wire. The implantation procedure for stent deployment is done with the usual technique. In case of stent deformation by pressure from the outside, it should be expanded through redilation (Figure 37.1).

Besides the evaluation of the clinical symptoms (reduction of diarrhea and weight gain), DSA is required after 6 and 12 months in order to rule out restenosing at an early stage when it is still reversible. This is repeated at 6-month intervals or when symptoms occur.

Results

There exist several case reports on stenting abdominal vessels in chronic mesenteric ischemia.[18,23–28,30–35] We know of only few sample studies on a comparably small number of patients.[14,25,26,36] In a study of Sheeran et al[34] on 12 patients, initial technical success was achieved in 11 of 12 cases, but one patient died post-procedurally due to bowel ischemia and infarction. Nyman et al[14] reported on PTA and stent placement in three of five patients who were admitted because of chronic mesenteric ischemia, showing clinical success in all cases.

In our own study sample of 12 patients (8 female, 4 male) with severe abdominal angina who underwent stent implantation after insufficient PTA, freedom from symptoms was achieved in all patients. In three cases there was an occlusion of the superior mesenteric artery with simultaneous stenosis of the celiac artery, with perfusion of the superior mesenteric artery's supply area via the pancreas arciform arteries. In the nine other cases, there were severe constrictions of the proximal superior mesenteric artery. The extent of the stenoses varied from 60% to 90%. The constricted segments varied from 1.5 to 2.5 cm in the case of the trunk, and from 1.0 to 3.5 cm in the case of the superior mesenteric artery. Nine stents were implanted in the superior mesenteric artery. Three stents were implanted in the constricted origin of the celiac artery upon occlusion of the superior mesenteric artery, in order to achieve better filling of the supply area of the superior mesenterica via the collateral circulation from the celiac artery through the pancreas arciform arteries. With a mean follow-up of 28 months, four restenoses that could be eliminated with PTA have occurred to date.

Two patients of our series showed an obvious discrepancy between the radiological finding of a deformed stent and absolute freedom from symptoms. The weakness of the stent design was insufficient rigidity, which made the prosthesis suscep-

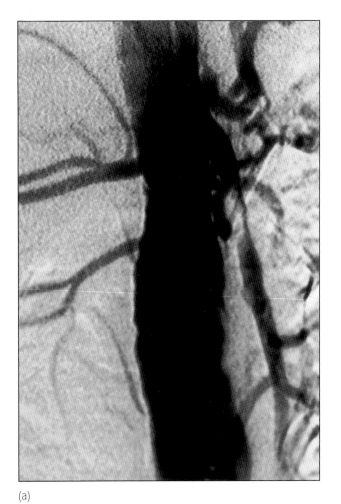

(a)

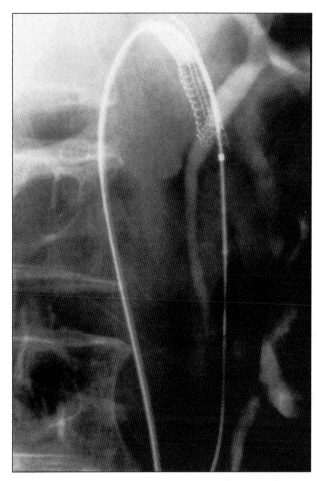

(b)

tible to denting from the outside. A higher rigidity could perhaps be achieved by selecting a thicker tantalum wire; however, the ability to remove those stents must still be demonstrated.

Conclusion

Implantation of endovascular stents in the mesenteric or celiac arteries provides an additional non-surgical therapy that can be used even when patients are not operable or are rated as a high operative risk because of generalized arteriosclerosis and a poor general condition. In contrast to other localizations, stent implantation in abdominal vessels is a not yet well-established additional expansion of interventional radiology. This especially risky application of endovascular stents was only considered because of the increasing experience in the use of stents in other vessel segments and in experimental investigations. Despite the absence of comparative studies with long-term follow-up, the feasibility of mesenteric and celiac angioplasty and stenting is becoming increasingly obvious owing to numerous case reports and small sample studies.

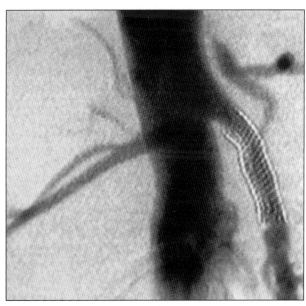

(c)

Figure 37.1
Implantation of a strecker-stent into the mesenteric artery.

References

1 Heberer G, Dostal G, Hoffmann K. Zur Erkennung und Behandlung der chronischen Mesenterialarterieninsuffizienz. *Dtsch Med Wschr* 1972; **97**: 750–4.

2 Liermann D, Kirschner J. *Angiographische Diagnostik und Therapie*. Stuttgart: Thieme, 1997.

3 Stanton Jr PE, Hollier PA, Seidel TW et al. Chronic intestinal ischemia: diagnosis and therapy. *J Vasc Surg* 1986; **4**: 338–44.

4 Kümmel R. Über die Sklerose der Eingeweidearterien in der Bauchhöhle. *Zbl Allg Path Anat* 1906; **17**: 129–31.

5 Litten M. Über die Folgen des Verschlusses der Arteria mesenterica superior. *Virchows Arch Path Anat* 1875; **63**: 289.

6 Derrick JR, Pollard HS, Moore RM. The pattern of atherosclerotic narrowing of the celiac and the superior mesenteric arteries. *Ann Surg* 1959; **149**: 685–9.

7 Cen M, Kämmerer K, Neef H. Verschluß der drei unpaaren Eingeweidearterien ohne klinische Symptomatik. *Dtsch Med Wschr* 1972; **97**: 197.

8 Chiene J. Complete obliteration of the celiac and the mesenteric arteries, the visceral receiving their blood supply through the extraperitoneal system of vessels. *J Anat Physiol* 1968; **69**: 65–7.

9 Jenson CB, Smith GA. A clinical study of 51 cases of mesenteric infarction. *Surgery* 1956; **40**: 930–7.

10 McCollum CH, Graham JM, DeBakey ME. Chronic mesenteric arterial insufficiency: results of revascularization in 33 cases. *South Med J* 1976; **69**: 1266–8.

11 Allen RC, Martin GH, Rees CR et al. Mesenteric angioplasty in the treatment of chronic intestinal ischemia. *J Vasc Surg* 1996; **24**: 415–21.

12 Hallisey MJ, Deschaine J, Illescas FF et al. Angioplasty for the treatment of visceral ischemia. *J Vasc Intervent Radiol* 1995; **6**: 785–91.

13 Maspes F, Mazzetti die Pietralata G, Gandini R et al. Percutaneous transluminal angioplasty in the treatment of chronic mesenteric ischemia: results and 3 years of follow-up in 23 patients. *Abdom Imaging* 1998; **23**: 358–63.

14 Nyman U, Ivancev K, Lindh M, Uher P. Endovascular treatment of chronic mesenteric ischemia: report of five cases. *Cardiovasc Intervent Radiol* 1998; **21**: 305–13.

15 Odurny A, Sniderman KW, Colapinto RF. Intestinal angina: percutaneous transluminal angioplasty of the celiac and superior mesenteric arteries. *Radiology* 1988; **167**: 59–62.

16 Roberts L Jr, Wertman DA Jr, Mills SR et al. Transluminal angioplasty of the superior mesenteric artery: an alternative to surgical revascularization. *Am J Roentgenol* 1983; **141**: 1039–42.

17 Warnock NG, Gaines PA, Beard JD, Cumberland DC. Treatment of intestinal angina by percutaneous transluminal angioplasty of a superior mesenteric artery occlusion. *Clin Radiol* 1992; **45**: 18–19.

18 Maleux G, Wilms G, Stockx L et al. Percutaneous recanalization and stent placement in chronic proximal superior mesenteric artery occlusion. *Eur Radiol* 1997; **7**: 1228–30.

19 Crotch-Harvey MA, Gould DA, Green AT. Case report: percutaneous transluminal angioplasty of the inferior mesenteric artery in the treatment of chronic mesenteric ischemia. *Clin Radiol* 1992; **46**: 408–9.

20 Castaneda-Zuniga WR, Gomes A, Weens C et al. Transluminal angioplasty in the treatment of abdominal angina. *Röfo* 1982; **137**: 330–2.

21 Furrer J, Gruentzig A, Kugelmeier J, Goebel N. Treatment of abdominal angina with percutaneous dilation of an arteriomesenteric superior stenosis. *Cardiovasc Intervent Radiol* 1980; **5**: 367–9.

22 Golden DA, Ring EJ, McLean GK, Freimann DB. Percutaneous transluminal angioplasty in the treatment of abdominal angina. *AJR* 1982; **139**: 247–9.

23 Saddenkni S, Sniderman KW, Hilton S, Sos TA. Percutaneous transluminal angioplasty of nonatherosclerotic lesions. *AJR* 1980; **135**: 975–82.

24 van Denise WH, Zawacki JK, Phillips D. Treatment of acute mesenteric ischemia by percutaneous transluminal angioplasty. *Gastroenterology* 1986; **91**: 475–8.

25 Liermann D, Strecker EP. Tantalum stents in the treatment of stenotic and occlusive diseases of abdominal vessels. In: Liermann D, ed. *Stents – State of the Art and Future Developments*. Morin Heights: Polyscience, 1995: 127–34.

26 Liermann D, Strecker EP, Jacobi V et al. Severe angina abdominalis treated by implantation of a highly flexible tantalum endoprosthesis. *Angiology* 1992; **43**: 275.

27 Liermann D, Strecker EP, Vallbracht C, Kollath J. Indikation und klinischer Einsatz des Streckerstents. In: Kollath J, Liermann D, eds. *Stents ein aktueller Überblick*. Konstantz: Schnetztor, 1990: 24–37.

28 Liermann D, Zegelman M, Kollath J et al. Is there a surgical contraindication against stents and is it possible to rescue a misplaced stent? *Eur Radiol* 1991; **1**: 76.

29 Kollath J, Liermann D. *Stents ein aktueller Überblick*. Konstanz: Schnetztor, 1990.

30 Forauer AR, McLean GK. Primary stenting of the superior mesenteric artery for treatment of chronic mesenteric ischemia – a case report. *Angiology* 1999; **50**: 63–7.

31 Waybill PN, Enea NA. Use of a Palmaz stent deployed in the superior mesenteric artery for chronic mesenteric ischemia. *J Vasc Intervent Radiol* 1997; **8**: 1069–71.

32 Finch IJ. Use of the Palmaz stent in ostial celiac artery stenosis. *J Vasc Intervent Radiol* 1992; **3**: 633–5.

33 Cohn JM, Molavi B, Collar A. Stenting of a superior mesenteric artery lesion via the right arm approach. *J Invas Cardiol* 1999; **11**: 503–5.

34 Khoo LA, Belli AM. Superior mesenteric artery stenting for mesenteric ischaemia in Sneddon's syndrome. *Br J Radiol* 1999; **72**: 607–9.

35 Peene P, Vanrusselt J, Coenegrachts JL et al. Strecker stent placement in the superior mesenteric artery for recurrent ischemic colitis. *J Belge Radiol* 1996; **79**: 168–9.

36 Sheeran SR, Murphy TP, Khwaja A et al. Stent placement for treatment of mesenteric artery stenoses or occlusions. *J Vasc Intervent Radiol* 1999; **10**: 861–7.

38

Percutaneous transluminal angioplasty of the subclavian arteries

Michel Henry, Isabelle Henry, Gérard Ethevenot and Michèle Hugel

Introduction

In recent years, percutaneous transluminal angioplasty (PTA) of the supra-aortic vessels, especially the subclavian (SA) and innominate arteries, has progressed from an experimental procedure to an accepted means of treatment with an outcome equal or superior to surgery in selected groups of patients.[1–4] Today, angioplasty is considered as the treatment of choice for the majority of cases by most interventionists.[3,5] Placement of endoprostheses broadens the indications towards total occlusions[1] and improves the results.[6] The first SA angioplasty was performed by Mathias et al[7] in 1980, and in the same year another case was reported by Bachman and Kim.[8] Since then many subsequent reports have confirmed its efficacy.[1,9–23] With experience of 135 consecutive patients who underwent PTA of subclavian or innominate arteries, we would like to discuss the technique, and the immediate and long-term results.

General considerations

Clinical signs

The subclavian and innominate arteries supply the brain as well as the arm with blood. Both vascular territories compete for the flow distribution in the case of a proximal stenosis or occlusion.

Therefore, the patient may suffer from symptoms of the arm or the brain,[24] and several clinical situations are encountered:

- The steal of blood from the vertebrobasilar circulation may be asymptomatic or symptomatic, with symptoms of impaired perfusion of the posterior cerebral circulation (subclavian steal syndrome). Clinically manifest verte-brobasilar insufficiency is caused by a unilateral obstruction, when the dominant vertebral artery (VA) is supplied by a stenotic SA. A stroke as a consequence of a SA obstruction is an unusual event when the carotid arteries are patent.

- Patients with acute arterial insufficiency of the upper extremity present with the same signs as with acute arterial insufficiency of the lower extremities: lack of pulse, pallor, paresthesia, pain and paralysis. A SA stenosis can be at the origin of thromboembolism with acute ischemia of the upper extremity.

- Chronic arterial insufficiency of the upper extremity is diagnosed when patients complain with disabling exertional arm discomfort.

- A coronary steal syndrome may have its origin in SA stenosis. Patients with mammary artery anastomosis will develop angina when the bloodflow in the SA is impaired.[25–31]

- Hemodialysis shunts and extraanatomical axillofemoral bypass grafts are endangered by a proximal SA obstruction.

Atherosclerotic disease is the most frequent etiology of subclavian and innominate obstructions, and the predilection site is the proximal part of the artery. The atherosclerotic plaques may extend to the aortic arch or involve the origin of the VA. The stenosis may be short, tubular, long, concentric or eccentric, ulcerated, or calcified. The occlusion always extends from the aortic arch to the origin of the VA. The arm symptoms are more severe when the obstruction is located distally to the origin of the VA because of the poor collateral circulation.[7]

Besides atherosclerotic disease, SA obstruction may be caused by the disease processes: fibromuscular dysplasia, neurofibromatosis, arteritis (Takayasu syndrome), radiation post-traumatic scarring and compression syndromes.[33–36]

Diagnosis

- Clinically, with a blood pressure difference greater than 20 mmHg between the two arms, we may suspect a SA obstruction.
- Duplex scan of the supra-aortic vessels enables the diagnosis of SA obstruction and subclavian steal syndrome and allows the diagnosis of associated lesions of other arteries like carotid arteries.
- The diagnostic imaging work-up of patients should include magnetic resonance imaging (MRI) with or without magnetic resonance angiography (MRA) or computed tomographic (CT) scan of the brain, with close evaluation of the posterior fossa and brainstem. MRA could be useful as a screening test to evaluate stenoses of both intracranial and extracranial vessels.
- A neurological examination by an independent neurologist is indispensable before and after the procedure and during the follow-up.
- A global arteriography and a selective arteriography of supra aortic vessels with multiple views allows us to assess the type, morphology and extent of the lesion, its relationship to the other arteries, and the origin of the internal mammary artery. We prefer to use the femoral approach for the angiographic diagnosis. The brachial approach using the contralateral access may be used, while the ipsilateral brachial approach is avoided for diagnostic purposes. Angiography is important not only for diagnosis of SA obstruction but also to diagnose associated lesions and particularly extracranial or intracranial carotid artery lesions.

Techniques of angioplasty (Figures 38.1–38.3)

A femoral or a brachial approach may be used interchangeably in most of the cases for the treatment of SA or innominate artery obstructions.[7,37] Sometimes it is helpful to use two arterial access points simultaneously to approach the lesion from both sides. This depends on the type of the lesion – stenosis or occlusion – and its location, as well as the patency of the iliac arteries.

In the majority of cases, SA angioplasty can be performed by the femoral route. Recanalization of an occluded SA or innominate artery normally requires a brachial approach, because the femoral route does not give sufficient support to the catheter to penetrate the occluded artery segment.[7,37,38] The brachial approach is also indicated in cases of severe tortuosity of aorta, iliac artery and SA or bilateral occlusion of the iliac arteries.

When the SA is occluded, the puncture of the humeral artery may be difficult. Sonographic or angiographic guidance may help the arterial puncture.

Technique by the femoral approach (Figure 38.1)

Femoral access may be used first in the majority of the cases. Several techniques can be used:

1. An 8F guiding catheter multipurpose type or, rarely, right coronary Judkins, is placed at the ostium of the SA. This

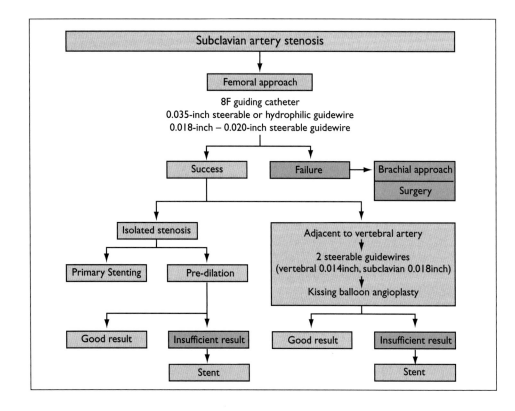

Figure 38.1

Femoral approach.

guiding catheter allows injections of the contrast medium and localization of the stenosis, which is crossed with a guidewire, either a 0.035-inch steerable or rarely a hydrophilic 0.035-inch, 0.020-inch or 0.018-inch guidewire for a very tight stenosis.

2. If the SA cannot be catheterized with a guiding catheter, the SA is selectively catheterized with a Vitek catheter or a Sidewinder or a Multipurpose catheter, generally 5F, and the stenosis is crossed with a 0.035-inch or 0.020-inch or 0.018-inch steerable guidewire, and rarely with a hydrophilic one in the presence of a very tight, irregular anfractuous stenosis. The catheter is then advanced into the axillary artery. Pressure gradients are then assessed. The guidewire is replaced by a rigid 0.035-inch Amplatz-type guidewire. The 5F catheter is withdrawn, and a 7F or 8F multipurpose-type guiding catheter advanced over the rigid guidewire up to the SA. As previously, selective injection of contrast medium enables us to locate the lesion. A balloon angioplasty is then performed (the diameter of the balloon is selected to be equal to that of the artery), the stenosis is dilated, the balloon is deflated and withdrawn, and a control angiography is performed, as well as an assessment of the pressure gradient. When possible, we avoid a balloon position over the origin of the VA to prevent VA occlusion by shifted atherosclerotic material. The risk of permanent VA occlusion is increased in patients with ostial stenosis of the VA. If the result is unsatisfactory (residual pressure gradient (5 mmHg or residual stenosis (20% on angiography), a stent is implanted. Stent implantation should be performed carefully, and covering the VA or the internal mammary artery must be avoided.

3. A third technique is currently used, particularly for direct stenting. It consists of the same technique as the one described above to catheterize the SA, but the 5F catheter used is previously placed in a guiding catheter, generally 7F or 8F (coaxial technique). Once the guidewire has crossed the lesion, both the 5F diagnostic catheter and the guiding catheter are advanced, and they usually cross the stenosis easily. The 5F catheter is then withdrawn and a stent is advanced over the guidewire, 'protected' by the guiding catheter, which is then progressively withdrawn and placed above the lesion. The endoprosthesis may then be deployed. Hard injection of contrast medium is performed to well place the stent.

Technique by the brachial approach (Figure 38.2)

By the brachial approach, we can place a long 6F or 7F sheath close to the lesion, which allows injection of contrast medium to locate the lesion. The technique is the same as the one described for the femoral approach with regard to crossing the lesion, balloon angioplasty and stenting.

Treatment of SA occlusion (Figure 38.3)

When the occlusion does not begin at the ostium of the SA and when there is a nipple, recanalization may be attempted with the femoral approach. In case of failure, the brachial approach is used.

When the occlusion begins at the ostium of the SA, it is usually impossible to cross the occlusion using the femoral

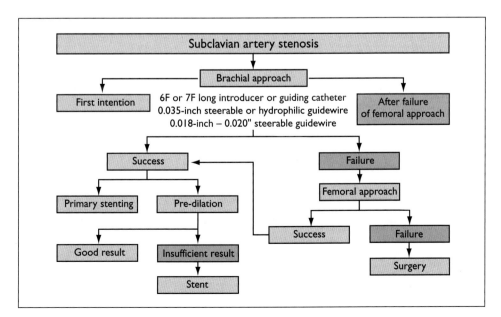

Figure 38.2
Brachial approach.

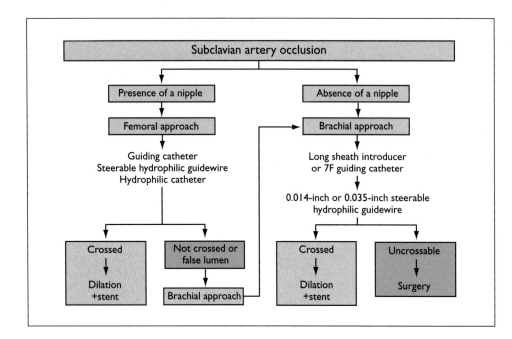

Figure 38.3
Treatment of SA occlusion.

approach. The brachial approach is then used. A catheter placed in the ascending aorta allows injection of contrast medium and localization of the lesion. Hydrophilic guidewires (0.035-inch Terumo J wire®) are then used to cross the lesion in combination with a multipurpose curved diagnostic catheter. Controlled force is often necessary to cross the occluded artery segment, especially in cases with calcified aortic arches.[7,37,39,40] After successful passage of the obstruction, the balloon is placed at the level of the occlusion, and inflated. Stenting is performed after using this access. In some cases (very tight calcified lesions), the guidewire is in the good lumen but it is impossible to progress and cross the lesion with the dilation balloon. We may try to exchange the hydrophobic wire for a stiff Amplatz wire inside a glide 4F or 5F Terumo catheter. This wire gives better support to cross the lesion with the balloon. In case of failure, once the guidewire has crossed the lesion, it may be advanced into the aorta and placed in a femoral artery. It may be caught back with a lasso through a femoral introducer, and the procedure (angioplasty + stenting) may be continued through either the femoral access or the brachial access point. By pulling the guidewire at its two extremities, crossing the lesion with the balloon is facilitated.

Associated VA stenosis

When the VA originates at the level of the stenosis, it is important to protect it with a 0.014-inch or a 0.018-inch coronary-type guidewire during the angioplasty procedure.

In the presence of an associated VA stenosis, the angioplasty may be performed using the kissing technique. Two balloons are placed at the site of the VA and SA stenoses, and simultaneously inflated. The decision regarding stent place-

ment is made by evaluation of the angioplasty results after deflation and withdrawal of the balloons.

The complication rate from embolization of plaque material is low,[10,41–43] and could be lowered by improving technique,[43–47] but brain embolization is always a possible complication of these procedures. Analyzing the site of plaques and stenoses in VA and SA, Staikov et al[48] described a special double-balloon PTA technique which may be helpful to avoid brain embolism in high-risk situations when a VA stenosis is associated with a SA stenosis. The double-balloon technique for PTA of the SA and VA has been employed previously.[45] Two selective PTA catheters are used simultaneously, one by the femoral approach and one by the brachial artery approach. The brachial catheter is exchanged over a coronary wire for a balloon catheter and the balloon is placed at the origin of the VA. The balloon in the VA is inflated to protect the vertebrobasilar territory from potential emboli when the SA stenosis is crossed by the guidewire and then by the dilation balloon. The SA stenosis is dilated while the VA dilation balloon is inflated. After dilation of the subclavian stenosis, the transfemoral balloon is deflated first and withdrawn to the origin of the SA. The restored bloodflow therefore flushes potential debris into the brachial artery. The VA balloon is then deflated. The result of the PTA of the SA and of the VA is evaluated by injection of contrast medium. If the result is not satisfactory, the procedure can be repeated or a stent can be placed by the transfemoral or transbrachial approach in the SA or the VA. When PTA has been successful, catheters and guidewires are removed.

The new cerebral protection devices, protection balloons like the PercuSurge Guardwire™ (Sunnyvale, USA) or filters (Angioguard, Mednova) could be used to protect the brain in some specific situations with patients at high-risk for brain embolism.

Stenting

Several type of stents may be implanted. For the prevertebral portion of the SA or the innominate artery, a balloon-expandable stent like a Palmaz (P154, P204, P304) stent seems a good option because of its excellent radial strength, radiopacity, accurate positioning and the possibility of flaring the proximal part which originates from the aorta.

The new Corinthian stent, which is more flexible, also seems promising. Other balloon-expandable stents may be used, e.g. Medtonic Ave, Megalink. Self-expandable stents have also been implanted in this location e.g. Wallstent, but with a lesion located at the offspring of the subclavian artery it is difficult to place the stent exactly without protrusion into the aortic arch or innominate artery.[49] For that reason, Nitinol self-expandable stents seem better, e.g. Optimed stent, Memotherm. Good results were also reported with the Strecker stent.[50]

For the post-vertebral location, we recommend self-expandable stents to avoid compression of the stents, e.g. Wallstent, Nitinol stents.

Medication

Before the procedure, the patients received 100 mg aspirin and 15 000 units of heparin per 24 h. 5000 units of heparin was also given as a bolus during the procedure, and heparin perfusion was continued for 24 h after the procedure. Aspirin at a dose of 100 mg/day was continued after that. In cases of stent implantation, ticlopidine 250 mg/day or clopidogrel 75 mg/day was given for 1 month.

Results

Patients

From January 1988 to October 1998, 135 patients (males 75, females 60) underwent PTA of the subclavian or innominate arteries: 19 right SAs (14%), 4 innominate arteries (3%), 112 left SAs (83%). The mean age of patients was 63 ± 11 years (range: 27–87 years). The mean age of males was: 63.7 ± 10.4 years (range: 40–81) and the mean age of females was 62.8 ± 12 years (range: 27–87). In the majority of cases (131 patients), the lesions were of atheromatous etiology. Dysplasia seemed to be the etiology in two patients, and post-radiation effects in two patients. In one of the patients treated for dysplasia, angioplasty was performed for severe restenosis which appeared 5 years after surgical endarterectomy. The locations were right SA, 112 (83%); left SA, 19 (14%) innominate artery, 4 (3%).

The main risk factors were: hypertension 55%, smoking 63%, dyslipidemia 37%, and diabetes 18%. Multivascular arterial disease was found in numerous cases: coronary disease 62%, peripheral arterial disease 38%, carotid artery stenosis 15%, and renal artery stenosis 5%.

In 110 cases, we found a tight stenosis (>70%), and in 25 cases a total occlusion. The mean percentage of stenosis was 80.9% ± 7.4% (range: 70–100), the mean lesion length 23.5 ± 8.7 mm (10–50), and the mean arterial diameter 7.2 ± 0.6 mm (5–9). Seventy lesions were calcified, 64 were eccentric, and 48 were ulcerated. Eight VAs were also stenosed on the side of the subclavian lesion, and three originated from the stenosed segment. Ninety-three lesions were pre-vertebral lesions, 29 were post-vertebral lesions and 13 were both pre- and post-vertebral lesions.

We found arterial blood pressure asymmetry in all patients on the diseased side. The difference for systolic blood pressure was always greater than 20 mmHg, mean 39 ± 17 mmHg.

The indications for angioplasty were: superior limb ischemia in 70 patients (subacute ischemia in 4 patients, chronic ischemia in 66 patients), and symptoms and signs of vertebrobasilar insufficiency in 72 patients. Vertebrobasilar insufficiency and superior limb ischemia were associated in 30 patients. Nine patients who had undergone a bypass procedure presented with signs of angina due to coronary steal. Fourteen asymptomatic patients were also treated because the lesion was very tight and because of the associated coronary arterial disease that may have required myocardial revascularization by internal mammary anastomosis.

The pre-angioplasty examination consisted of:

* duplex scan of all the supra-aortic vessels
* global and selective angiography of the supra-aortic vessels
* CT scan and neurological examination by an independent neurologist before the procedure.

We diagnosed:

* isolated stenoses, 67
* sub-clavian steal syndrome, 59
* coronary steal syndrome, 9
* associated vertebral stenoses, 12
* associated carotid stenoses, 20

Technique

The femoral approach was used in 99 patients with an 8F guiding catheter, according to the technique previously described.

The brachial approach was used in 26 patients with a 7F introducer, allowing easy stent placement. A combined brachial and femoral approach was used in 14 cases in the presence of a total occlusion.

It is worth noting that at the beginning of our experience we implanted stents (Palmaz P204 or P304) in cases of suboptimal results (residual pressure gradient >5 mmHg or residual stenosis >20% on the angiography), but we now tend to implant stents routinely, regardless of the result of angioplasty. Direct stenting may also be performed without pre-dilation, as we did in 15 patients.

Immediate technical results

Immediate technical success was obtained in 122 patients (94%). We were able to successfully treat stenoses of the SA (110 patients) with 100% success. However, we were able to treat only 12 total occlusions out of the 25 (48%). Thus, total occlusion of the SA remained a difficult problem. An isolated angioplasty was performed in 59 cases. A Palmaz stent was implanted in 66 patients (first case in 1989): 44 times for suboptimal result, 19 times for dissection and 3 times for restenosis. The mean length of the stents was 26.6 ± 11.5 mm, which indicated that the stents correctly covered the lesions. The mean diameter of the stents was 7.2 ± 0.7 mm, which is equal to the diameter of the treated artery. After the procedure, the mean residual pressure gradi-

ent was 3.5 ± 4 mmHg (Table 38.I). There was no longer any significant difference in the blood pressure between the two arms (Figures 38.4, 38.5 and 38.6 are examples of subclavian artery angioplasty and stenting.

Complications

- Local complications: we report two hematomas at the femoral puncture site without any significant consequences and one brachial thrombosis at the puncture site that required surgical treatment.
- Neurological complications, 2 (1.5%): we report one transient ischemic accident (TIA) with diplopia after treatment of a pre-vertebral lesion without subclavian steal syndrome and one major stroke with a hemiplegia occurring 2 h after the procedure in a patient presenting with bilateral carotid lesions. This patient died 4 days after the procedure.
- One subclavian thrombosis occurred after 24 h in a patient presenting with a dysplasic arterial lesion. The artery could not be recanalized. Since the patient refused surgery, he was treated medically.
- One subclavian thrombosis occurred on day 30 in a patient presenting with post-radiation stenosis, and was treated by a new PTA and stenting with success.

Table 38.1 Subclavian artery occlusive diseases, angioplasty and stenting: immediate results.[2]

	Mean % stenosis	Mean arterial diameter (mm)	Mean lesion length (mm)	Mean peak systolic gradient (mmHg)
Before PTA	80.9 ± 7.4	7.2 ± 0.6	23.5 ± 8.7	51 ± 33
After PTA	12.5 ± 3.5	7.1 ± 2.9	–	5 ± 4
After PTA and stent	4 ± 3.8	7.2 ± 0.7	26.6 ± 11.5	3.5 ± 4

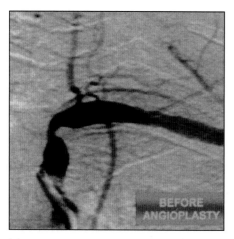

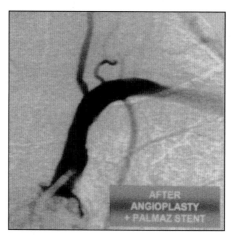

Figure 38.4
(a) Left prevertebral subclavian artery stenosis. (b) Results after angioplasty and stenting (Palmaz stents).

(a)

(b)

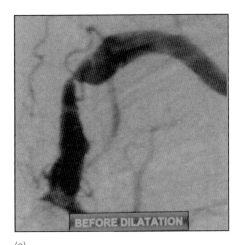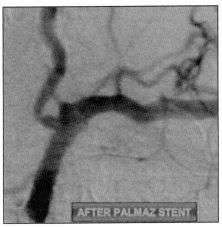

(a) (b)

Figure 38.5
(a) Left subclavian artery stenosis with subclavian steal syndrome. (b) Result after angioplasty and stenting (Palmaz stent).

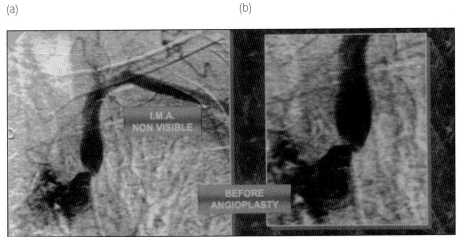

(a)

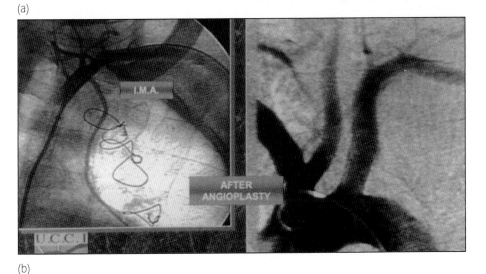

(b)

Figure 38.6
(a) Left subclavian artery stenosis with subclavian and coronary steal syndrome. (b) Results after angioplasty and stenting (Palmaz stent).

Follow-up

All our patients were followed up on duplex scan at 24 h. At 6 months, a duplex scan and an angiography were routinely performed. Then, a duplex scan was performed every 6 months, and an angiographic assessment was done only when restenosis was suspected.

Our mean follow-up was 51.8 ± 37.5 months, and the maximum follow-up was 10.9 years. We had 19 restenoses (14%): 13 occurred following angioplasty alone (18.8%), and 6 following angioplasty and stent implantation (9%). The difference is not statistically significant, but it seems that this is a tendency for a stent to lower the restenosis rate. Twelve of the restenoses occurred in pre-vertebral lesions, two in post-

Table 38.2   Subclavian artery occlusive disease patency rates.

| | All patients: 135 | | | | Recanalized patients: 122 | | |
	Global	Without stent	With stent		Global	Without stent	With stent
PI	76.1	67.5[a]	88.2[a]		83.1	79.1[b]	88.2[b]
PII	83.7	75.5[a]	96.1[a]		90.8	88.5[b]	96.1[b]
Follow up	8 years	8 years	4 years		8 years	8 years	4 years

[a] $p < 0.01$. [b] $p = 0.22$. 0

vertebral lesions, and three both in pre- and post-vertebral lesions. We treated these restenoses by another angioplasty (five cases), angioplasty and stent placement (seven cases) and surgery (carotido–sub-clavian bypass) (seven cases). In a post-vertebral tight restenosis inside a Palmaz stent (implanted for restenosis after surgical endarterectomy), we implanted another self-expandable stent (Optimed, Medcare, Conflans Ste Honorine, France) (Figure 38.7) with a very good result at 2 years. No restenosis appeared after treatment of an occlusion. Table 38.2 and Figures 38.8–38.13 indicate primary (PI) and secondary (PII) long-term patencies in all patients (135), and in the patients successfully treated (122), with and without stent placement.

According to Rutheford's criteria for all treated patients (135), PI is 76.1%, and PII is 83.7%. For all treated patients without and with stent respectively: PI 67.5%, 88.2% ($p < 0.01$); PII 75.5%, 96.1% ($p < 0.01$). Stents seem to improve long-term patency. And yet if we consider only recanalized patients (122), although there seems to be an improvement of the results after stent implantation, the difference is not statistically significant: PI 79.1%, 88.2% ($p = 0.22$); PII 88.5%, 96.1% ($p = 0.24$) (Table 38.2).

Discussion

SA stenosis is rare, with an incidence of 0.5% to 2%.[25] In most cases, the subclavian lesions are of atheromatous etiology and frequently form part of a multivascular arterial disease. Other etiologies may be found, such as fibromuscular dysplasia, post-radiation effects, Takayashu syndrome,[51] or other inflammatory arterial diseases. Until now, surgical treatment was considered as the reference. It involved either an intra- or extrathoracic bypass procedure. Although highly effective when successful, transthoracic surgical approaches carry a reported complications rate that could be as high as 23–25%. Complications included carotid embolization, cerebral ischemia, chylothorax, endarterectomy thrombosis, pneumothorax, pleural effusions, wound infection, neck lymph fistula, phrenic nerve palsy, and, most serious, Horner's syndrome, with a mortality of up to 8%.[52–53] The mortality of extraanatomical bypass is lower, but a complication rate of 8–15% is still present.[53–55] Subclavian balloon angioplasty offers a promising alternative, with low morbidity, shorter hospitalization, and a high rate of success.

The initial success rate is 97% in the series of Mathias et al,[37] 92% in the combined series of more than 400 cases reported by Becker et al,[56] 94% for Bogey et al,[57] and 94% in the data pooled from several studies.[19] These results are comparable to the initial results of surgery.[14]

The initial technical success rate depends on the status of the lesion. In the presence of a subclavian stenosis, the success rate is nearly 100%.[1,9,18,58] However, in the presence of an occlusion, the success rate is much lower in most of the series: 46% for Motarjeme,[1] 56% for Hebrang et al,[11] and 48% in our series. However, Mathias et al,[37] obtained a

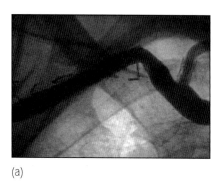

(a)

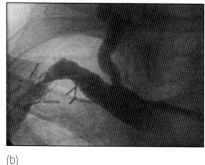

(b)

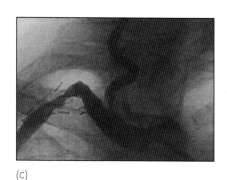

(c)

Figure 38.7

Figures 38.8–38.13

Primary (PI) and Secondary (PII) patencies for all patients with and without stents and for all recanalized patients with and without stents.

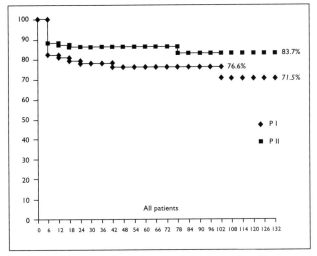

Figure 38.8

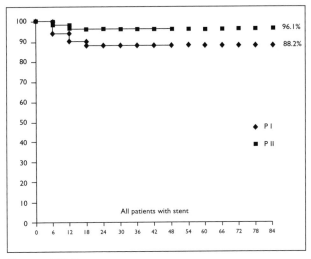

Figure 38.9

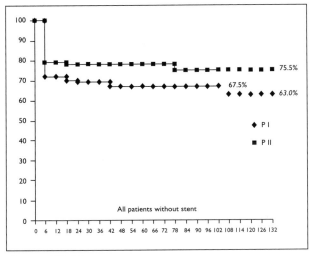

Figure 38.10

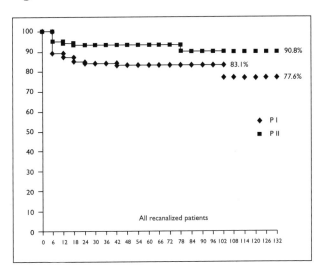

Figure 38.11

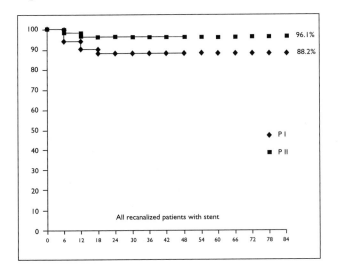

Figure 38.12

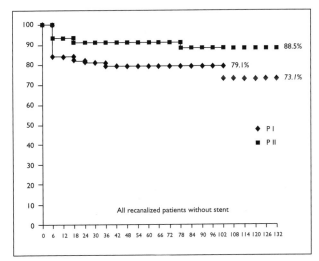

Figure 38.13

success rate of 83% in a series of 46 patients, and Kumar et al, 100%.[23] More recently Mathias and Jäger,[49] in a series of 416 patients with SA stenosis and 68 with SA occlusion obtained primary success rates of 98.8% in SA stenosis and 76.5% in SA occlusion. MacNamara et al,[59] in a review of 25 publications of SA stenoses in the literature (968 patients, 992 lesions), found an initial success rate of 95%, and in a review of six publications of SA occlusions (80 patients), found an initial success rate of 74%. A fibrinolysis performed before the procedure does not improve the recanalization rate.[1] Surgery is indicated in cases of failure of recanalization of a subclavian occlusion.

The results at the level of the innominate arteries seem similar to those obtained at the initial part of the SAs.[1,23]

The complication rate of these procedures remains low, particularly the embolic complications. Concern over the use of PTA in this disease has centered largely around the potential for the release of embolic debris during the procedure. However, significant embolic complications are relatively rare.[60] In addition, Ringelstein and Zeumer[61] have shown that it takes a significant period of time (20 s to 20 min or more) for flow in the VA to change from retrograde to antegrade after successful PTA, and they have postulated that this serves as a protective mechanism against cerebellar embolization. Becker et al[56] reported only three neurological complications and four peripheral embolizations in their series of more than 400 procedures. It also appears that the neurological ischemic accidents are mostly transient.[62,63] In a review of the literature with 1018 SA angioplasties, Kachel[50] reported a complication rate of 2.8% and an incidence of strokes of 0.2%.

Mathias and Jäger[49] observed in 3 of 484 procedures (0.6%) a TIA. All of them occurred in the carotid territory and were probably provoked by embolism from the aortic arch.

MacNamara et al,[59] with SA stenosis, reported a stroke rate of 0.4% and arm embolism in 0.3%, and with SA occlusion an arm embolism rate of 2.5%.

Mathias and Jäger[49] described three false SA aneurysms treated surgically (0.6%). This complication could now be treated by placing prosthetic graft–stents.

Vitek[10] has addressed the question of potential occlusion of the VA while performing subclavian PTA. In his experience, there have been no VA complications as long as the VA originates from a non-stenotic segment of the SA, including both normal-appearing segments and segments with post-stenotic dilation. In the presence of an associated vertebral stenosis, it is better to perform a simultaneous angioplasty procedure using the 'kissing' technique, or at least protect the artery with a guidewire kept in place in its lumen during the SA angioplasty procedure. The technique described by Staikov et al[48] may be useful in selected high-risk patients for embolism. The new techniques of brain protection could also be proposed for these patients.

The restenosis rate after subclavian angioplasty averages 13% after a mean follow-up period of 30 months.[22,56]

Duber et al[12] reported a higher restenosis rate after treatment of occlusions (50%), but Hebrang et al[11] reported results that were comparable to those achieved in PTA of stenoses. The combined series of Becker et al[56] suggest about a 19% recurrence rate. For MacNamara et al[59] the restenosis rate is 5.7% at a mean follow-up of 54 months for SA stenosis and 12% for SA occlusion at a mean follow-up of 33 months. If restenosis or reocclusion occurs, an additional stent may be successfully implanted.[12,37] In our series, the restenosis rate is 14% and a stent seems to limit it.

The long-term results of this procedure are satisfactory. Wilms et al[13] report an 86% clinical success rate at 25 months, while Hebrang et al[11] report 80% success at 4 years. In the Mathias and Jäger series,[49] after 2 years of follow-up a primary patency of 78.8% was found. The results of subgroups varied considerably between 76% and 84%, with the best outcome in the patients with SA stenosis and angioplasty combined with stent placement. The same subgroup also had the best patency rate after 5 years, at nearly 77%. The highest recurrence rate was observed in patients with SA occlusion treated only by angioplasty. Forty-six patients had a second angioplasty, with stent placement in 41% of them. The secondary patency after 5 years was 76%.

According to these results and our results, a prosthesis seems to improve the long-term patency rate but it is still difficult to achieve systematic stenting in all SA occlusive diseases. However, all SA occlusions should be treated with stents.[49]

The angioplasty technique of the SA has several peculiarities. The approach may be discussed. The femoral access site is usually used first in the presence of a stenosis. If crossing of the lesion fails, or if the femoral approach cannot be used, the brachial approach is used, or maybe the radial approach. This approach may also be used to decrease the risk of cerebral embolization during a right SA angioplasty. In the presence of an occlusion, the brachial approach is preferred to the femoral approach, more particularly if the occlusion begins at the origin of the SA.

Kumar et al[23] propose routine primary stenting because it achieves better results than balloon angioplasty, prevents intimal tear and abrupt vessel closures, theoretically could prevent debris embolization by trapping atherosclerotic material between the stent struts and the arterial wall, prevents possible particulate embolization into the VA and possibly lowers the restenosis rate.

As far as we are concerned, we currently tend to perform primary stenting in the presence of a subclavian lesion. Several types of stent may be implanted. The Wallstent stents are flexible, while the Palmaz stents are more rigid. Stenting should be restricted to the first part of the SA in order to avoid covering the origin of the VA and of the internal mammary artery. Because of the risk of compression of the stent, it may be better to implant a self-expandable stent for post-vertebral lesions.

Indications for PTA are the same as for surgery. However, because of its low risk, angioplasty is preferred. It seems appropriate in symptomatic patients with either neurological signs of vertebrobasilar insufficiency (e.g. syncope, ataxia, blurred vision, dizziness), or signs of ischemia of the upper limb, or both. The presence of a subclavian steal syndrome is a very favorable indication, since it prevents the risk of vertebral embolization. The subclavian steal is rarely bilateral (5% of cases).[64]

The isolated stenoses also represent a favorable indication, particularly in young patients, in whom the coronary risk is high, since the stenosis may render the bypass more difficult to start from the internal mammary artery. Recurrent angina following an internal mammary coronary bypass is also a good indication.[6,65–71] The incidence of this coronary subclavian steal syndrome has been reported to be 0.4%.[72] Marques et al[70] reported this incidence to be 0.7%. Treatment of the lesion (nine in our series) usually improves the symptoms. It is also indicated in patients presenting with lower limb ischemia secondary to a stenosis above an axillary–femoral bypass.

The indications are more debated in asymptomatic patients, because of their favorable evolution,[73,74] and low risk of aggravation of the neurological or ischemic signs. In these patients, we recommend subclavian angioplasty in the following two situations:

- Angioplasty of the subclavian stenoses before other cardiovascular intervention – coronary bypass, axillary-femoral bypass and preservation of the vasculature for other angioplasty procedures, particularly coronary procedures.
- Preservation of the cerebral perfusion. The treatment of subclavian lesions was proposed when there existed other arterial lesions at the level of the supra-aortic vessels, especially carotid vessels, so as to improve the cerebral flow.[14,15,18,75]

Conclusion

Angioplasty is currently the treatment of choice for lesions of the subclavian and innominate arteries. It should be proposed as the primary treatment, because it is associated with low risk, a high initial success rate and good long-term results.

Treatment of the total occlusions of the SAs remains difficult, and if crossing of the lesion fails, surgery should be opted for.

The indications for this procedure are still debated; and yet, the SA deserves to be preserved, because it is an axis of cerebral perfusion, and an access site for other angioplasty procedures. Also, the internal mammary artery, which is of the utmost importance as regards myocardial revascularization, originates from it.

Stenting seems to improve the long-term results and maybe we will have to recommend it for all lesions. We are awaiting controlled randomized studies, but SA occlusions, at least, should be treated with stents.

The Palmaz stent gives excellent results at the pre-vertebral level, and self-expandable stents are recommended at the post-vertebral level in order to avoid the possibility of post-vertebral compression.

References

1 Motarjeme A. Percutaneous transluminal angioplasty of supra-aortic vessels. *J Endovasc Surg* 1996; **3**: 171–81.

2 Vitek JJ, Raymon BC, Oh SJ. Innominate artery angioplasty. *Am J Neuroradiol* 1984; **5**: 113–14.

3 Motarjeme A, Gordon G. Percutaneous transluminal angioplasty of the brachiocephalic vessels: guidelines for therapy. *Int Angiol* 1993; **12**: 260–9.

4 Damuth HD, Diamond AB, Rappoport AS et al. Angioplasty of sub-clavian artery stenosis proximal to the vertebral origin. 1983; **4**: 1239–42.

5 Higashida RT, Ieshima GB, Halbach VV et al. Advances in the treatment of complex cerebrovascular disorders by interventional neurovascular techniques. *Circulation* 1991; **83**(suppl 1): 1196–206.

6 Diethrich EB, Cozacov JC. Sub-clavian stent implantation to alleviate coronary steal through a patient internal mammary artery graft. *J Endovasc Surg* 1995; **2**: 77–80.

7 Mathias VK, Schlosser V, Reimke M. Katheterrekanalisation eines Subklavianverschlusses. *Röfo* 1980; **132**: 346–7.

8 Bachman DM, Kim RH. Transluminal dilatation for subclavian steal syndrome. *AJR* 1980; **135**: 995–6.

9 Dorros G, Lewin PF, Jamnadas P et al. Peripheral transluminal angioplasty of the subclavian and innominate arteries utilizing the brachial approach: acute outcome and follow-up. *Cathet Cardiovasc Diagn* 1990; **19**: 71–6.

10 Vitek JJ. Subclavian artery angioplasty and the origin of the vertebral artery. *Radiology* 1989; **170**: 407–9.

11 Hebrang A, Maskovic J, Tomac B. Percutaneous transluminal angioplasty of the subclavian arteries: long-term results in 52 patients. *Am J Roentgenol* 1991; **156**: 1091–4.

12 Duber C, Klose KJ, Kopp H et al. Percutaneous transluminal angioplasty for occlusion of the subclavian artery: short and long-term results. *Cardiovasc Intervent Radiol* 1992; **15**: 205–10.

13 Wilms G, Baert A, Dewaele D et al. Percutaneous transluminal angioplasty of the subclavian artery: early and late results. *Cardiovasc Intervent Radiol* 1987; **10**: 123–8.

14 Farina C, Mingoli A, Schultz RD et al. Percutaneous transluminal angioplasty versus surgery for subclavian artery occlusive disease. *Am J Surg* 1989; **58**: 511–14.

15 Burke DR, Gordon RL, Mishkin JD et al. Percutaneous transluminal angioplasty of subclavian arteries. *Radiology* 1987; **164**: 699–704.

16 Toumade A, Zenglein JP, Braun JP et al. Angioplastie endoluminale percutane des artères vertébrales et sous-clavières. Confrontation angio-vélocimétrque. *J Neuroradiol* 1986; **13**: 95–110.

17 Mathias K. Percutaneous transluminal angioplasty of the supra-aortic arteries. In: Dondelinger RF, Rossi P, Kundziel JC, Wallace S, eds. *Interventional Radiology*. Stuttgart, New York: Georg Thieme Verlag, 1990: 564–83.

18   Boyer L, Canié D, Ribal JP et al. Angioplastie transluminale percutane des artères sous-clavière, axillaire et du tronc artériel brachiocéphalique. *Arch Mat Coeur* 1994; **87**: 371–8.

19   Graor RA, Gray BH. Interventional treatment of peripheral vascular disease. In: Young JR, Graor RA, Olin JW et al, eds. *Peripheral Vascular Disease.* St Louis: Mosby Year Book, 1991: 111–33.

20   Erbstein RA, Wholey NM, Smoot S. Sub-clavian artery steal syndrome: treatment by percutaneous transluminal angioplasty. *AJR* 1988; **151**: 291–4.

21   Selby JB Jr, Matsumoto AH, Tegtmeyer CJ et al. Balloon angioplasty above the aortic arch: immediate and long-term results. *AJR* 1993; **160**: 631–5.

22   Miliare A, Trinca M, Marbache P et al. Subclavian angioplasty: immediate and late results in 50 patients. *Cathet Cardiovasc Diagn* 1993; **29**: 8–17.

23   Kumar K, Dorros G, Bates MC et al. Primary stent deployment in occlusive subclavian artery disease. *Cathet Cardiovasc Diagn* 1995; **34**: 281–5.

24   Reivich M, Holling HE, Roberts B, Toole JT. Reversal of blood flow through the vertebral artery and its effect on cerebral circulation. *N Engl J Med* 1961; **265**: 878–85.

25   Perrault LP, Carrier M, Hudon G et al. Transluminal angioplasty of the subclavian artery in patients with internal mammary grafts. *Ann Thorac Surg* 1993; **56**: 927–30.

26   Crowe KA, Iannone LA. Percutaneous transluminal angioplasty for subclavian artery stenosis in patients with subclavian steal syndrome and coronary subclavian steal syndrome. *Am Heart J* 1993; **126**: 229–33.

27   Edwards WH. An unsuspected cause for recurrent angina: subclavian artery stenosis. *Am Surg* 1995; **61**: 1057–60.

28   Georges NP, Ferretti JA. Percutaneous transluminal angioplasty of subclavian artery occlusion for treatment of coronary–subclavian steal. *AJR* 1993; **161**: 399–400.

29   Kugelmass AD, Kim D, Kuntz RE et al. Endoluminal stenting subclavian artery stenosis to treat ischemia in the distribution of a patent left internal mammary graft. *Cathet Cardiovasc Diagn* 1994; **33**: 175–7.

30   Marques KM, Ernest SM, Mast EG et al. Percutaneous transluminal angioplasty of the left subclavian artery to prevent or treat the coronary-subclavian steal syndrome. *J Cardiol* 1996; **78**: 687–90.

31   Schulthesis T. Restenosis following subclavian artery angioplasty treatment of coronary-subclavian steal syndrome: definitive treatment with Palmaz-stent placement. *Cathet Cardiovasc Diagn* 1994; **33**: 172–4.

32   Andros G, Schneider PA, Harris RW et al. Management of arterial occlusive disease following radiation therapy. *Cardiovasc Surg* 1996; **4**: 135–42.

33   Hinchcliffe M, Ruttley MS, Carolan-Rees G. Case report: percutaneous transluminal angioplasty of irradiation induced bilateral subclavian artery occlusions. *Clin Radiol* 1995; **50**: 804–7.

34   Mathias K, Heiss HW, Gospos C. Subclavian-steal-syndrom – operieren oder dilatieren? *Langenbecks Arch Chir* 1982; **356**: 279–83.

35   Halbach VV, Fraser KW, Teitelbaum GP et al. Percutaneous transluminal angioplasty of subclavian stenosis from neurofibromatosis. *AJNR* 1995; **16**(4 suppl): 872–4.

36   Gambhir DS, Kaul UA, Verma P et al. A decade of subclavian angioplasty: aortoarteritis versus atherosclerosis. *Indian Heart J* 1996; **48**: 667–71.

37   Mathias KD, Luth I, Haarmann P. Percutaneous transluminal angioplasty of proximal subclavian artery occlusions. *Cardiovasc Intervent Radiol* 1993; **16**: 214–18.

38   Duber C, Klose KJ, Koop H et al. Percutaneous transluminal angioplasty for occlusion of the subclavian artery: short- and long-term results. *Cardiovasc Intervent Radiol* 1992; **15**: 205–10.

39   Dorros G, Bates MC, Palmer L et al. Primary stent deployment in occlusive subclavian artery disease. *Cathet Cardiovasc Diagn* 1995; **34**: 281–5.

40   Martinez R, Rodriguez-Lopez J, Torruella L et al. Stenting for occlusion of the subclavian arteries. Technical aspects and follow-up results. *Tex Heart Inst J* 1997; **24**: 23–7.

41   Motarjeme A, Keifer JW, Zuska AJ. Percutaneous transluminal angioplasty of the vertebral arteries. *Radiology* 1981; **139**: 715–17.

42   Théron J. Angioplasty of brachiocephalic vessels. In: Viñuela F, ed. *Interventional Neuroradiology: Endovascular Therapy of the Central Nervous System.* New York: Raven Press, 1992: 167–80.

43   Kachel R, Endert G, Basche S et al. Percutaneous transluminal angioplasty (dilatation) of carotid, vertebral, and innominate artery stenoses. *Cardiovasc Intervent Radiol* 1987; **10**: 142–6.

44   Nasim A, Sayers RD, Bell PRF et al. Protection against vertebral artery embolisation during proximal subclavian artery angioplasty. *Eur J Vasc Surg* 1994; **8**: 362–3.

45   Schroth G, Do DD, Remonda L et al. Spiezielle Techniken der Angioplastie brachiocephaler Gefässe. *Fortschr Röntgenstr* 1997; **167**: 165–73.

46   Sharma S, Kaul U, Rajani M. Identifying high-risk patients for percutaneous transluminal angioplasty of subclavian and innominate arteries. *Acta Radiol* 1991; **32**: 381–5.

47   Higashida TR, Tsai FY, Halbach VV et al. Transluminal angioplasty for atherosclerotic disease of the vertebral and basilar arteries. *J Neurosurg* 1993; **78**: 192–8.

48   Staikov IN, Daido D, Remonda I et al. The site of atheromatisis in the subclavian and vertebral arteries and its implication for angioplasty. *Neuroradiology* 1999; **41**: 537–42.

49   Mathias K, Jäger H. *PTA proximal subclavian artery obstruction. Tenth Internal Course Book of Peripheral Vascular Intervention ETC* 1999: 607–16.

50   Kachel R. Subclavian arteries and veins. In: Sigwart U, Bertrand, M, Serruys PW, eds. *Handbook of Cardiovascular Interventions.* New York: Churchill Livingstone, 1996: 855–69.

51   Hodgins GW, Dutton JW. Transluminal dilatation for Takayasu's arteries. *Can J Surg* 1984; **27**(4): 355–7.

52   Samoil D, Schwartz JL. Coronary subclavian steal syndrome. *Am Heart J* 1993; **126**: 1463–6.

53   Beebe HG, Stark R, Johnson ML et al. Choices of operation for subclavian–vertebral artery disease. *Am J Surg* 1980; **139**: 516–23.

54   Gerely RL, Andrus CH, May AG et al. Surgical treatment of occlusive subclavian artery disease. *Circulation* 1981; **64**(suppl 11): 228–30.

55   Aburahma AF, Robinson PA, Khan MZ et al. Brachiocephalic revascularization: a comparison between carotid–subclavian artery bypass and axilloaxillary artery bypass. *Surgery* 1992; **112**: 84–91.

56   Becker GJ, Katzen BT, Dake MD. Noncoronary angioplasty. *Radiology* 1989; **170**: 921–40.

57 Bogey WM, Demasi RJ, Tripp MD et al. Percutaneous trans-luminal angioplasty for subclavian artery stenosis. *Am Surgeon* 1994; **60**: 103–6.

58 Henry M, Amor M, Henry I et al. Endoluminal treatment of sub-clavian occlusive diseases. Percutaneous angioplasty and stenting. *Circulation* 1997; **96**(8): 1–284 (abstr).

59 MacNamara TO et al: Initial and long term results of treat-ment of brachiocephalic arterial stenoses and occlusions with balloon angioplasty, thrombolysis, stents. *J Invas Cardiol* 1997; **9**: 372–83.

60 Block PC, Elmer D. Release of atherosclerotic debris after transluminal angioplasty. *Circulation* 1982; **65**: 950–2.

61 Ringelstein EB, Zeumer H. Delayed reversal of vertebral artery blood flow following percutaneous transluminal angioplasty for subclavian steal syndrome. *Neuroradiology* 1984; **26**: 189–98.

62 Mathias K. Katheterbehandlung der arteriellen verschluss-krankheit supraaortaler Gefässe. *Radiologie* 1987; **27**: 547–54.

63 Jaschke W, Menges HW, Ockert D. PTA of the subclavian and innominate artery: short and long-term results. *Ann Radiol* 1989; **32**: 29–33.

64 Hennerici M, Klemm C, Rauntenberg W. The subclavian steal phenomenon: a common vascular disorder with rare neuro-logic deficits. *Neurology* 1988; **38**: 669–73.

65 Holmes JR, Crane R. Coronary steal through a patent inter-nal mammary artery graft: treatment by subclavian angioplasty. *Am Heart J* 1993; **125**: 1166–7.

66 Shapira S, Braun S, Puram B et al. Percutaneous transluminal angioplasty of proximal subclavian artery stenosis after left internal mammary to left anterior descending artery bypass surgery. *J Am Coll Cardiol* 1991; **18**: 1120–3.

67 Belz M, Marshall JJ, Cowley MJ et al. Subclavian balloon angioplasty in the management of the coronary subclavian steal syndrome. *Cathet Cardiovasc Diagn* 1992; **25**: 161–3.

68 Feld H, Nathan P, Raninga D et al. Symptomatic angina secondary to coronary subclavian steal syndrome treated successfully by percutaneous transluminal angioplasty of the subclavian artery. *Cathet Cardiovasc Diagn* 1992; **26**: 14.

69 Levitt RG, Sholey MH, Jarmolowski CR. Subclavian artery angioplasty for treatment of coronary artery steal syndrome. *J Vasc Intervent Radiol* 1992; **3**: 73–6.

70 Marques KMJ, Ernst SMPG, Mast EG et al. Percutaneous transluminal angioplasty of the left subclavian artery to prevent or treat the coronary subclavian steal syndrome. *Am J Cardiol* 1996; **78**: 687–90.

71 Schmitter SP, Marx M, Bernstein R et al. Angioplasty-induced subclavian artery dissection in a patient with internal mammary artery graft: treatment with endovascular stent and stent-graft. *AJR* 1995; **165**: 449–51.

72 Tyras DH, Bamer HB. Coronary subclavian steal. *Arch Surg* 1977; **112**: 1125–7.

73 Ackermann H, Diener HC, Seboldt H et al. Ultrasonographic follow-up of subclavian stenosis and occlusion: natural history and surgical treatment. *Stroke* 1988; **19**: 431–5.

74 Bornstein NM, Norris JW. Subclavian steal: a harmless hemo-dynamic phenomenon. *Lancet* 1986; **2**: 303–5.

75 Courtheoux P, Theron J, Maiza D et al. L'angioplastie endo-luminale percutanée des stenoses athéromateuses des troncs supra-aortiques proximaux. Tronc artériel brachiocéphalique, artères sous-clavières. *J Mal Vasc* 1986; **11**: 113–9.

39

Percutaneous transluminal angioplasty and stenting of extracranial vertebral artery stenosis

Michel Henry, Isabelle Henry, Christos Klonaris and Michèle Hugel

Introduction

Over the past decade percutaneous transluminal angioplasty (PTA) has been used to treat stenoses of the vertebral (VA) and basilar arteries for selected patients. In 1980, Sundt et al.[1] reported the first successful treatment of a basilar artery stenosis by PTA.

Since then a large number of centers have reported excellent clinical, angiographic, and hemodynamic improvement after treatment of extracranial and intracranial lesions.[2–15]

The risk of neurologic complications remains high for intracranial lesions. The reason for this is that the intracranial vertebral and basilar arteries are difficult to access and the PTA carries a high risk of damage to the perforating arteries that arise from this region.[6] PTA for this territory is still uncommon[16–18] and the outcome often not good.[19] Patients in the chronic stage who show no response to medical therapy should be considered for PTA.[19] There are only a few reports concerning the application of this procedure to these territories during the acute stage.[1,7,10,20,21]

The treatment of extracranial VA lesions is easier and can be proposed. A variety of surgical procedures have been described over the years but they are technically demanding and fraught with risks.[3–15,20]

However, PTA of these lesions and particularly ostial VA lesions can now be proposed with safety and efficacy for the treatment of vertebrobasilar ischemia or vertebrobasilar insufficiency (VBI). This is an under-diagnosed condition and the incidence of significant VA stenosis has been under-appreciated.[13] The complication rate from embolization of plaque material to the central nervous system can be lowered by improving technique in micro-balloon catheter technology, high-resolution radiographic imaging, proper neurologic monitoring, and patient selection.[8,9,19,22–25]

Balloon angioplasty alone has been limited by severe elastic recoil, poor improvement in the luminal area, high propensity for restenosis and failure to achieve less than 50% stenosis of the final lumen diameter.[2,13,19,22,26,–29] The use of stents seems to improve immediate and long-term results.

The vertebral artery is divided into four segments. The first segment, V_1 includes the origin of the VA (ostium) up to the level of entry into the *foramen* of the transverse process of the cervical vertebral body, usually C6. The second segment, V_2 or neck segment, courses up to the level of the *foramen* of the C2 transverse process. Distally to this level, up to the atlanto-occipital membrane, where the VA enters into the subarachnoidal space, is the V_3 segment. The V_4 segment is the intracranial portion of the VA.

Our report deals with the angioplasty and stenting of the extracranial portion of the VA and, particularly, the ostial segment.

General considerations

Vertebrobasilar insufficiency denotes global ischemia of the territory supplied by the basilar artery because of inadequate blood flow. This may result from central hypertension or from a drop in blood pressure within the vertebrobasilar system because of an occlusion or a stenosis in the proximal subclavian artery, the VA, or the basilar artery. Vertebrobasilar insufficiency embraces both the hemodynamic and embolic mechanisms responsible for the symptoms. But the majority of symptoms are related to hemodynamic impairment, in contrast to carotid disease in which emboli are the major source of anterior circulation stroke.

Arterial embolization is the underlying mechanism of VBI[12] in about 30% of cases and the relevance of embolization in the pathogenesis of transient ischemic attacks (TIAs) and strokes in the posterior circulation has been underestimated.

Atherosclerosis is the most common underlying problem in VBI. Plaque formation results in stenosing lesions that may affect the VA at any level but are most common at its origin from the subclavian artery. Plaques in the VA show the same degenerative features as plaques that appear elsewhere, such as ulceration, intra-plaque hemorrhage, and surface thrombus. The growth of a plaque may ultimately result in thrombosis of the VA.

One-quarter of all ischemic strokes occur in the territory of posterior circulation.[30] 20% of posterior circulation infarcts are thought to be cardioembolic in origin and a further 20% due to intra-arterial embolism, usually from the VA.[31] Seventy percent of vertebral and basilar occlusions are related to tight arterial stenoses.[32] In a series of 35 patients with occipital infarction, 6 had vertebral atheroma with presumed distal embolism.[33] So there is evidence that posterior circulation atherosclerosis is implicated in ischemic events.

Vertebrobasilar insufficiency may also be of hemodynamic origin. The symptoms appear only with rotation, extension, or flexion of the neck. The VA can be compressed by bone, mostly by osteophytes throughout its cervical trajectory. We have to differentiate this hemodynamic ischemia from the atherosclerosis ischemia.

Clinical findings

Clinically, patients may present with posterior fossa strokes and/or repetitive symptoms of vertebral and basilar insufficiency, including dizziness, diplopia, ataxia, nausea, vomiting, vascular headaches, bifacial numbness, cortical blindness, memory disturbance, nystagmus, and drop attacks. Other symptoms referable to posterior circulation ischemia include homonymous hemianopsia, poor eye-hand coordination, visual agnosia, vertical-gaze nystagmus, alternating hemiparesis and hemianesthesia, cranial nerve dysfunction, lethargy, and altered mental status.[34-36]

Two patterns of clinical presentation of VBI are recognized, depending on whether the patient has hemodynamic or embolic ischemia. Hemodynamic symptoms tend to be brief in duration and can generally be triggered by changes in the position of the patient's body or neck and can be relieved by lying down. Thromboembolic symptoms tend to last longer and to be varied in presentation, generally accompanied by findings of small infarctions in the magnetic resonance imaging (MRI) of the brainstem.

Prognoses associated with the two types of ischemia are also different. Strokes are uncommon in hemodynamic VBI patients, who experience complications derived from loss of balance. Thromboembolic disease carries a high risk of permanent neurologic deficit and may be life threatening.

Diagnostic imaging work-up

The diagnostic imaging workup of patients suspected of VBI may begin with a duplex examination and should include MRI with or without magnetic resonance angiography (MRA) or computed tomographic (CT) scanning of the brain with close evaluation of the posterior fossa and brainstem. For the prognosis it is important to determine whether the patient has suffered a stroke as opposed to an ischemic event, which can be reversible. It is also important to determine if the stroke is hemorrhagic or non-hemorrhagic. MRA could be useful as a screening test to evaluate stenoses of both intracranial and extracranial vessels.[37-41]

Angiography is essential with a complete four-vessel arteriogram as well as the intracranial portion of both the posterior and anterior circulation before deciding whether a patient is a suitable candidate for PTA. This is necessary to ascertain whether symptoms are secondary to ischemia from a hemodynamically critical stenosis or a thromboembolic stroke with occlusions of an intracranial vessel.

Angiography is also necessary to determine the extent of the lesion and evaluate it for evidence of ulceration, degree of stenosis, and the presence of fresh intraluminal thrombus. More than 90% of the VA pathology occurs at the origin of the VA, and this anatomy is involved in approximately 40% of all patients with symptoms of VBI.

Angiography is also essential to evaluate possible lesions in carotid and subclavian arteries.

Indications for vertebral angioplasty

Classically, patients should be managed initially by conventional medical therapy. Only for patients who fail to respond to this therapy should PTA be considered.[34,42-46]

A complete neurologic history and examination must be performed on all patients by an independent neurologist before and after the procedure and during the follow-up.

The current indications for the correction of extracranial VA lesions require:[13]

1. symptomatic (TIA or nondisabling ischemic stroke in the vertebral artery system) significant bilateral VA stenoses causing > 60% diameter reduction
2. a symptomatic unilateral significant stenosis of a dominant VA
3. significant unilateral lesions of a dominant VA when symptoms indicate ischemia in the ipsilateral posterior inferior cerebellar artery
4. significant stenoses in an asymptomatic patient who need collateral support (e.g. concurrent coronary artery (CA) occlusion).

In thromboembolic VBI, these considerations do not apply and PTA can be proposed. The smooth neointima that develop following a successful angioplasty may protect against future embolic events.

Angioplasty and stent placement

- *Access ways:*
  1. percutaneous access through the femoral artery is used in the majority of the cases[4,8,12,13]
  2. access through the brachial artery is used in case of severe lower extremity atherosclerosis, severe arterial tortuosities, and in case of failure by femoral access[13]
  3. the radial approach has been recently proposed.[47]
- *Techniques:*
  using the femoral approach a 6F to 8F sheath, depending on the artery, is inserted and a systemic anticoagulation is achieved by administrating intravenous heparin (5000 units) and checking an activated clotting time.

An appropriately-shaped guide catheter (Multipurpose, VBA catheter, right Judkins) is positioned in the subclavian artery just proximal to the ostium of the VA to be treated. For better control and support and to prevent the guide catheter from losing its position, an 0.018-inch extra-support wire can be placed in the ipsilateral axillary artery.[13]

Quantitative angiography is performed to evaluate the lesion, the degree of the stenosis, and to measure the diameter of the vessel to size balloons and stents. The degree of the stenosis is calculated in relation to the adjacent distal normal vessel diameter – analogous to the North American Symptomatic Carotid Endarterectomy Trial (NASCET) method for grading carotid artery stenosis – and calibration of the measurement is performed using the contrast-filled guide catheter as the reference.

The balloon diameter is determined by measuring the normal diameter of the vessel but below and above the site of the stenosis, so that it approximates but does not exceed this measurement. The diameter of the VA is variable, between 3 and 6 mm. The stenosis is crossed with an 0.014-inch or 0.018-inch coronary wire. Angioplasty is performed with a coronary balloon (Viva, Speedy. Bypass from Boston). We prefer to inflate the balloon no more than 10 seconds to avoid induction of further ischemia in an already compromised area.

Following angioplasty, an angiography control is performed to evaluate its results and choose the stent. The choice of the stent is largely governed by the location of the lesion and its anatomy. Balloon expandable stents are used to treat VA stenoses. For large vessels (> 4 mm in diameter) the Palmaz stent, Palmaz Corinthian, Medtronic AVE or other stents can be implanted and mounted on a Speedy balloon or on another low-profile balloon. For smaller vessels, any coronary stent can be used. Stents are deployed at high pressure (10–18 atm). Contrast media injection through the guide catheter facilitates the precise positioning of the stent. For ostial lesions, the stent must be placed at maximum 1 mm inside the lumen of the subclavian artery (SA). By the brachial approach, the same technique is used after insertion of a 6F or 7F sheath in the humeral artery.

Whatever the techniques, a post-procedure arteriogram is performed to evaluate the results of the procedure and the intracranial circulation for evidence of complications and distal embolization.

Close neurologic evaluation is performed during and immediately after the procedure and the day after. Patients are followed neurologically at 6 months post-procedure.

Doppler ultrasound is performed before the procedure, at day 1, and 6 months later. Angiographic control is also performed at 6 months, with CT scan evaluation.

In case of association of VA stenosis and SA stenosis, a kissing balloon technique can be performed by a femoral approach. A coronary wire is placed into the VA and a coronary balloon advanced over this wire. Another guide wire is placed in the SA with a dilatation balloon over it. The two balloons are placed at the site of the VA and SA stenoses and simultaneously inflated. Decision for stent placement is made by evaluation of the angioplasty results after deflation and withdrawal of the balloons.

With these techniques, the complication rate from embolization of plaque material is low[22,27,29,48] and could be lowered by improving techniques,[18, 22–25] but brain embolization is always a possible complication of these procedures. Analyzing the site of plaques and stenoses in VA and SA Staikov et al.[8] described a special double-balloon PTA technique which may be helpful in high-risk situations and particularly when a VA stenosis is associated with an SA stenosis to avoid brain embolism. The double-balloon technique for PTA of the SA and VA has been employed previously.[24] Two selective PTA catheters are used simultaneously, one by femoral approach and one by brachial artery approach. The brachial catheter is exchanged over a coronary wire for a balloon catheter and the balloon placed at the origin of the VA. The balloon in the VA is inflated to protect the vertebrobasilar territory from potential emboli when the SA stenosis is crossed by the guide wire and then by the dilatation balloon. The SA stenosis is dilated while the VA dilation balloon is inflated. After dilatation of the subclavian stenosis, the transfemoral balloon is deflated first and withdrawn to the origin of the SA. The restored blood flow therefore flushes potential debris into the brachial artery; then the VA balloon is deflated. The result of the PTA of the SA and the VA is evaluated by injection of contrast medium. If the result is not satisfactory, the procedure can be repeated or a stent can be placed by the transfemoral or transbrachial approach in the SA or the VA. When PTA has been successful, catheters and guide wires are removed.

The new cerebral protection devices, protection balloons the PercuSurge Guardwire™, (PercuSurge) or filters could be used to protect the brain in some specific situations with high-risk patients for brain embolism.

Medications

Aspirin (160 mg/day) and either ticlopidine (250–500 mg/day) or clopidogrel (75 mg/day) are given at least 3 days before the procedure and the same treatment is continued for 4 weeks. Thereafter, only aspirin is given.

Results

Patients' characteristics

Vertebral artery angioplasty was performed in 23 vessels in 22 patients (1 patient had bilateral VA stenosis). There were 12 males and 10 females, ranging in age from 57 to 80 years (mean 67.7 ± 6.9 years). All the lesions involved the ostium of the VA (left, 17; right, 6) and were symptomatic (diplopia, 2; dizziness, 22; TIA, 3). Three VA stenoses were associated with severe SA stenoses treated during the same procedure as the VA stenoses. Other associated diseases were carotid stenoses ($n = 18$), coronary diseases ($n = 12$), peripheral vascular diseases ($n = 8$), renal stenoses ($n = 2$), necessitating interventional procedures. Other comorbidities included hypertension ($n = 12$), elevated cholesterol > 200 mg/dl ($n = 13$), smoking ($n = 10$), diabetes mellitus ($n = 5$), obesity ($n = 4$), congestive heart failure ($n = 2$), atrial fibrillation ($n = 1$) and chronic renal failure ($n = 1$).

Technique

A femoral access way was used in all cases. We had 2 failures to access the VA due to severe tortuosities of iliac arteries and supra-aortic vessels. In these 2 cases, catheterization of the VA was attempted by a humeral approach but we also had a failure due to the same problem of vessel tortuosities. These high-risk patients were treated medically.

The first 3 patients were treated by PTA alone – the others (18 vessels), with stents after balloon predilatation. We implanted 9 Palmaz stents and 9 coronary stents. Three patients who had both SA stenosis and ostial VA stenosis were treated by double-balloon technique as previously described.

Angiographic results (Figures 39.1–39.3)

The VA reference size was 4.6 ± 0.6 mm (range 4–6). The mean stenosis before the procedure was 79.1 ± 7.4% (range 70–95), the mean lesion length 8.3 ± 2.4 mm (range 5–12). Minimum lumen diameter (MLD) was 1.12 ± 0.48 mm.

Of the cases, 21/23 achieved procedural success, defined as <20% diameter stenosis without any major neurological event, emergency surgery, or death after angioplasty and stent placement: MLD, 4.52 ± 0.8 mm; mean residual stenosis, 2.2 ± 3.7%; acute gain, 3.40 ± 0.7 mm (Table 39.1)

Table 39.1

Measurement	Baseline	Post-stent	p Value
MLD (mm)	1.12 ± 0.48	4.52 ± 0.8	< 0.001
Diameter stenosis (%)	79.1 ± 7.4	2.2 ± 3.7	< 0.001
Acute gain (mm)		3.40 ± 0.7	

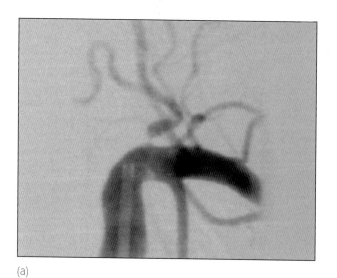

(a)

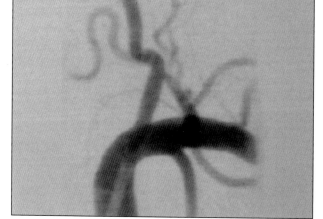

(b)

Figure 39.1
(a) Left ostial vertebral artery stenosis. (b) Final result after angioplasty and stenting.

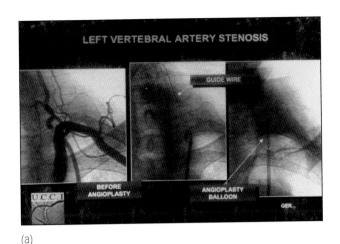

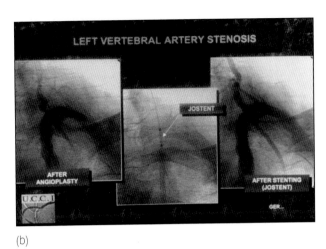

(a)   (b)

Figure 39.2
Left ostial vertebral artery stenosis procedure of angioplasty and stenting.

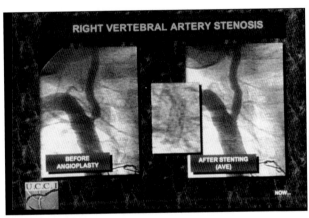

Figure 39.3
Right ostial vertebral artery stenoses angioplasty and stenting.

Procedure – related results and complications

There were no direct procedure-related myocardial infarction, stroke, or death during the 30-day post-procedure. None of the patients experienced cranial nerve palsies, wound infection, bleeding requiring transfusion or significant brachycardia, hypotension, or loss of consciousness after treatment with balloon inflations.

In all patients we observed a significant clinical improvement, with complete resolution of the clinical symptoms.

Follow-up

Results of a clinical follow-up are available for 20 patients at a mean of 31.3 ± 26.2 months: 4 patients have had neurologic symptoms during the follow-up due to a restenosis confirmed by Doppler scan and angiography (2 patients had been treated by angioplasty alone). Among these restenoses, we noticed 1 total occlusion of the VA and 3 tight restenoses (stenosis >70%) treated successfully with balloon angioplasty. The clinical symptoms resolved after the procedure.

Discussion

Vertebrobasilar system insufficiency is probably an underdiagnosed clinical condition,[13] due to several factors:

- The vertebrobasilar system is difficult to image with non-invasive methods.
- There has been a misperception that patients who have isolated dizziness or non specific symptoms do not have VBI.
- There has been a tendency to guide the diagnostic search in patients with ischemic stroke based on the need to find a surgical lesion. Thus, when patients are suspected of having an underlying lesion for which there is no popularly accepted surgical treatment in widespread use, angiographic evaluation has seldom been considered justifiable.

Stenoses and atherosclerotic lesion of the VA are frequently at its origin[27,49,50] as the internal carotid artery.[50] In general, the left VA is larger and is more often stenosed than the right. Using spiral CT angiography. Farres et al.[51] demonstrated plaques in the subclavian artery extending into the VA.

In the VA, plaques, stenosing and nonstenosing are more common on the medial than or the lateral wall. There is often a plaque extending from the superior wall of the subclavian artery into the orifice of the VA.

The generally accepted treatment for patients suffering from VBI includes platelet anti-aggregating factors, warfarin, or a combination of these.[52–54] Only in the most severe cases after failure of medical treatment, have surgical options been considered because of the potential complication and complexity of the procedure. A variety of surgical techniques has been developed for the treatment of the stenosis in the proximal VA, including endarterectomy, vertebral reimplantation into the common carotid artery or the subclavian arteries,[55,56] and bypass from the carotid or subclavian arteries using prosthetic grafts or autologous veins. Generally, a supraclavicular approach is used, although occasionally a transthoracic approach is necessary. In the largest reported series of VA operations, the Joint Study of Extracranial Arterial Occlusion,[57] 165 VA were treated with a mortality of 4.2% and an incidence of perioperative VA occlusion of 6%. In another series,[55] 109 vertebral operations were performed with 3% mortality rate and 2% rate of immediate thrombosis. In addition to the risk of stroke, these surgical procedures have a significant set of limitations, including an overall 10–20% risk of injury to the sympathetic fibers, the phrenic, the recurrent laryngeal, vagus, or thoracic nerves, as well as the potential for pulmonary complications from the thoracotomy.[55,56]

Given the difficulties operating on the VA, a percutaneous endovascular approach, angioplasty, has been proposed to treat a VA stenosis. The initial radiological and clinical results were uniformly reported beneficial to the patients.[2,3,26–29,58,59] However, in most of the cases, the stenosis was not fully dilated to the normal diameter of the VA.[29] If one carefully reviews previous reports on vertebral ostial angioplasties, most illustrate residual stenosis after the procedure. It has been well recognized that certain lesions, particularly those located at the ostia of coronary and renal arteries, have severe elastic recoil that limits the success of PTA.[13,60–62] At the ostial VA level, this may be due in part to adjacent subclavian plaque encroaching on the orifice of the VA. The stenosis at the ostium of a relatively small artery that originates from a significantly larger artery has a natural tendency for elastic recoil. This is exacerbated by the fact that the atherosclerotic plaques usually overlap the origin of the vessel and are extended into the wall of the larger artery, thus impeding the mechanism of PTA, such as sharing the intima and media and cracking the atherosclerotic plaque.

The use of larger balloons to gain greater luminal area has been proposed but often resulted in severe dissections that cause end-organ damage. Hence, there is the need for an endovascular scaffold or stent to hold back the elastic recoil and prevent restenosis. VA balloon angioplasty alone has been reported to be safe and is widely reported to help symptomatic patients.[2,3,13,27,59] The largest reported series is from Higashida et al.[59] who performed 34 vertebral angioplasties with an 8.8% incidence of transient neurologic complication and no permanent neurologic complications. Follow-up angiography revealed restenosis in 8.8% of patients within 2–5 months of angioplasty, with an undisclosed angiography follow-up rate. In fact a review of the illustration in previous VA angioplasty reports demonstrated significant residual post-procedure stenoses, probably emphasising the problem of elastic recoil.[13] With exceptions,[63] none of these reports included follow-up control angiographies. Because of the lack of angiographic follow-up, the exact restenosis rate is not known. Clinical data alone without follow-up angiography cannot predict the prevalence of anatomical restenosis.

The difficulty in obtaining images of the proximal VA by using non-invasive methods makes it almost imperative that angiographic studies be repeated during the follow-up period at least at 6 months, or better at 12 months follow-up.[13]

To overcome the problems of elastic recoil and atherosclerotic plaque overlap into the SA, and to improve long-term results, stenting was proposed for the treatment of VA stenoses, but the ideal stent for any segment of the VA has to be discussed. For the ostial lesions a P104 Palmaz stent seems a good option because of its excellent radial strength, short length, radiopacity, and accurate positioning. Other stents could be implanted, e.g. Corinthian, Medtronic AVE. When the proximal V_1 segment is very tortuous or kinked, more flexible stents may be used, particularly coronary stents (Cordis, Medtronic AVE, BeStent, Jostent). For lesions in the V_2 segment, the bone surrounding the vessel bone, self-expandable stents such as the Wallstent are better to avoid compression by the base during the neck movements.

For ostial lesions, the most important technical detail of this technique is proper, precise stent placement. The stent is intentionally placed minimally projecting into the SA. Meticulous attention to the precise relationship of the proximal edge of the stent to the SA is essential before deployment.

Procedure-related results in the majority of the published series are encouraging, with a low complication rate and good long-term results. Chastain et al.[13] treated 55 vessels in 50 patients with a technical success of 98%, no direct procedure-related myocardial infarction, stroke, or death. Clinical follow-up review performed at a mean of 25 ± 10 months revealed 2 patients with recurrence of VBI symptoms. Six months angiographic follow-up was completed in 90% of eligible patients, with a 10% incidence of restenosis.

Piotin et al.[11] treated 7 patients, with immediate resolution or improvements of symptoms in all patients.

Malek et al.[12] performed 13 VA angioplasties and stent placement, with improvements in symptoms in all patients except 1, who developed a stroke after the procedure due to a thrombotic occlusion of an untreated cavernous carotid artery stenosis. One patient had a TIA. Zhang et al.[64] treated 16 patients with an angiographic success of 100% and 1 post-procedure TIA. The restenosis rate was 6.2% at 6-month angiographic follow-up.

In a multicenter registry,[65] 54 patients were enrolled: 98% achieved procedural success without any major neurologic event, emergency surgery, or death; 3 patients (5.5%) developed restenosis with recurrent symptoms during follow-up (444 ± 353 days). The periprocedural complication rate is low, but potential complications include emboli originating from atheromatous plaques such as the carotid bifurcation location. When emboli are washed into the vertebrobasilar system, stroke may result. Most workers believe that the risk of embolization is low,[22,27] but some feel that the risk is substantial and that the PTA technique could be improved to lower the risk,[22–25,59] especially with plaques in the SA, close to the origin of the VA. The double-balloon technique, as described earlier, with the two approach ways seems useful. The new devices available on the market, used for brain protection for carotid angioplasty (occlusion balloon, filters), could also be used in this field for high-risk patients.

The antiplatelet and antithrombotic therapy before and during the procedure and after the stenting is very important to prevent thrombus formation and distal embolization. This is the rationale to premedicating the patients for 2–3 days with aspirin and ticlopidine or clopidogrel before the intervention and keeping them on this medication for 1 month after the procedure.

Abciximab was recently proposed in high-risk patients to reduce the risk of ischemic and embolic events.[66]

Three controversial issues remain. These are described by Chastain et al.[13]

- The need for intervention in asymptomatic patients found incidentally to have a stenotic VA lesion. These patients are treated because of the perceived need for the vertebrobasilar system to provide hemodynamic or collateral support. It is also necessary to consider that, although they are believed to be asymptomatic, many of these patients may have nonspecific symptoms such as dizziness[67,68] that may be alleviated by restoring adequate perfusion pressure to the vertebrobasilar system.
- The need for intervention in the case of a stenotic VA with a normal contralateral VA. Although the hemodynamic effect of the stenosis on brainstem perfusion can be easily compensated for by the normal contralateral vessel, the risk of in-situ thrombus formation and distal embolization is not eliminated. This pathogenic mechanism is reported to be a factor in approximately 25% of patients with VBI, more frequently in these with unilateral lesions.[69]
- Is the intervention reserved for patients in whom medical therapy has failed? We have no prospective randomized data. The treatment with both antiplatelet and anticoagulating drugs is at low risk, but does not treat the distal hemodynamic compromise caused by stenotic V.A lesions. This is significant enough to have been reported to cause VBI in 16% of the patients with this diagnosis.[69]

Conclusion

Percutaneous angioplasty and stent placement seem a useful technique for the treatment of VBI and the first treatment to be proposed. This technique is easy for experienced interventionists, safe, with a low complication rate and good long-term results.

Further prospective randomized studies are needed to demonstrate its clinical effectiveness in stroke prevention, its durability, and to define more clearly its indications.

References

1   Sundt TM, Smith HC, Campbell JK et al. Transluminal angioplasty for basilar artery stenosis. *Mayo Clinic Proc* 1980; **55**: 673–80.

2   Courtheoux P, Tournade A, Theron J et al. Transcutaneous angioplasty of vertebral artery atheromatous ostial stricture. *Neuroradiology* 1985; **27**: 259–64.

3   Theron J, Courtheoux P, Henriet JP et al. Angioplasty of supra-aortic arteries. *J Neuroradiol* 1984; **11**: 187–200.

4   Higashida RT, Hieshima GB, Tsai FY et al. Transluminal angioplasty of the vertebral and basilar artery. *AJNR* 1987; **8**: 745–9.

5   Schutz H, Yeung HP, TerBrugge K et al. Dilatation of vertebral artery stenosis. *N Engl J Med* 1981; **304**: 732.

6   Nomoura M, Hashimoto N, Nishi S et al. Percutaneous transluminal angioplasty for intracranial vertebral and/or basilar artery stenosis. *Clin Radiol* 1999; **54**: 521–7.

7   Lanzino G, Fessler R, Miletich R et al. Angioplasty and stenting of basilar artery stenosis: technical case report. *Neurosurgery* 1999; **45**: 404–8.

8   Staikov IN, Dai Do D, Remonda L et al. The site of atheromatosis in the subclavian and vertebral arteries and its implication for angioplasty. *Neuroradiology* 1999; **41**: 537–42.

9   Crawley F, Clifton A, Brown MM. Treatable lesions demonstrated on vertebral angiography for posterior circulation ischemic events. *Br J Radiol* 1998; **71**: 1266–70.

10 Kubis N, Houdart E, Merland J-J et al. Angioplastie des sténoses athéromateuses hémodynamiques des artères vertébrales intracrâniennes. *Rev Neurol* 1997; **153**: 6–7, 386–92.

11 Piotin M, Spelle L, Martin JB et al. Percutaneous transluminal angioplasty and stenting of the proximal vertebral artery for symptomatic stenosis. *AJNR* 2000; **4**: 727–31.

12 Malek AM, Higashida RT, Phatouros CC et al. Treatment of posterior circulation ischemia with extracranial percutaneous balloon angioplasty and stent placement. *Stroke* 1999; **30**: 2073–85.

13 Chastain H II, Campbell M, Iyer S et al. Extracranial vertebral artery stent placement: in-hospital and follow-up results. *J Neurosurg* 1999; **91**: 547–52.

14 Touho H, Karasawa J. Hemodynamic evaluation of the effect of percutaneous transluminal angioplasty for atherosclerotic disease of the vertebrobasilar arterial system. *Neurol Med Chir* 1998; **38**: 548–55.

15 Storey GS, Marks MP, Dake M et al. Vertebral artery stenting following percutaneous transluminal angioplasty. Technical note. *J Neurosurg* 1996; **84**: 883–7.

16 Honda S, Mori T, Fukuoka M et al. Successful percutaneous transluminal angioplasty of the intracranial vertebral artery 1 month after total occlusion – case report. *Neurol Med Chir* 1994; **34**: 551–4.

17 Nakano S, Yokogami K, Yamada R et al. Acute thrombolytic therapy and subsequent angioplasty for atherosclerotic stenosis of basilar artery – case report. *Neurol Med Chir* 1995; **35**: 674–7.

18 Nakatsuka H, Ueda T, Ohta S et al. Successful percutaneous transluminal angioplasty for basilar artery stenosis: technical case report. *Neurosurgery* 1996; **39**: 161–4.

19 Terada T, Yokote H, Tsuura M et al. Tissue plasminogen activator thrombolysis and transluminal angioplasty in the treatment of basilar artery thrombosis: Case report. *Surg Neurol* 1994; **41**: 358–61.

20 Touho H, Ohnishi H, Karasawa J et al. Percutaneous transluminal angioplasty for acute stroke due to stenosis of major cerebral vessels: Report of two cases. *Surg Neurol* 1994; **41**: 362–7.

21 Mori T, Kazitak, Mori K. Cerebral angioplasty and stenting for intracranial vertebral atherosclerotic stenosis. *AJNR* 1999; **20**: 787–9.

22 Kachel R, Endert G, Basche S et al. Percutaneous transluminal angioplasty (dilatation) of carotid, vertebral, and innominate artery stenoses. *Cardiovasc Intervent Radiol* 1987; **10**: 142–6.

23 Nasim A, Sayers RD, Bell PRF et al. Protection against vertebral artery embolization during proximal subclavian artery angioplasty. *Eur J Vasc Surg* 1994; **8**: 362–3.

24 Schroth G, Do DD, Remonda L et al. Spezielle Techniken der Angioplastie brachiocephaler Gefässe. *Fortschr Röntgenstr* 1997; **167**: 165–73.

25 Sharma S, Kaul U, Rajani M. Identifying high-risk patients for percutaneous transluminal angioplasty of subclavian and innominate arteries. *Acta Radiol* 1991; **32**: 381–5.

26 Mortarjeme A, Keifer JW, Zuska AJ. Percutaneous transluminal angioplasty of the brachiocephalic arteries. *AJR* 1982; **138**: 457–62.

27 Mortarjeme A, Keifer JW, Zuska AJ. Percutaneous transluminal angioplasty of the vertebral arteries. *Radiology* 1981; **139**: 715–7.

28 Vitek JJ. Subclavian artery angioplasty and the origin of the vertebral artery. *Radiology* 1989; **170**: 407–9.

29 Vitek JJ, Keller FS, Duvall ER et al. Brachiocephalic artery dilation by percutaneous transluminal angioplasty. *Radiology* 1986; **158**: 779–85.

30 Bamford J, Sandercock P, Dennis M et al. Classification and natural history of clinically identifiable subtypes of cerebral infarction. *Lancet* 1991; **337**: 1521–6.

31 Caplan LR. Brain embolism, revisited. *Neurology* 1993; **43**: 1281–7.

32 Castaigne P, Lhermitte F, Gautier JC et al. Arterial occlusions in the vertebrobasilar system, a study of 44 patients with post mortem data. *Brain* 1973; **96**: 133–54.

33 Pessin MS, Lathi ES, Cohen MB et al. Clinical features and mechanisms of occipital infarction. *Ann Neurol* 1987; **21**: 290–9.

34 Dyken ML. Anticoagulant and platelet-antiaggregating therapy in stroke and threatened stroke. Symposium on cerebrovascular disease. *Neurol Clin* 1983; **1**: 223.

35 Acheson J, Hutchinson EC. The natural history of focal cerebral vascular disease. *AMJ Med* 1971; **157**: 15.

36 Cartlidge NE, Whisnant JP, Elueback LR. Carotid and vertebral basilar transient cerebral ischemic attacks. *Mayo Clin Proc* 1978; **52**: 117.

37 Laub GA, Kaiser WA. MR angiography with gradient motion refocusing. *J Comput Assist Tomogr* 1988; **122**: 377.

38 Ruggieri PM, Laub GA, Masaryk TJ et al. Intracranial circulation: pulse sequence considerations in three-dimensional (volume) MR angiography. *Radiology* 1989; **171**: 785.

39 Hale JD, Valk PE, Watts JC et al. MR imaging of blood vessels using three-dimensional reconstruction: methodology. *Radiology* 1985; **157**: 727.

40 Masaryk TJ, Ross JS, Modic MT et al. Carotid bifurcations: MR imaging. *Radiology* 1988; **166**: 461.

41 Edelman RR, Mattle HP, Kleefield J et al. Quantification of blood flow with dynamic MR imaging and presaturation bolus tracking. *Radiology* 1989; **171**: 551.

42 Kistler JP, Roppor AH, Heros RC. Therapy of ischemic cerebral vascular disease due to atherothrombosis. *N Engl J Med* 1984; **311**: 100.

43 Weksler BB, Lewin ML. Anticoagulation in cerebral ischemia. *Stroke* 1983; **14**: 658.

44 Garde A, Samuelson K, Fahlgren H et al. Treatment after transient ischemic attacks: a comparison between anticoagulant drug and inhibition of platelet aggregation. *Stroke* 1983; **14**: 677.

45 Millikan CH. Treatment of occlusive cerebrovascular disease. In: Siekert RG (ed), *Cerebrovascular Survey Report for Joint Council Subcommittee on Cerebrovascular Disease*. Rochester, MN: Whiting Press, 1976: 141.

46 Sandok BA, Furtan AJ, Whisnant JP, Sundt TM. Guidelines for the management of transient ischemic attacks. *Mayo Clin Proc* 1978; **53**: 665.

47 Fessler RD, Wakhloo AK, Lanzino G et al. Transradial approach for vertebral artery stenting: technical case report. *Neurosurgery* 2000; **46**(6): 1524–7; discussion, 1527–8.

48 Théron J. Angioplasty of brachiocephalic vessels. In: Vinuela F (ed), *Interventional neuroradiology: endovascular therapy of the central nervous system*. New York: Raven Press, 1992: 167–80.

49 Tschammler VA, Landwehr P, Höhmann M et al. Farbkodierte Duplex-sonographie der extrakraniellen hirnversorgenden Arterien: diagnostische Aussegekraft und Fehlerquellen im Vergleich zur i.a DSA. *Fortschr Röntgenstr* 1991; **155**: 452–9.

50 Caplan LR. Bilateral distal vertebral artery occlusion. *Neurology* 1983; **33**: 552–8.

51 Farres MT, Grabenwöger F, Magometsching H et al. Spiral CT angiography: study of stenoses and calcification at the origin of the vertebral artery. *Neuroradiology* 1996; **38**: 738–43.

52 Caplan LR. Vertebrobasilar disease: should we continue the double standard of managing patients with brain ischemia? *Heart Dis Stroke* 1993; **2**: 377–83.

53 Caplan LR. Vertebrobasilar embolism. *Clin Exp Neurol* 1991; **28**: 1–22.

54 Caplan LR, Amarenco P, Rosengart A et al. Embolism from vertebral artery origin occlusive disease. *Neurology* 1992; **42**: 1502–12.

55   Imparato AM. Vertebral arterial reconstruction: a nineteen-year experience. *J Vasc Surg* 1985; **2**: 626–34.

56   Spetzler RF, Hadley MN, Martin NA et al. Vertebrobasilar insufficiency. Part 1: microsurgical treatment of extracranial vertebrobasilar disease. *J Neurosurg* 1987; **66**: 648–61.

57   Hass WK, Fields WS, North RR et al. Joint Study of Extracranial Arterial Occlusion. *JAMA* 1968; **203**: 961–8.

58   Schutz H, Yeung HP, Chiu MC et al. Dilatation of vertebral artery stenosis. *N Engl J Med* 1981; **304**: 732.

59   Higashida RT, Tsai FY, Halbach VV et al. Transluminal angioplasty for atherosclerotic disease of the vertebral and basilar arteries. *J Neurosurg* 1993; **78**: 192–8.

60   Zampieri P, Colombo A, Almagor Y et al. Results of coronary stenting of ostial lesions. *Am J Cardiol* 1994; **73**: 901–3.

61   Rees CR, Palmaz JC, Becker GI et al. Palmaz stent in atherosclerotic stenoses involving the ostia of the renal arteries: preliminary report of a multicenter study. *Radiology* 1991; **181**: 507–14.

62   Dorros G, Prince C, Mathiak L. Stenting of a renal artery stenosis achieves better relief of the obstructive lesion than balloon angioplasty. *Cathet Cardiovasc Diagn* 1993; **29**: 191–8.

63   Higashida RT, Hieshima GB, Tsai FY et al. Percutaneous transluminal angioplasty of the subclavian and vertebral arteries. *Acta Radiol* 1986; **369**: 124.

64   Zhang S, Jain S, Jeukins J et al. Aorta and long-term results of vertebral artery stenting. *Circulation* 1999; **100**:(Suppl I): I–674.

65   Jain S, Ramee S, White C et al. Treatment of atherosclerotic vertebral artery disease by endoluminal stenting: results from a US multicenter study. *JACC* 2000; **84A**:

66   Qureshi AI, Suri MF, Khan J et al. Abciximab as an adjunct to high risk carotid or vertebrobasilar angioplasty: preliminary experience. *Neurosurgery* 2000; **46**(6): 1316–24.

67   Baloh RW. Vertebrobasilar insufficiency and stroke. *Otolaryngol Head Neck Surg* 1995; **112**: 114–7.

68   Gomez CR, Cruz-Flores S, Malkoff MD et al. Isolated vertigo as a manifestation of vertebrobasilar ischemia. *Neurology* 1996; **47**: 94–7.

69   Wityk RJ, Chang HM, Rosengart A et al. Proximal extracranial vertebral artery disease in the New England Medical Center Posterior Circulation Registry. *Arch Neurol* 1998; **55**: 470–8.

40

Carotid angioplasty and stenting

Debabrata Mukherjee and Jay S Yadav

Introduction

Endovascular therapy has now expanded from the treatment of coronary and peripheral vascular diseases into the treatment of cerebrovascular diseases. Stroke remains a major public health problem, and carotid artery atherosclerotic disease causes a significant proportion of all strokes. Compared to endarterectomy, carotid stenting is a less invasive procedure that provides an attractive treatment alternative for some patients, particularly those with severe cardiac comorbidities. The feasibility and safety of the carotid stenting procedure as a treatment for severe carotid stenosis has improved with recent technological advances. This chapter outlines the current status of carotid angioplasty and stenting.

Percutaneous carotid intervention

Percutaneous transcatheter techniques have been used extensively in various vascular distributions. Although carotid angioplasty had been first attempted as early as 1977, the enthusiasm for this procedure has been limited by the fear of cerebral embolism.[1] Recent years have seen a rapid growth and increased interest in this procedure, due to the technological advances in endovascular procedures. Percutaneous intervention of the carotid arteries, when performed safely, has many advantages over surgical treatment. The potential risks of general anesthesia and the local surgical complications of endarterectomy, such as neck hematoma, infection, cervical strain, and cranial nerve damage, can be completely eliminated. Furthermore, this treatment approach is particularly appealing for higher-risk patients with coexistent coronary, myocardial or valvular heart disease.

Balloon angioplasty

Carotid angioplasty is of historical interest only as it has been almost completely replaced by stenting, which is a safer and more dependable procedure. Angioplasty was first reported by Mathias in 1977[2] and, in 1980, both Kerber et al[3] and Mullan et al[4] published case reports of successful carotid angioplasty during carotid endarterectomy. Since then, multiple case reports and observational series of angioplasty of the brachiocephalic vessels have been published, but these reports lack detailed outcome assessment and are only of historical value.[5-12] Procedural success ranged from 79% to 98%. Strokes occurred in 4–6% of patients, with no reported deaths during follow-up.

Carotid Stenting

In 1994, Marks et al[13] and Mathias[14] published the first reports of stent use in patients with high cervical carotid artery dissection and stenosis. Since then, several observational series reporting promising results of carotid stenting as a treatment option for carotid stenosis have been published.

Procedural details

Slightly different techniques of carotid stenting with similar basic principles have been reported. The goal is to access the

Table 40.1 Results of carotid stenting trials.

Study	Lesions (n)	Technical success	30-day outcome Stroke	MI	Death	Mean follow-up (months)	Stroke after 30 days	Restenosis
Diethrich et al[22]	117	116 (99.1%)	10 (8.3%)	0 (0.0%)	1 (0.9%)	7.6	2 (1.7%)	2 (1.7%)
Henry et al[18]	174	173 (99.4%)	5 (2.9%)	0 (0.0%)	0 (0.0%)	12.7	0 (0.0%)	4 (2.3%)
Laborde et al[19]	87	87 (100%)	4 (5.3%)	0 (0.0%)	1 (1.1%)	8.7	1 (1.1%)	2 (5.2%)
Wholey et al[21]	114	108 (95%)	4 (3.5%)	1 (0.9%)	2 (1.9%)	6	0 (0.0%)	1 (1.0%)
Shawl et al[17]	96	96 (100%)	3 (3.1%)	0 (0.0%)	0 (0.0%)	8	0 (0.0%)	1 (1.4%)
Yadav[20]	126	126 (100%)	8 (6.3%)	0 (0.0%)	1 (0.8%)	6	0 (0.0%)	4 (4.9%)
Wholey and Eles[23]	3129	3091 (98.9%)	121 (3.9%)	–	61 (2.0%)	6	14 (0.71%)	68 (2.2%)
Shawl et al[27]	192	190 (99%)	5 (2.9%)	0 (0.0%)	0 (0.0%)	19	5 (2.9%)	3 (2.0%)

MI, myocardial infarction.

carotid arteries with minimal manipulation of catheters, cross the lesion with the least possible trauma, gently pre-dilate the lesion, place a self-expandable stent to cover the lesion, and gently post-dilate the stent to achieve an acceptable lumen. A technique utilizing a telescoping apparatus with a long sheath is popular in North America. Various self-expandable stents are being investigated for this specific use (Figure 40.1). The safety and efficacy of adjuvant pharmacological therapy for platelet inhibition are also being actively studied.

Bradycardia and hypotension are not uncommon during carotid artery stenting procedures but are typically transient. Management of more prolonged hemodynamic alterations may involve temporary transvenous pacing and/or vasoactive medications.[15] In patients with severe left ventricular systolic dysfunction or valvular heart diseases, intraprocedural hemodynamic monitoring with a pulmonary artery catheter is helpful.

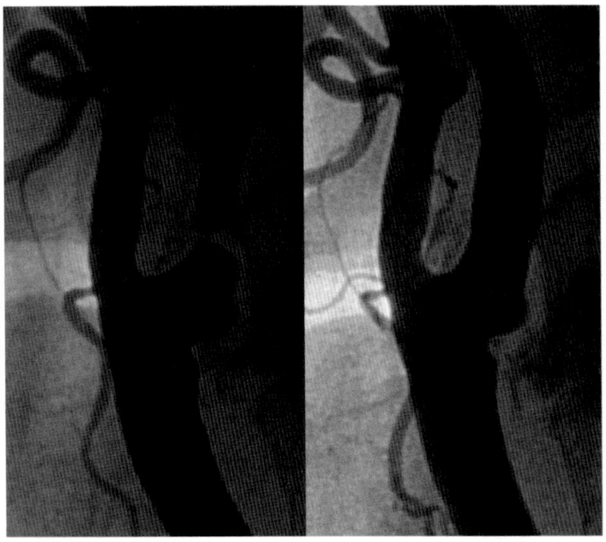

Outcome

Several reports of carotid stenting have been recently published (Table 40.1).[16–22] Wholey and Eles reviewed carotid artery stenting data from major interventional centers in Europe, South America, and North America.[23] The data were collected from surveys of the operators from various centers, and also from a review of published case series. The survey included questions on patient characteristics, procedural techniques, and the results of carotid stenting. This series reported on a total of 3129 carotid artery stent placement procedures as of October 1998, 46% of which were performed at 'high-volume' carotid stent centers in Europe and North America. One-third (37%) of the patients were asymptomatic. Technical success, defined as less than 30% residual stenosis covering a region no longer than the original lesion without any alteration of intracranial arterial anatomy, was achieved in 98.8% of patients. Various different stents were used, depending on the availability and operator preference. Stent deformation as detected by X-rays was seen in 28 instances (2% of all Palmaz stents), exclusively occurring with the balloon-expandable Palmaz stent (Cordis, Johnson and Johnson Interventional Systems, Warren, NJ, USA). Procedural and 30-day events were recorded. There were 74 (2.4%) reported transient ischemic events (TIAs). Minor strokes were defined as a new neurological event that resulted in slight functional impairment that either completely resolved within 7 days or caused an increase in the NIH stroke scale of less than four. Minor stroke rates ranged from 0% to 7% in different centers, with a total event rate of 78 (2.49%). Major stroke was defined as a new neurological deficit that persisted after 7 days and increased the NIH stroke scale by four or more. Major strokes were reported in

(a)   (b)

Figure 40.1
(a) Severe stenosis of internal carotid artery. (b) Angiogram after placement of the self-expanding SMART stent (Cordis).

43 patients with an event rate of 1.4% (range 0–4%). Procedure-related mortality at 30 days occurred in 30 (0.96%) patients. Post-procedure neurological sequelae occurred in 14 (0.79%) cases. Ultrasound studies were performed at 1 and 6 month post-stent placement at all 'high-volume' centers. Restenosis defined as diameter stenosis of >50% was approximately 2.5%.

The series reported by Yadav, Diethrich and Wholey have provided the most rigorous detail of carotid stenting techniques, procedural success, and patient outcomes.[20–22] Yadav et al[20] published their initial experience of carotid stenting in 107 consecutive patients. All procedures were successful. Patients had independent neurological examinations before and after the procedure. Periprocedural complications included one stent thrombosis, six minor strokes, and one major stroke. Clinical follow-up at 30 days showed one additional minor stroke, one major stroke, one myocardial infarction, and one death not due to cerebrovascular disease. The incidence of combined endpoint of all strokes and death was 7.9%, with 1.6% ipsilateral major stroke and death. In total, 81 (76%) patients underwent angiography or ultrasound evaluation 6 months after stenting. Four (4.9%) of these 81 patients had asymptomatic restenosis. Five asymptomatic patients had repeat interventions with angioplasty for restenosis in two, angioplasty for stent deformation in another two, and endarterectomy for restenosis in one. At 6-month follow-up, there were no strokes or deaths from cerebrovascular disease. The University of Alabama group extended their experience to 146 procedures, with similar results.[24] It is important to recognize that these results were obtained in a high-risk cohort and represent the initial, learning curve for carotid stenting. Seventy-seven percent of the patients treated with stenting in this series would have been ineligible for carotid endarterectomy on the basis of the ACAS and NASCET exclusion criteria.[25,26] The other major carotid stent series have included patients with a similar high-risk profile.

Diethrich et al[22] reported their experience in 110 patients with severe carotid stenosis. Stenting was successful in 99% of patients. There were seven (6.4%) strokes (two major, five minor), five (4.5%) TIAs and two asymptomatic stent occlusions in the first 30 days after the procedure. Overall, 89% of patients had successful procedures and were free from death, surgical intervention, stroke or stent occlusion at 30 days. During a mean of 7.6 months of follow-up, no additional neurological events were reported.

Wholey et al reported 114 lesions in 108 consecutive patients (58 men; mean age 70.1 years) with ≥70% carotid stenosis treated with percutaneous stent implantation. Forty-four percent were asymptomatic. Stents were successfully placed in 108 (95%) lesions. Of the six technical failures, five were access related and one was due to seizures during balloon dilation. Two major (1.8%) and two minor (1.8%) strokes occurred, all in symptomatic patients, one of whom died. There were five (4.4%) TIAs and two (1.8%) brief seizure episodes during dilation. The total stroke or death rate was 5.3%. At the mean 6-month follow-up, there was one restenosis (1.0%) from a stent compression, which was successfully dilated. There were no neurological sequelae, cranial palsies, or cases of stent or vessel thrombosis on follow-up.

Henry et al reported their experience of 174 stenting procedures in 163 patients.[18] This series differs from the others, as a cerebral emboli protection device was used in a small subset (n = 32, 18%). The majority (65%) of the patients were asymptomatic. Immediate technical success was achieved in all but one patient (99.4%). Eight (4.6%) neurological complications occurred in the periprocedural period: three TIAs, two minor strokes, and three major strokes. Two major complications developed despite cerebral protection. Over a mean follow-up of 1 year, no ipsilateral neurological complications were seen. Palmaz stent compression was seen in one patient, and four (2.3%) patients were identified with restenosis.

Recently, Shawl et al evaluated the safety and efficacy of carotid artery stenting in 170 consecutive high-risk patients who underwent the procedure in 192 carotid arteries.[27] The procedural success rate was 99%. During the initial hospital period and 30 days after carotid stenting, there was one major and there were two category 2 minor strokes, as well as two category 1 minor strokes (total 30-day stroke rate was 2.9%). There were no myocardial infarctions or death during or within 30 days of carotid stenting. None of the NASCET-eligible patients had a stroke. At a mean follow-up of 19 ± 11 months, three patients (2%) had asymptomatic restenosis. No other major strokes or neurological deaths occurred.

Owing to relatively small sample sizes and infrequent events in each series, independent predictors for procedural strokes have not been well studied. As in surgical trials, symptom status appears to correlate with the frequency of adverse neurological outcomes after carotid stenting. This was seen in the series reported by Yadav et al, where eight (11%) ipsilateral neurological deficits or deaths were encountered after 74 procedures for symptomatic carotid stenosis, and only two (4%) after 52 procedures in asymptomatic patients.[20] Similarly, Wholey et al observed a higher stroke rate in symptomatic patients.[21] However, in a multivariate analysis of 271 carotid procedures in 231 patients, Mathur et al found only advanced age and long or multiple stenosis to be independent predictors of procedural stroke.[28]

Restenosis, a long-term complication after carotid stenting, is fortunately rare. In the major carotid stent series, 33 (5%) of 655 carotid artery procedures were complicated by restenosis when systematically studied with either angiography or ultrasound follow-up evaluations. Stent deformation occurred in 10 (1.5%) patients, all occurring with the Palmaz stent. Even though only four (6.1%) cases of restenosis or stent deformation were symptomatic, 16 (37.2%) underwent treatment with repeat dilation, repeat stenting, endarterectomy, or bypass grafting. As balloon-expandable stents are replaced by self-expanding stents, stent deformation has become clinically irrelevant.

The field of carotid stenting is rapidly evolving with the advent of new pharmacological and technological advances. The availability of better, tailor-made instruments, emboli protection devices and advanced pharmacological adjuvant therapies will make carotid stenting a more attractive procedure.

Emboli protection devices

The major cause of stroke during carotid endarterectomy and percutaneous carotid intervention is the procedural embolization of plaque debris along with platelet and thrombin aggregates into the cerebral circulation. Transcranial Doppler monitoring, a non-invasive method to detect echogenic microemboli, has demonstrated frequent embolization during carotid endarterectomy and stenting.[29–32] Although data are limited, there appears to be a correlation between the number of emboli and neurological outcome after endarterectomy.[31,32] Consequently, various mechanical and pharmacological approaches to prevent distal embolization are currently under investigation to improve the safety of carotid stenting.[33–35]

Henry et al reported their experience in 58 carotid artery stent procedures using a prototype cerebral protection device and compared the results to 212 other patients treated without the emboli protection device.[35] This cerebral protection catheter is a low-profile, balloon-tipped device designed to block cerebral emboli when positioned in the internal carotid artery distal to the target lesion. Conceptually, the protection balloon occludes the run-off

circulation to the brain, trapping any particles dislodged following balloon angioplasty or stent delivery so that they can subsequently be extracted via aspiration into the guiding catheter. In this series, there was one immediate neurological complication (1.5%) compared to 11 (5.2%) in the group treated without the device. However, the feasibility of transient carotid occlusion without consequences and potential endothelial injury and embolization from the occlusion balloon itself are important concerns that need further evaluation. An alternative mechanical embolization device that allows continued perfusion while capturing emboli has been developed (Figures 40.2 and 40.3). This filter-type device has been recently tested in carotid, coronary and peripheral interventions, and should be available in the near future for rigorous randomized trials.[33]

Adjuvant pharmacological therapy

Pharmacological protection against embolization is based on randomized clinical trials utilizing platelet glycoprotein IIb/IIIa inhibitors during coronary interventions. Various Gp IIb/IIIa inhibitors, especially abciximab, have been shown to be effective in reducing the ischemic complications of death, myocardial infarction or urgent repeat revascularization after percutaneous coronary interventional procedures.[36–38]

The coronary experience has been extended to selected patients in 22 carotid stent procedures involving visible thrombus, total occlusion, or acute stroke. The preliminary data from these high-risk patients suggested relatively high bleeding complications, with two cases (7%) of central

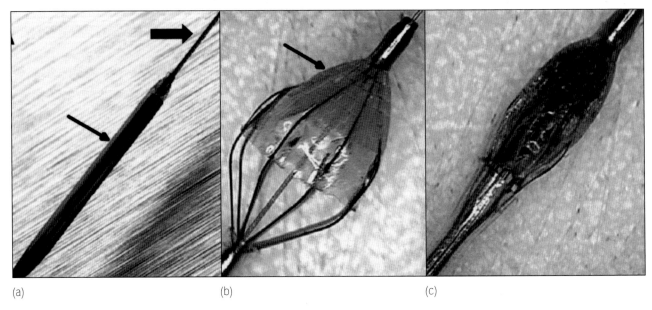

(a)   (b)   (c)

Figure 40.2
(a) An emboli protection device (Angioguard, Cordis) in closed state. The bold arrow represents a 0.014-inch wire that leads the device (4F) shown by the smaller arrow. (b) Open device with a filter with 100-μm pore size. (c) Closed filter with captured embolic debris.

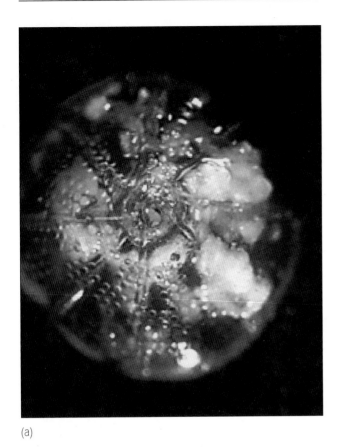

(a)

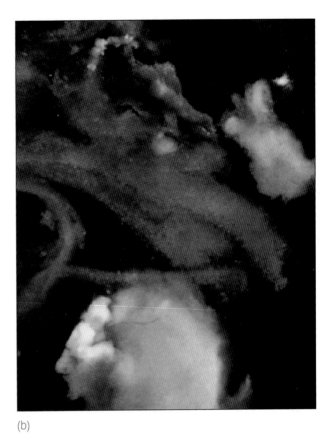

(b)

Figure 40.3
(a) Filter with atheromatous embolic debris. (b) Magnified view of typical atheromatous embolic particles retrieved during intervention.

nervous system bleeding, one hemorrhagic transformation of a previously ischemic stroke, and one subarachnoid hemorrhage from a ruptured aneurysm.[39] Periprocedural glycoprotein IIb/IIIa receptor inhibition may be safer and more effective when used in a routine prophylactic manner. This approach is being currently evaluated. Other potential therapies, including low molecular weight heparin or direct thrombin inhibitors, have not been studied in carotid stenting procedures. Only preliminary information on the efficacy and safety of clopidogrel therapy is available.[40]

Surgery versus percutaneous intervention

One randomized trial, CAVATAS, comparing surgery with percutaneous intervention, has been reported.[41] This study evaluated the safety and efficacy of percutaneous angioplasty versus endarterectomy of the carotid artery. Symptomatic patients with 70% stenosis were randomly assigned to angioplasty or surgery, or (if the patient was unsuitable for surgery) to angioplasty or best medical treatment. Preliminary data indicate that 253 patients were randomized to carotid

endarterectomy and 251 to carotid angioplasty (of whom 25% received stents). A major periprocedural complication was observed in 6.3% of patients in both groups (M. Brown, personal communication).[42] CAVATAS-2, with a larger sample size, should provide more insights into the role of percutaneous carotid intervention.

Two important trials comparing carotid artery stenting with endarterectomy have been planned. The CREST trial (Carotid Revascularization Endarterectomy versus Stent Trial) will randomize patients who are at low surgical risk to stenting or surgery. The primary endpoints for this trial are: (1) any stroke, myocardial infarction or death within 30 days; and (2) ipsilateral stroke after 30 days. This trial is planning to recruit 2500 patients, as event rate is likely to be low. A clinical events committee will adjudicate all events. The secondary endpoints for this study include comparisons of 30-day morbidity and mortality, long-term morbidity and mortality, restenosis rates, quality of life and cost-effectiveness for the two treatment alternatives. Multivariate analysis to identify subgroups of patients at differential risk for the two procedures will be performed.

The SAPPHIRE trial (Stenting and Angioplasty with Protection in Patients at High Risk for Endarterectomy) will randomize patients at high surgical risk to carotid endarterectomy or carotid artery stenting. The high-risk patient population is defined as patients with severe cardiac comorbidities (unstable angina, valvular heart disease, severe congestive heart failure), previous neck radiation, previous radical neck dissections, restenosis after endarterectomy, or presence of contralateral occlusion. Both de novo and restenotic lesions will be treated in symptomatic (>70% stenosis) or asymptomatic (>80% stenosis) patients. In total, 720 patients at 24 sites will be enrolled, and a parallel stent and surgical registries will be maintained for the non-randomized patients. The primary endpoint is a 30-day composite of any stroke, death, or myocardial infarction. The secondary endpoint is 1-year ipsilateral stroke and death rate. This trial will utilize the Cordis Nitinol carotid stent and Cordis Angioguard™ (Cordis, Warren, NJ), an emboli protection device.

References

1   Beebe HG, Archie JP, Baker WH et al. Concern about safety of carotid angioplasty. *Stroke* 1996; **27**: 197–8.

2   Mathias K. A new catheter system for percutaneous transluminal angioplasty (PTA) of carotid artery stenoses. *Fortschr Med* 1977; **95**: 1007–11.

3   Kerber CW, Cromwell LD, Loehden OL. Catheter dilatation of proximal carotid stenosis during distal bifurcation endarterectomy. *Am J Neuroradiol* 1980; **1**: 348–9.

4   Mullan S, Duda EE, Patronas NJ. Some examples of balloon technology in neurosurgery. *J Neurosurg* 1980; **52**: 321–9.

5   Brown MM, Butler P, Gibbs et al. Feasibility of percutaneous transluminal angioplasty for carotid artery stenosis. *J Neurol Neurosurg Psychiatry* 1990; **53**: 238–43.

6   Kachel R, Basche S, Heerklotz I et al. Percutaneous transluminal angioplasty (PTA) of supra-aortic arteries especially the internal carotid artery. *Neuroradiology* 1991; **33**: 191–4.

7   Tsai FY, Matovich V, Hieshima G et al. Percutaneous transluminal angioplasty of the carotid artery. *Am J Neuroradiol* 1986; **7**: 349–58.

8   Higashida RT, Tsai FY, Halbach W et al. Cerebral percutaneous transluminal angioplasty. *Heart Dis Stroke* 1993; **2**: 497–502.

9   Bergeron P, Chambran P, Hartung O, Bianca S. Cervical carotid artery stenosis: which technique, balloon angioplasty or surgery? *J Cardiovasc Surg (Torino)* 1996; **37**: 73–5.

10   Kachel R. Results of balloon angioplasty in the carotid arteries. *J Endovasc Surg* 1996; **3**: 22–30.

11   Gil-Peralta A, Mayol A, Marcos JR et al. Percutaneous transluminal angioplasty of the symptomatic atherosclerotic carotid arteries. Results, complications, and follow-up. *Stroke* 1996; **27**: 2271–3.

12   Motarjeme A, Keifer JW, Zuska AJ. Percutaneous transluminal angioplasty of the brachiocephalic arteries. *Am J Roentgenol* 1982; **138**: 457–62.

13   Marks MP, Dake MD, Steinberg GK et al, Lane B. Stent placement for arterial and venous cerebrovascular disease: preliminary experience. *Radiology* 1994; **191**: 441–6.

14   Mathias K. *Stent Placement in Arteriosclerotic Disease of the Internal Carotid Artery*. Oxford: Isis Medical Media, 1997.

15   Mendelsohn FO, Weissman NJ, Lederman RJ et al. Acute hemodynamic changes during carotid artery stenting. *Am J Cardiol* 1998; **82**: 1077–81.

16   Theron JG, Payelle GG, Coskun O et al. Carotid artery stenosis: treatment with protected balloon angioplasty and stent placement. *Radiology* 1996; **201**: 627–36.

17   Shawl FA, Efstratiou A, Lapetina FL et al. Stent supported carotid angioplasty (SSCA) in patients with symptomatic coronary artery disease: acute and long term results. *J Am Coll Cardiol* 1998; **31** (Suppl): 454A.

18   Henry M, Amor M, Masson I et al. Angioplasty and stenting of the extracranial carotid arteries. *J Endovasc Surg* 1998; **5**: 293–304.

19   Laborde JC, Fajadet J, Cassagneau B et al. Carotid stenting in patients at risk for surgery: immediate and long-term results. *J Am Coll Cardiol* 1998; **31** (Suppl): 63A.

20   Yadav JS, Roubin GS, Iyer S et al. Elective stenting of the extracranial carotid arteries. *Circulation* 1997; **95**: 376–81.

21   Wholey MH, Jarmolowski CR, Eles G et al. Endovascular stents for carotid artery occlusive disease. *J Endovasc Surg* 1997; **4**: 326–38.

22   Diethrich EB, Ndiaye M, Reid DB. Stenting in the carotid artery: initial experience in 110 patients. *J Endovasc Surg* 1996; **3**: 42–62.

23   Wholey MH, Eles G. Cervical carotid artery stent placement. *Semin Intervent Cardiol* 1998; **3**: 105–15.

24   Roubin GS, Yadav S, Iyer SS, Vitek J. Carotid stent-supported angioplasty: a neurovascular intervention to prevent stroke. *Am J Cardiol* 1996; **78**: 8–12.

25   North American Symptomatic Carotid Endarterectomy Trial Collaborators. Beneficial effect of carotid endarterectomy in symptomatic patients with high-grade carotid stenosis. *N Engl J Med* 1991; **325**: 445–53.

26   Executive Committee for the Asymptomatic Carotid Atherosclerosis Study. Endarterectomy for asymptomatic carotid artery stenosis. *JAMA* 1995; **273**: 1421–8.

27   Shawl F, Kadro W, Domanski MJ et al. Safety and efficacy of elective carotid artery stenting in high-risk patients. *J Am Coll Cardiol* 2000; **35**: 1721–8.

28   Mathur A, Roubin GS, Iyer SS et al. Predictors of stroke complicating carotid artery stenting. *Circulation* 1998; **97**: 1239–45.

29   McCleary AJ, Nelson M, Dearden NM et al. Cerebral haemodynamics and embolization during carotid angioplasty in high-risk patients. *Br J Surg* 1998; **85**: 771–4.

30   Markus HS, Clifton A, Buckenham T, Brown MM. Carotid angioplasty. Detection of embolic signals during and after the procedure. *Stroke* 1994; **25**: 2403–6.

31   Gaunt ME, Martin PJ, Smith JL et al. Clinical relevance of intraoperative embolization detected by transcranial Doppler ultrasonography during carotid endarterectomy: a prospective study of 100 patients. *Br J Surg* 1994; **81**: 1435–9.

32   Ackerstaff RG, Jansen C, Moll FL et al. The significance of microemboli detection by means of transcranial Doppler ultrasonography monitoring in carotid endarterectomy. *J Vasc Surg* 1995; **21**: 963–9.

33   Yadav JS, Grube E, Rowold S et al. Detection and characterization of emboli during coronary intervention. *Circulation* 1999; **100**: I-780.

34   Whitlow PL, Lylyk P, Parodi P. Protected carotid stenting: preliminary results of a multicenter trial. *Circulation* 1999; **100**: I–436.

35   Henry M, Amor M, Henry I et al. Carotid angioplasty and stenting with a new cerebral protection device: the Percusurge Guardwire Device. Circulation 1999; **100**: I–674.

36   The EPISTENT Investigators. Randomised placebo-controlled and balloon-angioplasty-controlled trial to assess safety of coronary stenting with use of platelet glycoprotein-IIb/IIIa blockade. Evaluation of platelet IIb/IIIa inhibitor for stenting. *Lancet* 1998; **352**: 87–92.

37   The EPILOG Investigators. Platelet glycoprotein IIb/IIIa receptor blockade and low-dose heparin during percutaneous coronary revascularization. *N Engl J Med* 1997; **336**: 1689–96.

38   Tcheng JE. Glycoprotein IIb/IIIa receptor inhibitors: putting the EPIC, IMPACT II, RESTORE, and EPILOG trials into perspective. *Am J Cardiol* 1996; **78**: 35–40.

39   Chastain HDI, Mt Wong P, Mathur A et al. Does abciximab reduce complications of cerebral vascular stenting in high risk lesions? *Circulation* 1997; **96**: I–283.

40   Bajzer CT, Kapadia SR, Yadav JS. Clopidogrel use in carotid artery stenting. *Am J Cardiol* 1999; 22 September: **84** (abstr 15).

41   Sivaguru A, Venables GS, Beard JD, Gaines PA. European carotid angioplasty trial. *J Endovasc Surg* 1996; **3**: 16–20.

42   Mendelsohn FO, Mahaffey KW, Yadav JS. Management of Atherosclerotic Carotid Disease: Medical, Surgical and Interventional Aspects, 2nd edn. New Jersey: Lippincott Williams & Wilkins Healthcare, 1999.

41

Carotid angioplasty under cerebral protection with the PercuSurge device

Michel Henry, Isabelle Henry, Christos Klonaris and Michèle Hugel

Introduction

Cerebrovascular accidents occur each year in 500 000 Americans and result in 150 000 deaths and in substantial morbidity.[1] Although antiplatelet agents have a continuing role in reducing cerebrovascular risk, randomized controlled trials have shown that a reduction in carotid artery stenosis by carotid endarterectomy (CE) is superior to that of medical therapy alone.[2–4]

CE, however, has certain limitations. In the North American Symptomatic Carotid Endarterectomy Trial (NASCET), 5.8% of patients had perioperative stroke or death.[2] In the Asymptomatic Carotid Atherosclerosis Study (ACAS), the perioperative stroke rate was 2.8%.[4] In higher-risk patients, particularly those with severe coronary artery disease, perioperative morbidity and mortality have been reported in up to 18% of patients.[1,5–14] Cranial nerve palsies have been reported in up to 27% of patients.[1,10] Also, restenosis occurs in 5–19% of patients, and scarring from the initial operation can make repeat CE difficult.[9,15] Independent predictors of adverse outcome include contralateral occlusion, previous ipsilateral CE and combined coronary and carotid artery disease.[2,5–14] Further, CE is limited to the cervical portion of the carotid artery.

Based on the encouraging results obtained in the coronary and peripheral circulation with percutaneous interventional techniques, a natural evolutionary step was their application at the cerebrovascular level. Several recent studies suggest that carotid angioplasty and stenting (CAS) can be performed with a perioperative combined stroke and death rate of 2.9–8.2%.[16–22] Shawl et al[21] recently showed the safety and efficacy of elective carotid artery stenting in a series of 170 high-risk patients (192 carotid arteries stented). The total 30-day stroke rates were 2.9% for treated patients and 2.6% for treated arteries. This procedure may prove to be safer, less traumatic and more cost-effective than CE. Moreover, the risk/benefit ratio may be greatest in patients at highest risk for CE.[5,6,12–14] Furthermore, carotid artery stenting is not limited to the cervical portion of the carotid artery.

However, embolic stroke, even with a meticulous technique and experienced operators, represents the major drawback of the procedure. The majority of the neurological complications are due to the intracerebral embolism of plaque fragments or thrombus during different procedural steps. Cerebral protection devices have been developed to reduce the incidence of embolic events during carotid angioplasty.[23]

We therefore prospectively examined the outcome of 184 carotid angioplasties and stenting under cerebral protection using a new device, the PercuSurge Guardwire™ System (PercuSurge Inc., Sunnyvale, CA, USA), in 167 patients to assess whether this therapy is comparable to historical controls of both CE and angioplasty without cerebral protection.

Methods

Study population

Between February 1998 and September 2000, 167 patients (184 carotid stenoses) met the inclusion criteria and underwent CAS under protection using the PercuSurge Guardwire™ device. All patients were required to agree to regular follow-up and sign an informed consent statement.

Patient selection criteria

Patients were eligible for the study if they presented a ≥ 70% diameter stenosis of the internal carotid artery (ICA) documented on intra-arterial digital subtraction angiography and evaluated according to the Nascet criteria.[2] Patients were excluded if any of the following occurred: multiple stenoses in the ICA, intracranial pathology, presence of angiographically visible thrombus, gastrointestinal bleeding in the last 6 months, hemorrhagic disorders, participation in another study during the last 3 months, and inability to give informed consent.

Description of the protection device (Figure 41.1)

The device, described elsewhere,[24] briefly consists of three main components:

1. The GuardWire temporary occlusion catheter: a 0.014-inch or 0.018-inch wire constructed of hollow nitinol hypotube incorporating into its distal segment an inflatable compliant balloon capable of occluding vessel outflow. The choice of balloon diameter (3–6 mm) depends on the artery diameter.
2. A MicroSeal incorporated at the proximal end of the wire, allowing inflation and deflation of the distal protection balloon (PB) utilizing a MicroSeal adapter. The MicroSeal keeps the elastomeric balloon inflated while allowing catheter exchange at the proximal end, similar to commonly used guidewires.
3. The aspiration catheter placed over the Guardwire to aspirate generated debris and flush the ICA.

Protected CAS technique (Figure 41.2)

An 8F or 9F multipurpose guide catheter is initially placed into the common carotid artery (CCA) by femoral approach. The Guardwire is then gently advanced through the guide catheter, the lesion crossed and the marker of the PB placed 2 or 3 cm beyond it. The MicroSeal adapter is then attached and the PB slowly inflated with a fixed volume of dilute contrast, occluding the ICA and diverting vessel outflow towards the external carotid artery (ECA). On detachment of the MicroSeal adapter, the occlusion balloon remains inflated. Pre-dilation of the lesion or direct stenting are then performed under protection. Any generated debris is removed from the ICA by aspiration alone or aspiration and flushing techniques.

Two techniques have been used:

- Technique 1. The PB remains inflated during the whole procedure and the aspiration is performed once after stent placement and post-dilation.

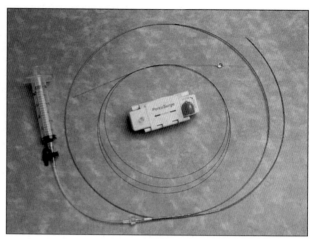

Figure 41.1
Guardwire™ temporary occlusion and aspiration system.

- Technique 2. The PB is deflated between predilation and stent placement to restore the cerebral flow. Aspiration is performed after each of these two stages.

The technique used depends on the tolerance of the occlusion, the cerebral collateral circulation, the status of the contralateral artery, the duration of the procedure and the technical problems encountered.

In both scenarios, the aspiration catheter is advanced over the wire into the dilated area, and a 20-ml syringe is connected to it to aspirate debris. Additionally, in our initial 40 cases, flushing of the treated area was performed using saline injections through the guide catheter to 'drive' the particles towards the ECA. The injection was performed with an injection pump at a rate of 2 ml/s for 10 s.

Finally, the MicroSeal adapter is reattached to the Guardwire, and the PB deflated, allowing normal flow to be restored. If the angiographic result is satisfactory, the device is removed.

All patients were prescribed aspirin 250 mg/day indefinitely, and received ticlopidine 250-to 500 mg/day or clopidogrel 75 mg/day, for at least 2 days and preferably for 1 week before the procedure and for 1 month after it. Unfractionated intravenous heparin (5000 IU) and atropine (1 mg) were routinely administered just after the introducer sheath placement. A temporary pacemaker was never used. Heparin was continued until the following day at doses sufficient to keep the activated clotting time (ACT) >200 s. In five patients, abciximab was given in conjunction with the procedure, based on clinical judgement because of the presence of subocclusive lesions and/or suspicion of thrombi. The introducer sheaths were removed after the procedure when the ACT was ≤180 s, and no further anticoagulation was given. Patients were usually discharged the day after the procedure.

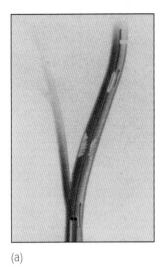 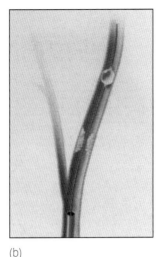 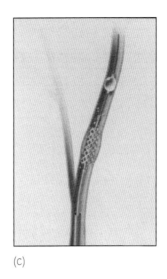 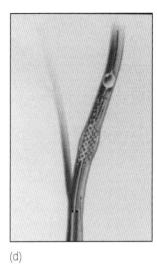

(a)   (b)   (c)   (d)

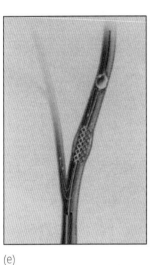 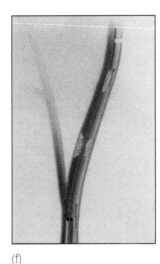

(e)   (f)

Figure 41.2

(a) Severe right internal carotid artery stenosis above the bifurcation. Selective DSA after the MP-1 guiding catheter has been placed in the common carotid artery. (b) The lesion has been crossed by the Guardwire, the protection balloon inflated and the angioplasty balloon (proximal marker) placed at the location of the carotid stenosis. (c) Inflation of the angioplasty balloon under cerebral protection. (d) Stent deployment under cerebral protection (Palmaz stent P204). (e) Aspiration of generated debris under cerebral protection with the aspiration catheter (proximal marker). (f) Final result after balloon angioplasty and stenting of the right carotid artery.

Periprocedural assessment

A neurological assessment by an independent neurologist using the N-score clinical examination scale,[25] baseline blood and chemistry values, coagulation profile, electrocardiogram, brain CT scan or magnetic resonance imaging (MRI) and duplex studies were routinely performed.

During duplex study, a characterization of plaque echodensity was made in a subgroup of 20 patients according to Nicolaides' method,[26,27] which consists of a gray-scale analysis of the overall plaque echogenicity. The gray-scale median density value (MDV) was determined for the different plaques. The MDV was compared to the number and the size of the particles released during CAS, and the relationship between the degree of stenosis evaluated by the pic systolic velocity and the importance of embolism was studied.

Computerized digital subtraction angiography with at least two orthogonal projections of the carotid bifurcation and images of the intracranial circulation were performed and recorded for each patient before and after the procedure. The NASCET angiographic criteria[2] were used to calculate the degree of stenosis before and after angioplasty and stenting, with the distal, non-tapering portion of the ICA serving as the reference segment.

During and after carotid artery stenting, neurological status was continuously monitored by simple contralateral hand-gripping maneuvers.

Follow-up

All patients underwent a neurological examination, a duplex scan and a CT scan the day after CAS, a neurological examination and a duplex scan at day 30 and every 6 months thereafter, and an angiogram at 6 months. Any change in neurological status after CAS required repeated CT brain scan. Quantitative analysis was performed by an independent observer who did not know the patient outcome.

Study endpoints

The *primary clinical endpoints* assessed included any major/minor stroke, death or myocardial infarction (MI) within the first 30 days post-procedure. Among them, the periprocedural complications were defined as any major/minor stroke, death or MI occurring in the first 48 h.

The *secondary clinical endpoints* were the need for new intervention, angioplasty or endarterectomy at 6 months.

The *angiographic endpoints* were: angiographic success rate, defined as achieving a <30% residual stenosis, and angiographic restenosis, defined as a reduction of the arterial lumen diameter >50%. The procedural success was defined as a reduction in the stenosis to ≥30% and absence of any neurological complication, MI or death.

Data collection, statistical methods

Clinical, angiographic and procedural data were prospectively recorded on a standardized form. The clinical and demographic variables collected included age, gender, symptoms, associated cardiac or peripheral artery disease, presence or absence of diabetes mellitus, hypertension, hyperlipidemia, history of smoking, bilateral carotid artery stenosis or occlusion and whether the patient was randomizable into NASCET or ACAS.

All data are expressed as the mean value ±SD or as numbers of patients or percentages for categorical variables.

The comparisons between the types of plaque, the number and the size of particles, the degree of stenosis and the importance of embolism were performed with regression test analysis.

The survival curve was drawn on an actuarial basis using the Kaplan–Meier method.

Definitions

- *Myocardial infarction*: Development of new Q-waves on the electrocardiogram (ECG) and/or creatine kinase elevation to at least twice the normal level, accompanied by above-normal elevation of the MB band.
- *Transient ischemic accident (TIA)*: A new neurological deficit that completely resolved within 24 h.
- *Minor stroke*: A new neurological deficit that persisted for >24 h, but completely resolved or returned to baseline within 7 days. By definition, minor strokes are non-disabling neurological events.
- *Major stroke*: A new neurological deficit that persisted after 7 days.

Results

Patient characteristics (Table 41.1)

One hundred and eighty-four procedures were attempted in 167 consecutive patients (129 males, 38 females; age 70.5 ± 9.2 years, range 40–91 years). Seventeen patients had bilateral procedures.

Ninety-three patients were asymptomatic (50.5%), and 91 were symptomatic (49.5%). Cardiovascular risk factors were: hypertension in 125 patients (74.8%), diabetes in 32 (19.2%), hyperlipidemia in 101 (60.5%), smoking in 100 (59.9%), and obesity in 22 (13.2%). Associated diseases were: stable coronary artery disease in 79 patients (47.3%), unstable angina in 7 (4.2%), cardiac failure in 14 (8.4%), peripheral arterial disease in 38 (22.8%), renal artery stenosis in 19 (11.4%), renal insufficiency in 12 (7.2%), and respiratory failure in 13 (7.8%). One hundred and twenty-two patients (73%) would have been excluded from the NASCET or ACAS entry criteria.

Lesion characteristics (Table 41.2)

One hundred and fifty-seven lesions were atherosclerotic, 18 were restenoses (postsurgical 15, post-angioplasty 3) and 7 were post-radiation stenoses. One lesion was an inflammatory

Table 41.1 Baseline clinical and demographic characteristics (n = 167).

Number of patients/Number of procedures	167/184
Male/Female	129/38
Age (years)	
Mean ± SD	70.5 ± 9.2
Range	40–91
Bilateral procedure	17/167 (10.2%)
Contralateral ICA	
Stenosis	36/167 (21.6%)
Occlusion	11/167 (6.6%)
Previously stented contralateral ICA	24/167 (14.4%)
Hypertension	125/167 (74.8%)
Diabetes mellitus	32/167 (19.2%)
Hyperlipidemia	101/167 (60.5%)
Smoking	100/167 (59.9%)
Obesity	22/167 (13.2%)
Stable coronary artery disease	79/167 (47.3%)
Unstable angina	7/167 (4.2%)
Cardiac failure	14/167 (8.4%)
Peripheral artery disease	38/167 (22.8%)
Renal artery stenosis	19/167 (11.4%)
Renal insufficiency	12/167 (7.2%)
Respiratory failure	13/167 (7.8%)

Table 41.2	Lesion characteristics.
Symptomatic	91 (49.5%)
Asymptomatic	93 (50.5%)
Atherosclerotic	157/184 (85.3%)
Restenoses	18/184 (9.8%)
Postsurgical	15
Post-angioplasty	3
Post-radiation	7/184 (3.8%)
Inflammatory arteritis	1/184 (0.5%)
Post-traumatic aneurysm	1/184 (0.5%)
Mean % stenosis	81.5±9.3% (70–99)
Mean lesion length	14.5±6.2 mm (5–50)
Mean arterial diameter	5.0±1.2 mm (4.1–7.1)
Calcification	85/184 (46.2%)
Ulceration	135/184 (73.4%)
Hyperechogenic	87/184 (47.3%)
Echolucent	96/184 (52.2%)

arteritis, and another was a post-traumatic aneurysm. The mean percentage of stenosis was 81.5 ± 9.3 % (70–99%). Mean lesion length was 14.5 ± 6.2 mm (5–50 mm) and the mean arterial diameter was 5.0 ± 1.2 mm (4.1–7.1%). Eighty-five lesions (46.2%) were calcified, 135 were ulcerated (73.4%), 87 were hyperechogenic (47.3%), and 96 were echolucent (52.2%). Thirty-six patients had a contralateral ICA stenosis, and 11 had a contralateral ICA occlusion. Twenty-four patients had a previously stented contralateral ICA.

Techniques of cerebral protection

One hundred and forty-nine lesions were treated using the continuous occlusion technique. The mean occlusion time (s) was 378 ± 180 (149–1479).

Thirty-four lesions were treated by the second, staged technique. The mean dilation occlusion time (s) was 323 ± 149 (109–762), and the mean stent implantation occlusion time (s) was 299 ± 140 (125–717).

The mean occlusion time for all lesions (s) was 422 ± 220 (125–1479).

Immediate technical success (Figures 41.3–41.5)

Technical success was achieved in 183 of 184 cases (99.5%).

There was one failure to cross the lesion with the Guardwire because of excessive tortuousity of the CCA and ICA. This procedure was successfully performed without cerebral protection.

In one patient, after completion of the procedure, deflation of the occlusion balloon using the MicroSeal adapter was impossible, due to a kink at the MicroSeal junction. This problem was managed by cutting the hypotube section of the Guardwire distally to the MicroSeal area, using scissors; the balloon was then immediately deflated.

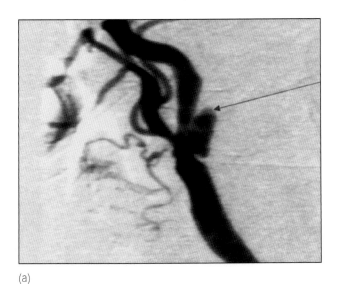

(a)

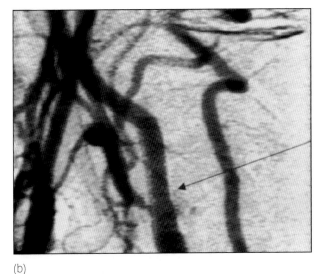

(b)

Figure 41.3
(a) Left ulcerated carotid artery stenosis. (b) Result after angioplasty and stenting (Palmaz stents).

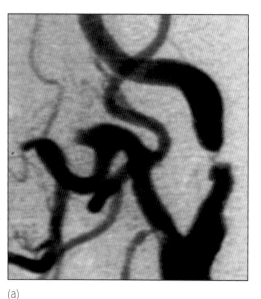

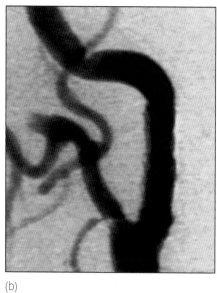

Figure 41.4
Left internal carotid artery stenosis. (a) before angioplasty. (b) Final result after stenting.

(a)

(b)

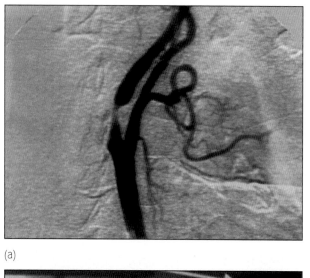

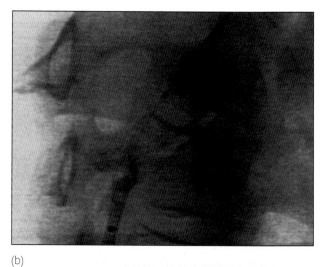

(a)

(b)

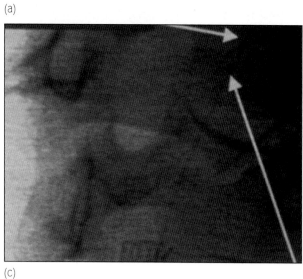

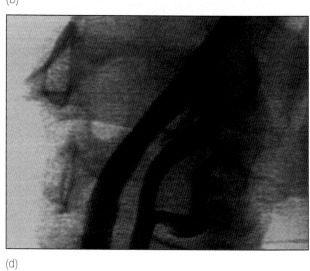

(c)

(d)

Figure 41.5
(a) Right carotid artery stenosis. (b) Stent implantation under protection. (c) Aspiration of the debris with aspiration catheter. (d) Final result.

Stents implanted

All lesions were treated with endoprostheses except three post-angioplasty restenoses. We implanted 127 Palmaz stents (P204, 73; P154, 52; Corinthian, 2), 31 Wallstents, 28 Nitinol self-expandable stents (Expander – Bolton Medical), and one Jostent-covered stent to treat the aneurysm. The Nitinol and Wallstent stents covered the bifurcation without jeopardizing the flow in the ECA. All stents were well deployed.

The mean stent diameter was 5.6 ± 1.4 mm at the proximal part, and 5.2 ± 0.7 mm at the distal part. The mean stented lesion length was 22.8 ± 9.6 mm (15–57 mm). The mean percentage residual stenosis was $3.5 \pm 4.5\%$.

Tolerance to occlusion balloon

The occlusion during PB inflation was well tolerated in 176 cases (95.7%), of who 47 had significant contralateral ICA disease (stenosis or occlusion). Two types of intolerance were observed:

- *Complete intolerance* (two patients, 1.1%) immediately after inflation of the protection balloon. One with total occlusion of the contralateral ICA developed loss of consciousness and seizures. The patient totally recovered after rapid balloon deflation. CAS was successfully completed without cerebral protection. One with poor collateral circulation by the Willis circle also developed rapid loss of consciousness. However, the procedure could be completed under protection. The patient totally recovered rapidly after deflation of the PB.

- *Partial transient intolerance* (six patients, 3.3%): beginning approximately 2 min after flow interruption, with transient symptoms such as agitation, brief loss of consciousness or transient neurological deficit. The procedure was completed under protection. All patients had rapid and complete recovery while the PB was still inflated. Four of them had a hypotensive response to dilation with bradycardia which could have promoted this intolerance.

Six patients developed a spasm of the ICA above the dilated area at the location of the PB which rapidly responded to vasodilator therapy.

Collected debris

Aspiration of the debris was performed in all patients.

The aspirated blood samples were collected in filters (pores of 40μm) and analyzed using optic and electron microscopic techniques. Visible debris was extracted from all patients (mean diameter 250μm (56–2652μm), mean number per procedure 74 (7–145)). Different types of particles were found: atheromatous plaques, cholesterol crystals, calcified crystals, necrotic cores, fibrin, recent and old thrombi, platelets, macrophage foam cells, lipoid masses and acellular material.

Figure 41.6 shows the distribution of particles for one patient, and Figure 41.7 the images of the debris in the electronic microscope.

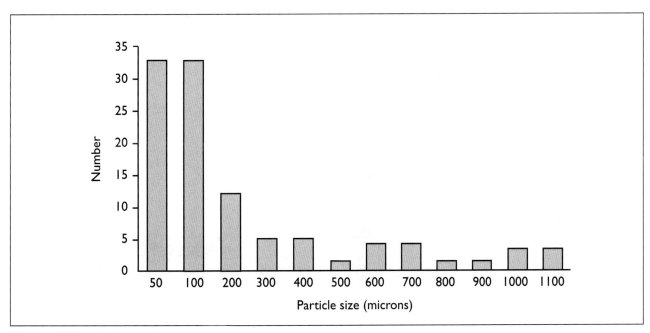

Figure 41.6
The distribution of particles in one patient.

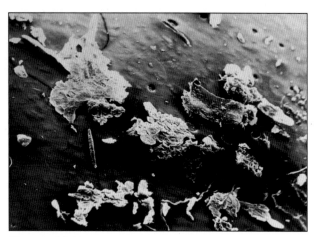

Figure 41.7
The images of debris as seen under an electron microscope.

Carotid duplex scan

The MDVs of the atheromatous plaques having induced a carotid stenosis, evaluated by echoscanning in a subgroup of 20 patients, are shown in Figure 41.8.

Low values of MDV were related to hypoechoic plaques, and high values to hyperechoic plaques. The hypoechoic plaques were related to a greater number of particles, with a correlation between the MDV and the number of particles of 0.72.

There was a good correlation between the MDV and the mean size of the debris (0.75), indicating that hyperechoic plaques produced larger debris.

Hypoechoic plaques were producing a great number of small particles, and hyperechoic plaques less but larger debris.

No relationship between the degree of stenosis and the importance of embolism was found. The risk of embolization during CAS seems to be independent of the nature and severity of the plaque.

30-Day complications

Four neurological complications occurred (2.2%), of which three were periprocedural complications (1.6%):

- One *amaurosis* in a symptomatic patient having a tight ulcerated right ICA stenosis, after a Wallstent acute thrombosis during the procedure. The thrombosis was seen on the angiogram after deflation of the PB. This balloon was quickly reinflated and abciximab injected (bolus of 0.25 mg/kg and 10 μg/min continuous infusion for 12 h thereafter). Thromboaspiration and flushing through the guide catheter were performed 10 min later, and the PB finally deflated. The final angiogram showed no residual thrombus inside the stent. Nevertheless, the patient developed an amaurosis, which was probably the consequence of an embolism from the ECA through a communication between the ECA and the ophthalmic circulation. Indeed, a communication between the ECA and the ophthalmic circulation was diagnosed after careful angiographic inspection.
- One TIA with transient hemiparesis after a procedure of CAS of a tight asymptomatic left ICA stenosis in a patient

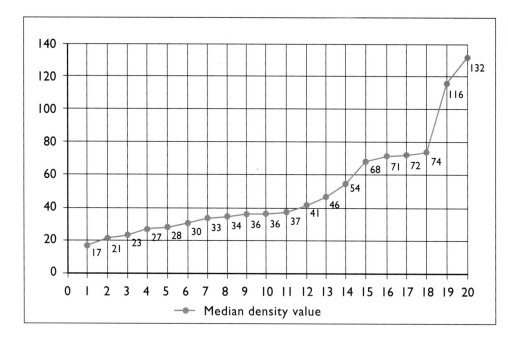

Figure 41.8
Mean density value.

who had a prolonged occlusion time (19 min). No evidence of ischemia was detected at subsequent serial CT examinations.

- One TIA with brachial monoparesis in a symptomatic patient.

The other neurological complication was one intracerebral hemorrhage with hemiparesis on the third day after a CAS procedure under abciximab (same protocol as previously described), in a patient having a symptomatic subocclusion of the right ICA. The patient partially recovered 2 months later.
Cardiac events (0.6%):

- One symptomatic patient died from cardiac failure 3 weeks after the CAS procedure.
- No MI occurred during the hospital period or in the 30 days after CAS.

The overall 30-day incidence of stroke and death was 2.7% (major stroke 1.1%, TIA 1.1%, death 0.5%) per patient.
No episode of cranial nerve palsy occurred.

Follow-up

The mean follow-up was 335 ± 165 days (30–940 days).
Three deaths occurred:

- One patient died from a major stroke located at the contralateral side of the previously treated ICA. at 6 months.
- Two other patients died from MI.

No other minor or major stroke occurred.

One asymptomatic restenosis observed at 6 months was treated successfully by new angioplasty.
The event-free survival was 97% at 20 months (Figure 41.9).

Discussion

Recent randomized trials[2–4,28,29] have proved the efficacy of surgical endarterectomy for severe symptomatic and asymptomatic extracranial carotid artery stenosis and its superiority over medical treatment. However, the benefits of the procedure are critically dependent on the rate of perioperative complications.[10,12,13] If CAS is to be considered as an alternative to surgery, its complication rate should parallel that of endarterectomy.

CAS could be proposed in an increasing number of patients with carotid artery stenosis if an acceptable risk of perioperative stroke/death rate can be provided.[16–23,31–34] However, even with experienced interventionalists, the risk of embolic stroke, a devastating complication, remains the main limitation of the procedure.

The frequency of debris migration and distal embolism has been demonstrated by ex vivo human carotid stenting techniques[35] and confirmed by clinical studies.[12,36]

The number of embolic particles generated by percutaneous techniques seems to far exceed that of endarterectomy.[33,35,36] Although their clinical significance has not yet been documented,[36,37] it is known that their presence could not have any beneficial effect for the brain.

Furthermore, the minimum particle size capable of producing ischemic events has not been determined.

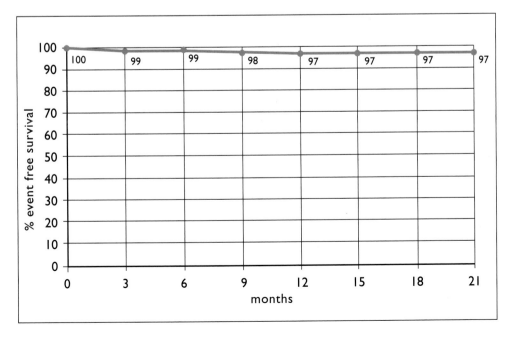

Figure 41.9
Kaplan–Meier actuarial curve demonstrating event-free survival (MI, any stroke, death).

Various patient and plaque characteristics have been suggested as predictors of debris generation and embolic events[35,38] to define high-risk groups for CAS procedure. In our study, debris was extracted from all patients, even in lesions theoretically at low risk of cerebral embolism (restenosis, echogenic plaques, concentric lesions), suggesting that the risk of embolization is independent of the nature of the plaques. Additionally, stent deployment does not provide sufficient protection against embolic plaque debris migration. In all series of CAS, the embolic risk exists regardless of the implantation technique and the stent characteristics. Manninen et al[38] compared endovascular stent placement with percutaneous transluminal angioplasty of carotid arteries in cadavers in situ and found no difference with respect to distal embolization.

Vitek et al, in 1984, first reported[39] a case of successful innominate artery angioplasty where the risk of cerebral embolization was reduced by temporary occlusion of the origin of the right CCA with a second balloon catheter. In the last decade, as a testimony to suboptimal results and the need for embolic risk elimination, several protection techniques during carotid angioplasty have been proposed.[40,41]

The Percusurge Guardwire device was first tested in animals by Oesterle et al,[42] and this was followed by clinical use[43] in 27 saphenous vein graft coronary angioplasties. It has been shown that the system is compatible with routine angioplasty procedures, is capable of containing and retrieving atherosclerotic debris, and might aid in the prevention of distal embolization.

The device has been proposed for cerebral protection during carotid angioplasty. One of its advantages is that it behaves similarly to the steerable coronary guidewires, allowing it to cross the stenosis easily and reducing the number of technical failures. We have experienced only one failure to cross a tight stenosis in a tortuous CCA and ICA. Additionally, the Guardwire provides efficient support to advance the dilation balloon and the stent. The deflation time of the occlusion balloon is fast, approximately 15 s.

Limitation of the technique

This study shows that protected CAS is a feasible and safe procedure with a very low 30-day neurological complication rate (2.2%). These results are favorable when compared with series using brain-unprotected techniques,[16,18,21,37,44,45] and reach the levels of historical surgical controls.

However, cerebral protection cannot prevent all plaque debris migration and embolic events that may occur at all steps of the procedure. The balloon protection device offers protection against embolism only after the lesion has been crossed by the wire, but this maneuver, as well the initial positioning of the guide catheter in the CCA are also capable of releasing embolic material. Utilization of smaller tools and adaptation of coronary techniques may limit the risks and give a better outcome.

Table 41.3   Transcranial Doppler: number of HITS per patient during the different steps of carotid angioplasty stenting.

	Unprotected	Protected
Probing of CCA	3	2
Introduction of long sheath	7	7
Passage of stenosis	9	3
Pre-dilation	78	9
Stent placement	89	8
In–stent dilation	146	11

Table 41.4   MRI and clinical.

	Unprotected (%)	Protected (%)
New signal-intense lesions	28.5	8.2
TIAs	6.9	3.2
Minor stroke	2.2	1.9
Major stroke	1.3	0

Recently, Mathias and Jaeger[46] published a very interesting study. They studied 70 carotid angioplasties without protection, 102 carotid angioplasties with protection (Percusurge 78%, Angioguard 22%) by transcranial Doppler monitoring (TCD) during the procedure and by MRI of the brain before and 24 h after carotid angioplasty stenting.

By TCD the number of HITS for the patient was calculated during the different steps of carotid angioplasty (Table 41.3). Even with protection, HITS were registered, but the number of HITS is much greater without protection, and the more critical step for brain embolism is pre-dilation, stent placement and in-stent dilation.

By MRI, Mathias and Jaeger noticed that new signal intense lesions are more frequent with unprotected angioplasties (28.5% versus 8.2%). (Table 41.4.)

This study demonstrated that cerebral protection reduced the rate of embolization during carotid angioplasty stenting. A major stroke was not seen after cerebral protection.

Tolerance of occlusion

Before the procedure, complete angiographic assessment of the four supra-aortic vessels is mandatory for determination of the collateral supply through the circle of Willis, vertebrobasilar and contralateral carotid flow. Patients with congenital absence or acquired disease of these structures may not tolerate flow occlusion. This problem is similar but not identical to surgical clamping during carotid endarterectomy, since flow through the ECA is unaffected with PB inflation. This vessel also provides collateral flow to both the anterior and posterior cerebral circulation, which is useful when the ICA is occluded but potentially harmful in cases where flushing is used to clean the treated area. In this study, occlusion of the ICA was well tolerated in the majority of cases. We had eight cases of intolerance, but only one case of complete intolerance (rapid development of symptoms immediately after flow interruption) in which cerebral protection was not used to complete the procedure.

More commonly, a delayed intolerance of brief duration started while the procedure was well advanced, usually after stent deployment and before debris aspiration. In these cases, the procedure could be completed with aspiration and re-establishment of the cerebral flow, thus keeping the benefits of the protection.

Flushing

After aspiration, potential remaining debris may be flushed towards the ECA and lead to ischemic complications in cases of distal anastomosis between the ECA and the ICA or vertebrobasilar artery territory through the meningeal or occipital arteries. Diagnostic angiography prior to treatment is mandatory for diagnosis of these particularities, which rule out the flushing step and restrict the debris removal to aspiration. In our series, one neurological complication appeared after flushing. We stopped flushing after this occurrence.

Flushing vigorously at high pressure during the cleaning procedures may lead to reflux to the origin of the CCA (more critical on the right side, since the length of the CCA is usually less) and/or to the right vertebral artery, with the risk of neurological deficit in this territory.

We now believe that aspiration is sufficient to clean up the treated area.

The different protection devices

Various cerebral protection devices, especially filters, are proposed. Their most remarkable advantage is that they do not stop cerebral flow. Nevertheless, the size of the pores ($\geq 100\,\mu m$ today) unfortunately allows the flow of microparticles,[47,48] which could lead to ischemic cerebral, particularly ocular, complications.

These devices have to be evaluated to define their respective indications. No result has been published yet.

Filters may have a more specific indication in patients with insufficient cerebral supply, hardly capable of tolerating a balloon occlusion. Nevertheless, in our series, we have seen that even with contralateral carotid disease, the occlusion balloon was well tolerated in most of the cases.

Procedural considerations and late outcome

The importance of pretreatment with aspirin and ticlopidine or clopidogrel, as well as its duration, in preventing complications seem important but not proved. A randomized trial is needed to rigorously examine this issue. However, given the demonstrated importance of these agents in coronary stenting, such a trial seems unlikely to be undertaken.

Abciximab has been proposed[49] as an adjunctive therapy. Its potential benefit and indications remain to be evaluated.

Clinical implications and future studies

In the low-risk patients randomized into NASCET and ACAS, relief of obstruction has been shown to lower the risk of cerebrovascular events.

Whether relief of the obstruction in other patient groups with different baseline characteristics would have the same treatment advantage is not known with certainty, and nor is the relative effectiveness of CAS and CE in preventing cerebrovascular accidents and death in the high-risk patients. In the series of Shawl et al,[21] during the 19–month follow-up of patients, there were very few neurological events, suggesting that the effectiveness of obstruction relief may well be reflected in long-term clinical benefit. The results of our CAS under cerebral protection series are similar and very promising.

For this reason, randomized controlled trials of CE versus CAS are now the next step in evaluating CAS. Until randomized trials are available, caution should be exercised in discarding CE in patient groups in which it has been proven effective.

One randomized trial – the Carotid and Vertebral Artery Transluminal Angioplasty Study (CAVATAS), which examined the role of angioplasty versus CE – has been completed.[50] This trial, although underpowered, suggested that balloon angioplasty without routine stenting has a similar safety profile to elective CE. These data suggest that routine stent implantation will further improve the percutaneous management of carotid artery disease.

A second trial comparing CE and CAS – the Carotid Revascularization Endarterectomy Trial (CREST), sponsored by the NIH – is planned.[51] The final results of CREST will not be available for at least 5–6 years.

In the interim, there are sufficient published reports to support the use of CAS by experienced operators in patients known to be at high risk for CE.[16–18,37,44,45] Such procedures require an experienced team of neurologists and interventionalists.

Patients at high risk for CE include patients with carotid artery lesions above the C2 or C3 cervical vertebrae or at the ostium of the common carotid artery and patients with cervical spine disease or fixation, previous radical neck dissection, fibromuscular dysplasia, previous cervical radiation, previous CE, and the presence of important comorbid conditions, including unstable angina, recent MI and severe congestive heart failure.

In addition, there will be continuing evolution of new stents, dilation and post-dilation strategies and distal neuro-protection devices that will require evaluation.[52]

Study limitations

This is a prospective non-randomized monocentric study where CAS under cerebral protection was performed by highly experienced operators.

Whether similar results will be obtained by less experienced operators is not known.

This study represents early clinical experience with equipment designed for coronary and peripheral vascular interventions. Devices designed specifically for carotid artery intervention may improve outcome.

Randomized studies comparing the gold standard procedure of CE versus protected CAS, and CAS with and without cerebral protection, are awaited, as well as randomized studies to evaluate and compare different neuroprotection devices (filters, PB and others).

Conclusion

Carotid artery stenting has been demonstrated to be feasible and safe, even in high-risk patients, with a complication rate comparable to that of patients in the ACAS and NASCET trials.

However, CAS without cerebral protection is associated with the risk of brain embolism. The addition of protection devices may decrease this risk, and their application to all cerebral angioplasty procedures might widen the indications and offer complication rates at least equal to or even smaller than those obtained with CE.

Multicenter randomized studies (CAS versus CE) are awaited, but is it ethical to now set up a study without cerebral protection?

In the interim, there are sufficient published reports to support the use of CAS by experienced operators in patients considered to be at high risk for surgery, and higher-risk patients could be treated because of the availability of protection.

The cost of these different techniques has to be evaluated.

References

1   American Heart Association. *Heart and Stroke facts: 1996 Statistical Supplement*. Dallas: AHA, 1996.

2   North American Symptomatic Carotid Endarterectomy Trial Collaborators. Beneficial effect of carotid endarterectomy in symptomatic patients with high-grade carotid stenosis. *N Engl J Med* 1991; **325**: 445–53.

3   European Carotid Surgery Trialists' Collaborative Group. MRC European Carotid Surgery Trial: Interim results for symptomatic patients with severe (70–99%) or with mild (0–29%) carotid stenosis. *Lancet* 1991; **337**: 1235–43.

4   Executive Committee for the Asymptomatic Carotid Atherosclerosis Study. Endarterectomy for asymptomatic carotid artery stenosis. *JAMA* 1995; **273**: 1421–8.

5   Graor RA, Hetzler NR. Management of coexistent carotid artery and coronary artery disease. *Curr Concepts Cerebrovasc Dis Stroke* 1988; **23**: 19–23.

6   Newman DC, Hicks RG. Combined carotid and coronary artery surgery: a review of the literature. *Ann Thorac Surg* 1988; **45**: 574–81.

7   Sundt TM Jr, Meyer FB, Piepgras DG et al. Risk factors and operative results. In: Meyer FB, ed. *Sundt's Occlusive Cerebrovascular Disease*, 2nd edn. Philadelphia: WB Saunders, 1994: 241–7.

8   Link MJ, Meyer FB, Cherry KJ et al. Combined carotid and coronary revascularization. In: Meyer FB, ed. *Sundt's Occlusive Cerebrovascular Disease*, 2nd edn. Philadelphia: WB Saunders, 1994: 323–31.

9   Zierler RE, Brandyk DF, Thiele BL, Strandness ED. Carotid artery stenosis following endarterectomy. *Arch Surg* 1982; **117**: 1408–15.

10 Lusby RJ, Wylie EJ. Complications of carotid endarterectomy. *Surg Clin North Am* 1983; **63**: 1293–301.

11 Winslow CM, Solomon DH, Chassin MR et al. The appropriateness of carotid endarterectomy. *N Engl J Med* 1988; **318**: 721–7.

12 Rothwell PM, Slatterg J, Waslow CP. A systematic review of the risks of stroke or death due to endarterectomy for symptomatic carotid stenosis. *Stroke* 1996; **27**: 260–5.

13 McCrory DC, Goldstein LB, Samsa GP et al. Predicting complications of carotid endarterectomy. *Stroke* 1993; **24**: 1285–91.

14 Gaseeki AP, Eliaszio M, Ferguson GG et al. Long term prognosis and effect of endarterectomy in patients with symptomatic severe carotid stenosis and contralateral stenosis or occlusion. Results from North American Symptomatic Carotid Endarterectomy Trial (NASCET) group. *J Neurosurg* 1995; **83**: 778–82.

15 Das MB, Hertzer NR, Ratcliff J et al. Recurrent carotid stenosis: a five year series of 65 operations. *Ann Surg* 1985; **202**: 28–35.

16 Yadav JS, Roubin GS, Iyers SS et al. Elective stenting of the extracranial carotid arteries. *Circulation* 1997; **95**: 376–81.

17 Diethrich EB, Ndiaye M, Reid DB. Stenting in the carotid artery: initial experience in 110 patients. *J Endovasc Surg* 1996; **3**: 42–6.

18 Roubin GS, Yadav S, Iyer SS, Vitek J. Carotid stent-supported angioplasty: a neurovascular intervention to prevent stroke. *Am J Cardiol* 1996; **78**(suppl 3A): 8–12.

19 Henry M, Amor M, Masson I et al. Angioplasty and stenting of the extracranial carotid arteries. *J Endovasc Surg* 1998; **5**: 293–304.

20 Henry M, Amor M, Klonaris C et al. Angioplasty and stenting of the extra-cranial carotid arteries. *Tex Heart Inst J* 2000; **27**: 150–8.

21 Shawl F, Kadro W, Domanski MJ et al. Safety and efficacy of elective carotid artery stenting in high-risk patients. *J Am Coll Cardiol* 2000; **35**: 1721–8.

22 Henry M, Amor M, Masson I et al. Endovascular treatment of atherosclerotic stenosis of the internal carotid artery. *J Cardiovasc Surg* 1998; **39** suppl 1: 141–50.

23 Theron J, Payelle G, Coskun O et al. Carotid artery stenosis: treatment with protected balloon angioplasty and stent placement. *Radiology* 1996; **201**: 627–36.

24 Henry M, Amor M, Henry I et al. Carotid stenting with cerebral protection: first clinical experience using the Percusurge Guardwire System. *J Endovasc Surg* 1999; **6**: 321–31.

25 Orgogozo JM, Calpideo R, Anagnostou CN et al. Mise au point d'un score neurologique pour l'évaluation clinique des infarctus sylviens. *Presse Med* 1983; **12**: 3039–44.

26 Biasi GM, Mingazzini PM, Baronio L et al. Carotid plaque characterization using digital image processing and its potential in future studies of carotid endarterectomy and angioplasty. *J Endovasc Surg* 1998; **5**(3): 240–6.

27 Biasi GM, Sampaolo A, Mingazzini et al. Computer analysis of ultrasonic plaque echolucency in identifying high risk carotid bifurcations lesions. *Eur J Vasc Endovasc Surg* 1999; **17**(6) 476–9.

28 North American Symptomatic Carotid Endarterectomy Trial Collaborators. Benefit of carotid endarterectomy in patients with symptomatic moderate or severe stenosis. *N Engl J Med* 1998; **339**: 1415–25.

29 European Carotid Surgery Trialists Collaborative Group. Randomized trial of endarterectomy for recently symptomatic carotid stenosis: final results of the MRC European Carotid Study Trial (ECST). *Lancet* 1998; **351**: 1379–87.

30 Grotta J. Elective stenting of extracranial carotid arteries. *Circulation* 1997; **95**: 303–5.

31 Bergeron P, Chambran P, Bianca S. Traitement endovasculaire des artères à destinée cérébrale : échecs et limites. *J Mal Vasc* 1996; **21**: 123–31.

32 Bergeron P, Chambran P, Hartung O et al. Cervical carotid artery stenosis: which technique, balloon angioplasty or surgery? *J Cardiovasc Surg* 1996; **37**(suppl 1–5): 73–5.

33 Gil Peralta A, Mayol A, Gonzalez M Jr et al. Percutaneous transluminal angioplasty of the symptomatic atherosclerotic carotid arteries. Results, complications and follow-up. *Stroke* 1996; **27**: 2271–3.

34 Wholey MH, Wholey M, Jarmolowski CR. Endovascular stents for carotid occlusive disease. *J Endovasc Surg* 1997; **4**: 326–38.

35 Ohki T, Marin ML, Lyon RT et al. Ex vivo human carotid artery bifurcation stenting: correlation of lesion characteristics with embolic potential. *J Vasc Surg* 1998; **27**: 463–71.

36 Jordan WD, Voellinger DC, Doblar DD et al. Microemboli detected by transcranial doppler monitoring in patients during carotid angioplasty versus carotid endarterectomy. *Cardiovasc Surg* 1999; **7**: 33–8.

37 Mathur A, Roubin GS, Iyer SS et al. Predictors of stroke complicating carotid artery stenting. *Circulation* 1998; **97**: 1239–45.

38 Manninen HI, Rasanen HT, Vanninen RL et al. Stent placement versus percutaneous transluminal angioplasty of human carotid arteries in cadavers in situ: distal embolization and findings at intravascular US, MR imaging and histopathologic analysis. *Radiology* 1999; **212**: 483–92.

39 Vitek JJ, Raymon BC, Oh SJ. Innominate artery angioplasty. *AJNR* 1984; **5**: 113–14.

40 Kachel R. Results of balloon angioplasty in the carotid arteries. *J Endovasc Surg* 1996; **3**: 22–30.

41 Theron J. Angioplastie carotidienne protégée et stents carotidiens. *J Mal Vasc* 1996; **21**: 113–22.

42 Oesterle SN, Hayase M, Baim DS et al. An embolization containment device. *Catheter Cardiovasc Intervent* 1999; **47**: 243–50.

43 Webb JG, Carere RG, Virmani R et al. Retrieval and analysis of particulate debris after saphenous vein graft intervention. *J Am Coll Cardiol* 1999; **34**: 468–75.

44 Shawl FA, Efstratiou A, Hoff S, Dougherty K. Combined percutaneous carotid stenting and coronary angioplasty during acute ischemic neurologic and coronary syndromes. *Am J Cardiol* 1996; **77**: 1109–12.

45 Wholey MH, Wholey M, Bergeron P et al. Current global status of carotid artery stent placement. *Cathet Cardiovasc Diagn* 1998; **44**: 1–6.

46 Mathias K, Jaeger M. How much cerebral embolization occurs during CAS? In: *International Symposium on Endovascular Therapy, Miami*, 2001: 73–5.

47 Ohki T, Veith FJ. Carotid stenting with and without protection devices: should protection be useful in all patients? *Semin Vasc Surg* 2000; **13**(2): 144–52.

48 Ohki T, Roubin GS, Veith FJ et al. Efficacy of a filter device in the prevention of embolic events during carotid angioplasty and stenting. An ex-vivo analysis. *J Vasc Surg* 1999; **30**(6): 1034–44.

49 Bhatt DL, Kapadia SR, Yadav JS, Topol EJ. Update on clinical trials of antiplatelet therapy for cerebrovascular diseases. *Cerebrovasc Dis* 2000; **10**(suppl 5): 34–40.

50 CAVATAS Investigators. Endovascular venous surgical treatment in patients with carotid stenosis in the Carotid and Vertebral Artery Transluminal Angioplasty Study. (CAVATAS). *Lancet* 2001; **357**: 1729–37.

51 Hobson RW, Brott R, Ferguson G et al. CREST: Carotid Revascularization Endarterectomy versus Stent Trial. *Cardiovasc Surg* 1997; **5**: 457–8.

52 Hanley HG, Sheridan FM, Rivera E. Carotid stenting: a technology in evolution. *J La State Med Soc* 2000; **152**(5): 235–8.

42

Clinical trials in carotid angioplasty and stenting

Walter A Tan and Mark H Wholey

Background

Carotid angioplasty and stenting (CAS) is an emerging alternative therapy, especially in patients who are poor surgical candidates. The resurgent interest in carotid stenting from both industry and the medical community is based on nonrandomized series from independent experienced centers across the world and one large randomized clinical trial (RCT) that suggest comparable benefit-to-risk ratios with these percutaneous methods.[1–6] Data from a retrospective world registry of more than 5000 patients who have undergone CAS since June 1997 indicate a 98.4% technical success rate, and an acceptable combined incidence of stroke and death of 5.76% and 3.38% for symptomatic and asymptomatic patients, respectively.[7] These complication rates appear to be competitive with those seen with surgery in the benchmark trials of the North American Symptomatic Carotid Endarterectomy Trial (NASCET), and the Asymptomatic Carotid Atherosclerosis Study (ACAS) (Table 42.1).[8,9]

In addition, there have been improvements in equipment (emboli protection devices or EPDs, brachiocephalic guide catheters) and standardization of technique (small balloon predilation and routine stenting) that have good potential for enhancing both the procedural safety and the durability of the results.[10,11]

Randomized clinical trials

The prospective, blinded RCT is the gold standard fair arbiter for comparing treatments or therapeutic strategies. Randomization minimizes both obvious and intangible differences between treatment groups, thereby executing the scientific method of reducing an experiment to only one variable – in this case, the treatment assigned.

Two early RCTs of carotid stenting were terminated prematurely because of unexpected high death and stroke rates.[12,13] These studies were done in the context of early

Table 42.1 Benchmarks from RCTs of surgery versus medical therapy for symptomatic and asymptomatic carotid artery stenosis

RCT	Stroke rate at 2 years		Absolute risk reduction (%)	30-day death + stroke (%) after CEA
	Drug treatment (%)	CEA (%)		
NASCET				
Severe (70–90%) stenosis	21.4	8.6*	12.8	5.8*
Moderate (50–69%) stenosis	14.2	9.2*	5.0	6.9*
ACAS	5	3.8*	1.2	2.6*

ACAS = Asymptomatic Carotid Atherosclerosis Study; CEA = carotid endarterectomy; NASCET = North American Symptomatic Carotid Endarterectomy Trial; RCT = Randomized clinical trial.
*Perioperative strokes included.

Table 42.2 Contemporary randomized clinical trials of surgery versus endovascular therapy for symptomatic and asymptomatic carotid artery stenosis

Trial (No.)	Study population	Sponsor	Treatments	Primary end point	Comment
CAVATAS-1 (504)[1]	Sxtic ICA ≥ 70%, 1992–97; exclusion criteria per investigator discretion	British Heart Foundation; National Health Service	PTA vs CEA	PTA vs CEA: (a) 30-day death + stroke: 6.4% vs 5.9% (P= NS) (b) Restenosis (US > 70%) at 1 year: 12% vs 5% (p < 0.001)	Significantly more CN palsy with CEA; survival curves similar at 3 years
CREST (2,500)[26]	Sxtic < 180 days ICA ≥ 50% (approx. NASCET criteria)	NIH and Guidant	CAS ± EPD vs CEA	30-day events (D/MI/ stroke) plus ipsilateral stroke > 30 days	First patient (lead-in) 12/00
SAPPHIRE (600–900)	High surgical risk patients (e.g. sxtic CAD, unfavorable anatomy, post XRT)	Cordis	SMART/ Precise Stent + Angioguard vs CEA	30-day D/MI/stroke; 12-month death/ipsilateral stroke	As of 4 April, 2001, 132 patients randomized; 105 patients in registry
ICSS/CAVATAS-2 (2000)	Similar to CAVATAS-1	Stroke Association (England) ± Medical Research Council	Stenting + EPD vs CEA	Long-term stroke-free survival	Anticipate enrollment to commence May 2001

Abbreviations and terms:
CAD = coronary artery disease; CAVATAS = Carotid and Vertebral Artery Transluminal Angioplasty Study; CEA = carotid endarterectomy; CN = cranial nerve; CREST = Carotid Revascularization Endarterectomy vs Stent Trial; D = death; EPD = emboli protection device; ICA = internal carotid artery; ICSS = International Carotid Stenting Study; MI = myocardial infarction; PTA = percutaneous transluminal angioplasty; SAPPHIRE = Stenting and Angioplasty with Protection in Patients at High Risk for Endarterectomy; SMART = shape memory alloy recoverable technique; Sxtic = symptomatic; US = ultrasound; XRT = radiation therapy.

operator learning curves and non-customized catheter-based equipment and devices that were suboptimal for brachiocephalic arterial applications. On the other hand, the Carotid and Vertebral Artery Transluminal Angioplasty Study (CAVATAS–I), a European trial, is the largest RCT to date and showed no difference in hard clinical end points of short-term death or stroke.[1] Specifically, the 30-day post-procedure combined death and stroke rate for the initial strategy using percutaneous (balloon) transluminal angioplasty (PTA) was 6.4%, and not statistically different from the 5.9% for carotid endarterectomy (CEA). As might be expected, there was a higher procedure-related complication rate in the form of cranial nerve paralysis with CEA, but most of these facial or vocal cord dysfunctions were transient. However, there was a higher restenosis (renarrowing) for the PTA group at 1 year (18% vs 5%, $p < 0.001$).

RCTs that employ contemporary procedural techniques comparing CAS versus CEA are the Carotid Revascularization Endarterectomy versus Stent Trial (CREST), Stenting and Angioplasty with Protection in Patients at High Risk for Endarterectomy (SAPPHIRE), and the International Carotid Stenting Study (ICSS/CAVATAS-2) (Table 42.2).[10]

The study population in the National Institutes of Health (NIH) sponsored CREST is restricted to low-to-moderate surgical risk patients who do not have major comorbid medical or anatomic features that would interfere with the evaluation of outcomes, or substantially reduce the likelihood of long-term follow-up. For example, patients with diabetes or previous myocardial infarction (MI) may be eligible but not patients with atrial fibrillation or cardiomyopathy, or previous CEA. The study entry criteria are similar to the NASCET but with more specifically defined medical exclusions. As of April, 2001, there were 44 centers selected, 3 approved for the lead-in phase, and 1 approved for the randomization phase. The use of an EPD is under consideration.

On the other hand, the industry-sponsored SAPPHIRE trial seeks to evaluate the differential benefit of the surgical versus endovascular strategies in high-risk patients. This is the traditional target population for assessing novel technologies, since high event rates with conventional therapy make it reasonable to seek better alternatives. From a trial design standpoint, higher expected rates of the outcome of interest (i.e. death, MI, or stroke) mean a higher likelihood of detecting a therapeutic benefit with smaller and more affordable study sample sizes. Whereas there are many other observational studies (Tables 42.3a and 42.3b), that evaluate the safety and feasibility (phase I and II clinical trials) of other stents and EPDs, this is the only RCT for the high-risk

Table 42.3a   Observational studies and registries of carotid angioplasty and stenting (CAS) with or without distal embolic protection devices: comparison of definition of high risk

Qualifying criteria	ARCHeR (ongoing)	SHELTER (ongoing)	MAVErIC (pending)
Degree of carotid stenosis Symptomatic ≥50% Asx ≥80%	Y	Y	Y
Days since last symptom	180	120	Not specified
Ultrasound alone can qualify	N (QCA required)	N (QCA required)	Not specified
Inclusion criteria: High-risk feature			
I. Anatomic/surgical consideration			
Contralateral occlusion	0.5	Y	Excludes any contralateral lesion ≥70%
Bilateral significant stenosis requiring treatment		Y	
Previous neck radiation	Y	Y	Y
Prior radical neck dissection	Y	Y	Y
Spinal immobility (e.g. cervical arthritis, kyphosis)	Y	Y	Y
Carotid lesion above C2	Y	Y	Y
Low carotid lesion	Y	Y	Y
Presence of tracheotomy stoma	Y	Y	Y
Restenosis after prior CEA	Y	Y	Y
Failed CEA		Y	
At risk for surgical wound infection			Y
Severe tandem lesions			Y (if ≥70% stenosis)
Carotid artery dissection			Y
II. Demographic			
Elderly (years)	≥75 requires 2 other '0.5' inclusion criteria	≥80 (0.5)	≥80 (0.5)
III. Cardiovascular comorbidity			
MI within ___ (time period)	30 days (0.5)	≥3 and ≥30 days (0.5)	≥3 days and <6 weeks (0.5)
Rest angina with ECG changes	0.5	Y	Y (0.5)
CAD definition	≥2 proximal or major CAD >70% stenosis (0.5)	≥2 proximal or major CAD >70% stenosis without angina (0.5)	
Need for CABG or valve surgery	Y (0.5)	Y (within 30 days)	Excludes
Need for other procedures		AAA repair or other peripheral vascular surgery within 30 days (0.5)	Excludes
CHF definition	EF <30% or NYHA III/IV	EF <30% or NYHA III/IV	NYHA III/IV
IV. Other comorbidities			
Contralateral laryngeal nerve palsy	Y	Y	Y
Dialysis dependent	Y	Allows	
Abnormal pulmonary function: FEV₁ <30% of predicted	Y	Y	Y
Uncontrolled DM	Fasting glucose >400 mg/dl or ketones >2+		
Listed for organ transplantation (heart, lung, liver, kidney)	Y		History of liver failure with elevated PT

Abbreviations and terms: (0.5) = meets only $\frac{1}{2}$ of a criterion, i.e. needs another factor that carries a weight of 0.5 to allow inclusion; AAA = abdominal aortic aneurysm; Asx = asymptomatic; CABG = coronary artery bypass grafting; CAD = coronary artery disease; CAS = carotid angioplasty and stenting; CEA = carotid endarterectomy; CHF = congestive heart failure; DM = diabetes mellitus; ECG = electrocardiogram; EF = ejection fraction; FEV = forced expiratory volume in 1 second; MI = myocardial infarction; NYHA = New York Heart Association classification; PT = prothrombin time; QCA = quantitative carotid angiography; Y = yes.

Table 42.3b   Observational studies of carotid angioplasty and stenting (CAS) with or without distal embolic protection devices: comparison of exclusion criteria

Exclusion criteria	ARCHeR	SHELTER	MAVErIC
I. Anatomic/angiographic characteristic			
Pure CCA lesion	Y		
Target ICA diameter < 4 or > 9 mm	Y	Y (≤ 3 or ≥ 6 mm for Guardwire Plus)	< 5.5 mm or > 7.5 mm
Carotid artery dissection		Y	
Severe vessel tortuosity	Y	Y	
Intraluminal filling defect/thrombus	Y	Y	
Long lesion			> 35 mm
Occluded or 'string sign' > 1 cm	Y	Y	Y
Ipsilateral intracranial or extracranial stenosis > target lesion	Y	Y	
Intracerebral aneurysm	≥ 5 mm	Y	
Cerebral mass (e.g. tumor, abscess, infection)	Y	Y	
Cerebral arteriovenous malformation	Y	Ipsilateral	
Prior carotid stent or stent–graft ipsilaterally	Y	Y	Y
Lesion requires > one stent			Y
Severe aortic arch/proximal CCA disease	Y		
II. Neurologic			
Recent stroke within ___ (time period)	7 days	< 3 weeks	neuro symptoms < 4 weeks, including TIAs
Hemorraghic transformation of stroke within 60 days	Y	Stroke in evolution	
Spontaneous intracranial hemorrhage	Y	Y	
History of major ipsilateral stroke likely to confound study end points	Y	NIHSS ≥ 15	
Stroke and TIA mimics (e.g. seizures, tumor)	Y (within 24 months)		
Vertebrobasilar insufficiency symptoms only	Y		
Cardiac sources of emboli (e.g. atrial fibrillation, atrial septal defect)	Y	Y	Y
Severe dementia	Y	Y	
III. Life-threatening comorbidity			
Life expectancy	< 2 years	< 1 year	< 1 year
Acute MI within ___ (time period)		2 days	72 hours
Abnormal creatinine level		> 2.5 mg/dl (but allows dialysis-dependent patients)	
Infection or immunocompromised state		WBC > 15 000; + bld culture; immunocompromised	WBC > 3000
Requires high-risk procedures			Planned CABG, AAA repair or other peripheral vascular surgery-pre- or post-CAS
Allergy to heparin, ASA, nitinol or X-ray contrast	Y		Y
Active bleeding diathesis or coagulopathy	Y	Y	Significant gastrointestinal bleed within 6 months

Table 42.3b   Continued

Exclusion criteria	ARCHeR	SHELTER	MAVErIC
Hemoglobin < 8 g/dl (unless on dialysis) plt < 50 K; INR > 1.5 (irreversible); heparin-associated thrombocytopenia			Plt < 100 000 or > 700 000
Won't consider blood transfusion if needed	Y		Y
Contraindications to both clopidogrel and ticlopidine	Y	Y	
Percutaneous arterial access unsafe (morbid obesity or sustained SBP > 180), or proper angiographic assessment unfeasible	Y		Y
Unable or unwilling to sign consent, or understand/comply with study procedures	Y	Y	Y
Unable/unwilling to return for follow-up	Y	Y	Y
Active participation in other drug/device trial	Y	Y	Y (within 30 days of enrollment)

Abbreviations and terms: AAA = abdominal aortic aneurysm; CABG = coronary artery bypass grafting; CAS = carotid angioplasty and stenting; CCA = common carotid artery; ICA = internal carotid artery; INR = international normalized ratio; MI = myocardial infarction; plt = platelet count; TIA = transient ischemic attack; WBC = white blood cell count; Y = yes (excluded from study).

population of patients. The entry criteria for SAPPHIRE are relatively more permissive than those for the other high-risk studies, including allowing duplex carotid ultrasound estimates of lesion severity to qualify patients for entry into the trial.

The final key RCT is the Stroke Association (England) sponsored ICSS (MM Brown, pers. comm.) This is the carotid stenting follow-up study to their RCT on balloon angioplasty versus CEA (CAVATAS). This is an important study because of the more generalized and practical entry criteria (low, moderate, and high-risk patients) – essentially any symptomatic patient with a 70% stenosis (as measured by the common carotid method or ultrasound equivalent) deemed suitable for either stenting or CEA. The main differences from CAVATAS are the requirement for enrolling centers to first demonstrate a good procedural safety record and that cerebral protection devices are now advocated.

Prospective observational studies

Prospective study designs mandate prior specification of objective patient entry criteria and end-point assessments which mitigates (but does not totally eliminate) both investigator and patient biases.

Study subjects can be conceptually divided along two broad categories that stratify risk: (1) symptomatic versus asymptomatic neurologic presentation and (2) projected risk for perioperative complications. The first classification is based on historical studies and NASCET that established the poor natural history of patients presenting with a stroke or transient ischemic attack (TIA) within the last 6 months. The second classification is a complex amalgamation of different subpopulations of patients who historically have suffered greater than 10% death or stroke rates with a carotid surgical strategy. These diverse subgroups include cardiovascular comorbidity (severe heart failure, synchronous coronary artery disease or acute coronary syndrome), anatomically inaccessible carotid artery lesion (above the mandible or intrathoracic), hostile surgical bed (redo CEA or history of neck irradiation), or other severe organ system dysfunction (pulmonary or renal failure).

Multicenter consecutive series for carotid stent efficacy and safety have been conducted to fulfill US regulatory requirements. These were for the SMART (shape memory alloy recoverable technology) stent (Cordis Johnson & Johnson Interventional Systems, Warren, NJ), the Acculink stent (Guidant, Santa Clara, CA), and the EndoTex NEXT-STENT (EndoTex, Cupertino, CA): the latter two series have completed enrollment and are accruing long-term follow-up data.

A larger planned study that has relatively open-entry criteria is the Carotid Revascularization with Endarterectomy or Stenting Systems (CARESS) Registry. This is a cohort study that plans to monitor contemporaneous CAS and CEA cases prospectively. Besides the permissive inclusion criteria, the distinguishing aspects of this planned study are its long-term primary end point of death and stroke (48 months), a higher proportion of surgeons as endovascular operators than in other trials, and the availability of different stents or EPD that is left to the discretion of the study interventionalist. Duplex ultrasound estimates to qualify for entry into the trial are allowed, and there is a slightly lower entry threshold stenosis (75%) for the asymptomatic population.

There are three prospective large observational clinical trials that will evaluate the performance of stents with EPD in the high-risk population. The differences between the definitions of 'high risk' amongst these trials are listed in Table 42.3a and 42.3b. The Acculink for Revasularization of Carotids in High-Risk Patients (ARCHeR, Guidant) was designed as the parallel study to complement the low-risk study population of CREST, since both studies utilize the same stent system. Plans are also under way to use the Accunet EPD in ARCHeR. This trial has the most detailed study design and restrictive inclusion criteria. It is the only trial that specifically proscribes treatment of pure common carotid artery target lesions, and will probably have the least number of very elderly (> 75 years old) patients of all these studies. Whereas most other large-scale studies prohibit CAS in patients with a history of stroke within the last 3–4 weeks, SAPPHIRE and ARCHeR allow more acute endovascular intervention (beyond the 2- and 7-day stroke time windows, respectively). Therefore, these latter two studies will hopefully provide some secondary data, evaluating a strategy of early neurovascular intervention after an acute event.

The Stenting of High-Risk Extracranial Lesion Trial with Emboli Removal (SHELTER), has recently begun enrollment. This study will evaluate the balloon occluder class of emboli protection devices (PercuSurge, Inc.) in conjunction with the Wall Stent (Boston Scientific Corp., Natick, MA).[14] It will also be one of few studies that allows dialysis-dependent patients and those who are scheduled to have peripheral vascular surgery (e.g., abdominal aortic aneurysm repair). SHELTER permits patients with acute MI (AMI) to be treated relatively early, and is the only study that protocolizes the initial heparin bolus on a weight basis.

The Evaluation of the Medtronic AVE Self-Expanding Carotid Stent System with Distal Protection in the Treatment of Carotid Stenosis Study (MAVErIC, Medtronic AVE, Inc., Santa Rosa, CA) plans to evaluate their own carotid stent system with the EPD device their company recently acquired that is being used in the SHELTER trial. This is the PercuSurge Guardwire Plus temporary occlusion and aspiration system (PercuSurge, Inc., Sunnyvale, CA).[15] It specifically excludes patients with carotid stenosis ≥ 70% in the internal carotid artery (ICA) contralateral to the target lesion, in part in anticipation of later broader use with less experienced operators. This is to further enhance

the safety of this device, since procedural time is critical in the context of attenuated collateral cerebral flow. MAVErIC is the only study that lists carotid artery dissection as an inclusion criteria, and, similar to SHELTER, will allow AMI patients to be treated fairly early (beyond 72 hours post-MI). Similar to CARESS, thus far there is no prohibition of patients who have intracranial stenosis ipsilateral to the target lesion. Of note, the study does exclude patients with neurologic symptoms, including TIAs, within the 4 weeks prior to presentation.

Multiplicity of studies – raison d'être

It is a reasonable perspective to not assume that all stents and delivery systems have equal safety characteristics, given the different device system profiles, designs, deployment precision, and operational simplicity. For example, each new passenger airplane is expected to pass safety standards notwithstanding the addition of newer and presumptively better technology.[16] Wider general usage not infrequently brings out obscure system weaknesses, or even unforeseen device–device or product–consumer interactions.[17,18] Even the 'perfect' product for safety, automobile airbags, are now well documented to have untoward outcomes for an important subpopulation of commuters – toddlers. In the United States, each new device is mandated by the Food and Drugs Administration (FDA) to provide prospective clinical safety and feasibility data.[19–21]

It is also obvious that the absolute incremental advantage of carotid stenting will be different across the different high-risk subgroups. For instance, while CAS is relatively unaffected by carotid lesion location, the risks of systemic comorbidity is global and pertain to both surgical and endovascular approaches.[22] Moreover, the risk of exacerbating renal failure may be similar or even worse for CAS (due to contrast load) than for CEA. This justifies the existence of multiple prospective registries that have minimal exclusion criteria, in order to gather real-world and real-time data amongst different clusters of operators and patients.

However, patients with carotid artery disease comprise a very heterogeneous group, with a wide range of risks in terms of both natural history and periprocedural complications. This is predominantly because of demographic characteristics: the mean age of these patients is close to 70 years, compared to about 60 years for patients in acute MI trials. The expected 1-year death rate for the typical septuagenarian is already 2.6% to start with, based on the latest life tables from the *National Vital Statistics Report* (Vol. 48, No. 18, February 7, 2001). In the population with atherosclerosis, many other competing comorbidities may confound long-term cause-specific mortality outcome analysis. Deaths attributable to cardiac causes for this population are well documented in the literature. Moreover, there is a higher prevalence of other conditions that predispose these patients to stroke, such as atrial fibrillation, lipohyalinosis, aortic arch atheroma, left ventricular dysfunction, and concomitant requirements for chronic anticoagulation or antiplatelet therapy. Thus, to be able to define the incremental value of any therapeutic intervention in these difficult populations, a control group is imperative, such as that provided by randomized trials.

It must be pointed out that none of the current randomized attempts to test the real-world utility of EDPs or to evaluate whether adjunctive therapies which are useful in other vascular beds (e.g. glycoprotein IIb/IIIa inhibitors), apply to CAS, in spite of growing utilization of both. There needs to be at least one study wherein the use of EPD and stent is uncoupled, since there is probably a subgroup of patients in whom no benefits can be expected to justify the extra procedural time, intravascular manipulation, and costs imposed by EPDs.

Nonetheless, lessons must be learned from the history of CEA. Carotid endarterectomy is currently the established standard of care for the prevention of stroke from carotid artery stenosis. While this had been the sentiment of vascular and neurosurgeons for more than two decades, it took RCTs to validate the efficacy of this procedure for symptomatic and asymptomatic patients in the eyes of the wider medical community.[8,9,23,24] For better or for worse, this is the standard that CAS must also pass.

Summary

The current standard for assessing new medical strategies and technologies is the clinical trial. Both randomized clinical trials and prospective observational studies play important roles in providing complementary information to help understand the appropriate role of carotid angioplasty and stenting in stroke prevention.

Large scale-randomized trials (CREST, SAPPHIRE, and ICSS) are under way that assess the spectrum of low to high surgical risk patients. Prospective observational studies and registries that are weighted toward specific subgroups are also discussed in detail.

Acknowledgments

The authors would like to express their gratitude for the continued support and efforts of Michele Klein-Fedyshin, Michelle Burda, Marge Codispoti, Debbie Downey, and Ray Tate of the UPMC Shadyside Medical Library, and Doris Cavlovich and the PVI Research Section.

References

1. Sivaguru A, Venables GS, Beard JD, Gaines PA. European carotid angioplasty trial. *J Endovasc Surg* 1996; **3**: 16–20.

2. Wholey MH, Jarmolowski CR, Eles G et al. Endovascular stents for carotid artery occlusive disease. *J Endovasc Surg* 1997; **4**: 326–38.

3. Roubin GS, Yadav S, Iyer SS, Vitek, J. Carotid stent-supported angioplasty: a neurovascular intervention to prevent stroke. *Am J Cardiol* 1996; **78**: 8–12.

4. Wholey MH, Wholey M, Bergeron P et al. Current global status of carotid artery stent placement [see comments]. *Cathet Cardiovasc Diagn* 1998; **44**: 1–6.

5. Henry M, Amor M, Masson I et al. Angioplasty and stenting of the extracranial carotid arteries. *J Endovasc Surg* 1998; **5**: 293–304.

6. Henry M, Klonaris C, Amor M et al. Stent supported carotid artery angioplasty: the beneficial effect of cerebral protection. *Circulation* 2000; **102** (suppl) II–476.

7. Wholey MH, Wholey M, Mathias K et al. Global experience in cervical carotid artery stent placement. *Cathet Cardiovasc Intervent* 2000; **50**: 160–7.

8. Anonymous. Beneficial effect of carotid endarterectomy in symptomatic patients with high-grade carotid stenosis. North American Symptomatic Carotid Endarterectomy Trial Collaborators. *N Engl J Med* 1991; **325**: 445–53.

9. Anonymous. Randomised trial of endarterectomy for recently symptomatic carotid stenosis: final results of the MRC European Carotid Surgery Trial (ECST). *Lancet* 1988; **351**: 1379–87.

10. Tan WA, Jarmolowski CR, Wechsler LR, Wholey MH. New developments in endovascular interventions for extracranial carotid stenosis. *Tex Heart Inst J* 2000; **27**: 273–80.

11. Heuser RR. Endovascular haute couture revisited; ready-to-wear comes of age. *Cathet Cardiovasc Diagn* 1998; **45**: 314.

12. Alberts MJ, McCann R, Smith TP. A Randomized Trial of Carotid Stenting vs. Endarterectomy in Patients with Symptomatic Carotid Stenosis: study design. *J Neurovascular Dis* 1997; **2**: 228–34.

13. Naylor AR, Bolia A, Abbott RJ et al. Randomized study of carotid angioplasty and stenting versus carotid endarterectomy: a stopped trial. *J Vasc Surg* 1998; **28**: 326–34.

14. Tan WA, Jarmolowski CR, Bates M et al. Cerebral protection systems for distal emboli during carotid artery interventions. *J Intervent Cardiol* 2001; **14**: 465–74.

15. Henry M, Amor M, Henry I et al. Carotid stenting with cerebral protection: first clinical experience using the PercuSurge GuardWire system. *J Endovasc Surg* 1999; **6** 321–31.

16. Federal Aviation Administration. FAA proposes actions on in-flight entertainment systems. *FAA* 2001; **2001**.

17. Aeppel T. Mounting pressure: under the glare of recall, tire makers are giving new technology a spin. *Wall Street J* 2001; A1.

18. Reuters. Ford faces safety lawsuits: automaker faces multibillion dollar suits from Firestone recall, other issues. CNN.com. Atlanta, GA, 2001.

19 Donawa ME. Working draft of the FDA GMP final rule (Part I). *Med Device Technol* 1995; **6**: 13–22.

20 Donawa ME. A US FDA medical device update. Part II. *Med Device Technol* 1996; **7**: 12–16, 18.

21 Donawa ME. New FDA draft guidance on premarket submissions. *Med Device Technol* 1999; **10**: 12–14.

22 Tan WA, Tamai H, Park SJ et al. Long-term outcomes after unprotected left main trunk percutaneous revascularization in 279 patients. *Circulation* 2001; **104**: 1609–14.

23 Anonymous. Study design for randomized prospective trial of carotid endarterectomy for asymptomatic atherosclerosis. The Asymptomatic Carotid Atherosclerosis Study Group. *Stroke* 1989; **20**: 844–9.

24 Warlow CP. Symptomatic patients: the European Carotid Surgery Trial (ECST). *J Mal Vasc* 1993; **18**: 198–201.

25 Hobson RW 2nd, Brott T, Ferguson R et al. CREST: Carotid Revascularization Endarterectomy versus Stent Trial [editorial]. *Cardiovasc Surg* 1997; **5**: 457–8.

43

Endovascular surgery in multivascular atherosclerosis

LA Bockeria, BG Alekyan, AA Spiridonov, Yul Buziashvili, EB Kuperberg, AV Ter-Akopyan, VF Kharpunov and MD Kirnus

Introduction

Treatment of patients with multivascular atherosclerosis is one of the most difficult problems in cardiovascular surgery and, particularly, in endovascular surgery. This group is represented by patients with atherosclerotic disease of different areas of the vascular bed (coronary arteries, brachiocephalic vessels, renal arteries, limb arteries).

Treatment of stroke is one of the most important problems. This is due to the great extent of cerebrovascular disease, where the leading role belongs to ischemic stroke of atherosclerotic origin. The mortality due to ischemic stroke in modern countries varies from 12% to 20% of the total, and is second to the mortality due to heart diseases and tumors.[1]

Cerebrovascular pathology in Russia accounted for 27.3% in 1995 and 29.2% in 1998 of all the vascular diseases. The number of cerebrovascular cases in Russia increased by 5.3% per year and first revealed cases by 5.5%, and the mortality exceeded 37% of all the deaths resulting from cardiovascular causes. About 26 000 patients died in Russian hospitals of cerebral ischemic events in 1998.[2]

Treatment of brachiocephalic artery disease was only by surgery before 1980, but since 1980 many hospitals have developed the less traumatic endovascular methods of treatment of cerebrovascular pathology.

Symptoms of chronic inferior limb ischemia may be due to the involvement of limb arteries, isolated and combined abdominal aorta and aortic bifurcation, and iliac and femoral artery occlusions.

Abdominal aorta occlusion as a cause of inferior limb ischemia was first described by Gaham.[3] Leriche described in 1923,[4] and analysed in detail in 1940,[5] a series of clinical cases of young patients with symptoms of abdominal aorta occlusion.

Reconstructive surgical procedures such as superior resection of abdominal aorta with aortofemoral bifurcational bypass, aortofemoral bypass grafting, and thrombo-endarterectomy from aortoiliac segment, are currently in wide use. The mortality after such procedures is 2–13% and the amputation rate up to 10%.

The failure to achieve satisfactory results with surgical reconstructive procedures, especially in patients with concomitant coronary, renal or brachiocephalic artery involvement, led to the development of endovascular methods of treatment in abdominal aorta occlusion.

The use of thrombolytics and, later, interventional procedures, provided a success rate of 93–100%.

Concerning the patterns of arterial bed involvement, the patients with multivascular atherosclerosis represent the most severe cases. The optimal strategies for their treatment have not been developed yet. There are no united principles of treatment; the order of performance of both surgical and interventional procedures has not been developed yet.

The aim of this study was to show the possibilities of combination of surgical and endovascular methods of treatment as well as endovascular surgery alone in the treatment of patients with multivascular atherosclerosis.

Materials and methods

In this report we share our experience of the treatment of patients with multivascular atherosclerosis. We have treated 251 patients with atherosclerotic disease of different arteries. Surgical and interventional procedures were carried out in 121 (48.2%) patients, and endovascular procedures alone in 130 (51.8%) patients (Figure 43.1). The patients' age varied from 43 to 71 years. At least two arterial beds or distant segments of one arterial bed were affected.

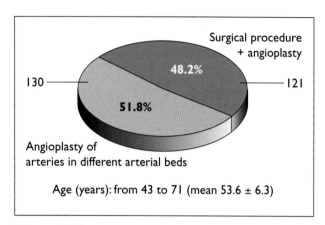

Surgical procedure
+ angioplasty

48.2%

130 ——— 121

51.8%

Angioplasty of
arteries in different arterial beds

Age (years): from 43 to 71 (mean 53.6 ± 6.3)

Figure 43.1
Distribution of patients with multivessel disease (n=251).

Seventy-four (61.2%) of the group of patients with combined treatment underwent coronary artery bypass grafting (CABG) and percutaneous transluminal angioplasty or stenting of different arterial bed segments; 35 (28.9%) patients underwent surgical procedures on inferior limb arteries and interventions on other arterial bed vessels, or a combination of the two above methods on inferior limb arteries; 9 (7.4%) patients underwent surgical procedures on brachiocephalic arteries and percutaneous transluminal angioplasty (PTA) of other arterial beds as well as surgical procedures in combination with endovascular procedures on different aortic branches; and 3 (2.5%) patients underwent surgery on renal arteries combined with endovascular procedures on different arterial beds.

In 42 (56.8%) patients CABG was performed as a first step, and as a second step PTA or stenting. Thirty-two (43.2%) patients underwent endovascular procedures first with further CABG. They were distributed as follows: in 38 (51.4%), CABG combined with PTA of inferior limb arteries; in 9 (12.2%), CABG combined with PTA (7 patients) or stenting (2 patients) of brachiocephalic arteries; and in 27 (36.5%), CABG combined with endovascular procedures on renal arteries.

Among 38 patients undergoing CABG and PTA of inferior limb arteries, the order of the above procedures was as follows: CABG was carried out first in 25 (65.8%) patients, and in 13 (34.2%) patients the endovascular procedure on different stenosed or occluded segments of inferior limbs was done first. We have to emphasize that this group included the patients with severely diseased coronary and iliac arteries. All of these patients needed the CABG with IABP support. Twenty-six (65.6%) of 38 patients underwent endovascular procedures on one artery only, and 12 PTA of two leg arteries. Fifteen (55.6%) of 27 patients with severe coronary artery disease and vasorenal hypertension underwent CABG as a first step and PTA of the renal artery as a second step. Twelve (44.4%) of 27 patients underwent the renal PTA first, which allowed the performance of CABG as the next step of

treatment. In 22 (77.3%) of 27 patients, a disease of one renal artery was noted, and in five (22.7%) patients both renal arteries were stenosed. Nine patients with severe atherosclerotic disease of the brachiocephalic arteries in combination with other artery involvement underwent both surgical and endovascular procedures. Four (44.4%) of 9 patients underwent surgical procedures in combination with PTA on different aortic branches. Two (22.2%) of 9 patients with brachiocephalic artery involvement in combination with inferior limb artery pathology underwent surgical procedures on different aortic branches in combination with PTA of leg arteries. Three (33.3%) of 9 patients underwent a combination of surgery on brachiocephalic arteries and PTA of diseased renal arteries.

In a group of 35 patients, 22 (62.9%) underwent a combination of surgical and endovascular procedures for pathologies of different segments of inferior limb arteries; 7 (20%) patients had both surgery on leg arteries and intervention on brachiocephalic arteries, in 4 (11.4%) patients the surgical procedure on leg arteries was combined with PTA on renal arteries, and in 2 (5.7%) patients the surgical procedure on leg arteries was combined with PTCA.

The patients who underwent endovascular procedures only (n = 130) due to multivascular atherosclerosis were subdivided into two groups. The first group included 123 (94.6%) patients with two arterial beds involved, and the second group included 7 (5.4%) patients with the involvement of three arterial beds.

Among 123 patients with the involvement of two arterial beds, 25 (20.3%) underwent endovascular procedures both on coronary and brachiocephalic arteries. Of 25 patients, 19 had subclavian artery pathology, 5 had internal carotid artery disease (CAD), and one had CAD with brachiocephalic trunk involvement (Figure 43.2).

Among 19 patients with CAD in combination with subclavian artery pathology, occlusion of the left subclavian artery was revealed in 7 patients. There was an absence of radial pulse in those with subclavian artery occlusion, and it was diminished in the rest. Doppler ultrasound showed collateral or altered laminar patterns of bloodflow in arm arteries in cases of subclavian artery disease. The systolic pressure gradient in the upper extremities was 50.4 ± 4.7 mmHg. The patients complained of headache, dizziness, and coordination disturbances; ophthalmoscopy revealed transient changes in retinal blood supply. Symptoms of arm ischemia were also present (pain, loss of feeling, muscular weakness).

In 57 (46%) patients, coronary percutaneous intervention was combined with endovascular treatment of different arterial segments of the lower extremities (65 (47%) procedures) (Figure 43.3); in one patient with a high occlusion of the abdominal aorta, we performed right coronary artery (RCA) stenting with thrombolysis and stenting of both iliac arteries. Twenty-five (20%) patients underwent endovascular procedures on coronary and renal

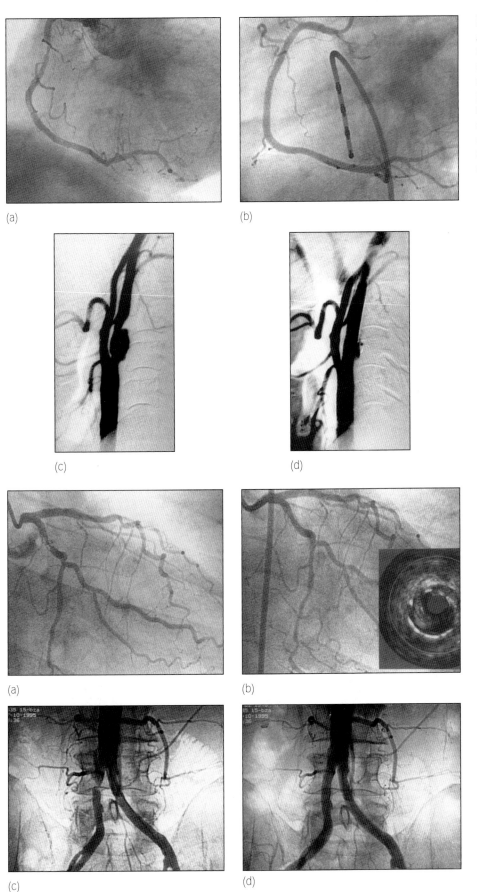

Figure 43.2
Angiogram of the patient with right coronary artery lesion: (a) before stenting; (b) after stenting. Angiograms of the same patient with right internal carotid artery lesion: (c) before stenting of the right internal carotid artery; (d) after implantation of the self-expanding 'Easy Wallstent' (Boston Scientific Corp.).

(a)

(b)

(c)

(d)

Figure 43.3
Angiograms of the patient with left circumflex artery disease: (a) before stenting; (b) after Bx Velocity (Cordis, J&J) stent implantation. Angiograms of the same patient with right common iliac artery pathology: (c) before percutaneous transluminal angioplasty (PTA) of right common iliac artery: (d) after PTA of right common iliac artery.

(a)

(b)

(c)

(d)

Figure 43.4
Angiograms of the patient with
LAD disease: (a) before PTCA; (b)
after PTCA. Angiograms of the
same patient with left renal artery
lesion: (c) before stenting; (d) after
Corinthian (Cordis, J&J) stent
implantation.

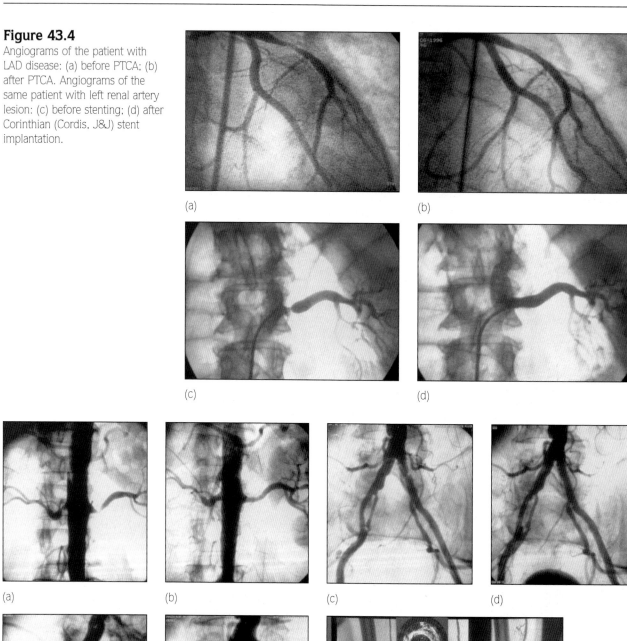

(a)

(b)

(c)

(d)

(a)

(b)

(c)

(d)

(e)

(f)

(g) & (h)

Figure 43.5
Angiograms of the patient with atherosclerotic disease of both renal arteries: (a) before stenting of renal arteries; (b) after Palmaz
(Cordis, J&J) stent implantation to the right and left renal arteries. Angiograms of the same patient with left common iliac artery
pathology: (c) before stenting; (d) after Jostent (Jomed) implantation to the left common iliac artery. Angiograms of the same patient
with right external iliac artery stenosis: (e) before its stenting; (f) after Jostent (Jomed) implantation. Angiograms of the same patient
with right superficial femoral artery occlusion: (g) before recanalization and stent implantation to the right superficial femoral artery; (h)
after stenting and PTA of the segment distal to the stented area. Complete stent deployment is confirmed with intravascular ultrasound.

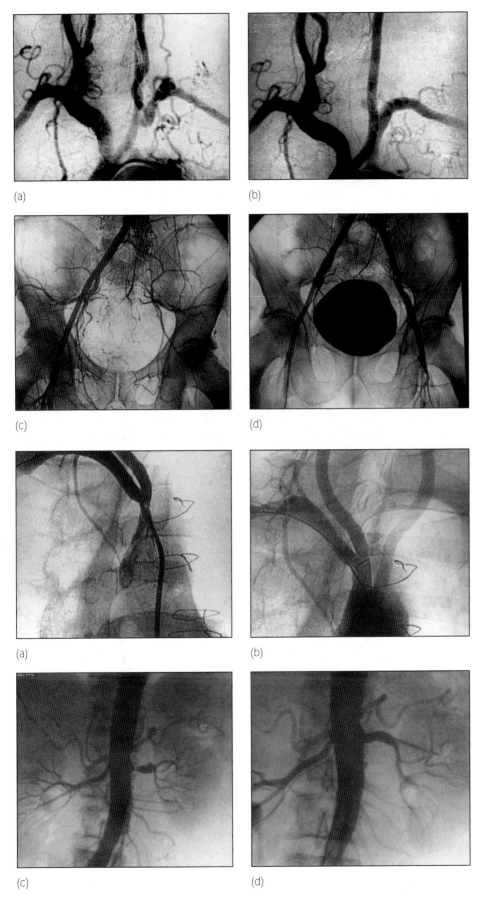

(a)

(b)

(c)

(d)

(a)

(b)

(c)

(d)

Figure 43.6
Angiograms of the patient with multivascular atherosclerosis. Right subclavian artery occlusion: (a) before wire recanalization and self-expanding Easy Wallstent (Boston Scientific) implantation to the right subclavian artery; (b) after stenting. Angiograms of the same patient with left common and external iliac artery occlusion: (c) before recanalization and percutaneous transluminal angioplasty; (d) after successful procedure.

Figure 43.7
Angiograms of the patient with multivascular atherosclerosis. Status post-coronary artery bypass graft. Stenosis of brachiocephalic trunk: (a) before balloon pre-dilation and Palmaz stent implantation to the brachiocephalic trunk; (b) after successful procedure. Angiograms of the same patient with left renal artery stenosis: (c) before Corinthian (Cordis, J&J) stent implantation; (d) after stenting.

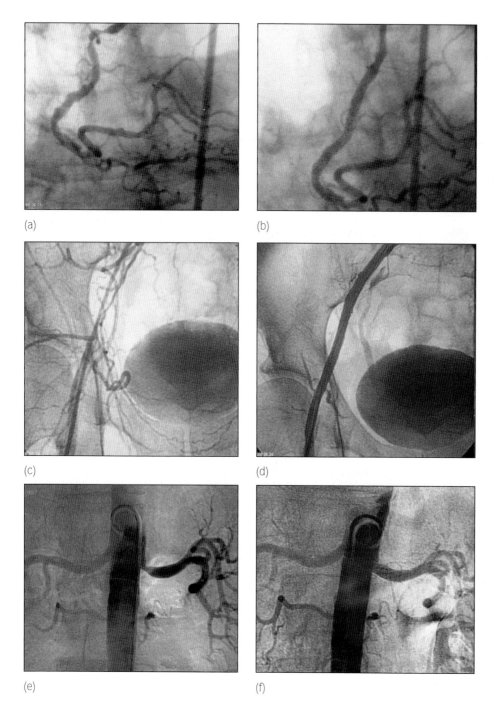

(a)

(b)

(c)

(d)

(e)

(f)

Figure 43.8
Angiograms of the patients with involvement of three arterial beds: carotid artery disease. Right coronary artery (RCA) stenosis: (a) before stenting; (b) after RCA stenting. Angiograms of the same patient with right common and external iliac artery occlusion: (c) before wire recanalization and Jostent (Jomed) implantation; (d) after stenting. Angiograms of the same patient with left renal artery stenosis: (e) before Perflex (Cordis, J&J) stent implantation; (f) after the procedure.

arteries (30 (22%)) (Figure 43.4), 5 (4%) patients underwent balloon angioplasty or stenting of different segments of leg arteries and PTA or stenting of renal arteries (9 (6%) procedures) (Figure 43.5), 7 (5.7%) patients underwent PTA of brachiocephalic arteries with PTA of lower limb arteries (Figure 43.6), and 2 (1%) patients underwent PTA of brachiocephalic and renal arteries (Figure 43.7).

Among patients with three vascular beds involved, there were 14 endovascular procedures done. Two (28%) patients with coronary, brachiocephalic and lower extremity arteries

affected underwent 10 (73%) procedures and 5 (72%) with coronary, renal and lower extremity arteries involved underwent 4 (27%) endovascular procedures (Figure 43.8).

All of the endovascular procedures were performed under local anesthesia. To perform the endovascular procedure in a patient with high abdominal aorta occlusion we chose the radial approach, and in all other cases the femoral approach. The patients received aspirin 325 mg once daily and ticlopidine 250 mg twice daily 2 days before the procedure, and intravenous heparin 5000 IU was given at the beginning of the procedure for antithrombotic purposes. In three cases with brachiocephalic artery pathology, we faced difficulties when advancing the balloon catheter through the severely stenosed areas, so in these cases we chose the two-step dilation, with a coronary balloon being used first with subsequent replacement by the appropriate balloon catheter.

We usually used balloons of the same diameter as the non-affected arterial segment. The diameter of the balloons used varied from 3 to 10 mm. The balloons used were from Bard and Cordis, USA. The stents used were SMART, Palmaz, Perflex and Corinthian by Cordis. After interventions, the patients received intravenous dextran 400 ml and pentoxyphylline 100 mg for 24 h, and aspirin 325 mg once daily with ticlopidine 250 mg twice daily for 2 months.

After interventions such as PTA and/or stenting, the patients have usually been discharged from the hospital by the second or third day.

Results

To assess the immediate results, we used the data on clinical findings, non-invasive data and angiographic data. After the procedures, the symptoms of cerebral, vertebral and limb ischemia were controlled; in seven patients after recanalization and PTA of a chronically occluded subclavian artery, the antegrade vertebral arterial bloodflow was restored with control of vertebral-to-subclavian steal syndrome.

After the completion of interventions on inferior limb arteries in the patients, Doppler ultrasound showed an increase of ankle index from 0.4 ± 0.03 to 0.97 ± 0.06; the symptoms of chronic ischemia were also well controlled.

After completion of endovascular procedures on renal arteries, the degree of arterial narrowing decreased from 50–90% to 10–35%; also the systolic arterial blood pressure decreased from 240–180 mmHg to 160–140 mmHg, and diastolic pressure from 150–100 mmHg to 100–80 mmHg.

Complications

After the endovascular procedures, we noted the following complications: femoral artery thrombosis in six (4.6%) patients, pseudoaneurysm in one (0.8%) patient, and renal artery dissection in one (0.8%) patient. The patients with femoral artery thrombosis and pseudoaneurysm underwent surgical procedures, and the patient with renal artery dissection was managed on therapy. Two deaths have taken place after stentings of brachiocephalic trunk and internal carotid artery.

Conclusions

1. Endovascular surgery is a safe and effective method of treatment in patients with stenotic and occlusive lesions of coronary, brachiocephalic, renal and peripheral arteries in multivascular atherosclerosis.

2. The use of endovascular methods of treatment in patients with multivascular atherosclerosis allows them to be prepared for open cardiovascular surgical procedures, and, in selected cases, may serve as the only suitable method of treatment.

3. Gaining clinical experience and obtaining the follow-up results will define the order of performance of endovascular and surgical procedures in multivascular atherosclerotic disease.

References

1   Alekyan BG, Henry M, Spiridonov AA, Ter-Akopyan AV. *Endovascular Surgery in a treatment of patients with the pathology of brachiocephalic arteries.* Moscow, 2001.

2   Bockeria LA, Alekyan BG, Spiridonov AA et al. Endovascular methods of treatment for patients with multivascular atherosclerosis. *Serdechno-sosudistiaya Chirurgia (Thoracic and Cardiovascular Surgery)* 2001; **2**: 150.

3   Ashida K, Imaizumi M, Isaka Y et al. Complete recanalization of total occlusions in abdominal aorta by intra-aortic infusion of thrombolytic agent – a case report. *Angiology* 1993; Jul; 574-9.

4   Marin ML, Veith FJ, Sanches LA et al. Endovascular repair of aortoiliac occlusive disease. *World J Surg* 1996; **20**: 679-86.

5   Nyman U, Uher P, Lindh M et al. Primary stenting in infrarenal aortic occlusive disease. *Cardiovasc Intervent Radiol* 2000; **23**: 97-108.

44

Endovascular treatment of descending thoracic aortic aneurysms and dissections

Patrice Bergeron, Thierry De Chaumaray, Erica Taube, Nicola Mangialardi and Joël Gay

Introduction

Although there has been considerable progress in surgical techniques and in anesthesia and intensive care, the surgical treatment of descending thoracic aortic aneurysms still suffers from a high rate of morbidity and mortality. Nevertheless, the natural history taken by aneurysm lesions involving the vital prognosis makes it necessary to propose a therapeutic solution to the patients concerned. Imaging techniques are constantly improving and, with the new technological advances, a less-invasive approach in treating thoracic aortic aneurysms can be expected from endovascular techniques. For selected indications, the mid-term results with endovascular therapy are very encouraging, since there is a significant drop in morbidity and mortality. Moreover, it seems possible to apply these techniques not only to thoracic aortic aneurysms but also to dissections and traumatic ruptures as well as to rarer disorders such as emboligenic ulcers of the aorta. Our objective is to review the state of the art in endovascular treatment of descending thoracic aortic aneurysms and to compare it to surgical treatment in terms of feasibility, indications, and results.

Epidemiology

The incidence of aneurysms involving the descending thoracic aorta is estimated at approximately 6 to 10.4 cases per 100 000 inhabitants per year.[1,2] The aneurysms we are discussing involve the distal part of the thoracic aorta from the left subclavian to the diaphragm and represent 20–35% of aortic locations. The ascending aorta is affected in 45% of cases; the aortic arch and the celiac aorta in 10% of cases each. Between the 1970s and the 1990s the global incidence doubled, mainly due to improved diagnosis techniques and

particularly due to the diffusion of computed tomography (CT) scans, but also because the population is aging through increased life expectancy. During this period, the incidence adjusted to age was three times higher in men than in women. Average age at diagnosis was 69 years and it was higher in women (76 years vs 62 years in men). The main risk factors are the same as in atheromatous diseases (age, gender, smoking, high blood pressure, and hypercholesterolemia). The risk of rupture increases when the aneurysm is larger than 6 cm.

Etiology

There are a variety of etiologies for descending thoracic aortic aneurysms:

- Atherosclerotic aneurysms are by far the most frequent. All types are possible, ranging from limited aneurysms to extended aneurysmal disease of the descending aorta from the left subclavian to the diaphragm. These aneurysms are usually fusiform. This etiology usually concerns older patients (60–70 years old), predominantly males with associated comorbidity – high blood pressure, coronary disease, brain disorders, and chronic obstructive pulmonary disease (COPD). These lesions are associated with infra-abdominal aortic aneurysms in 32.5% of cases;[3] thus representing an increased risk.

- Dissecting aneurysms rank second. They occur after acute type B dissections or represent residual complications of type A aortic dissections after previous ascending aorta repair.[4,5] Unless they complicate vascular dysplasia, these dissections occur in older patients with high blood pressure who easily experience associated lesions similar to those observed in atheromatous aneurysms. The origin of the dissection is usually an intimal tear located just below the left subclavian artery. The aortic wall is split along its circumference following a spiral-shaped path, which creates a false channel with an outer wall consisting only of the adventitia and of a small portion of the media. If circulation continues inside this false channel – which is the most common form of evolution – the aorta gradually expands and this results in the occurrence of an aneurysm. These lesions often concern the entire thoracoabdominal aorta, but they may be limited to the descending thoracic aorta, especially if the abdominal aorta is affected by atheromatous calcified lesions that prevent its extension.

- Post-traumatic aneurysms are often located at the isthmic portion of the aorta (Figure 44.1). They result from thoracic traumatisms with deceleration.[6–9] The aneurysms are usually fusiform due to the aortic split along their circumference. Mural thrombosis is rare. The peculiarity with these aneurysms is that they occur in young subjects with a safe aorta above and below the aneurysm, particularly favorable to graft fixation.
- For dystrophic aneurysms which can be true or secondary dissecting aneurysms there is often a family disposition. They are usually cases of Marfan's syndrome.[10] In rarer cases, they can concern Ehlers–Danlos syndrome, tuberous sclerosis,[11] or other connective tissue diseases.
- False aneurysms are located at the surgical anastomosis. However, true aneurysms can develop on the natural aortic wall with a patch left in place; e.g. for reimplantation of visceral arteries.
- Congenital aneurysms are usually associated with isthmic coarctation.[12]
- Inflammatory aneurysms are secondary to aortitis. They are usually cases of Takayasu's disease,[13] sometimes Horton's disease, Behçet's syndrome,[14] or giant cell aortitis.
- Infectious aneurysms – which are a priori not indications for endovascular therapy – have become exceptional.[15]
- Intramural hematomas and penetrating aortic ulcers are less common but can lead to rupture in 26% and 40% respectively.

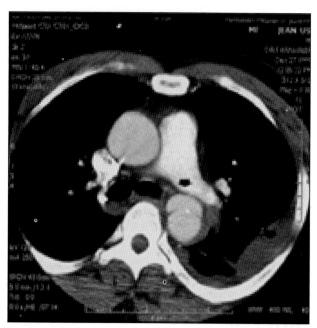

Figure 44.1
Acute traumatic aortic dissection (arrow).

aneurysms who were not operated, usually due to old age and/or the great number of associated comorbidities,[16,17] the actuarial 5-year survival rate was approximately 20%. Death is caused by aneurysm rupture in 50% of cases. These ruptures concern voluminous aneurysms (> 60 mm in diameter) or those having drastically increased in size between two successive examinations. Lastly, these ruptures seem more frequent in dissecting aneurysms. Other complications may occur, such as compression of neighboring organs (lungs, nerves, bronchi, or esophagus), thromboembolic events (lower limbs, digestive tract, kidneys, or spinal cord) by aortic branch occlusion due to extended wall thrombosis or by cruoric, atheromatous or cholesterol thrombus migration. The severity of this spontaneous evolution justifies an aggressive approach, although efforts must be made to limit the number of complications and the vital risk. Up until a few years ago, only surgical therapy was able to achieve this goal.

Natural history

The spontaneous evolution of descending thoracic aortic aneurysms is less well known than that of abdominal aortic aneurysms, since most studies are old, but the condition seems at least as severe. The main threat is rupture due to the gradual increase of parietal constraints, as the aneurysm increases in diameter and the wall becomes thinner according to Laplace's law.[3] Once the rupture occurs in the pleural cavity, it rapidly leads to death, except in cases of pleural symphysis. Mediastinal rupture is more common and can be contained during several hours or days.

In different series of patients with descending thoracic aortic

Surgical therapy and results

From an intellectual point of view the surgical concept is straightforward because it consists in simply removing the damaged segment of the aorta with graft interposition. In practice the situation is different, since this type of surgery addresses mostly older patients presenting multiple associated deleterious disorders (or comorbidities). The operation involves respiratory constraints (extensive surgical approach, exclusion of left lung) and major hemodynamic problems due to aortic clamping (sudden increase of left ventricular post-charge and decreased ejection fraction, redistribution of circulating blood volume in favor of the upper portion of the organism, decreased local circulation below the clamp, particularly to kidneys and spinal cord between 80 and 85%). These modifications are particularly difficult to endure by patients whose cardiac and coronary reserves are often amputated at their basal state. This explains the origin of practically all complications and morbidity and mortality associated with surgical therapy (respiratory insufficiency, myocardial infarction, renal insufficiency, and medullar complications), which is why a complete preliminary examination is necessary to eliminate any possible contraindication.[18–21]

Immediate results

Mortality at the hospital varies between 3 and 15% for planned surgery. It can reach 50% in emergency cases. Death is primarily due to cardiac and lung failure. Even for very well-trained teams it still appears difficult to improve on these rates at this point. Medullar complications vary between 0 and 19% but they are usually around 5% no matter which protection technique is used. Prolonged respiratory assistance is needed for at least 15% of patients. The rate of renal failure varies between 3 and 20%.[22–27]

Long-term results

The 5-year actuarial survival rate is estimated at around 60%. Delayed death is usually due to cardiac complications (39%), although aneurysm rupture at a different location occurs in 1 out of 5 cases. Redo operations for residual or recurring aneurysms appear frequent.[21,28] The rates of postoperative morbidity and mortality have clearly decreased over the last 20 years; however, their toll is still heavy enough to justify the introduction of new therapeutic techniques derived from past experience with abdominal aortic aneurysms stent-grafting. There appear to be a number of theoretical advantages: no aortic clamping, superficial and less-invasive surgical approach, no need for circulatory assistance. For more detailed information, the reader is advised to consult the reference literature. The aim of this chapter is to briefly review surgical treatment, while developing on endovascular therapy.

Endovascular repair of thoracic aortic aneurysms

Endovascular treatment of thoracic aorta aneurysms is a relatively recent technique[29] derived from procedures developed to treat the abdominal aorta. This represents a major benefit for a pathology in which the rate of natural or post-surgical morbidity and mortality is extremely high.

Anatomical and pathological classification

This is an essential tool to help standardize the medical literature – the classification by the medical team from Amsterdam[30] takes into account medullar ischemia, which is the primary potential complication of thoracic aorta aneurysms exclusion. The proximal (P) and distal (D) position of the extremities of the stent–graft are defined. The supra-aortic trunks and the intercostal arteries are used as anatomical boundaries (Figure 44.2). P_1, P_2, or P_3 indicate that the stent begins at the first, second, or third vessel of the aortic arch. D_n indicates where the stent–graft ends or which pair of intercostal arteries is covered last. A fourth type, P_4 completes this classification, referring to the sixth dorsal vertebra (D6) and the sixth intercostal artery pair, indicating that beyond this limit covering the aorta presents an increased risk of medullar ischemia. Thus, an endoluminal stent–graft (ELG) located between D_5 and D_8 is defined as P_3D_8; a location between D_7 and D_{12} is defined as $P_4D_7D_{12}$.

For stent–grafts covering D_6 to D_{12} the authors suggest applying a clamping test and recording the motor-evoked potentials (MEPs). If the MEPs indicate signs of medullar ischemia, then surgical treatment must be undertaken with re-implantation of intercostal arteries. Fortunately, the intercostal arteries are rather frequently obstructed by mural thrombi, which reduces this ischemia risk. In cases of thoracic

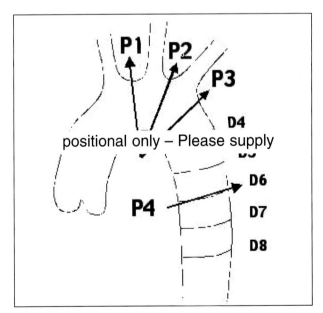

Figure 44.2

Anatomical classification of thoracic aortic stent–graft locations. P = proximal extremity according to supra-aortic trunk; D = distal extremity according to intercostal artery covered. P4 indicates a stent–graft placed beyond D6, with associated increased risk of medullar ischemia.

aorta dissections the most widely accepted classification is Stanford's, which identifies two types: A and B. Type A indicates that the aortic dissection involves the ascending aorta. In type B the dissection concerns only the descending thoracic aorta. The immediate prognosis is different in each case. Type A requires emergency treatment (surgical at present), due to the risk of intrapericardium rupture and tamponade. Type B is usually treated medically, mainly by blood pressure control and, currently, ELG treatment is being proposed. The same PD nomenclature is used.

Endoluminal stent–grafts

Following the same pattern as in abdominal aortic aneurysms, thoracic stent–grafts were initially homemade.[31] The current industrial stent–grafts respect higher mechanical testing criteria and are far more reliable. Given the medicolegal requirements, we do not recommend the use of the former stent–grafts, except in compassionate cases where industrial ELGs do not fit. There are a wide variety of industrial stent–grafts available on the market: most are self-expanding (Ancure®, Aneurx®, Talent®, Excluder®, Zenith®, Endofit®), and only the Lifepath® is balloon-expandable. The Talent® and Excluder® stent–grafts (Figure 44.3a,b) are the most widely used. Prosthetic fabrics are either Dacron or polytetrafluorethylene (PTFE). The device is more or less rigid and thus more or less flexible in crossing the iliac axes and the aortic arch. Simplicity of the delivery system is variable also. We invite the reader to refer to the descriptions by the different companies for more details. Stent-grafts are available

in different diameters and, especially, in different lengths. However, sometimes, several segments of stent–grafts have to be used overlapping to cover longer aneurysms.

Case selection

Case selection is a major problem: it determines immediate results and long-term outcome. There are multiple criteria regarding the patient, the aneurysm and the stent–graft:

1. Patient selection must take into account the surgical risk attached to comorbidity and to medullar ischemia but also to the results of endovascular treatment. The long-term results of aortic stent–grafts are still unknown and there are no studies comparing stent–grafting to medical and surgical options. It appears logical to suggest a conventional surgical procedure with lasting results for low-risk subjects. Conversely, patients at higher risk could be treated using ELG.

2. It is essential to take into account anatomical criteria. Here, too, there are good cases that meet the right conditions and bad candidates when ill-chosen anatomical criteria are used; if criteria are not respected, a high rate of failure can be expected. The length of the neck above and below the aneurysm is critical. A minimum length of 20 mm is recommended for adequate stent–graft anchorage. Covering the subclavian artery and even the left common carotid artery following transposition or bypass operation allows for a wider range of indications if necessary. Regarding the inferior neck, the celiac trunk distance is the determining factor. Stent–graft diameter should be 2–4 mm

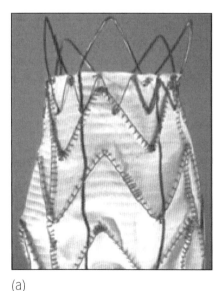
(a)

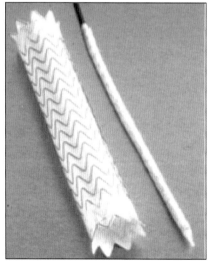
(b)

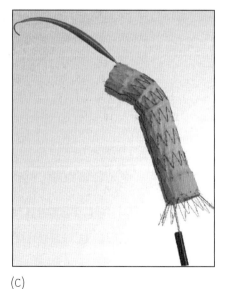
(c)

Figure 44.3
The Talent (a) Excluder (b) and (c) Zenith self-expanding stent–grafts.

larger than the aorta. Precise measurements of the aneurysm are necessary: CT scanning is the best preoperative examination for measuring diameters. Arteriography using a calibrated catheter (Figure 44.4) provides a measurement of the length of the aneurysm. It is important to take into account the tortuosities of the aneurysm which increase the required stent length. The lately released CT station (EasyVision, Philips) allows accurate measurement of the center line length. It must be kept in mind that a junction between two stent segments represents a zone of weakness where endoleaks can occur. The length of the overlap must exceed 2 cm. The condition of the iliac arteries must be considered since the diameter of the introducer is important and may in certain cases not cross a tortuous, calcified and narrow iliac artery.

3. Lastly, stent–graft criteria should also be taken into consideration. Some stents have a bare zone by which vessel ostia can be covered, thus increasing the anchorage surface. Most of all, flexibility and size of the delivery system determine the choice of a stent–graft. For thoracic aortic dissections, there is general agreement that coverage of the entry point is sufficient. Complete coverage of the aneurysm is considered only in cases of chronic dissections.

Implantation technique

The best imaging systems are found in catheterization rooms, although the mobile C-arm systems found in operating theaters are appropriate. We use Philips BV300

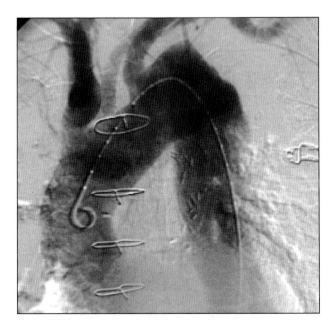

Figure 44.4
Calibrated catheters are useful to measure the length of the aneurysm and/or the necks.

and BV Pulsera. A large field must be visible and road mapping is necessary. Landmarks on the patient or on the operating table are marked with a pen on the screen if the screen must be moved. The operating table should not be moved, if possible. The angle of the C-arm is particularly important to avoid parallax errors, especially with short necks. The left oblique anterior (LOA) view is usually the most advantageous angle.

Access. Femoral access is the most common, a small horizontal incision in the inguinal fold is sufficient to expose the common femoral artery. A more advanced dissection involving the external iliac artery can facilitate insertion of the system. Other subperitoneal approaches from the iliac artery or even from the abdominal aorta have also been used, as well as access from the left common carotid artery or from the right axillary artery. The best access should be used, and additional dilatation can eventually be administered in the case of iliac stenosis.

An additional percutaneous approach from the left (most frequent) or right humeral artery may be necessary when the origin of the supra-aortic vessels has to be marked. This approach allows angiography and insertion of a guide wire from subclavian to femoral arteries. Superstiff guides are used in such cases. This additional approach is not used for distal thoracic aortic aneurysms.

Steps

- A femoral arterial puncture is made on the best side selected for stent–graft insertion (ipsilateral). A 280-cm hydrophilic guide wire is inserted into the thoracic aorta and a 7 French (7F) introducer is put into place.
- A 7F introducer is also placed on the contralateral femoral artery to allow arteriography with a calibrated pigtail catheter over an hydrophilic guide wire. This provides a global left oblique view of the thoracic aorto aneurysm to evaluate the length of the stent needed. Precise diameter determination may be supplemented with intravascular ultrasound (IVUS), which allows the neck quality to be assessed (calcification, irregularity, thrombus) or by transesophagal echocardiography (TEE).
- A super stiff guide replaces the hydrophilic guide wire on the ipsilateral side.
- The ascension of the delivery system follows the removal of the 7F introducer and a transverse arteriotomy of the femoral artery is made.
- Positioning at the upper neck can be assisted by injecting a complementary contrast through humeral access, centered on this landmark for a more accurate deployment.
- The stent–graft is deployed according to each manufacturer's specific system (Figure 44.5). It appears useful to reduce the blood pressure down to 80 mmHg in order to avoid displacement. Some authors have used adenosine-induced transient cardiac asystole.[32] Post-

deployment ballooning may be used in some cases. A three-leaf balloon has the advantage of allowing continued blood flow in the aorta, thus avoiding displacement of the stent–graft.

- For graft extension, one or more complementary stent–grafts are deployed and made to overlap by at least 2 cm.
- Global angiographic control to check for any endoleaks in the aneurysm sac. Additional balloon inflation or additional cuff extension may be necessary for complete sealing.
- Removal of the delivery system, suture of arteriotomy and closing of surgical approach.
- Totally percutaneous systems using the Perclose device are also possible and allow for 1-day hospital stay.

The same criteria apply to the treatment of aortic dissections. The ELG is deployed in the true channel and covers the proximal damaged area. Covering only the intimal tear of the dissection is an accepted procedure; the rest of the false channel is then no longer under pressure and is expected to thrombose and evolve favorably. Use of perioperative TEE is extremely useful to confirm false channel exclusion. Further associated manipulations are often needed.

Associated procedures

For atheromatous aneurysms the main objective is to facilitate placement of the stent–graft when access appears difficult, and to ensure proper anchorage of the ELG when the neck is short. For dissections of the thoracic aorta, the main associated procedures are fenestration or stenting to treat associated malperfusion.

Procedures to facilitate access

1. Set free the common femoral artery and the external iliac artery. Their extension corrects the aortic axis and thus facilitates introduction of the stent–graft.
2. Subperitoneal iliac access. This allows for implantation of a prosthetic tube on the external or common iliac artery – in certain cases even on the distal aorta if the iliac arteries are not exploitable. The larger vessel diameter and straightness of the prosthetic tube emerging from the cut-down are particularly convenient for introducing the stent–graft.

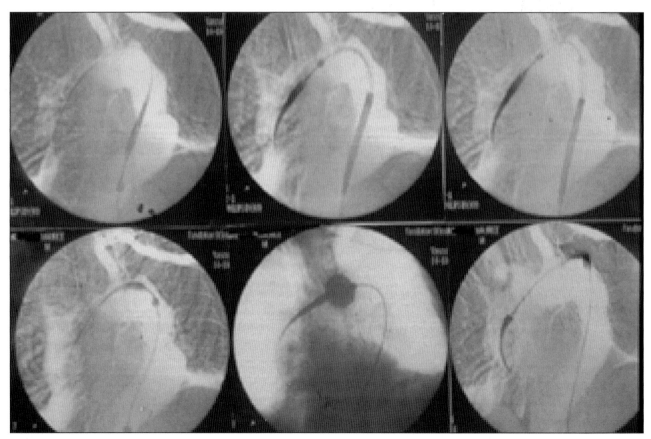

Figure 44.5
Different steps of stent–graft deployment. Reproduced with permission from *Minerva Medica* 2003; 44: 349–61.

3. Access through the supra-aortic trunks. Access through the common carotid artery has already been used.[34] This requires clamping of the artery in question and can cause cerebral emboli or ischemia. We have experience with access through the right axilary artery, particularly in women, in order to introduce Excluder stent–grafts without using an introducer.

4. The combined femoro-subclavian access. This consists in introducing a stiff guide wire – through the left or right subclavian artery – which comes out through the femoral artery after capture with a loop. Use of such a super stiff guide can straighten the artery axis and facilitate insertion of the ELG. Some accidental ruptures of the subclavian artery have been reported, which justifies the use of a guiding catheter to protect the artery.

5. Short, oblique necks, calcified or overloaded with thrombus deposit, are weak spots for prosthesis fixation. Stent–grafts with beveled tips are currently under study and could avoid tilting of the prosthesis once the neck of the aneurysm resumes its oblique position after withdrawal of the introducer.

Correction of malperfusion syndrome during aortic dissections

Malperfusion syndrome has to be diagnosed early during angiography to avoid clinical complications. When an aortic false channel is under pressure, this can give rise to severe ischemic complications to the abdominal visceral organs by dissection of the visceral arteries (renal, superior mesenteric arteries) or by tearing the intima (Figures 44.6–44.10). Such lesions can be further complicated by visceral artery thrombosis and infarction. The same mechanism applies to ischemia of the medulla or of the lower limbs through iliac compression.

Specific complementary endovascular tools can treat these complications. A stent placed at the origin of the visceral artery can reopen the compressed artery or treat a flap of the intima. Fenestration results in communication between the true and the false channel in order to balance the blood pressures on either side, thus also releasing the compression of the true channel. This is a difficult technique, requiring a great deal of skill. Both channels have to be accessed through one or both femoral arteries. Fenestration of the membrane separating the two channels is done using a balloon after perforation. Cardiac trans-septal kits can be used, and they are usually introduced into the smaller channel (often the true channel). The perforating needle is inserted into the false channel, where a balloon or lasso marking system is placed, or even an IVUS. A much simpler 'scissors technique' has been proposed by Beregi (pers. comm.), which consists of a longitudinal section of the

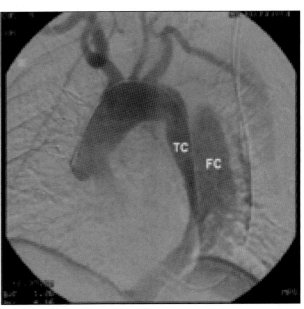

Figure 44.6
Acute type B dissection. Note the true (TC) and the false channel (FC).

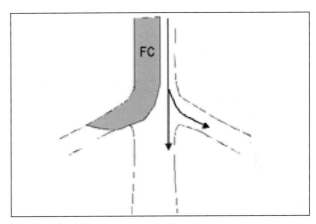

Figure 44.7
Occlusion of the right renal artery by the false channel (FC).

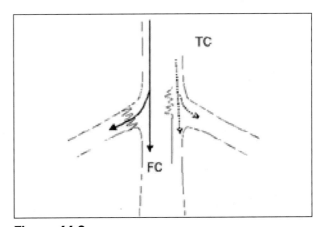

Figure 44.8
False occlusion of the left renal artery by compression of the true channel (TC). The intima on the right renal artery is torn.

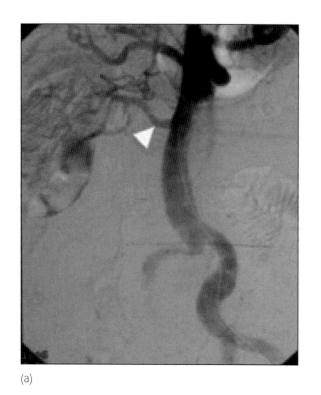

(a)

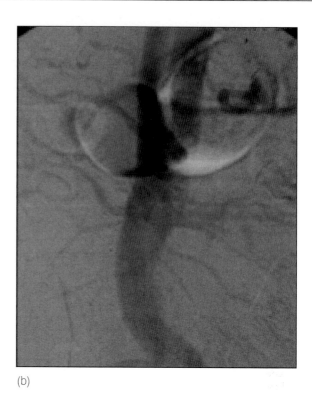

(b)

Figure 44.9
Malperfusion syndrome. (a) The true channel gives the right renal artery (arrow). (b) The left renal artery arises from the false channel.

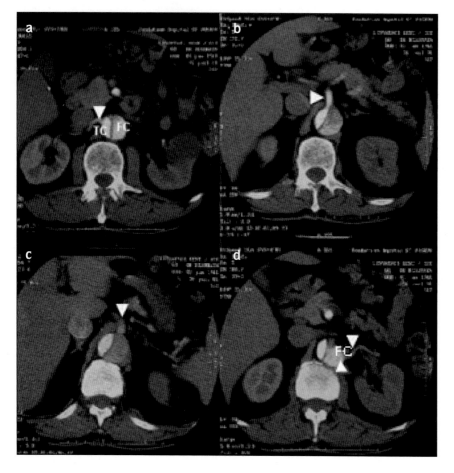

Figure 44.10
(a) The right renal artery (arrow) arises from the true channel (TC). (b) Same for SMA (arrow). (c) The celiac artery (arrow) arises from the false channel (FC). (d) The left renal artery (arrow head) arises from the false channel (FC).

membrane separating the false channel from the true one. This can be done by placing one guide wire in each channel, placing the two guide wires in the same guiding catheter, and pushing on the guiding catheter to cut the membrane.

Other complementary treatments

Among other complementary treatments, spinal liquid drainage may be very useful in the case of paraplegia, allowing quick recovery. Also, epi-aortic and visceral vessels transposition may be required to make the proximal (Figure 44.11) or distal aortic neck suitable.

Surveillance and follow-up

Successful implantation of a thoracic ELG requires regular surveillance. This is justified by the risk of secondary endoleaks due to possible stent migration or modifications of the *excluded* aneurysm. Upon discharge of the patient, a contrast-enhanced CT scan serves as a reference for future evaluation. Later surveillance is based mainly on CT scan investigations. The first follow-up control is done at 6 months and serves two research purposes:

1. to detect secondary endoleaks around the ELG

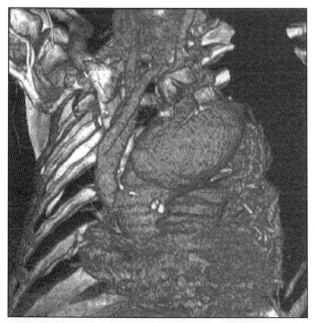

Figure 44.11
This patient suffering from an extended thoracic aortic aneurysm underwent a total transposition of the supra-aortic vessels in order to exclude the aortic arch with stent-grafts.

2. to measure the diameter of the aneurysm sac for comparison with the reference CT scan.

Volumetric assessment techniques are also a means of measuring the volume in the aneurysm sac and are more reliable in determining whether the aneurysm decreased; however, only few centers have access to the software. In general, if the exclusion is successful, i.e. eliminating all blood circulation and endotension within the aneurysm, it must regress. In this case, CT scan controls are done on an annual basis. A stable aneurysm does not mean that it is cured, and the physicians must remain watchful. This aspect of endoluminal stent–grafting is essential because it raises the question of how valid this technique is in the long term. While surgery takes care of the problem once and for all by resection of the aneurysm and ligation of the collaterals, ELG only excludes the aneurysm. In certain cases, this exclusion can be only temporary and, indeed, several examples of re-established circulation and pressure within the aneurysm have been reported, sometimes ending in fatal ruptures. This technique is satisfying when applied to patients with high surgical risk whose life expectancy is often limited. Yet its application to patients in good condition poses the problem of their definitive recovery. To date there is no means of ensuring that there will be no secondary flow in the aneurysm. As a matter of fact, the mechanisms underlying late recirculations are multiple and complex, and often unexplained.

The following principles should be emphasized:

- It is not possible to affirm that an aneurysm has been definitely cured by endoluminal stent–grafting. Its corollary is therefore that regular surveillance using CT scan or ultrasound is required.
- The schedule of control visits is determined by the initial result and the evolution.
- Unstable aneurysms that increase in volume must be reoperated on as soon as possible, either by endovascular or surgical technique, regardless of whether there is an endoleak and no matter what its type.
- Stable aneurysms presenting a noticeable type I endoleak must also be corrected rapidly.
- Stable abdominal aortic aneurysms presenting a type II endoleak must be watched very closely by ultrasound or CT scan at 6-month intervals. Search for an associated type I endoleak must be done systematically at every control. A type II endoleak does not preclude the possibility of an undiagnosed type I endoleak.
- Excluded and stable aneurysms without evident type I or II endoleaks must be monitored by CT scan once per year.
- Spontaneous disappearance of a type I endoleak is not proof of complete exclusion of the aneurysm from endotension.
- Any new thoracic event occurring in a patient carrying an endoluminal stent–graft for aneurysm must be documented by a new aortic CT scan.

Personal experience

In 1996, we had an experience with home-made devices, which proved unsatisfactory and was abandoned. Then from October 1999 to February 2003, 38 patients had endoluminal treatment of the descending thoracic aorta using industrial stent–grafts. The average age was 70 years old (35-88) and the male/female ratio was 5:3. Thirty-three patients were suffering from thoracic aortic aneurysms or chronic thoracic aortic dissection, of which one emergency case of aorto–pulmonary fistula with hemoptysis, and one patient with ruptured TAA who died intra-operatively. Three patients presented with associated abdominal aortic aneurysm, of which one was surgically repaired and the other ones with stent–grafting technique. Nine patients (9/33 = 27%) required adjunctive procedures for proximal or distal neck management: 3 complete transpositions of the supra-aortic vessels, 1 transposition of the left SCA + CCA, 2 isolated transpositions of the sub-clavian artery, 1 over-stenting of the celiac artery and 1 surgical management of the celiac aorta. One patient required aortic valve repair + replacement of the ascending aorta + total transposition of the supra-aortic vessels. WL. Gore endoprostheses were used in 11 patients, Talent endoprostheses were used in 21 patients. The number of stent–graft segments per patient varied between 1 to 6 (Figure 41.12).

For elective stent–grafting of 32 TAA, 2 patients (6.2%) died at 2 and 3 days, one from aneurysm rupture due to partial covering, and the other from coagulation problems after rupture of the iliac artery during stent placement. The in-hospital death rate was 3/33 = 9%. One patient (3.1%) had a stroke after 4 days, which partially resolved (non-disabling stroke). Two patients died within 6 months after procedure of respiratory insufficiency and cardiac infarction respectively. There were no other complications, in particular no case of paraplegia. All patients were controlled before discharge by 3-D CT scan and x-rays. All aneurysmal sacs were successfully excluded, without endoleak. During the follow-up period (mean: 2 years; 1-40 months) one patient had a fatal major stroke at 15 months post-procedure. Late death rate is 3/30 = 10%. Follow-up controls by CT scan and x-rays were performed at 6 and 12 months post-procedure and then yearly. They confirmed the exclusion of the aneurysms (Figure 41.13) without late endoleaks or stent migration.

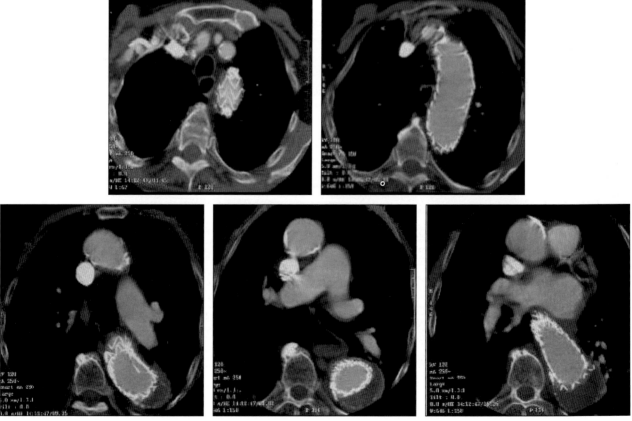

Figure 44.12
Extensive thoracic aneurysm treated by four endoluminal grafts (Excluder).

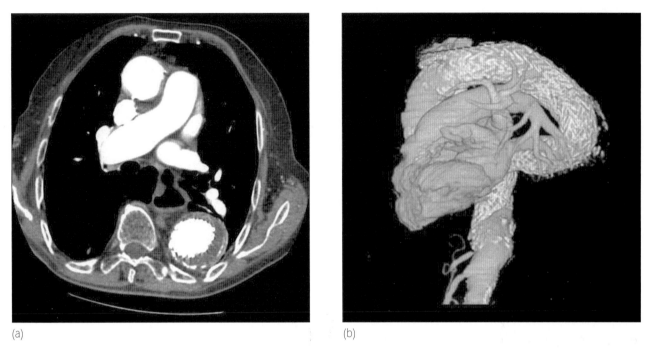

(a)   (b)

Figure 44.13
Endovascular exclusion of an extended thoracic aortic aneurysm at 3 years of follow-up. (Same patient as in Figure 41.12.)

Table 44.1	Results from the literature for thoracic aortic aneurysms only					
First author Senior author (Year, ref)	Nb thoracic aortic stent–grafting	Nb TAA	Early mortality (%)	Conversion (%)	Paraplegia (%)	Long-term survival (%)
Mitchell R. Dake M. 1999[34]	103	103	9 (30 days)	4.8	2.9	73±5 (actuarial 2yrs)
Greenberg R. 2000[35]	25	25	20 (30 days)	12	12	NA
Buffolo E. 2002[36]	191	61	10.4 (in-hospital)	9.8	0	87.4±29 (actuarial)
Criado F. 2002[37]	47	31	2.1 (30 days)	0	0	87.2 mean FU : 18mths
Heijmen R. Moll F. 2002[38]	28	28	0 (in-hospital)	3.6	0	36.4 mean FU : 21mths
Herold U. 2002[39]	34	7	2.9 (in-hospital)	0	0	91.2 mean FU : 8mths
Najibi S. Lumsden A. 2002[40]	19	19	5.3 (in-hospital)	5.3	0	94.7 12 M
Orend K. Sunder-Plassmann L. 2003[41]	74	40	9.5 (30 days)	8	0	91.7 mean FU : 22mths
Bergeron P. 2003[42]	38	33	6.2 (in-hospital)	0	0	75.8 mean FU : 24mths

Table 44.2   Results from the literature for combined thoracic aortic aneurysms and dissections

Author (Year, ref)	Nb TAA	Nb TAD	Total	Mortality (%)	Paraplegia (%)	Technical success (%)
Shimono 1999[43]	10	18	28	7.1	0	93
Won 2001[44]	11	12	23	0	0	91
Bortone 2001[45]	11	5	16	6.2	0	100
Totaro 2002[46]	7	25	32	0	0	97
Guo 2002[47]	6	6	12	0	0	75
Brunkwall 2003[48]	36	6	42	2.4	4.8	92

Results from the literature

We have summarized the results from the literature in Tables 44.1 and 44.2, although this is in no way an exhaustive overview. The results are difficult to analyze because aortic dissections and aneurysms are often mixed. Only a few are comparative studies between endovascular therapy, medication, or surgery. We lack long-term results. Comparative prospective studies are expected to provide more formal proof.

Conclusion

Endovascular treatment of thoracic aortic aneurysms and dissections is clearly an important breakthrough in the management of this serious pathology. It is largely justified to continue investigating this domain since the surgical alternative is very difficult. Mid-term results are extremely encouraging and authorize implantation in high-risk patients with limited life expectancy. Scientific literature providing long-term results is insufficient, and therefore the technique should not be applied to patients in good general condition who are able to handle a planned conventional intervention. Acute type B dissections may benefit from covering the aortic tear with a stent–graft. This must be randomized with medical therapy before wide application can be considered.

References

1   Bickerstaff K, Pairdero PC, Hollier LH et al. Thoracic aortic aneurysms: a population based study. *Surgery* 1982; **92**: 1103–8.

2   Clous WD, Hallet JW Jr, Scaff HV et al. Improved prognosis of thoracic aortic aneurysms. *JAMA* 1998; **280**: 1926–9.

3   Pressler V, McNamara JJ. Thoracic aortic aneurysms: natural history and treatment. *J Thorac Cardiovasc Surg* 1980; **79**: 489–98.

4   Hirst AE, Gore I. The etiology and pathology of aortic dissection. In: Doroghazi RM, Slater ES (eds), *Aortic dissection*. New York: McGraw-Hill, 1983: 13–53.

5   Asfoura JY, Vigt DG. Acute aortic dissection. *Chest* 1991; **99**: 724–9.

6   Gundry SR, Burney RE, Mackenzie JR et al. Traumatic pseudo-aneurysms of the thoracic aorta: anatomic and radiologic correlations. *Arch Surg* 1984; **119**: 1055–60.

7   Parmley LF, Mattingly TX, Manion WC, Jahnke EJ. Non penetrating traumatic injury of the aorta. *Circulation* 1958; **17**: 1086–101.

8   Vlahakes GJ, Warren RL. Traumatic rupture of the aorta. *New Engl J Med* 1995; **332**: 389–90.

9   Duhaylongsod FG, Glower DD, Wolfe WG. Acute traumatic aortic aneurysm: the Duke experience from 1970–1990. *J Vasc Surg* 1992; **15**: 331–43.

10   Mohr R, Adar R, Rubinstein Z. Multiple aortic aneurysms in Marfan's syndrome: case report and review of literature. *J Cardiovasc Surg* 1984; **25**: 566–70.

11   Larbre F, Loire R, Guibaud P et al. Observation clinique et anatomique d'un anévrisme de l'aorte au cours d'une sclérose tubéreuse de Bourneville. *Arch Fr Pédiatr* 1971; **28**: 975–84.

12   Edwards JE. Aneurysm of the thoracic aorta complicating coarctation. *Circulation* 1973; **48**: 195–201.

13   Toure MK, Pasquier G, Herreman F et al. Anévrismes au cours de la maladie de Takayasu. *Arch Mal Cœur* 1982; **75**: 695–700.

14   Hills EA. Behçet's syndrome with aortic aneurysms. *Br Med J* 1967; **53**: 572–7.

15   Parkhurst GF, Decker JP. Bacterial aortitis and mycotic aneurysm of the aorta. *J Pathol* 1955; **31**: 831–5.

16   Perko MJ, Norgaard M, Herzog TM et al. Unoperated aortic aneurysm: a survey of 170 patients. *Ann Thorac Surg* 1995; **59**: 1204–9.

17 Coady MA, Rizzo JA, Hammond GL et al. What is the appropriate size criterion for resection of thoracic aneurysms? *J Thoracic Cardiovasc Surg* 1997; **113**: 476–91.

18 Cartier R, Orszulak TA, Pairolero PC et al. Circulatory support during crossclamping of the descending thoracic aorta. *J Thoracic Cardiovasc Surg* 1990; **99**: 1038–47.

19 Svensson LG, Crawford ES, Hess KR et al. Variables predictive of outcome in 832 patients undergoing repairs of the descending thoracic aorta. *Chest* 1993; **104**: 1248–53.

20 Borst HG, Jurmann M, Bühner B et al. Risk of replacement of descending aorta with a standardized left heart bypass technique. *J Thoracic Cardiovasc Surg* 1994; **107**: 126–33.

21 Lawrie GM, Earle N, Debakey ME et al. Evolution of surgical techniques for aneurysms of the descending thoracic aorta: twenty-nine years experience with 659 patients. *J Card Surg* 1994; **9**: 648–61.

22 Verdant A, Cossette R, Pagé A et al. Aneurysms of descending thoracic aorta: three hundred sixty-six consecutive cases resected without paraplegia. *J Vasc Surg* 1995; **21**: 385–91.

23 Coselli JS, Konstadinos AP, La Francesca S, Cohen S. Results of contemporary surgical treatment of descending thoracic aortic aneurysms: experience with 198 patients. *Ann Vasc Surg* 1996; **10**: 131–7.

24 Hayashi J, Eguchi S, Yasuda K et al. Operation for non dissecting aneurysm in the descending thoracic aorta. *Ann Thorac Surg* 1997; **63**: 93–7.

25 Mercier F, Fabiani JN. Chirurgie des anévrismes de l'aorte thoracique descendante: traitement chirurgical moderne et résultats. *J Thoracic Cardiovasc Surg* 1998; **39**(Suppl 1): 11–14.

26 Biglioli P, Spirito R, Porqueddu M et al. Quick, simple clamping technique in descending thoracic aneurysm repair. *Ann Thorac Surg* 1999; **67**: 1038–44.

27 Safi HJ, Winnerkvist A, Miller CC et al. Effect of extended cross-clamp time during thoraco-abdominal aortic aneurysm repair. *Ann Thorac Surg* 1998; **66**: 1204–9.

28 Galloway AC, Schwartz DS, Culliford AT et al. Selective approach to descending thoracic aortic aneurysm repair: a ten-year experience. *Ann Thorac Surg* 1996; **62**: 1152–7.

29 Volodos NL, Karpovich IP, Troyan VI et al. Clinical experience of the use of self-fixing synthetic prostheses for remote endoprosthetics of the thoracic and abdominal aorta and iliac arteries through the femoral artery and as intraoperative endoprosthesis for aorta reconstruction. *Vasa* 1991; **33**(Suppl): 93–5.

30 Balm R, Reekers JA, Jacobs MJHM. Classification des procédures endovasculaires dans le traitement des anévrysmes de l'aorte thoracique. In: Branchereau A, Jacobs M (eds), *Traitement chirurgical et endovasculaire des anévrysmes aortiques*. Futura, Armonk, NY, 2000, 19–26.

31 Dake MD, Miller DC, Semba CP et al. Transluminal placement of endovascular stent–grafts for the treatment of descending thoracic aortic aneurysms. *N Engl J Med* 1994; **331**: 1729–34.

32 Dorros G. Adenosine-induced transient cardiac asystole enhances precise deployment of stent–grafts in the thoracic or abdominal aorta. *J Endovasc Surg* 1996; **3**: 270–2.

33 May J. Common carotid artery access for aortic endografting. When and how should it be done? *Abstract book 27th Global Veith Symposium*, New York, 2000.

34 Mitchell RS, Miller DC, Dake MD et al. Thoracic aortic aneurysm repair with an endovascular stent graft: the 'first generation'. *Ann Thorac Surg* 1999; **67**:1971–4;discussion, 1979–80.

35 Greenberg R, Resch T, Nyman U et al. Endovascular repair of descending thoracic aortic aneurysms: an early experience with intermediate-term follow-up. *J Vasc Surg* 2000; **31**: 147–56.

36 Buffolo E, da Fonseca JH, de Souza JA, Alves CM. Revolutionary treatment of aneurysms and dissections of descending aorta: the endovascular approach. *Ann Thorac Surg* 2002; **74**: S1815–7;discussion S1825–32.

37 Criado FJ, Clark NS, Banatan MF. Stent graft repair in the aortic arch and descending thoracic aorta: a 4-year experience. *J Vasc Surg* 2002; **36**: 1121–8.

38 Heijmen RH, Deblier IG, Moll FL et al. Endovascular stent–grafting for descending thoracic aortic aneurysms. *Eur J Cardiothorac Surg* 2002; **21**: 5–9.

39 Herold U, Piotrowski J, Baumgart D et al. Endolumial stent graft repair for acute and chronic type B aortic dissection and atherosclerotic aneurysm of the thoracic aorta: an interdisciplinary task. *Eur J Cardiothorac Surg* 2002; **22**: 891–7.

40 Najibi S, Terramani TT, Weiss VJ et al. Endoluminal versus open treatment of descending thoracic aortic aneurysms. *J Vasc Surg* 2002; **36**: 732–7.

41 Orend KH, Scharrer-Pamler R, Kapfer X et al. Endovascular treatment in diseases of the descending thoracic aorta: 6-year results of a single center. *J Vasc Surg* 2003; **37**: 91–9.

42 Bergeron P, de Chaumaray T, Gay J, Douillez V. Endovascular treatment of thoracic aortic aneurysms. *J Cardiovasc Surg* 2003; **44**: 349–61.

43 Shimono T, Kato N, Hirano T, Takeda K, Yada I. Early and mid-term results of endovascular stent grafting for aortic aneurysms. *Nippon Geka Gakkai Zasshi* 1999; **100**: 500–5.

44 Won JY, Lee DY, Shim WH et al. Elective endovascular treatment of descending thoracic aortic aneurysms and chronic dissections with stent-grafts. *J Vasc Interv Radiol.* 2001; **12**: 575–82.

45 Bortone AS, Schena S, Mannatrizio G et al. Endovascular stent–graft treatment for diseases of the descending thoracic aorta. *Eur J Cardiothorac Surg* 2001; **20**: 514–9.

46 Totaro M, Mazzesi G, Marullo AG et al. Endoluminal stent grafting of the descending thoracic aorta. *Ital Heart J.* 2002; **3**: 366–9.

47 Guo W, Gai L, Liu X. Endovascular stent–grafting of descending thoracic aortic lesions. *Zhonghua Wai Ke Za Zhi.* 2001; **39**: 838–41.

48 Brunkwall J, Gawenda M, Südkamp M, Zähringer M. Current indication for endovascular treatment of thoracic aneurysms. *J Cardiovasc Surg* 2003; **44**: 465–70.

45

Abdominal aortic aneurysm: interventional treatment

Juan Carlos Parodi and Claudio J Schönholz

Introduction

Endoluminal treatment of aneurysms has emerged as a potential therapeutic alternative since its introduction in 1991.[1] Although initial and mid-term results of endoluminal aneurysm exclusion are very encouraging, late adverse events still represent a big limitation for the widespread use of the technique.[2–7]

To obtain information about the long-term results, we retrospectively reviewed the available data on 30 consecutive patients followed for more than 5 years after the endoluminal treatment of abdominal aortic aneurysms (AAA) using the home-made Parodi endograft (PE). In addition, prospectively gathered information on 136 consecutive patients treated using the Vanguard endograft (Boston Scientific Corp., Natick, MA) was analyzed. Only mid-term results (mean 28 months, range 7–53 months) were available for evaluation in the latter group (VE). The information served as a basis of comparison with the results of the PE group.

Material and methods

We collected information on the outcome of 30 consecutive patients whose AAA was excluded using the initial endograft design created by Parodi. All patients had at least a contrast-enhanced computed tomography (CT) scan, complete medical examination, and color duplex studies before treatment. The PE essentially consisted of a tubular or tapered fabric graft (aorto-aortic or aorto-uni-iliac configurations) attached at both ends by large Palmaz stents (Figure 45.1). Also, the aorto-uni-iliac exclusion was completed by performing a femorofemoral bypass and occluding the contralateral common iliac artery with a stent plug, as described in detail previously.[8] Mean follow-up in this

group of patients was 59 months (range 32–119 months). All patients were males; the average age was 71.3 years. The average size of the AAA was 59 mm in diameter at the time of treatment. All patients had at least one CT scan with contrast enhancement after the fifth year of the procedure.

One hundred and thirty-six patients were treated using the Vanguard device in its three versions (I, II, and III). Of these patients, 100 consecutive patients with a complete follow-up were included in this study. The Vanguard endograft was a thin-walled Dacron (polyethylene terephthalate) graft fully supported over its entire length by a diamond-shaped nitinol stent, which provides radial and longitudinal force to maintain its conformability. The final length of the endograft can be tailored, adding or omitting extensions. Mean follow-up was 28 months (range 7–53 months). Eighty seven percent of the patients were males, the age average was 70.4 years, and the average size of the AAA was 56 mm. Patients were followed every 6 months with clinical examination, plain X-ray of the abdomen, color duplex, and contrast-enhanced CT. Additional conventional 5-mm thick sections through the device were obtained with a 3-min delay to detect endoleaks.

Results

Parodi endograft (PE)

Of 103 patients treated from September 1990 to March 1996 in our institution, 51 patients underwent aortic tube graft replacement, with eight patients having only one proximal stent, and 45 aorto-iliac stent grafting. However, the following description refers to the results after 5 years of implantation. Patients with acute and mid-term failures were not included. This limitation produced a case selection. Only the survivors are analyzed; even patients whose cause of

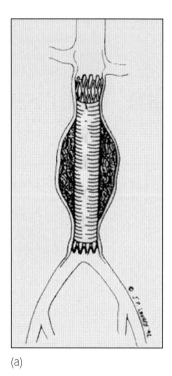

Figure 45.1
(a) Aorto-aortic stent graft. (b) Aorto-uni-iliac configuration. The procedure is completed by performing a femorofemoral bypass. The contralateral common iliac artery is occluded by a covered stent.

(a)

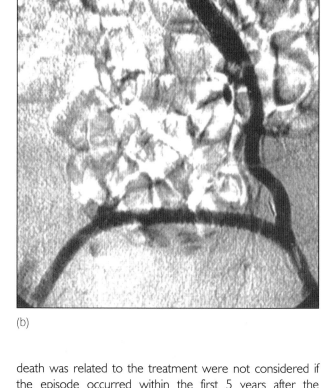

(b)

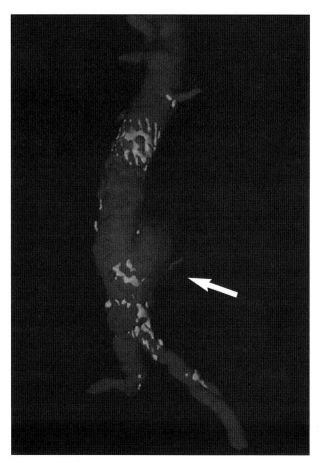

Figure 45.2
CT (computed tomography) reconstruction of a type I distal endoleak (arrow).

death was related to the treatment were not considered if the episode occurred within the first 5 years after the treatment. The aorto-aortic endograft design failed in 12 patients out of 15 (80% failure rate). All failures were due to the development of a distal endoleak (Figure 45.2). The aneurysm increased in size in eight patients (43.7 ± 6.3 mm vs 52.8 ± 11.9 mm, $p = 0.08$); the aneurysm sac remained the same size in three and decreased in another four patients (44.3 ± 8.6 mm vs 36.7 ± 6.1 mm, $p = 0.2$). Two patients with aneurysm shrinkage presented distal endoleaks, whereas three patients (20%) had a successful durable exclusion: the size of the aneurysm decreased in two of them and the other patient did not register any diameter change. The aorto-aortic design was abandoned in 1994.

The aorto-uni-iliac design of the PE was successful in 10 out of 15 patients in the long term. The size of the aneurysm decreased in size in all 10 cases and no endoleak developed (46.6 ± 5.9 mm vs 40.3 ± 5.1 mm, $p = 0.02$). Five patients developed late endoleaks. There were type I endoleaks, one a proximal and the others distal (iliac) endoleaks, and two patients had persistent type II endoleaks. All five patients with endoleaks had their aneurysms enlarged (70.6 ± 12.3 mm vs. 80.2 ± 14.3 mm).

Careful measurement of the proximal neck indicated that neck dilatation did not take place using the PE, regardless of the final outcome. In the 15 patients who had the aorto-aortic design, excluding their aneurysm, the initial neck diameter was 23.9 ± 2.4 mm and after 78 months 24.2 ± 2.9 mm ($p = 0.7$). In the aorto-uni-iliac design, the initial neck diameter was 25.3 ± 2.2 mm and after 78 months was 25.7 ± 2.6 mm ($p = 0.6$).

Vanguard endograft

Twenty two percent of the 100 patients developed adverse events during a mean follow-up of 28 months. No proximal or distal type I endoleaks were registered. Four of the five causes of failures were device-related. The only non-device-related failure was the development of a type II endoleak (25p.) that caused enlargement of the aneurysm in five patients (5%) and infection of the endograft (2%). Device related failures were:

- occlusion of one limb   8%
- dislocation of segments   3%
- wearing of the graft   3%
- fracture + migration   3%.

The three aneurysm ruptures were related to the development of acute type III endoleaks: one of the patients suffered a dislocation of segments and in the other two patients wearing of the graft ended in aneurysm rupture. Infection occurred in two patients, the first after 2 years of implantation related to a surgical drainage of a kidney abscess. The second patient had an inflammatory aneurysm. Six months after a successful exclusion, the patient developed an abscess involving the right psoas muscle. The endograft was removed. The proximal and distal necks were suture ligated and an axillobifemoral bypass was constructed. *Streptococcus bovis* was isolated from the surgical samples. The patient is still alive 10 months after the endograft explantation.

The aneurysm increased in size in 13 patients (3.9 ± 1.9 mm). In all of them, an endoleak was detected. The aneurysm sac remained the same size in 14 patients and decreased in another 73 patients (6.97 ± 5.94 mm.). Eleven patients with aneurysm shrinkage presented a type II endoleak (6.33 ± 4.5 mm).

Fifty-three patients were evaluated with plain abdominal radiographs: thirteen endografts demonstrated increased distance between stents struts, indicating broken sutures. In six patients we found broken sutures, leading to separation of the first two rows of nitinol. In three patients significant separation occurred between the first two rows of nitinol and the rest of the device. The distal segment migrated caudally, resulting in a type III endoleak.

Discussion

Interesting data emerged from the present study that deserves comment and elaboration. Several findings will be discussed.

Neck dilatation

Neck dilatation is the main concern of several investigators in the field.[9,10] No neck dilatation was found in the initial group of patients (PE). Only one case (3.33%) of proximal endoleak resulted in the long term, in a patient in whom the proximal stent was placed far from the renal arteries and in contact with the mural thrombus. Lack of neck dilatation was also found by James May in a recently published study.[11–15] In two of our long-term cases, even a reduction of the diameter of the proximal neck was evident (Figure 45.3). Encapsulation of the proximal bare segment of the proximal stent was seen in the two patients in whom we performed a post-mortem examination (Figure 45.4). It seems reasonable to think that balloon expandable stents behave in a different way to self-expandable stents. Balloon expandable stents stretch the wall from the beginning but no further increase of the diameter of the stent takes place over time. By contrast, self-expandable stents continue to expand until the nominal diameter is reached unless tissue resistance limits its expansion. When the expandable force is concentrated in reduced surfaces, dilatation takes place very rapidly, producing migration of devices; an example of this was the initial experience using the Anaconda device in Europe (Benedetti Valentini, pers comm). The anchoring mechanism in the Anaconda device is a single ring with a shape that resembles the mouth of an anaconda snake. In spite of the lack of conclusive evidence, the limited data available indicate that the bare stent segment (balloon and self-expandable) when it is embedded in the vessel wall is regularly covered by a layer of myointimal hyperplasia. Stents actually become part of the architecture of the arterial wall.

The distal neck of an abdominal aortic aneurysm had a quite different behavior when an endograft was fixed to it: almost regularly, the distal neck of the aorta dilated over time. Eighty percent of the aorto-aortic endografts failed by this mechanism, resulting in distal endoleak. The difference in behavior of the proximal and distal neck is most probably due to the different composition of the wall. The proximal neck is richer in elastic fibers and seldom calcified. Mural thrombus in the proximal neck exists in a small proportion of patients and apparently does not have a significant impact in results.[16] In addition, strong inter-crossing fibers in the adventitia coming from the visceral branches give strength and stability to the proximal neck adjacent to the renal arteries' ostia.

The data mentioned above refers to cases of the PE group. Results using the Vanguard device are somewhat different but, at least in the mean term, no significant neck dilatation resulted. During the first 12 months the neck had the tendency to dilate in a very discrete manner (24.1 ± 2.9 mm vs 24.4 ± 2.9 mm); subsequently, the neck stabilized (24.2 ± 2.9 mm vs 24.3 ± 2.8 mm). The late caudal migration of the separated distal segment of the device in the VE group (three patients) was produced by fracture of the metal skeleton of the endograft. As the mean follow-up in this group is just 28 months, no further conclusions can be drawn in terms of long-term neck dilatation.

Our policy of deploying the proximal end of the endograft crossing the renal arteries' ostium or flush to them is probably

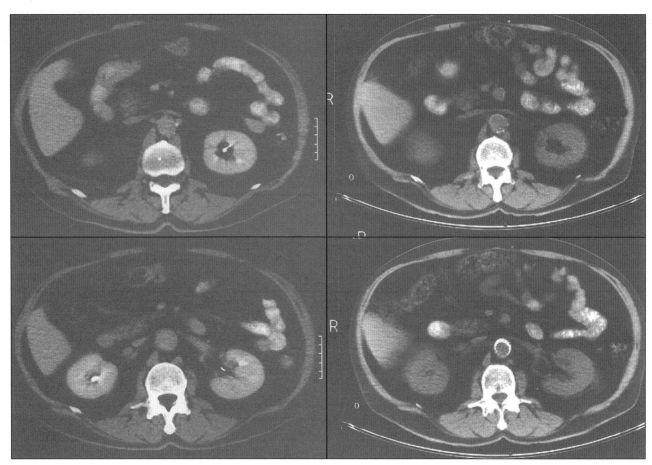

Figure 45.3
No changes in the aorta at the level of the renal arteries were registered in this patient. However, reduction of the diameter of the proximal neck was evident after 10 years.

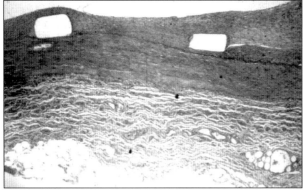

Figure 45.4
Encapsulation of the proximal bare segment of the proximal stent was seen in the two patients in whom we performed a post-mortem examination.

responsible for the secure fixation of the endograft. With regard to the iliac arteries as landing zones for endograft fixation, 13% of the PE cases showed late type I endoleak after 5 years. Those iliac arteries were dilated (more than 15 mm in diameter) before the treatment. In the two cases of

late endoleak from the iliac arteries after 5 years, only the proximal iliac artery was covered by the endograft. The region of the iliac bifurcation, which has the maximum strength, was not reached by the endografts. We adopted a policy of covering the whole common iliac artery in 1992. No other iliac dilatation was registered.

Shrinkage of aneurysms and endoleaks

Shrinkage of aneurysm was constant during follow-up when the aneurysm was effectively excluded with the PE (47 ± 5.5 mm vs 40.3 ± 4.7 mm, $p = 0.004$). The presence of type I endoleaks resulted in aneurysmal growth in two-thirds of cases (49.7 ± 13.1 mm vs 59.5 ± 17.5 mm, $p = 0.1$). Only two out of 30 patients of the PE group had persistent type II endoleaks, seen in the follow-up CT scans. These two patients suffered aneurysmal growth (78 ± 5.6 mm vs 84 ± 8.5 mm, $p = 0.4$). The fact that one-third of the patients with type I endoleaks had no aneurysmal growth is intriguing. The probable explanation for this finding is the following: small-flow type I endoleaks with an appropriate outflow (several lumbar arteries) have a low pressure inside the sac; conversely, high-flow endoleaks with no outflow result in rapid aneurysmal growth and rupture.[17–21]

There were three ruptures of the aneurysm in the Vanguard endograft group. Interestingly, those patients were free of endoleaks for more than 2 years, and the development of an acute type III endoleak resulted in aneurysmal rupture within the following 48 hours. The cause of an acute type III endoleak was a dislocation of the contralateral limb in one patient and perforation of the fabric graft in the other two patients. Those patients had no type II endoleaks and the size of the aneurysm had decreased before the late complication. Post-mortem study in one patient disclosed an atrophic wall of the remnant aneurysm. Speculation can be made in terms that if a late endoleak occurs it will find an atrophic wall to contain it. Resistance to dilatation would be decreased, as well as the strength of the wall. One could conclude that a late-onset endoleak in a free of endoleak sac represents a great risk for rupture. Thus, durable, material fatigue-free, reliable endografts are mandatory.

Type II endoleaks

Type II endoleaks were present in 6.6% of the aneurysms after 5 years in the PE group. The two cases of long-term type II endoleaks resulted in a very discrete increase in the size of the aneurysm.

In 11 of the 100 cases of VE, type II endoleaks provoked aneurysmal growth. Of those patients, five were successfully treated by embolization or clipping of the offending branches after aneurysm enlargement more than 4 mm.

Persistent type II endoleak and infection were the only causes of long-term failure that were not device-related in the Vanguard group. Long-term type II endoleaks can, in theory, induce or facilitate device failure. We demonstrated in a model that hemodynamic changes inside the aneurysmal sac in the presence of type II endoleaks could be the following. Systolic pressure is always lower inside the aneurysmal sac. In the presence of an endoleak, diastolic and mean pressure are higher inside the sac in comparison to the systemic pressure. As an explanation, we can speculate that the blind end of the aneurysm sac has an inappropriate outflow for the blood that enters the sac during systole. This explanation seems reasonable, since the diastolic and mean pressures dropped as the outflow of the aneurysm increased. These pressure changes produced extra stress on the endograft, which expanded during systole and collapsed during diastole.[22]

It is gaining general acceptance that a large inferior mesenteric artery (IMA) should be coil embolized during the initial treatment, providing that the superior mesenteric artery

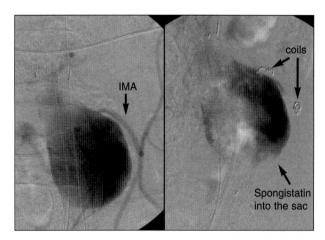

Figure 45.5
Coil embolization of the inferior mesenteric artery (IMA) and sac filling with Spongostan.

(SMA) and at least one hypogastric artery are wide open. Opinion on what to do with open lumbar arteries is divided. The most common approach is to leave them alone and treat those patients that after 6 months still have backflow from the arteries which results in aneurysmal growth. Our empiric approach is to coil embolize the IMA and fill the sac with Spongostan when the IMA and several lumbar arteries are open (Figure 45.5).[23] Long term outcome of patients treated in this way is still unknown.

Alternatives to treating type II endoleaks after 6 months when the aneurysm increases its size are laparoscopic clipping of the branches (Figure 45.6), coil embolization of the IMA through micro-catheters introduced through the SMA, and coil embolization of lumbar arteries through the iliolumbar branch. Direct puncture of the aneurysm with coil and thrombin injection is also an alternative.[24] Conversion to an open procedure is the last alternative to be considered.

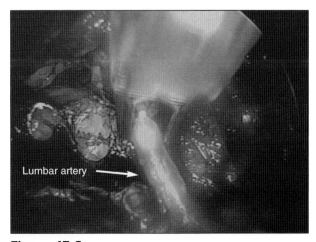

Figure 45.6
Video-assisted clipping of the collateral branches.

Occlusion of one limb of the endograft

No limb occlusion resulted in the long-term follow-up in the 15 cases of aorto-uni-iliac endografting (PE).

Occlusion of one of the limbs of the VE group occurred in eight patients, being the main cause of failure. Occlusion of the limbs in the VE group mostly occurred after 18 months of implantation. Remodeling of the aneurysm and angulation of the limbs was evident in most.

Dislocation of segments

In three cases, dislocation of segments occurred in the VE group, all after 2 years of the initial treatment. One case ended with rupture of the aneurysm. Dislocation was the result of extreme angulation of the device after remodeling.

Fracture of wires and sutures

In 24.5% of the VE cases, we visualized separation of segments or fracture of metal components. In spite of this, only three patients suffered the consequences of this loss of integrity of the endograft. Fracture and separation of the two initial rows of the endograft produced migration of the device caudally with the occurrence of an endoleak.

These findings are evidence that preclinical testing of the devices performed by the medical industry was incomplete and insufficient. The complexity and multiplicity of vectors of forces acting permanently and dynamically inside the aneurysmal sac, in addition to the foreign body reaction of the recipient of the endograft, may explain the loss of integrity of the devices.

Pulsation and external forces acting on the endograft produce complex movement of the endograft component as a whole and also motion and micro motion among components. Friction among metals removes the protective oxide layer covering the endograft, facilitating corrosion and fracture.

Wearing of the fabric graft

The most vulnerable spot in endografts is where the metal component interacts with the fabric graft. Wearing results from friction and is aggravated when a metal component protrudes, concentrating the friction to a small area of the fabric graft. Angulation and fracture of the metal skeleton further facilitate wearing of the fabric graft.

In the VE group three cases of wearing of the fabric graft were detected. Two patients suffered an aneurysm rupture.

Migration of the endograft

Migration of the endograft is a subject very often seen in the surgical literature, mostly related to neck dilatation.[25–28] There are obvious variables related to migration: radial force of the device, length of the proximal neck, angulation of the neck, area in which the proximal end is positioned (crossing the renal arteries, flush or far from them), utilization of hooks and barbs, and angulation of the endograft. Traction force from the proximal end was calculated to be about 10 newtons (1 kg).

In the PE group no migration was observed. In the VE group three endografts migrated caudally when the first two rows of the metal skeleton separated.

Summary of the analysis of long and mid-term failures in both groups

Adverse events in the Parodi endograft group (PE) were related to:

- dilatation of the distal aortic neck
- persistent type II endoleak
- late type I endoleak probably due to implantation of the endograft far from the renal artery take-off
- dilatation of a previously ectatic iliac artery.

There were no device-related failures in the long term in the PE group.

Adverse events in the VE group were mostly related to device failure: occlusion of one limb (8%), dislocation of a segment (3%), wearing of the fabric graft (3%), proximal migration (3%). Non-device-related failures were persistent type II endoleak with enlargement of the aneurysm (5%) and infection (2%).

Four of the five causes of adverse events in the Vanguard endograft group were related to device failure. Persistent type II endoleak and infection were the only non-device-related complications.

Re-design of the Vanguard device is mandatory and should take into account the lessons learned in the clinical setting.

There are potential solutions to offer to a new design of a totally supported endograft:

1. Occlusion of the limbs, the most common cause of late failure, can be solved using kink-resistant limbs (like the Wallgraft).
2. Dislocations of segments: reliable locking mechanisms can be included in the design.
3. Fractures: stronger structures resistant to fatigue and carefully tested using appropriate testing models could eventually solve the problems.

4. Wearing of the fabric graft: stronger graft and metal skeleton designed and incorporated into the system in such a way that friction with the fabric graft becomes less critical. A non-totally supported system such as the PE or the Ancure device should be considered as a valid alternative.

Conclusions

1. Aorto-aortic endografts have a high failure rate due to distal neck dilatation.
2. The aorto-uni-iliac configuration using the Parodi endograft had acceptable results in the long term. A few conditions should be fulfilled, however, to achieve good results: the proximal stent should be crossing or flush to the renal arteries ostia and the common iliac arteries should be completely covered by the endograft. As this is our current practice, it is reasonable to assume that this endograft could be extremely useful in the treatment of aneurysms. Further studies are necessary to confirm our observation.
3. Type II endoleaks produce aneurysmal growth in a small proportion of patients of both groups analyzed.
4. The totally supported Vanguard device had a high rate of failure in the mid-term: 22% of the patients needed a secondary procedure after a mean follow-up of 28 months. Four of the five causes of failures were device-related.
5. It is clear that the endoluminal treatment of aneurysms is a complex matter and further developments are needed before its widespread use is recommended.

Perspectives for the future of endoluminal treatment of aneurysms

Analysis of failures is providing valuable information, suggesting new directions or resuming old directions abandoned in the past.

Application of existing technology is still in its infancy. Application of future technology is warranted.

Going back to the initial concept when the first endograft was created is extremely useful.

The first design resembled the proven surgical aortic replacement with a fabric graft using surgical sutures. Instead of suture, a stent attached and sealed the fabric graft.

Simplifying the concept, all we have to achieve is the replacement of the surgical suture by a mechanical device as reliable, or perhaps more reliable.

Totally supported devices have several advantages over the non-supported systems but also many drawbacks.

Both ways should be explored, perhaps using them in different situations and anatomic conditions.

In the mean time, application of endografts should be limited to centers with large experience and just offering treatment to high-risk patients with a short life expectancy, harboring a large (more than 5.5 cm) or symptomatic aneurysm. Encouraging experiences treating endoluminally ruptured aneurysms are being reported and probably will represent a good indication in the future.[29,30] Aortic dissections and thoracic aneurysms are emerging as indications for endoluminal treatment, accounting for their high complication and mortality rates resulting from standard surgical treatment.

References

1. Parodi JC, Palmaz JC, Barone HD. Transfemoral intraluminal graft implantation for abdominal aortic aneurysms. *Ann Vasc Surg* 1991; **5**: 491–9.
2. Parodi JC. Endoluminal stent grafts: overview. *J Invasive Cardiol* 1997; **9**: 227–9.
3. May J, White GH, Waugh R et al. Improved survival after endoluminal repair with second-generation prostheses compared with open repair in the treatment of abdominal aortic aneurysms: a 5-year concurrent comparison using life table method. *J Vasc Surg* 2001; **33**(2 suppl): S21–6.
4. Greenberg RK, Lawrence-Brown M, Bhandari G et al. An update of the Zenith endovascular graft for abdominal aortic aneurysms: initial implantation and mid-term follow-up data. *J Vasc Surg* 2001; **33**(2 suppl): S157–64.
5. White RA. Clinical and design update on the development and testing of a one-piece, bifurcated, polytetra-fluoroethylene endovascular graft for abdominal aortic aneurysm exclusion: the Endologix device. *J Vasc Surg* 2001; **33**(2 suppl): S154–6.
6. Matsumura JS, Katzen BT, Hollier LH, Dake MD. Update on the bifurcated EXCLUDER endoprosthesis: phase I results. *J Vasc Surg* 2001; **33**(2 suppl): S150–3.
7. Zarins CK, White RA, Moll FL et al. The AneuRx stent graft: four-year results and worldwide experience 2000. *J Vasc Surg* 2001; **33**(2 suppl): S135–45. [Review]
8. Parodi JC, Criado FJ, Barone HD, Schonholz C, Queral LA. Endoluminal aortic aneurysm repair using a balloon-expandable stent–graft device: a progress report. *Ann Vasc Surg* 1994; **8**: 523–9.
9. May J. Symposium on distortion and structural deterioration of endovascular grafts used to repair abdominal aortic aneurysms. Introduction. *J Endovasc Surg* 1999; **6**: 1–3.
10. Harris P, Brennan J, Martin et al. Longitudinal aneurysm shrinkage following endovascular aortic aneurysm repair: a source of intermediate and late complications. *J Endovasc Surg* 1999; **6**: 11–16.
11. Chaikof EL, Matsumura JS. Endovascular repair of abdominal aortic aneurysms: problems and progress. *Semin Vasc Surg* 1999; **12**: 163–4.
12. Albertini J, Kalliafas S, Travis S et al. Anatomical risk factors for proximal perigraft endoleak and graft migration following endovascular repair of abdominal aortic aneurysms. *Eur J Vasc Endovasc Surg* 2000; **19**: 308–12.

13   Walker SR, Macierewicz J, Elmarasy NM, Gregson RH, Whitaker SC, Hopkinson BR. A prospective study to assess changes in proximal aortic neck dimensions after endovascular repair of abdominal aortic aneurysms. *J Vasc Surg* 1999; **29**: 625–30.

14   Sonesson B, Malina M, Ivancev K, Lindh M, Lindblad B, Brunkwall J. Dilatation of the infrarenal aneurysm neck after endovascular exclusion of abdominal aortic aneurysm. *J Endovasc Surg* 1998; **5**: 195–200.

15   May J. The outcome of endoluminal repair of AAA with short proximal necks. *Cardiovasc Surg* 2000; **8**: 329–30.

16   Gitlitz DB, Ramaswami G, Kaplan D, Hollier LH, Marin ML. Endovascular stent grafting in the presence of aortic neck filling defects: early clinical experience. *J Vasc Surg* 2001; **33**: 340–4.

17   May J, White GH, Waugh R et al. Rupture of abdominal aortic aneurysms: a concurrent comparison of outcome of those occurring after endoluminal repair versus those occurring de novo. *Eur J Vasc Endovasc Surg* 1999; **18**: 344–8.

18   White RA, Donayre C, Wallot I et al. Abdominal aortic aneurysm rupture following endoluminal graft deployment. *J Endovasc Ther* 2000; **7**: 257–62.

19   Lumsden AB, Allen RC, Chaikot EL et al. Delayed rupture of aortic aneurysms following endovascular stent grafting. *Am J Surg* 1995; **170**: 174–8.

20   Torsello GB, Klenk E, Kasprzak B et al. Rupture of abdominal aortic aneurysm previously treated by endograft stent–graft. *J Vasc Surg* 1998; **28**: 184–7.

21   Umscheid T, Stelter WJ. Time-related alterations in shape, position, and structure of self-expanding, modular aortic stent–grafts: a 4-year single-center follow-up. *J Endovasc Surg* 1999; **6**: 17–32.

22   Parodi JC, Berguer R, Ferreira LM, La Mura R, Schermerhorn ML. Intra-aneurysmal pressure after incomplete endovascular exclusion. *J Vasc Surg* 2001; **34**: 909–14.

23   Lehmann JM, Macierewicz JA, Davidson IR, Whitaker SC, Wenham PW, Hopkinson BR. Prevention of side branch endoleaks with thrombogenic sponge: one-year follow-up. *J Endovasc Ther* 2000; **7**: 431–3.

24   van den Berg JC, Nolthenius RP, Casparie JW, Moll FL. CT-guided thrombin injection into aneurysm sac in a patient with endoleak after endovascular abdominal aortic aneurysm repair. *AJR Am J Roentgenol* 2000; **175**: 1649–51.

25   Makaroun MS, Deaton DH. Is proximal aortic neck dilatation after endovascular aneurysm exclusion a cause for concern? *J Vasc Surg* 2001; **33**(2 suppl): S39–45.

26   Albertini J, Kalliafas S, Travis S et al. Anatomical risk factors for proximal perigraft endoleak and graft migration following endovascular repair of abdominal aortic aneurysms. *Eur J Vasc Endovasc Surg* 2000; **19**: 308–12.

27   Harris PL, Vallabhaneni SR, Desgranges P, Becquemin JP, van Marrewijk C, Laheij RJ. Incidence and risk factors of late rupture, conversion, and death after endovascular repair of infrarenal aortic aneurysms: the EUROSTAR experience. European Collaborators on stent/graft techniques for aortic aneurysm repair. *J Vasc Surg* 2000; **32**: 739–49.

28   Broeders IA, Blankensteijn JD, Wever JJ, Eikelboom BC. Mid-term fixation stability of the EndoVascular Technologies endograft. EVT Investigators. *Eur J Vasc Endovasc Surg* 1999; **18**: 300–7.

29   Ohki T, Veith FJ. Patient selection for endovascular repair of abdominal aortic aneurysms: changing the threshold for intervention. *Semin Vasc Surg* 1999; **12**:226–34.

30   Armon MP, Wenham PW, Hopkinson BR. Suitability for endovascular aneurysm repair in an unselected population (*Br J Surg* 2001; **88**: 77–81). *Br J Surg* 2001; **88**: 889–90.

46

Complications of interventional treatment of aortic aneurysms

Luigi Inglese and Emilio Calabrese

Endovascular exclusion of an aortic aneurysm through EVG (endovascular graft) insertion is a demanding and complex procedure. One may expect complications to occur both early (Table 46.1) and late (Table 46.2).

Early complications

Early complications occur immediately, or within the first 30 days. The most common are primary endoleaks, thrombosis, fever, and inappropriate positioning of the EVG. Problems may arise due to access complications, poor patient selection, or inappropriate technique.

Access complications

The common femoral artery (CFA) is the usual access for insertion of EVG. A transverse incision is made proximal to the takeoff of the profunda to utilize an artery of suitable dimensions and to avoid tackling with the area of bifurcation where hard calcific plaques may sometimes be found. The EVG should be inserted gently, avoiding going subintimal.

Damage to the intima is most often produced when small diameter vessels are entered. Careful arterial repair should be undertaken at the end of the procedure with interrupted 6/0 Prolene sutures and, only if unavoidable, with the application of a patch. The environment where EVG insertion is performed may have inferior sterility standards when compared to an operating room and synthetic materials should be avoided in the groin, where the infection rate is the highest. Hematoma, lymphocele, and wound dehiscence promote infection and they are best prevented with impeccable surgical technique.

Table 46.1 Early complications after endovascular graft for abdominal aortic aneurysm

Endoleak (primary)
Graft thrombosis
Fever and post-implantation syndrome
Failed graft delivery
Malpositioning of graft
Femoral artery damage
Lymphocele
Hematoma
Wound dehiscence
Iliac artery damage
Renal artery occlusion or embolization
Renal failure
Hemorrhage
Embolism
Cardiac event
Anesthesia-related problems
Intestinal ischemia

Table 46.2 Late complications after endovascular graft for abdominal aortic aneurysm

Endoleak (secondary)
Thrombus apposition into the graft
Displacement of EVG
Graft failure
Progression of native aneurysm
Rupture of aneurysm
Stenosis distal to the graft
Infection
Buttock claudication
Erosion through aortic wall
Aortoenteric fistula

Distal intimal tears should be fixed with U-type 7/0 sutures inserted from inside out to fix any flap prior to closure of the arterial incision.

During isolation of the profunda femuris, one must be careful not to injure the vessel posteriorly or to damage other smaller branches, because severe bleeding may ensue.

Small femoral arteries should not be utilized for insertion of EVG, especially for those grafts that have larger French sizing. In cases where the CFA is of inadequate diameter, a retroperitoneal suprainguinal incision should be made to access the external iliac artery.

Effective anesthesia is essential during passage of the prosthesis, to limit the possibility of pain and arterial spasm.

When a 'trolley-cab' technique is performed through the radial or brachial artery in difficult cases, one must avoid pulling too hard on the guide going from the arm to the groin, in order to prevent damage to the inferior part of the subclavian artery. To limit this risk, the guide should always be surrounded by a guiding catheter, which will reduce the shear and tear on the vessel wall at the critical takeoff point of the subclavian artery.

The axillary artery just below the clavicle could also be an alternate access site for EVG insertion. This vessel has suitable dimensions but it is extremely fragile and difficult to repair.

Anesthesia

Under epidural or spinal anesthesia, sudden initial hypotension may occur because many patients are kept NPO (nothing by mouth) for several hours while waiting their turn. Most patients should be started on intravenous fluid administration whenever they are kept NPO for over 6 hours and they should be given a fluid load prior to anesthesia. Epidural anesthesia is more technically demanding than spinal anesthesia, and the operator must be careful not to puncture the dura. Should this happen, then spinal fluid leak will be best treated with bed rest, hydration, or a 'blood patch' technique if indicated.

Venous bleeding in the epidural space is a possibility, aggravated by antiplatelet medications and heparin. Significant bleeding in the epidural space may produce thecal compression and neural damage. Laminectomy as a decompression procedure may be required to address the problem because neurological damage follows delay in treatment.

Renal complications

Several patients are selected for EVG insertion because their renal failure makes them poor candidates for standard bypass surgery. The administration of large quantities of iodinated contrast medium may aggravate their problem. In addition, cholesterol emboli and plaque disruption during the procedure may produce further damage. Limiting the amount and concentration of the contrast media used during the procedure helps reduce adverse effects due to toxicity and overload. The use of carbon dioxide as contrast medium is being recommended to entirely avoid renal damage from contrast agents. CO_2 has several advantages, such as administering several repeated injections with no risk of tubular damage, or insufflating through an introducer in the femoral artery without the need to pass a pig-tail into the aorta. The gaseous contrast will rise, reaching the abdominal aorta and will clear up rapidly through the lungs. Disadvantages derive from occasional poor visualization and from the fact that substantial experience is needed to obtain good images. A high-quality, high-speed and high KV angiographic DSA suite is needed to obtain good CO_2 imaging.

The risk of cholesterol emboli is best reduced by careful manipulation of the catheter and the graft in the suprarenal area. Postoperative surveillance to detect progressive rises in serum potassium and serum creatinine levels will help address the problem with temporary dialysis if needed.

Plaque dislodgement may sometimes be resolved with immediate selective renal artery catheterization and stent-supported angioplasty.

A too highly placed graft may partially or totally cover one or both the renal arteries. This severe complication may require immediate surgery. Endovascular catheter-guided perforation and cross-renal ballooning of the graft may be considered as an emergency procedure to achieve immediate perfusion of the occluded renal artery, but there are risks of further damage in performing this procedure.

When the bare struts of the proximal end of the EVG cross the renal arteries, a procedure employed in repairing short neck aneurysm, the renal flow is not usually reduced, but thrombosis may sporadically occur and requires immediate intervention.

Failed EVG delivery

Tortuous iliac arteries may hamper the safe passage of the graft, and several tips and tricks may be needed. Very stiff guides will straighten most iliac arteries and facilitate the passage. In other cases, a 'trolley car' technique, with a long 300-cm guide running from the arm to the groin, being pulled on to straighten the vessel, will address the problem. Sometimes, a direct axillary approach or retroperitoneal suprainguinal incision to access the external iliac artery may be needed. Choosing an appropriate device may simplify the delivery, as more pliable insertion systems could facilitate the passage through tortuous vessels.

Faulty positioning of the EVG

Delivery above the renal arteries is a serious complication to be avoided by repeated angiographic controls with a sentinel catheter, before completing the proximal opening of the prosthesis. A graft inserted too far below the renal arteries may expand against a dilated segment of the abdominal aorta, masked as normal because of an inner thrombus ring. In this situation the graft does not achieve an effective seal and may migrate or produce a massive endoleak. Attempting to position the graft just below the renal artery is desirable in most cases.

After the initial delivery is completed, the proximal part of the EVG should be gently dilated with a highly compliant balloon, to ensure proper adhesion to the aortic and iliac walls. The first dilatation must be performed with the balloon bridging between the proximal end of the EVG and the distal part of the aorta overlapping the renal ostia. If the balloon instead is inflated first against the middle section of the prosthesis, the prosthesis may be dislodged and be pulled back from the aneurysmal neck. Even after proper initial dilatation at the neck, all other ballooning of the graft must be done gently to avoid dislodging the prosthesis.

At the bifurcation of the prosthesis and along the iliac arteries, gentle inflation of the balloon under strict fluoroscopic control is essential to avoid damage to the struts and rupture of the iliac artery. Problems may be caused by aortic bifurcations where the two iliac arteries arise at a very wide angle. In these cases, the distal branches of most endoprostheses may kink. Inserting the prosthesis with an inverted leg position gives a better pattern to the limbs of the EVG and achieves advantageous hemodynamics. Nevertheless, wide iliac artery bifurcation angles remain a relative contraindication to EVG aortoiliac procedures.

Endoleaks

Resolution of the aneurysmal problem depends largely of the elimination of blood flow within the aneurysmal sac, obtained by perfect sealing of the proximal and distal necks and curtailing of the branch flow to the excluded sac. Endoleaks represent persistent residual flow into the aneurysmal sac: they are signs of imperfectly performed procedures and should never be underestimated.

Endoleaks are defined as primary if they occur immediately or within the first 30 days and as secondary if they occur subsequently.

Primary endoleak

Their incidence varies between 0% and 40% in the literature and it seems that some of them might regress spontaneously.

Type I: leak at the proximal or distal attachment point. The most frequent leak, the type I leak is due to a failure of the graft in sealing the proximal aortic rim or the distal iliac rim. Causes include a short aortic neck, inappropriate positioning of a graft, wrong measurement of the aortic neck or iliac artery diameter, or a kinked aorta.

Valuable techniques in preventing type I leaks are excluding patients without appropriate neck anatomy; using devices whose bare struts bridge the renal arteries when tackling short aortic necks; oversizing liberally (over 20%) the diameter of the prosthesis; measuring aortic and iliac artery diameters on a properly performed helical computed tomography (CT) scan; double checking repeatedly graft positioning before delivery.

Treatment of a recognized type I leak entails gentle ballooning of the proximal end of the prosthesis, adding a second cuff at the aortic neck proximally when possible, and adding an additional limb to prolong the distal graft if the leak is at the iliac end.

If the iliac artery is severely oversized, one may apply, through an extraperitoneal supra-inguinal incision, a tape surrounding the iliac artery, to reduce the diameter of the vessel and seal it around the endograft: this is a controversial procedure.

One should always refer all type I endoleaks to surgery if attempts at an endovascular solution fail.

Type II: leak due to sustained flow from branch vessels. A type II leak is due to back-filling of the aneurysm from one or more lumbar arteries and/or from the inferior mesenteric artery through collaterals coming from the superior mesenteric artery. It is caused by a large patent IMA or by lumbar vessels draining into the aneurysm sac, or by a failed embolization of the internal iliac artery when an iliac aneurysm is covered by the EVG.

Prevention requires selective catheterization and coil embolization of large branches prior to endograft insertion. The proximal IMA or any prominent lumbar artery should be embolized with coils. The hypogastric artery should also be embolized if it is to be covered with the endograft, or it can be reimplanted more distally onto the external iliac artery.

Treatment of type II leaks can be cumbersome, requiring laparoscopic clipping of the inferior mesenteric artery or endoscopic clipping or TAC-guided glue injection into the aneurysmal sac at the lumbar artery drainage site. Selective catheterization of IMA through SMA collaterals and embolization with coils has also been described.

Type III: leaks due to structural failure of the endovascular graft. Type III leaks are due to tears in the polytetrafluorethylene (PTFE) or Dacron fabric, failure at the connection of limbs, or to strut failure. Causes include defects in graft construction, poor handling of the graft during delivery, inappropriate choice of the diameter of the additional iliac limb, and faulty insertion of the additional limb.

Prevention requires improvement in design and construction of the prosthesis, and treatment may demand surgical removal of the graft.

Type IV: leaks due to porosity of graft material. Type IV leaks are due to leak of contrast through the pores of the Dacron and seem to be produced by excessive porosity of the fabric due to insufficient thickness. They should be seen rarely, only with higher porosity Dacron grafts. It is important not to confuse this leak with tears in the fabric, which are a much more severe problem. The problem should be self-limited after administration of protamine at the end of the procedure.

When evaluating microleaks, Doppler ultrasound and balloon occlusion arteriography can sometimes pinpoint endoleaks better than a CT scan, differentiating between excessive porosity and microtears.

Intestinal ischemia

Interfering with free blood flow in the inferior mesenteric artery may produce sigmoid colon ischemia when collateral flow is insufficient. The problem may be aggravated by the simultaneous occlusion of one or both internal iliac arteries. This is a problem shared by both EVG insertion procedures and open aortic surgery. Symptoms do not appear before the third postoperative day, when blood-tinged stools will alert to possible intestinal problems. Rectosigmoidoscopy performed at the third or fourth day will show mucosal changes and provide guidance for appropriate treatment. In mild cases, which is the most common occurrence, close observation and intravenous feeding to protect the bowel may suffice and help heal the lesions. In more severe cases, prolonged total parenteral nutrition and strict observation will be needed, because of the risk of perforation and sepsis. Surgeons should be on the alert for impending perforation, in which case intestinal resection, with or without diverting colostomy, should be performed.

Because the prosthesis is entirely protected within the natural aortoiliac wall, risks of contamination of the prosthetic material are limited. Another rare intestinal complication may arise from distal cholesterol emboli, producing focal ischemia. It may be due to dislodgement of material during attempts at embolization of the IMA or during suprarenal transit and manipulation of intravascular devices. This complication needs to be followed with frequent intestinal endoscopies and treated according to the severity of symptoms and mucosal findings.

Thrombosis

Immediate or delayed occlusion of the graft, the most commonly encountered complication, usually affects one iliac branch. It may be caused by inappropriate anticoagulation during the procedure, faulty positioning, kinking of the limbs of the graft, stenosis, or dislodgement of thrombus.

Prevention measures include pre-treatment with antiplatelet drugs and administration of 0.75–1 mg/kg intravenous heparin, followed by activated clotting time control. Patients with coagulation disturbances, such as those with factor V Leiden or factor II chromosomal anomalies could be at risk, especially those who are homozygote or have combined anomalies. Low antithrombin III levels significantly decrease the efficacy of heparin and can be associated with severe thrombotic complications. Preoperative control on the resistance to activated protein C and of the serum levels of antithrombin III will alert to such cases. Resistance to activated protein C and antithrombin III preoperative tests should always be performed prior to EVG insertion.

Treatment of this complication requires, at first, a good control of the coagulation process and adequate heparinization, followed by clot removal coupled with judicious urokinase administration. Urokinase, albeit useful and often effective, is a dangerous drug to use and cases of severe hemorrhage have been reported, both in the aneurysmal field and in the femoral artery exposure field. Mechanical thrombectomy is a more reasonable approach using endovascular devices such as Boston Scientific's Oasis or Fogarty catheters.

Fogarty catheters need to be used with extreme gentleness, avoiding overdistension of the balloon and trauma to the native artery, during thrombus pullout maneuvers. Previously thrombosed segments should be considered for coverage with a second stent graft.

What absolutely needs to be addressed is the underlying cause of the thrombus formation. Stenosis or kinking should be adjusted if present. The potential for re-thrombosis is always high and patients should be carefully monitored in the postoperative period. When there is recurrent unilateral thrombosis or underlying non-repairable kinking or stenosis, then a surgical femorofemoral crossover will provide appropriate palliation with good distal blood flow to the limb.

Embolism

Distal embolism may be caused by intra-arterial manipulation and dislodgement of plaque material. Renal artery and mesenteric artery embolism have been already addressed elsewhere. Femoral artery embolism may be difficult to identify if pre-procedural Doppler evaluation and an arteriogram have not been performed. Chronic superficial femoral artery occlusion may be then misdiagnosed as acute embolism and treated accordingly, with poor results. When distal embolism is diagnosed in the lower limb, embolectomy is the procedure of choice, performed with the help of a Fogarty catheter. Trash foot, due to distal microemboli, is a more difficult problem to address and may require urokinase, with its associated problems. Urokinase may not dissolve particulate thrombi, and necrosis of significant parts of the toes and foot may ensue in spite of fibrinolytic treatment. Trash foot treatment should follow the same guidelines usually employed in conventional open aortic surgery.

Clamping the distal femoral artery during the endovascular procedure helps reduce the incidence of distal embolism but proper purging procedures should also be enacted when opening up the femoral flow.

Hemorrhage

Bleeding may be due to damage or complete rupture of the arterial wall during positioning of the graft or during final dilatation of the limbs. Dissection and vessel damage during introduction of the graft along the femoral and external iliac arteries may be a cause of hemorrhage, especially when there is vessel spasm. In addition, the use of balloons that are extremely compliant and may be inadvertently dilated to very large diameters could cause severe damage to the vessels, specifically at the distal end point of the iliac limbs where ruptures may develop at the bifurcation of external and internal iliac arteries. At the iliac bifurcation, prompt recognition of the problem and immediate action are paramount to avoid life-threatening hemorrhage. Internal iliac embolization rapidly followed by sealing with a covered stent graft may solve the problem; otherwise, emergency surgery will be needed. Temporary control of the bleeding site may be obtained by gently inflating a long balloon inside the vessel. Administering protamine to reverse the heparin effect in case of vessel rupture can only compound the problem, because the bleeding may not stop and thrombosis will develop inside the vessel, making a patent repair more difficult to achieve.

In the external iliac tract, symptoms and initial signs of damage could be minimal and one often sees self-contained hematomas in postoperative CT scans. When one detects signs of external iliac damage during EVG insertion, stent graft external iliac coverage should be performed.

Fever and post-implantation syndrome

Post-procedure fever is commonplace, when Dacron-covered stents are utilized. The fever may appear 2–3 days after the procedure and may persist for 2–3 weeks. It is best treated with reassurance and NSAIDs (non-steroidal anti-inflammatory drugs) such as ibuprofen at a dosage of 400 mg three times a day by mouth.

Patients often report a temperature above 38°C, leukocytosis > 10 000, elevated C-reactive protein and interleukin-6 levels. There is also a higher release of tumor necrosis factor-alpha when compared to conventional aortic repair.

It is essential to differentiate benign hyperthermia produced by graft insertion from massive intraoperative bacterial contamination and consequent sepsis. This may require a very aggressive approach, with blood cultures, antibiotics administration and, in some cases, graft removal.

While simple percutaneous transluminal angioplasty (PTA) may require limited, but still reasonable aseptic measures, the use of tissue-covered stents needs strict sterility. Breaks in aseptic technique seem to be more common among non-surgical operators, and antibiotics are no substitute for proper asepsis.

Late complications

Thrombosis and endoleaks are the most common late complications. Inappropriate initial procedures may cause delayed complications, but some problems arise from subsequent deformation of the aorta and progression of disease.

Endoleaks (secondary)

Delayed endoleaks may be type I, II, or III and may derive from progressive enlargement of the aortic neck, dislodgement of the prosthesis and deformations due to shortening or elongation of the aorta itself, and persistent nourishing flow from patent branch vessels

Type I endoleaks require surgical intervention either with replacement of the EVG and surgical insertion of a new graft or, as reported in some series, with the application of a tape around the aortic neck: results with this technique are considered controversial. Sometimes, type I endoleaks can be sealed with the endovascular insertion of a more proximal adjunct to the original endoprosthesis. In no case should a type I endoleak be left alone, as it will most probably produce enlargement of the aneurysm and subsequent rupture and death. Dislodgement and consequent migration of a stent–graft may produce a severe type I endoleak and will require urgent surgery. Short necks and severe neck angulations are frequent causes of delayed type I endoleaks and initial patient selection is the best way to reduce the incidence of this late problem.

Type II endoleaks, when identified at a later time, may require simple observation if not severe; or they may require embolization or clipping, if associated with a severe leak and/or enlargement of the aneurysm, or with an increase of metalloproteinase MMP-9 and MMP-3 levels.

Type III endoleaks are more common in the long term and, improvement in the construction of the devices is constantly reducing their incidence. Strut fatigue and slipping of the connection between iliac and aortic limb require endovascular repair and insertion of additional stents or surgery.

Type IV endoleaks occurring late could be the result of an inaccurate CT scan diagnosis missing well-defined microleaks that can be detected by balloon occlusive arteriogram and Doppler ultrasound.

Thrombosis

One or both limbs of the graft may progressively or suddenly occlude. When one branch only occludes, options are embolectomy, urokinase, and concomitant resolution of underlying causes. Crossover bypass is a good alternative solution. When both limbs occlude, embolectomy is a first approach. Sometimes, axillofemoral, toracofemoral, or aortobifemoral bypass may be needed.

Whenever late thrombosis occurs, the status of the distal runoff vessels should be investigated, because progression of distal occlusive disease may be responsible for the graft occlusion.

If the EVG prosthesis is removed due to thrombosis, through a surgical approach, the surgeon should be informed as to the type of device that had been implanted: grafts that have struts located externally to the PTFE or Dacron are more difficult to remove than those which have internal struts and externally placed Gore-Tex.

Aneurysmal sac complications

Progressive dilatation of the aneurysmal sac may occur in spite of no identifiable endoleak at CT scan. Exhaustive workup to rule out any leak should be completed, including ultrasound, nuclear magnetic resonance (NMR) with gadolinium, spiral CT scan with contrast, and multiple projection arteriogram. A CO_2 arteriogram may help detect otherwise invisible low-volume endoleaks.

In the presence of progressive dilatation of the aneurysm and no treatable endoleak, surgery should be immediately performed to prevent rupture.

Serial determinations of metalloproteinase in the serum (MMP-3 and MMP-9) by the ELISA (enzyme-linked immunosorbent assay) method may help detect progression of a clinically stable aneurysm and prompt further studies and treatment.

Stenosis distal to the graft

Some degree of stenosis may be observed just distal to the iliac limb of the graft and, if stable over time and hemodynamically non-significant, it may not require invasive treatment. Close monitoring is necessary and additional angioplasty and stenting may be required only in the face of progression, or when critical and symptomatic stenoses are present.

Buttock claudication and ischemic sciatic neuropathy

Occlusion of the internal iliac artery may occasionally produce pain in the gluteus when walking or even at rest. This is rarely incapacitating and may improve with time. Distal implantation of the hypogastric artery in the external iliac artery prevents this complication but adds complexity and potential complications to the original procedure.

Aortic wall erosion

This rare complication has been associated with migration of the prosthesis and kinking at the aortic neck. Erosion through the aortic wall may produce a dangerous aortoenteric fistula at the duodenal level, but only anecdotal reports in the literature have occurred so far. Thinning of the aortic wall is a common report after long-term successful EVG implantation: it should be closely monitored over time.

Infection

Infection of the EVG is a serious complication, and intractable sepsis may ensue. Depending on the type of bacteria involved, symptoms and findings may be more or less dramatic. Cultures are essential, as certain types of bacteria can usually be eradicated with long-term antibiotic treatment, while others demand immediate removal of the foreign body.

Bacteremia will pose risks even for the newly re-implanted prosthesis, requiring complex surgical planning, microbiological evaluation and treatment, and staged procedures.

Complex procedures entail complications that experience and technical progress may often reduce. The future of EVGs will largely depend on the reduction of long-term complications, so that they may favorably compete with the time-proven surgical approach. Accurate patient selection, careful planning, and operator expertise are still the most valuable means of preventing complications.

References

1 Yamashita A, Wakamatsu H, Kawata R et al. Perioperative management of endovascular stent graft placement for abdominal aortic aneurysm. *Jap J Anaesthesiol* 2000; **49**(9): 987–94.

2 Schumacher H, Richter GM, Hansmann J et al. Carbon dioxide angiography for endovascular grafting in high-risk patients with infrarenal abdominal aortic aneurysms *J Vasc Surg* 2001; **33**(3): 646–9.

3 May J, White GH, Yu W et al. Conversion from endoluminal to open repair of abdominal aortic aneurysms: a hazardous procedure. *Eur J Vasc Endovasc Surg* 1997; **14**(1): 4–11.

4 May J, White GH, Harris JP. Technique for surgical conversion of aortic endoprosthesis. *Eur J Vasc Endovasc Surg* 1999; **18**(4): 284–9.

5 Kopchok H, Whire R, Donayre C. Troubleshooting maldeployed aortic endografts. *J Endovasc Surg* 1998; **5**(3): 266–8.

6 White GH, Yu W, Maj J et al. Endoleak as a complication of endoluminal grafting of abdominal aortic aneurysms: classification, incidence, diagnosis and management. *J Endovasc Surg* 1997; **4**(2): 152–68.

7 Buth J, Laheij RJ. Early complications and endoleaks after endovascular abdominal aortic aneurysm repair: report of a multicenter study. *J Vasc Surg* 2000; **31**(1 Pt 1): 134–46.

8 Puech-Leao P. Banding of the common iliac artery: an expedient in endoluminal correction of aortoiliac aneurysms. *J Vasc Surg* 2000; **32**(6):1232–4.

9 Barker C, Wellons E, Abul-Khoudoud O et al. Safety of coil embolization of the internal iliac artery in endovascular grafting of abdominal aortic aneurysms. *J Vasc Surg* 2000; **32**(4): 684–8.

10 Rilinger N, Sokiranski R et al. Treatment of leaks after endovascular repair of aortic aneurysms. *Radiology* 2000; **215**(2): 414–20.

11 Koussa M, Gaxotte V, Beregi JP et al. Diagnosis and treatment of Type II endoleak after stent placement for exclusion of abdominal aortic aneurysm. *Ann Vasc Surg* 2001; **15**(2): 148–54.

12 White GH, Maj J, Waugh RC et al. Type III and Type IV endoleak: toward a complete definition of blood flow in the sac after endoluminal AAA repair. *J Vasc Surg* 1998; **5**(4):305–9.

13 Hausegger KA, Schedlbauer P, Deutschmann HA, Tiesenhausen K. Complications in endoluminal repair of abdominal aorta aneurysms. *Eur J Radiol* 2001; **39**: 22–33.

14 Jaeger HJ, Mathias KD, Gissler HM, Wather LD. Rectum and sigmoid colon necrosis due to cholesterol embolization after implantation of an aortic stent-graft. *J Vasc Intervent Radiol* 1999; **10**(6):751–5.

15 Karch LA, Hodgson KJ, Mattos MA et al. Adverse consequences of internal iliac artery occlusion during endovascular repair of abdominal aortic aneurysms. *J Vasc Surg* 2000; **32**(4): 676–83.

16 Resch T, Ivancev K, Lindblad B et al. Aneurysm expansion and retroperitoneal haematoma after thrombolysis for stent-graft limb occlusion caused by distal endograft migration. *J Endovasc Ther* 2000; **7**(6): 446–50.

17 Norgren L, Swartbol P. Biological responses to endovascular treatment of abdominal aortic aneurysms. *J Endovasc Surg* 1997; **4**: 169–73.

18 Harris P, Brennan J, Martin J et al. Longitudinal aneurysm shrinkage following endovascular aortic aneurysm repair: a source of intermediate and late complications. *J Endovasc Surg* 1999; **6**(1): 11–16.

19 Gould DA, Edwards RD, McWilliams RG et al. Graft distortion after endovascular repair of abdominal aortic aneurysm: association with sac morphology and mid-term complications. *Cardiovasc Intervent Radiol* 2000; **23**(5): 358–63.

20 Harris PL, Vallabhaneni SR, Desgranges P et al. Incidence and risk factor of late rupture, conversion and death after endovascular repair of infrarenal aortic aneurysms: the EUROSTAR experience. *J Vasc Surg* 2000; **32**(4): 739–49.

21 White GH, Maj J, Petrasek et al. Endotension: an explanation for continued AAA growth after successful endoluminal repair. *J Endovasc Surg* 1999; **6**(4):308–15.

22 Maj J, White GH, Waugh R et al. Rupture of abdominal aortic aneurysms: a concurrent comparison of outcome of those occurring after endoluminal repair versus those occurring de novo. *Eur J Vasc Endovasc Surg* 1999; **18**(4):344–8 .

23 Ramaiah VG, Thompson CS, Rodriguez-Lopez JA et al. Endovascular repair of AAA rupture 20 months after endoluminal stent-grafting. *J Endovasc Surg* 2001; **8**(2): 125–30.

24 Sangiorgi G, D'Averio R, Mauriello A et al. Plasma level of MMP3 and MMP-9 as markers of successful AAA exclusion after EVG treatment. *Circulation* 2001 **104**: 288–95.

25 Lindholt JS, Ashton HA, Scott R. Indicators of infection with Chlamydia pneumoniae are associated with expansion of abdominal aortic aneurysms. *J Vasc Surg* 2001; **34**: 212–15.

26 Kibria SG, Gough MJ. Ischaemic sciatic neuropathy: a complication of endovascular repair of abdominal aortic aneurysm. *Eur J Vasc Endovasc Surg* 1999; **17**(3): 266–7.

27 Janne d'Othee B, Soula P, Otal P et al. Aortoduodenal fistula after endovascular stent-graft of and abdominal aortic aneurysm. *J Vasc Surg* 2000; **31**(1) 190–5.

28 De Virgilio C, Bui H, Donayre C et al. Endovascular vs. open abdominal aortic aneurysm repair: a comparison of cardiac morbidity and mortality. *Arch Surg* 1999; **134**(9): 947–50, discussion, 950–1.

47

Percutaneous endovascular treatment of peripheral aneurysms

Michel Henry, Isabelle Henry, Christos Klonaris and Michèle Hugel

Introduction

Peripheral arterial aneurysms are relatively uncommon diseases.[1,2] They may present incidentally and asymptomatic (discovery for example on echography or on a computed tomography (CT) scan carried out for another disease) or following complications such as rupture, compression, or thromboembolism.

Until now, their treatment has been exclusively surgical, but the operative risks are high, particularly when surgery is required on an emergency basis.[3,4]

An endovascular treatment has been recently proposed. It usually involves the following two techniques:

- placement of a stent–graft following arteriotomy due to the large size of the prosthesis[5,6]
- percutaneous implantation of an endoprosthesis (mostly covered).[7–14]

This minimally invasive technique avoids surgical incision and should reduce morbidity and mortality associated with surgical repair of peripheral aneurysms.

We are reporting our experience of percutaneous endoluminal treatment of 50 peripheral aneurysms (48 patients) using covered stents in the majority of the cases.

Patients and methods

Between October 1993 and October 1998, 48 patients underwent elective percutaneous endovascular treatment of 50 peripheral aneurysms. Two patients had bilateral aneurysms (femoral 1 and iliac 1). Forty-one patients were males, 7 were females, with a mean age of 65.7 ± 10 years (range 47–85 years). The risk factors were smoking in 35 patients, hypertension in 28, dyslipidemia in 28, and diabetes in 12.

Twenty-three patients also had concomitant coronary artery disease, 7 presented with severe respiratory insufficiency, and 2 had renal failure.

All patients presented with clinical arterial defects of the lower limbs (mean arterial brachial pressure index 0.62 ± 0.16). According to Rutherford's classification, 16 patients were in category 1, 24 were in category 2/3, and 8 in category 4.

With regards to the distal runoff, 7 patients had one, 22 had two, and 21 had three distal patent arteries.

Nine patients also had an associated aneurysm of the abdominal aorta, but these aneurysms were not large enough to be referred to surgery.

In all patients the clinical assessment consisted of an arterial duplex scan examination, a front and profile arteriography of the abdominal aorta and distal arteries, and a computed tomography (CT) scan. This was to determine the precise localization of the aneurysm, its size (length, diameter), shape, the presence of a major arterial branch within the aneurysm (problem of the internal iliac artery for the iliac localizations), and position as compared to the healthy artery (important for fixation of the prosthesis in the healthy artery).

The aneurysms involved the following arteries:

- iliac: 25 cases involved the common iliac artery and 1 involved the internal iliac artery
- femoral: 12 cases
- popliteal: 12 cases.

The lesion characteristics are summarized in Table 47.1.

The aneurysms were atheromatous in 46 cases. Two were false aneurysms that developed at the distal extremity of a Cragg Endopro System 1 stent, which had been placed after recanalization of the femoral artery ($n = 1$) and popliteal artery ($n = 1$). Two aneurysms were of infectious origin (post-angioplasty and stenting of common iliac arteries). The endovascular therapy was decided 3 months after a prolonged treatment with antibiotics and disappearance of the infection.

Table 47.1   IFPA lesion characteristics

Location	No.	Mean lesion length (mm)	Mean lesion diameter (mm)
Iliac	26	55.6 ± 28.8 (10–150)	30 ± 13.4 (13–80)
Femoral	12	95.4 ± 95.2 (20–290)	20 ± 9.5 (8–40)
Popliteal	12	75 ± 72.1 (20–260)	19.9 ± 8 (12–35)

Indication for treatment of the aneurysm depended on clinical criteria (severity of intermittent claudication due to associated stenoses), or on anatomical criteria (diameter of the aneurysm, estimated on angiography or on CT scan, with risks of rupture).

Different prostheses were used to treat these aneurysms. Table 47.2 summarizes the different prostheses and the sites of their implantation.

The first aneurysm we treated was located in the common iliac artery. It was treated with a stent graft consisting of a polytetrafluorethylene (PTFE) prosthesis (IMPRA) sutured on two P204 Palmaz stents (Cordis/J&J, Warren, NJ), placed by the percutaneous approach through a 12F introducer sheath.

Four aneurysms were treated with non-covered stents:

- One pseudoaneurysm, associated with a stenosis, developed in the distal part of a Cragg Endopro System 1 stent which had been implanted 2 years earlier for treatment of a popliteal occlusion. A Wallstent stent (7 mm in diameter, 3 cm in length) was then implanted with an excellent result.
- One isolated aneurysm was situated in the internal iliac artery. The ostium of this artery presented a very tight stenosis. Adjacent to it, there was a tight stenosis in the external iliac artery. A selective catheterization of the internal iliac artery was performed by a contralateral approach, and embolization was done using several coils (Cook Inc., Bloomington, IN). The angioplasty of the initial

part of the external iliac artery led to total occlusion of the internal iliac artery, thereby excluding the aneurysm. A P304 Palmaz stent was then placed, covering the ostium of the internal iliac artery and the initial part of the external iliac artery, providing an excellent result. The exclusion of the aneurysm was confirmed on the CT scan.

- One aneurysm in the common iliac artery, adjacent to a tight stenosis, was treated with a self-expandable nitinol stent (Optimed, Medcare, Franconville, France) with a very good result.
- One aneurysm in the popliteal artery was treated with the new self-expandable nitinol Expander stent (Bolton Medical) with a very good result. This stent is very flexible and seems well adapted to this location.

All the other aneurysms were treated with covered stents. To avoid migration, the size of the stents used was 10–20 % larger than the normal size of the artery. We have used four types of prostheses:

The Cragg Endopro System 1 or Passager (Boston Scientific, Natick, MA). The technical characteristics of this prosthesis have been described.[7,9–13] It was often used in the treatment of occlusive iliofemoropopliteal lesions.[11–13] Twenty-two aneurysms were treated with this endoprosthesis (8 at the iliac level, 7 at the femoral level and 7 at the popliteal level).

The origin of the internal iliac artery was involved in one patient presenting with an iliac aneurysm. To prevent retrograde filling of the aneurysm, transcatheter coil embolization of the internal iliac artery was performed prior to the placement of the covered stent.

The Corvita prosthesis (Schneider/Boston Scientific, Bülach, Switzerland). This new prosthesis is still at the experimental stage. It consists of two main components:

- a self-expanding cylindrical wire structure
- a highly porous and elastic coating consisting of polycarbonate urethane.

This prosthesis exists in various lengths and sizes and can be cut to the required length by the user.

Twenty-one aneurysms were treated by Corvita prosthesis implantation using either the percutaneous retrograde approach (n = 13), the antegrade approach (n = 6), or the contralateral approach (n = 1). The popliteal approach was used in one case. The introducer size ranged between 7F and 12F.

Table 47.2.   IFPA – type of stents

Stents	Iliac	Femoral	Popliteal	Total
Covered stents	**32**	**18**	**15**	**65**
Cragg/Passager	9	13	12	34
Corvita	20	5	3	28
Endotex	1	–	–	1
Wallgraft	1	–	–	1
Stent graft	1	–	–	1
Non-covered stents	**2**	**–**	**3**	**5**
Palmaz	1	–	–	1
Optimed	1	–	–	1
Expander	–	–	2	2
Wallstent	–	–	1	1
Total	**34**	**18**	**18**	**70**

The Wallgraft (Schneider/Boston Scientific, Bülach, Switzerland). This prostheses was once used to treat an aneurysm in the common iliac artery, with success.

The new Endotex prosthesis (in experiment). This prosthesis was also used once to treat a common iliac aneurysm with immediate success. This stent consists of a flat sheet of nitinol covered with polyester.

The JOSTENT-covered stent (JOMED AB, Helsingborg, Sweden). This balloon expandable prosthesis is available in lengths ranging from 28 to 58 mm and its expansion diameter ranges from 5 to 10 mm. It consists of a double thin stainless steel prosthesis. There is a PTFE coating between the two prostheses. It may be used to treat peripheral aneurysms but a flexion area such as the popliteal artery should be avoided due to potential compression.

Table 47.3 shows the number of stents used to treat the 50 aneurysms. Seventy prostheses were used. In certain cases, several prostheses were implanted in the same artery in order to completely cover the aneurysm.

Any associated stenosis is dilated with a balloon that has a diameter equal to that of the artery. During the entire procedure, repeated angiographies are performed to make sure that the positioning of the prosthesis is correct and there is no residual leakage. An intravascular ultrasound examination (IVUS) was performed in 4 patients, and it confirmed a good intravascular result.

The procedures were performed under local anesthesia and mild neuroleptanalgesia. At the beginning of the procedure, 1 g of aspirin and 5000 units of intravenous heparin was given as bolus. Heparin was then given for 24 hours and the patient's coagulation was checked regularly. Thereafter, the patients received ticlopidine (500 mg/day) and aspirin (100 mg/day) for 1 month. (aspirin 250 mg/day) was then continued thereafter. Patients also routinely received 3 mg of Kefadol (cefamandole) following the procedure, as prophylaxis against infection.

Strict follow-up of these patients was performed:

- duplex scan, echo-Doppler, and CT scan were performed the day after the procedure.
- at 6 months, the patients were followed-up by duplex scan, angiography, and CT scan
- thereafter, a duplex scan was performed every 6 months. Arteriography and a CT scan were performed only if a problem was suspected.

Immediate results

Results are shown in Figures 47.1–47.4.

An immediate technical success with total exclusion of the aneurysm was obtained in all cases except 2 (96%). In one case of a long, tortuous and calcified femoropopliteal aneurysm, which was associated with a severe stenosis, it was impossible to cover its lower part due to the stiffness of the introduction device of the Cragg Endopro System 1, and a mild leakage persisted at the lower part.

In the second case of large iliac aneurysm (8 cm in diameter) we had an incomplete exclusion of the aneurysmal sac despite placement of a Corvita endoprosthesis. Placement of coils in the aneurysmal sac, using the contralateral approach, allowed a total exclusion of the aneurysm, and this was confirmed on angiogram and CT scan. All other aneurysms were perfectly excluded, and the results were confirmed by a follow-up echo-doppler and/or CT scan performed after the procedure.

Table 47.3 indicates the mean length of the prostheses as compared to the mean length of the lesions at the different levels. It indicates a good coverage of the lesions.

Table 47.4 shows the mean arterial diameter obtained as compared to the mean diameter of the aneurysms at the different sites.

The mean Doppler index at 24 hours was 0.92 ± 0.10.

Table 47.3 IFPA – immediate results: length of prosthesis

Location	No.	Mean lesion length (mm)	Mean length of prosthesis (mm)
Iliac	26	55.6 ± 28.8 (10–150)	68.7 ± 28.4 (13–80)
Femoral	12	95.4 ± 95.2 (20–290)	117 ± 95.4 (25–300)
Popliteal	12	75 ± 72.1 (20–260)	105.8 ± 94.1 (30–300)

Table 47.4 IFPA – immediate results: diameter

Location	No.	Mean lesion diameter before stent (mm)	Mean arterial diameter after stent (mm)
Iliac	26	30.9 ± 13.3 (13–80)	9.1 ± 2.0 (6–14)
Femoral	12	20.0 ± 9.5 (8–40)	7.5 ± 1.6 (6–10)
Popliteal	12	19.9 ± 7.9 (12–35)	7.8 ± 2.0 (6–14)

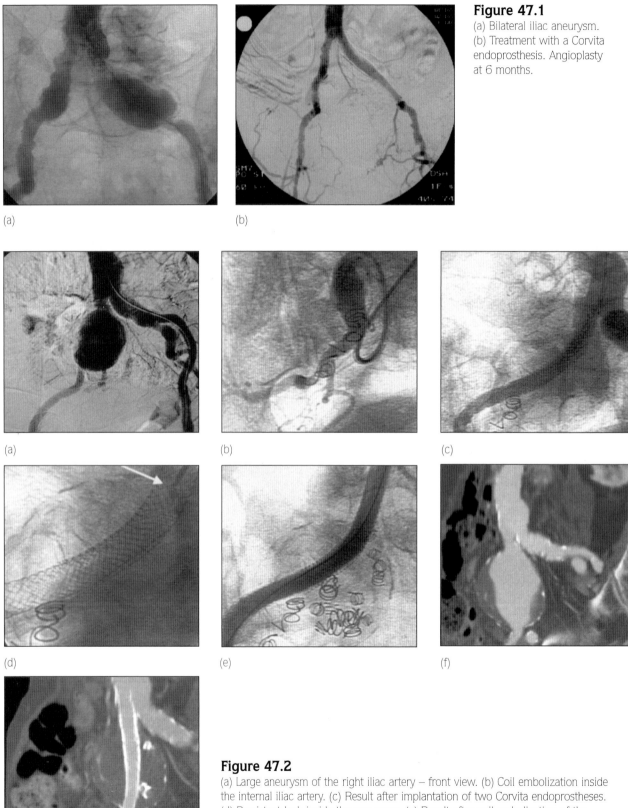

Figure 47.1
(a) Bilateral iliac aneurysm.
(b) Treatment with a Corvita endoprosthesis. Angioplasty at 6 months.

Figure 47.2
(a) Large aneurysm of the right iliac artery – front view. (b) Coil embolization inside the internal iliac artery. (c) Result after implantation of two Corvita endoprostheses. (d) Persistent leak inside the aneurysm. (e) Result after coil embolization of the aneurysmal sac by contralateral approach. (f) Spiral CT scan – large iliac aneurysm. (g) Immediate post-procedure result. Total exclusion of the aneurysm after coils embolization inside the sac.

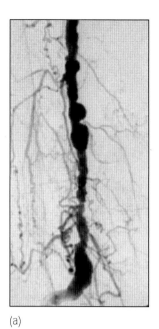
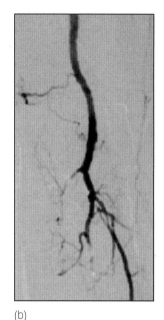

(a)   (b)

Figure 47.3

(a) Long femoro-popliteal aneurysm. (b) Result after implantation of a Corvita endoprosthesis.

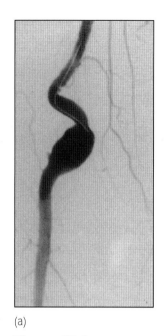
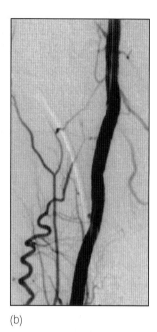

(a)   (b)

Figure 47.4

(a) Aneurysm of the upper part of the popliteal artery. Treatment with Cragg Endopro System 1 prosthesis (or Passager). (b) Result after treatment.

Complications

1. Thrombosis of the prosthesis: 8/50 (16%)

- *4 early thromboses* between day 1 and day 15: 2 at the iliac level (1 with a Corvita prosthesis, successfully treated using Fogarty's technique, 1 with an Endotex prosthesis requiring a bypass); 2 at the popliteal level (1 with a Corvita prosthesis, successfully treated by repeat angioplasty, and 1 with a Cragg Endopro System 1/Passager stent requiring a bypass)
- *3 thromboses* which appeared between 3 and 6 months; 1 at the femoral level (Cragg Endopro System 1/Passager), requiring bypass surgery; 2 at the popliteal level (1 Cragg Endopro System 1/Passager, 1 Corvita endoluminal graft), treated medically (the patients had refused surgery)
- *1 thrombosis* appeared at 2 years at the popliteal level (Corvita prosthesis). The prosthesis was recanalized by the percutaneous approach.

The thrombosis rate seems more frequent in the popliteal artery, but it is worth mentioning that no serious problem arose after stent thrombosis and there was no need for amputation.

2. Distal embolism.
A distal embolism occurred at the deep femoral artery level, following exclusion of an iliac aneurysm. It was successfully treated by surgical embolectomy.

3. Fever and pain syndrome.
This syndrome was observed in 4 patients following implantation of Cragg stents at the femoral level. We found no infectious etiology. Everything returned to normal within a few days.

4. One hematoma at the puncture site.
This did not require surgery.

5. Two deaths.
One patient died at 6 days and the other one at 6 months (patients who been treated for bilateral femoral aneurysms) of myocardial infarction.

Follow-up

A strict follow-up of these patients is important to detect any problem, restenosis, or leakage, and to evaluate the patency rate of these prostheses.

Restenosis

At 6 months follow-up the mean ankle brachial index (ABI) was 0.87 ± 0.11. Two restenoses appeared outside the stent:

- 1 at the iliac level (Cragg stent) associated with a small leakage successfully treated by angioplasty and implantation of another Cragg stent
- 1 at the popliteal level (Corvita stent) treated by angioplasty and implantation of a Vascucoil stent (Medtronic, Boulogne Billancourt, France).

Long-term follow-up

The mean follow-up was 20.6 ± 13.2 months. Our maximum follow-up was 61 months. Figures 47.5–47.9 summarize the different primary (PI) and secondary (PII) patency rates at the different levels. In our series, the patencies were very good at the iliac level (PI = 92.1%, PII = 96%) and less good but satisfactory at the femoralopopliteal level (PI = 78.3%, PII = 86.9%).

Discussion

The most common etiology of iliofemoropopliteal aneurysms is atherosclerosis. Other causes include infection, dissection, trauma, postoperative injury, and collagen diseases such as Marfan syndrome. Among our patients, the etiology was atherosclerosis in 46 cases, infection in 2 cases, and anastomosis in 2 cases. These aneurysms are easily identified by ultrasonography, contrast-enhanced CT scanning, or angiography.

Popliteal artery aneurysms are the most common peripheral aneurysm (70%),[15–18] and they are very often bilateral. They occur with a frequency that is second only to that of aneurysms of the abdominal aorta. A review[19] of a large series of popliteal aneurysms showed that they are associated with abdominal aortic aneurysms in 28% and with iliac and femoral aneurysms in 35% of cases.[20] They have a high incidence of thromboembolic and limb-threatening complications (36–69% of the cases).[21–30] They are sometimes diagnosed by symptoms produced by neurological compression or venous compression with phlebitis. Rupture at this level is rare. An aneurysmal diameter of 15 mm or more should be an indication for intervention.

Femoral aneurysms are the second most common form of peripheral artery aneurysms. They are also usually bilateral. Eighty-five percent of them are associated with aortoiliac aneurysms and 44% with popliteal aneurysms.[31] They are usually asymptomatic and they can be diagnosed by palpation of a pulsatile mass in the groin. However, sometimes they present with a distal embolization or an acute thrombosis threatening the limb. Pseudoaneurysms are frequent at this level, secondary to a trauma, arterial rupture or rupture at the level of an anastomosis of a bypass graft. An arterial diameter of more than 20 mm should be an indication for intervention.

Isolated aneurysms of the iliac arteries are rather uncommon, accounting for only 2–7% of atherosclerotic aneurysms of the aortoiliac segment.[32–35] They may rupture, embolize, thrombose, or produce pressure symptoms. The natural course of an iliac aneurysm is one of progressive expansion, which eventually leads to rupture. The rate of rupture, which increases with aneurysm size, has been estimated to be 31%.[3] Other clinicians estimate the rate to be 14–70%.[4,28,36–40] The mean diameter of ruptured iliac aneurysms was 5.6 cm,[3] but ruptures of 3 cm aneurysms have been reported.[2]

The signs and symptoms of iliac aneurysms are produced by the mass effect or erosion into adjacent organs.[3] Symptoms are usually related to gastrointestinal, genitourinary, neurological or venous structures.[8] Internal iliac artery aneurysms have a very poor prognosis. The largest surgical series by Brin and Busuttil[41] reported a 67% incidence of rupture with a 90% mortality in untreated patients. Treatment is recommended for iliac aneurysms larger than 3 cm in diameter.[41,42]

Until recently, peripheral aneurysms were treated surgically.

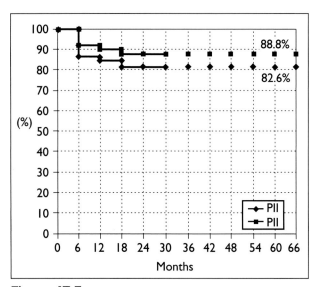

Figure 47.5
IFPA: all lesions.

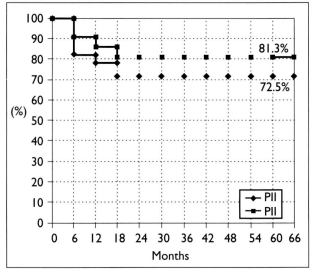

Figure 47.6
IFPA: iliac.

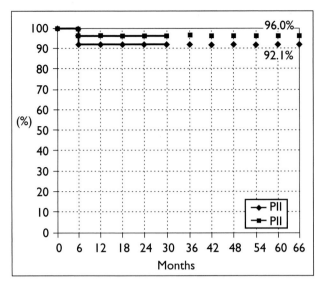

Figure 47.7
IFPA: femoropopliteal.

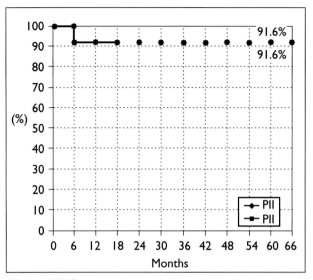

Figure 47.8
IFPA: femoral.

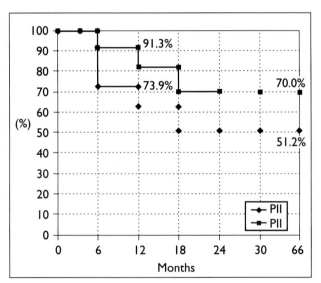

Figure 47.9
IFPA: popliteal.

At the popliteal level, the risk of untreated disease is high (30% risk of amputation) but operative repair in patients without symptoms is relatively safe.[18,21,23,43] Good long-term patency rates have been achieved, especially when the runoff vessels have not been occluded by embolization.[44] Exclusion of the aneurysm and bypass or resection bypass can be performed,[17,18] but morbidity and risks of amputation in patients undergoing elective repair have been reported.[15,25,43,45] The mortality was 3–5% and the risk of amputation was 7–15% in patients without symptoms and 80% in the patients presenting with thrombosis. The patency rate at 5 years has been reported to be 91% in asymptomatic patients and 54% in symptomatic patients.[29]

At the femoral level, the same technique of exclusion of

the aneurysm and performed can be performed with excellent results. The mortality was 2%, the risk of amputation 2–5%, but 30% in the case of an extensive femoropopliteal thrombosis.[46]

For iliac aneurysms, the current recommended treatment is surgical repair but this is associated with a mortality rate of 7–11% for elective operations and 33–50% when surgery is required on an emergency basis.[3]

The technical complexities of operating on vessels deep within the pelvis, especially after previous aortic surgery, have made standard elective surgical management of iliac aneurysms more difficult than for aortic aneurysms.[5] Exclusion of the aneurysm or alternative therapies using simple aneurysm ligation, coil embolization have therefore been attempted to treat these aneurysms.[47–49] Whereas radiographic exclusion of flow in the aneurysms has been successfully achieved with these techniques, continued growth and rupture of the apparently excluded lesions is well documented.[50–53] The lower extremity arterial flow may also be compromised.[5]

With an internal iliac artery aneurysm, the origin of the aneurysm may be easily oversewn, but the anterior and posterior divisions of the internal iliac artery usually arise deep in the pelvis and may be difficult or impossible to ligate or oversew from within. Without occlusion of these vessels, the aneurysm can remain patent by filling itself from contralateral pelvic collateral branches and the potential for aneurysm rupture remains.[6]

Hollis et al[54] described a technique of percutaneous occlusion of the entire iliac system, and cross femoral bypass to revascularize the lower extremity on the affected site. With this technique, proximal ligation is not performed and, theoretically, the iliac system could recanalize and rupture of the internal iliac artery aneurysm can occur.[6]

Endoluminal graft placement is an alternative approach to conventional surgical repair of peripheral aneurysms. This new technique is less invasive and avoids the need for incision, general anesthesia and prolonged hospitalization; also, there is minimal blood loss. These advantages are particularly important in patients who are high-risk surgical candidates because of associated comorbid medical conditions. This concept was initially proposed by Dotter.[55] In 1985, Cragg et al.[56] reported the first percutaneous graft placement procedure with the use of a nitinol stent. The experimental feasibility of treating aneurysms with Dacron or PTFE grafts was demonstrated by several authors.[57–60] Parodi et al. performed the first percutaneous treatment of an aortoiliac aneurysm.[28]

Since then, endovascular stented grafts have been used effectively to treat aneurysms of the thoracic and abdominal aorta as well as other vessels, pseudoaneurysms, and arteriovenous fistulas.[28,36,38,59,61–65] This technique of stent–graft placement was also developed to treat peripheral aneurysms. Marin et al.[5,44] used a stent composed of PTFE grafts combined with balloon-expandable Palmaz stents at both extremities. Although this technique fosters good results, it also has certain drawbacks:

- since the stent is in a 14F introducer, it requires a surgical arteriotomy
- there is a possibility of a narrowing or kinking of the uncovered midgraft segment because of the absence of metallic reinforcement.

Marin et al. observed one case of kinking after treatment of an iliac aneurysm with this technique.[5] Laborde et al.[59] also observed kinking of the prosthesis in 6 out of 8 cases and 2 acute thromboses in an experimental model. Recently, Dorros et al.[66] reported 11 isolated iliac artery aneurysms treated by the same stent graft as described by Marin. The devices were delivered percutaneously through standard 14F sheaths and deployed by balloon dilation.

Non-covered stents have also been proposed for the treatment of peripheral aneurysms. Vorwerk et al.[49] used non-covered self-expanding stents to treat ulcerated plaques and focal aneurysms involving the iliac arteries. Blais and Bonneau[67] successfully used a non-covered stent to thrombose an iliac pseudoaneurysm next to a stenotic lesion. We treated 4 aneurysms with this type of non-covered stent. These non-covered stents may only be used in a limited number of small aneurysms with a narrow neck, in the lower third of the femoral artery, and in the popliteal artery, in the case of focal lesions; these prostheses are more flexible and better adapted to these locations. Some interventionalists have treated large-neck iliac aneurysms percutaneously by placing stents across the neck, followed by coil embolization through the struts of the stent.[68] However, the use of covered stents seems to be the easiest technique since it allows the treatment of most of the lesions using a percutaneous approach.

Razavi et al.[8] reported a series of 7 iliac aneurysms treated with Z-covered stents, coated either with polyester material (3 cases) or ultrathin PTFE graft material (4 cases). These stent grafts were introduced through 12–16F angiographic sheaths placed percutaneously, but a surgical suture of the artery was necessary in 4 cases after withdrawal of the introducer. Therefore, this limits the interest in these stents.

Covered stents, such as Cragg Endopro System 1/Passager, Corvita and Wallgraft, have the advantage of being implantable percutaneously through introducers that usually range from 7F to 9F. Several limited series have been published,[7,9,10–14] and have reported promising results. The Corvita endoluminal graft may be cut to the required length by the user. It is soft, and therefore the operator can place it using the contralateral approach. These covered stents have a metallic self-expandable support on their entire length: this avoids external compression or kinking of the prosthesis that could reduce arterial flow, as has been seen with stent grafts.

Recently, Curti et al.[12] reported a series of 13 procedures for 11 iliac pseudoaneurysms and 2 true iliac aneurysms with a 92% technical success and found the self-expanding Passager stent more useful in treating these patients, due to its good radial strength.

Beregi et al.[13] reported a series of 19 aneurysms (7 iliac, 5 subclavian, 3 femoral, 3 popliteal, 1 carotid) treated with Cragg Endopro System 1 or Passager with a 95% technical success. The 1-year patencies for iliac, head and neck, femoral, and popliteal arteries are 86%, 50% 33%, and 100%, respectively. The authors describe local puncture site complication (thrombosis or hemorrhage) due to the large introducer size (12F) needed to implant a stent of 10 mm in diameter. The brachial access is a potential for this technique.

To treat aneurysms originating near a major collateral vessel, the embolization of that vessel seems essential prior to stent placement to prevent retrograde filling of the aneurysm and to reduce the risk of rupture of this aneurysm. Special care should be given for the treatment of internal iliac aneurysms. Indeed, it should first be excluded with a stent placed in the iliac artery, usually using the retrograde ipsilateral approach, and it should then be embolized with coils that will stop the arterial flow coming from afferent arteries originating at the pelvis. These coils are usually placed using the contralateral approach. However, embolization of such vessels exclude a bilateral procedure that avoids complications such as pelvis ischemia[7] (bowel or urinary tract).

At the popliteal level, good results have been reported with endovascular therapy.[28,39,44,55–60,63,69–76] However, it seems that the treatment of such aneurysms leads to a higher thrombosis rate. Movements of the knee may lead to kinking of the prosthesis, which may be responsible for thromboses. It is worth mentioning that, in our series, even after thombosis of the prothesis, the limb never had threatening ischemia and did not require amputation. Rousseau et al.[7] believe that this procedure should not be performed for aneurysmal lesions extending distally to the origin of the anterior tibial artery to avoid obstruction of this vessel by the prosthesis.

Dorffner et al.[9] suggest that implantation in vessels subject to mechanical stress such as the popliteal segments 2 (from the branches of the superior genicular arteries to the branches of the inferior genicular arteries) and 3 (from the branches of the inferior genicular arteries to the arcus tendineus m. solei) is not recommended because disintegration of stent filaments may occur. However, implantation of covered stents to treat aneurysms of the distal femoral artery and popliteal segment 1 can be performed safely.

When treating long aneurysms, it is safer to place the distal stent first and then the proximal stent(s), overlapping each other at least 1 cm, to avoid the stents separating from each other and falling into the aneurysmal sac, leading to leakage.

Several types of complications may arise in treating these aneurysms:

- The initial arteriogram obtained after placement of the stent–graft may reveal small leaks into the aneurysms from proximal and distal communication. The leaks can be corrected by placement of additional identical stent graft or by transcatheter embolization with coils.[8] One patient in our series presented a stent leak that was successfully corrected by the placement of coils in the aneurysmal sac. Leaks may appear later, thus indicating the importance of a strict follow-up with echo-Doppler and CT scan.
- Early thrombosis may be observed, particularly at the popliteal level.[7] A fibrinolytic drug treatment may then be implemented. It is difficult to know if an anticoagulant therapy would have been better than antiaggregant drugs, as in our protocol.
- Restenosis is described at the extremities of the prostheses (2 cases in our series), similar to the bypass stenoses observed by the surgeons. This justifies a regular surveillance of these prostheses so as to detect and treat them with an angioplasty or placement of another prosthesis.[7,11]
- Distal embolizations may occur during the treatment of these aneurysms.[5] This may require other interventional procedures (thromboaspiration, mechanical thrombectomy) or surgical embolectomy.
- Appearance of a leakage can occur during the follow-up (1 case in our series) demonstrating the importance of follow-up.

The indications for the interventional treatment of peripheral aneurysms are still debated. The interventional treatment seems to be an alternative to surgery for iliac and femoral lesions. Iliac aneurysms are often associated with distended arteries that are too large for currently available stents. Forcing the indications for endovascular repair entails the risk of converting to operation or using a large number of stents to obtain complete exclusion of the aneurysm. The state of the abdominal aorta should also be considered if it shows signs of aneurysmal disease; treating the isolated iliac aneurysm may be only a temporary measure, since subsequent aortic repair will become necessary.[66] For popliteal aneurysms an interventional treatment may be proposed for patients with high surgical risks. The thrombosis rate seems to be higher with covered stents and may limit the indications at this level.

There were no guidelines for choosing one stent rather than another: choice mainly depends on the operator's decision. In our experience we observed no difference in terms of complications between the different covered stents. These stents seem also equivalent in terms of mid- and long-term patencies. The Corvita prosthesis may be easier to implant in long lesions and using the contralateral approach (these prostheses are available in longer lengths than the other stents and they can be cut to the desired length). Compressive forms of aneurysms, particularly in the iliac artery, are still treated surgically. The signs of compression usually persist after the interventional treatment. Only very high surgical risk patients should undergo an endoluminal treatment.

This technique could also be useful in the case of aneurysmal ruptures that have high operative mortality, such as aneurysmal ruptures of traumatic origins.[38,69]

Conclusion

Percutaneous interventional treatment of peripheral aneurysms currently seems to be an alternative to surgery. The implantation of covered stents using the percutaneous approach is easy and efficient, and immediate success is obtained in most cases. And yet, the thrombosis rate obtained with these prostheses is high, and it may limit their indications, particularly in the popliteal artery. The mid-term patency in the iliac and femoral arteries is good. The popliteal artery is still a surgical indication, except for high-risk patients.

Technical improvements are awaited, to make it a safer and more efficient treatment.

References

1 Lucke B, Rea MH. Studies on aneurysms. *JAMA* 1921; **77**: 935–40.
2 Brunkwall J, Hauksson H, Bengtsson H et al. Solitary aneurysms of the iliac artery system: an estimate of their frequency of occurrence. *J Vasc Surg* 1989; **10**: 381–4.
3 Richardson JW, Greenfield LJ. Natural history and management of iliac aneurysms. *J Vasc Surg* 1988; **8**: 165–71.
4 McCready RA, Pairolero PC, Gilmore JC et al. Isolated iliac artery aneurysms. *Surgery* 1983; **93**: 699–703.
5 Marin ML, Veith FJ, Lyon RT et al. Transfemoral endovascular repair of iliac artery aneurysms. *Am J Surg* 1995; **170**: 179–82.
6 Cynamon J, Marin ML, Veith FJ et al. Endovascular repair of an internal iliac artery aneurysm with use of a stented graft and embolization coils. *JVIR* 1995; **6**: 509–12.

7   Rousseau H, Gieskes L, Joffre F et al. Percutaneous treatment of peripheral aneurysms with the Cragg Endopro System1. *JVIR* 1996; **7**: 35–9.

8   Razavi MK, Dake MD, Semba CP et al. Percutaneous endoluminal placement of stent-grafts for the treatment of isolated iliac artery aneurysms. *Radiology* 1995; **197**: 801–4.

9   Dorffner R, Winkelbauer F, Kettenbach J et al. Successful exclusion of a large femoropopliteal aneurysm with a covered nitinol stent. *Cardiovasc Intervent Radiol* 1996; **19**: 117–9.

10 Gieskes L, Rousseau H, Otal P et al. Traitement percutané par endoprothèse couverte des anévrismes poplités: expérience clinique préliminaire. *J Mal Vasc* 1995; **20**: 264–7.

11 Henry M, Amor M, Cragg A et al. Occlusive and aneurysmal peripheral arterial disease: assessment of a stent-graft system. *Radiology* 1996; **201**: 717–24.

12 Curti T, Stella A, Rossi C. Endovascular repair as first-choice treatment for anastomatic and true iliac aneurysms. *J Endovasc Ther* 2001; **8**: 139–43.

13 Beregi JP, Prat A, Willoteaux S. Covered stents in the treatment of peripheral aneurysms: procedural results and midterm follow up. *Cardiovasc Intervent Radiol* 1999; **22**: 13–19.

14 Krajcer Z, Khoshnevis R, Leachman DR. Endoluminal exclusion of an iliac artery aneurysm by wallstent endoprosthesis and PTFE vascular graft. *Tesc Heart Inst J* 1997; **24**: 11–14.

15 Halliday AW, Wolfe JH, Taylor PR et al. The management of popliteal aneurysm: the importance of early surgical repair. *Ann R Coll Surg* 1991; **73**: 253–7.

16 MacGowan GW, Saif MF, O'Neil G et al. Ultrasound examination in the diagnosis of popliteal artery aneurysms. *Br J Surg* 1985; **72**: 528–9.

17 Lowell R, Gloviczki P. Anévrismes de l'artère poplitée, les risques de l'abstention chirurgicale. *Ann Chir Vasc* 1994; **8**: 14–23.

18 Szilagyi DE, Schwartz RL, Reddy HD. Popliteal arterial aneurysms: their natural history and management. *Arch Surg* 1981; **116**: 724–8.

19 Cole CW, Thijssen AM, Barber GG et al. Popliteal aneurysms: an index of generalized vascular disease. *Can J Surg* 1989; **32**: 65–8.

20 Breslin DJ, Jewell ER. Peripheral aneurysms. *Cardiol Clin* 1991; **9**: 489–96.

21 Vermilion BD, Kimmins SA, Pace WG et al. A review of 147 popliteal aneurysms with long term follow-up. *Surgery* 1981; **90**: 1009–14.

22 Baird JR, Sivasankar R, Hayward R et al. Popliteal aneurysm: a review and analysis of sixty-one cases. *Surgery* 1966; **59**: 911–17.

23 Whitehouse WM Jr, Wakefield TW, Graham LM et al. Limb-threatening potential of atherosclerotic popliteal artery aneurysms. *Surgery* 1983; **93**: 694–9.

24 Evans WE, Hayes JP. Popliteal and femoral aneurysms. In: Rutherford RB, (ed.), Vascular Surgery, Vol 2, 3rd edn. Philadelphia: WB Saunders, 1989: 951–7.

25 Anton GE, Hertzer NR, Beven EG et al. Surgical management of popliteal aneurysms: trends in presentation treatment, and results from 1952 to 1984. *J Vasc Surg* 1986; **3**: 125–34.

26 Evans WE, Bernhard VM, Kauffman HM. Femorotibial bypass in patients with popliteal aneurysms. *Am J Surg* 1971; **122**: 555–7.

27 Linton RR. The arteriosclerotic popliteal aneurysm: report of fourteen patients treated by preliminary lumbar sympathetic ganglionectomy and aneurysmectomy. *Surgery* 1949; **26**: 41–58.

28 Parodi JC, Palmaz MD, Barone HD. Transfemoral intraluminal graft implantation for abdominal aortic aneurysm. *Ann Vasc Surg* 1991; **5**: 491–9.

29 Shortell CK, DeWeese JA, Ouriel K et al. Popliteal artery aneurysms: a twenty-five-year surgical experience. *J Vasc Surg* 1991; **14**: 771–9.

30 Bouhouros J, Martin P. Popliteal aneurysm: a review of 116 cases. *Br J Surg* 1974; **61**: 469–75.

31 Graham LM, Zelenock GB, Whitehouse WM Jr et al. Clinical significance of arteriosclerotic femoral artery aneurysms. *Arch Surg* 1980; **115**: 502–7.

32 Nachbur BH, Inderbitzi RG, Bar W. Isolated iliac aneurysms. *Eur J Vasc Surg* 1991; **5**: 375–81.

33 McCready RA, Pairolero PC, Gilmore JC et al. Isolated iliac artery aneurysms. *Surgery* 1983; **93**: 688–93.

34 Lowry SF, Kraft RO. Isolated aneurysms of the iliac artery. *Arch Surg* 1978; **113**: 1289–93.

35 Sacks NPM, Huddy SPJ, Wegner T et al. Management of solitary iliac aneurysms. *J Cardiovasc Surg* 1992; **33**: 679–83.

36 Dake MD, Miller C, Semba CP et al. Transluminal placement of endovascular stent-grafts for the treatment of descending thoracic aortic aneurysms. *N Engl J Med* 1994; **331**: 1729–34.

37 May J, White G, Waugh R et al. Transluminal placement of a prosthetic graft-stent device for treatment of subclavian artery aneurysm. *J Vasc Surg* 1993; **18**: 1056–9.

38 Marin ML, Veith FJ, Panetta TF et al. Transluminally placed endovascular stented graft repair for arterial trauma. *J Vasc Surg* 1994; **20**: 466–73.

39 Cragg AH, Dake MD. Percutaneous femoropopliteal graft placement. *Radiology* 1993; **187**: 643–8.

40 Schuler JJ, Flanigan DP. Iliac artery aneurysms. In: Bergan JJ, Yao JST (eds), Aneurysms: Diagnosis and Treatment. New York: Grune & Stratton, 1982: 469–85.

41 Brin B, Busuttil R. Isolated hypogastric artery aneurysms. *Arch Surg* 1982; **117**: 1329–33.

42 Kasulke RJ, Clifford A, Nichols W et al. Isolated atherosclerotic aneurysms of the internal iliac arteries. *Arch Surg* 1982; **117**: 73–7.

43 Reilly MK, Abbott WM, Darling RC. Aggressive surgical management of popliteal artery aneurysms. *Am J Surg* 1983; **145**: 498–502.

44 Marin ML, Veith FJ, Panetta TF et al. Transfemoral endoluminal stented graft repair of a popliteal artery aneurysm. *J Vasc Surg* 1994; **19**: 754–7.

45 Schellack J, Smith RB III, Perdue GD. Nonoperative management of selected popliteal aneurysms. *Arch Surg* 1987; **122**: 372–5.

46 Morris GC, Edwards W, Cooley DA et al. Surgical importance of profunda femoris artery: analysis of 102 cases with combined aorto-iliac and femoro-popliteal occlusive disease treated by revascularization of deep femoral artery. *Arch Surg* 1961; **82**: 52–7.

47 Reuter SR, Carson SN. Thrombosis of a common iliac artery aneurysm by selective embolization and extraanatomic bypass. *Am J Roentgenol* 1980; **134**: 1248–50.

48   Michaels JA, McWhinnie D, Hands LJ et al. Iliac aneurysm treated by percutaneous occlusion and femorofemoral crossover grafting. *Fr J Surg* 1994; **81**: 37–8.

49   Vorwerk D, Gunther RW, Wendt G et al. Ulcerated plaques and focal aneurysms of iliac arteries: treatment with noncovered, self-expanding stents. *Am J Roentgenol* 1994; **162**: 1421–4.

50   Deb B, Benjamin M, Comerota AJ. Delayed rupture of an internal iliac artery aneurysm following proximal ligation for abdominal aortic aneurysm repair. *Ann Vasc Surg* 1992; **6**: 537–40.

51   Kwaan JHM, Dahl RK. Fatal rupture after successful surgical thrombosis of an abdominal aortic aneurysm. *Surgery* 1984; **95**: 235–7.

52   Schanzer H, Papa MC, Miller CM. Rupture of surgically thrombosed abdominal aortic aneurysm. *J Vasc Surg* 1985; **2**: 278–80.

53   Cho SI, Johnson WC, Bush HL Jr et al. Lethal complications associated with nonrestrictive treatment of abdominal aortic aneurysms. *Arch Surg* 1982; **117**: 1214–7.

54   Hollis HW Jr, Luethke JM, Yakes WF et al. Percutaneous embolization of an internal iliac artery aneurysm: technical considerations and literature review. *JVIR* 1994; **5**: 449–51.

55   Dotter CT. Transluminally placed coil spring endarterial tube grafts: long term patency in canine popliteal artery. *Invest Radiol* 1969; **4**: 329–32.

56   Cragg AH, Lund G, Rysavy JA et al. Percutaneous arterial grafting. *Radiology* 1985; **150**: 45–9.

57   Balko B, Piasceck GJ, Dhiraj MS et al. Transfemoral placement of intraluminal polyurethane prosthesis for abdominal aneurysm. *J Surg Res* 1986; **40**: 305–9.

58   Lawrence DD, Charnsangevej C, Wright KC et al. Percutaneous endovascular graft: experimental evaluation. *Radiology* 1987; **163**: 357–60.

59   Laborde JC, Parodi JC, Clem MF et al. Intraluminal bypass of abdominal aortic aneurysm: feasibility study. *Radiology* 1992; **184**: 185–90.

60   Boudghene F, Anidjar S, Allaire E et al. Endovascular grafting in elastase-induced experimental aortic aneurysms in dogs: feasibility and preliminary results. *JVIR* 1993; **4**: 497–504.

61   Mirich D, Wright KC, Wallace S et al. Percutaneously placed endovascular grafts for aortic aneurysms: feasibility study. *Radiology* 1989; **170**: 1033–7.

62   Parodi JC. Endovascular repair of abdominal aortic aneurysms. *Adv Vasc Surg* 1993; **1**: 85–106.

63   Chuter TAM, Green RM, Ouriel K et al. Transfemoral endovascular aortic graft placement. *J Vasc Surg* 1993; **18**: 185–97.

64   Marin ML, Veith FJ. Transfemoral repair of abdominal aortic aneurysms. *N Engl J Med* 1994; **331**: 1751.

65   Marin ML, Veith FJ, Panetta TF et al. Percutaneous transfemoral stented graft repair of a traumatic femoral arteriovenous fistula. *J Vasc Surg* 1993; **18**: 298–301.

66   Dorros G, Cohn JM, Jaff M. Percutaneous endovascular stent graft repair of iliac artery aneurysms. *J Endovasc Surg* 1997; **4**: 370–5.

67   Blais C, Bonneau D. Postangioplasty pseudoaneurysm treated with a vascular stent. *Am J Roentgenol* 1994; **162**: 238–9.

68   O'Brien CJM, Rankin RN. Percutaneous management of large-neck aneurysms with arterial stent placement and coils embolization. *JVIR* 1994; **5**: 443–8.

69   Parodi JC. Endovascular repair of abdominal aortic aneurysms and other arterial lesions. *J Vasc Surg* 1995; **21**: 549–57.

70   Cragg AH, DeJong S, Barnhart W et al. Nitinol intravascular stent: results of preclinical evaluation. *Radiology* 1993; **189**: 775–8.

71   Hausseger KA, Cragg AH, Lammer J et al. Iliac artery stenting: clinical experience with a nitinol stent. *Radiology* 1994; **190**: 199–202.

72   Lee JH, Park JB, Andreasen GF et al. Thermomechanical study of Ni-Ti alloys. *J Biomed Mater Res* 1988; **22**: 573–88.

73   Chalmers RTA, Hoballah JJ, Sharp WJ et al. Effect of an endovascular stent on healing of an end-to-end polytetrafluoroethylene artery anastomosis in a canine model. *Br J Surg* 1994; **81**: 1443–7.

74   Henry M, Amor M, Ethevenot G et al. Initial experience with the Cragg Endopro System 1 for intraluminal treatment of peripheral vascular disease. *J Endovasc Surg* 1994; **1**: 31–43.

75   Becker GJ, Benenati JF, Zemel G et al. Percutaneous placement of a balloon-expandable intraluminal graft for life threatening subclavian arterial hemorrhage. *JVIR* 1991; **2**: 225–9.

76   Marin ML, Veith FJ, Cynamon J et al. Transfemoral endovascular stented graft treatment of aortoiliac and femoropopliteal occlusive disease for limb salvage. *Am J Surg* 1994; **168**: 156–262.

48

Endovascular stent–grafts for the treatment of arterial disease

Nicholas J Morrissey and Michael L Marin

Introduction

Covered stents have gained widespread applicability in the treatment of arterial disease since the introduction of this technology by Parodi in 1991.[1] The treatment of aortic and iliac artery aneurysms with endovascular devices has progressed rapidly with a number of commercially made devices approved or undergoing clinical trials. Early devices were 'homemade' by surgeons or interventionalists specifically for the case at hand. Out of this early manufacturing, a number of principles of stent–graft design were developed. The use of stent–grafts has reached beyond treatment of aneurysms to applications in occlusive disease as well as trauma. This review will focus on the devices used in treatment of a variety of arterial diseases and the prospects for future application of covered stents.

The earliest stent–grafts for treatment of abdominal aortic aneurysms (AAAs) were made by suturing graft material to balloon-expandable stents. The first report of AAA repair with stent–grafts in humans was published by Parodi in 1991.[1] Early device design was simple and consisted of a thin-walled Dacron graft sutured to a stainless steel Palmaz stent (Figure 48.1). The devices used in these first reports consisted of simple tube graft designed for aneurysms limited to the infrarenal aorta with sufficient proximal and distal normal aorta to allow for implantation (Figure 48.2). The more versatile aortouniiliac design allows for extension of the device into one of the iliac or femoral arteries. The contralateral common iliac artery is then occluded endoluminally to prevent retrograde perfusion of the aneurysm sac. Flow to the contralateral lower limb and pelvis is restored by performing a femoral–femoral bypass (Figure 48.3). Early results with tube devices revealed

Figure 48.1
Modified Parodi endovascular device. The dilated proximal portion of the device is used to seat the graft in the infrarenal aorta. The device then tapers to a caliber appropriate for implantation into the iliac or femoral artery.

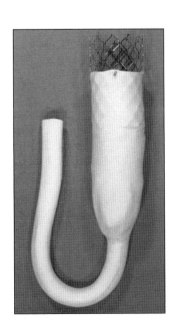

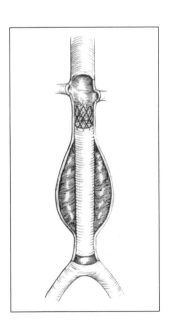

Figure 48.2
A tube device for treatment of infrarenal aortic aneurysm, showing a graft with only a proximal stent. Later versions of tube devices have a stent at both the proximal and distal ends.

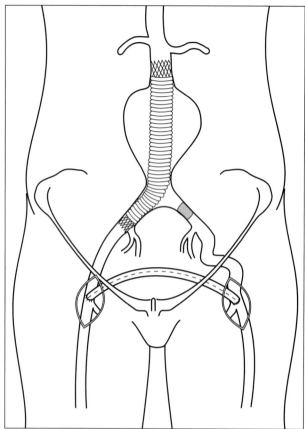

Figure 48.3
Aortouniiliac stent–graft for exclusion of infrarenal AAA. An occluder device in the left iliac artery prevents retrograde perfusion of the aneurysm sac. A femoral–femoral bypass restores flow to the left pelvis and lower extremity.

a relatively high rate of type I endoleak due to attachment site failure.[2] The preferred design for endoluminal devices became a bifurcated system, either modular or unibody.[3] There are a number of devices either approved by the US Food and Drug Administration (FDA) or undergoing clinical trials for use in treatment of AAA. A brief description of a number of representative devices that demonstrate the ongoing evolution of this technology is appropriate.

Endovascular stent–grafts

Guidant (Ancure™) endovascular device

This device was approved for use in the United States in 1999. The Ancure is a bifurcated unibody system. There are stents only at the proximal and distal attachment points, with the rest of the graft unsupported. The proximal and distal stents have

hooks that are designed to enhance attachment at these crucial points. Results of clinical trials were published in 1997[3] and an update has been recently published.[4] There was a 1.5% mortality rate, and a 9% initial endoleak rate, with 50% of these resolving with observation alone. Only 20 patients out of 669 required conversion to open repair.[3] There have been no reports of aneurysm rupture in patients treated with the Ancure stent–graft. The current delivery system for the Ancure is 27F, which requires open exposure of the common femoral artery for placement. In addition, smaller arteries may not accommodate this size delivery sheath, in which case placement via the iliac artery may be necessary.

This device has recently been removed from the market due to delivery system issues.

Medtronic AneuRx™ device

A second device which was approved by the US FDA in 1999 is the AneuRx system (Figure 48.4).[5] This bifurcated device is modular, requiring separate implantation of the second limb through the contralateral femoral artery. The second limb is docked within the main body device (Figure 48.4). The modular design introduces the risk of leak at this junction (type III endoleak), which is reduced by mandatory overlap between the second limb and the main body. The AneuRx features a woven polyester graft that is fully supported externally by nitinol stents (Figure 48.4). The early design of the stent–graft was felt to be too rigid to adjust to changes in the aneurysm morphology and was blamed for early cases of device migration and delayed rupture.[6] The device design was altered to allow more flexibility of the whole system and theoretically decrease the risk of migration. The Ancure and AneuRx are the only products currently approved by the FDA for use in the United States.

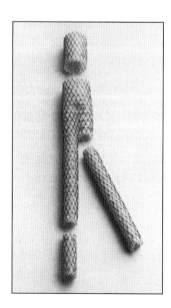

Figure 48.4
Medtronic AneuRx™ bifurcated stent–graft. The modular system also has proximal and distal extensions if needed to fully reconstruct the aortoiliac segment.

Figure 48.5

Proximal aspect of Talent™ aortic stent–graft. This view demonstrates the proximal bare stent that secures the device across the renal segment.

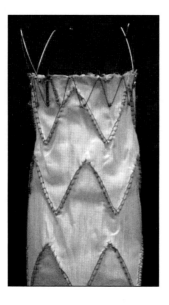

The Talent™ (Medtronic) endovascular stent–graft

This device is also a modular bifurcated system, although tube and aortouniiliac systems are also available. The device is made of Dacron, fully supported by internal nitinol stents. A notable feature of the Talent device is the long bare stent segment at the proximal end of the device (Figure 48.5). This bare stent is situated across the renal artery orifices following deployment. Such a transrenal segment allows fixation of the device along a longer segment of normal aorta and may improve the quality of the seal between the aorta and the stent–graft.[7] The ends of the limb segments may be made with the fabric cut flush with the stents (closed web) or with the fabric shaped to the configuration of the stent (open web). Alternatively, the distal stents may be uncovered (bare spring). The flexibility in distal limb configurations allows custom design of the iliac limbs so iliac aneurysms can be excluded while maintaining patency of the internal iliac arteries. The Talent stent–graft has undergone phase I and II trials in the United States, and has been used extensively in Europe and the United States.[8] The initial endoleak rate was 19%, with 75% of these leaks sealing spontaneously within 30 days. Approval for use in the United States is pending.

The Cook Zenith™ endovascular stent–graft

The Zenith system from Cook consists of woven polyester graft material supported throughout its length with self-expanding Z-stents. The device is a modular bifurcated design, but is also available in aortouniiliac configuration (Figure 48.6). The introducer tip is tapered to minimize

trauma to the artery at the insertion site and there are side holes to allow for angiography through the tip. The Zenith stent–graft has a proximal bare stent that expands radially upon deployment. There are hooks at the proximal aspect of the bare stent to secure the device suprarenally (Figure 48.6) The proximal bare stent is deployed after pulling a trigger wire that holds the stent in place to prevent premature deployment. A recent review of 528 patients treated with the Zenith device was reported.[9] The early endoleak rate was 15%, and there were three late conversions, two due to aneurysm rupture. The Cook Zenith device has recently been approved for use in the United States.

Gore Excluder™ endoprosthesis

The Excluder stent–graft system is a modular bifurcated system. It is made of thin-walled ePTFE (polytetrafluoroethylene), externally supported throughout its length with nitinol stents (Figure 48.7). The main body is delivered through an 18F sheath, while the contralateral limb is delivered through a 12F sheath (Figure 48.8). There are no transrenal stents, but there is an external sealing cuff of PTFE at the proximal stent to increase sealing at the proximal attachment site. This device is deployed rapidly by pulling a PTFE fiber line after confirming the proper position angiographically. Results in the first 29 cases have been reported and phase II data are being analyzed at present.[10]

The excluder was recently approved for use in the US.

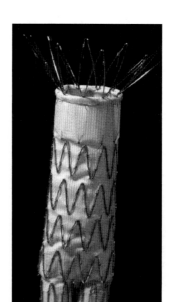

Figure 48.6

Proximal aspect of the Cook Zenith™ endovascular graft. Note the proximal bare stent with attachment barbs and the Z-stents supporting the graft.

Figure 48.7
Gore Excluder™ AAA endovascular prosthesis. This modular device is composed of ePTFE, supported by a nitinol stent framework.

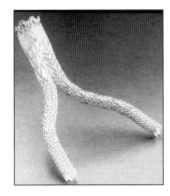

More advanced features being developed by Teramed include renal and iliac artery side branch technology. A bifurcated iliac limb is currently being studied which allows for stent–grafting of the internal and external iliac arteries. The Teramed Tributary™ system allows the device to exclude common iliac aneurysms that extend up to the bifurcation and also to exclude internal iliac aneurysms. A device with renal artery side branches has also been developed. This stent–graft will allow coverage of the aorta at and above the renal arteries, while maintaining renal artery perfusion. Such innovations in stent–graft technology will make endovascular therapy of AAA applicable to more challenging lesions.

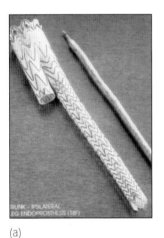

(a)

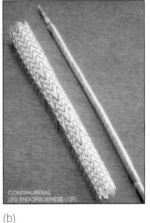

(b)

Figure 48.8
Main body (a) and contralateral limb (b) of Gore Excluder endoprosthesis with delivery sheaths shown.

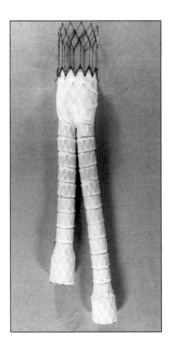

Figure 48.9
Cordis–Quantum™ AAA stent–graft. Note the long transrenal bare stent with large interstices. There are attachment hooks at the distal aspect of the bare stent. The graft is fully supported internally with a nitinol stent framework.

Cordis–Quantum™ endovascular stent–graft

The Quantum (Cordis Endovascular)™ is a bifurcated modular device with an internal nitinol framework supporting the entire graft. There is a long suprarenal bare stent with large interstices to maintain renal and visceral arterial flow. In addition, the large openings in the bare stent portion make it possible to perform catheter-based interventions through the stent (Figure 48.9). The limbs of the Quantum™ device feature variable overlap so that each limb can be lengthened or shortened *in situ* to most accurately position the device in the iliac artery (Figure 48.10). This custom in-situ sizing allows one device size to be used for nearly all iliac artery configurations. Another feature of the limbs is the relatively narrow long segment that flares out to a distal 'bell-bottom' shape (Figure 48.10). This configuration allows easy passage of both limbs of the device through even narrow distal aortic bifurcations, while the distal wider segment can form a seal in larger-diameter common iliac segments.

Figure 48.10
Cordis–Quantum™ bifurcated stent–graft. Note the different lengths of the iliac limbs. Each limb may be overlapped a variable amount in order to size the device *in situ*. Also note the 'bell-bottom' configuration of the distal ends of the device. The device is modular.

Stent–grafts in the treatment of thoracic aneurysms

The thoracic aorta poses special challenges for endovascular techniques. Lesions are often near the angulated aortic arch and its major branch vessels, making secure sealing of a device challenging. Visceral and spinal cord vessels are a factor when dealing with extensive thoracic and thoracoabdominal lesions, and device delivery systems may be too large to navigate access vessels. An early series of thoracic aorta aneurysms (TAAs) treated with 'homemade' devices was reported by Dake and colleagues.[11] Endoleaks, paraplegia, and stroke were significant complications. Greenberg et al. also reported a smaller series of 25 cases.[12] Once again, endoleak and paralysis were significant issues. Paraplegia seemed to be related to the amount of thoracic aorta that was covered by the device.[12]

Currently, the Gore Thoracic Excluder and Talent thoracic stent–graft are under investigation in high-risk patients (Figure 48.11). Development of devices that allow for stent grafting of branch vessels of the arch and visceral aorta appear to be the next stage of development in thoracic aortic endografting.

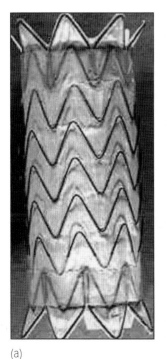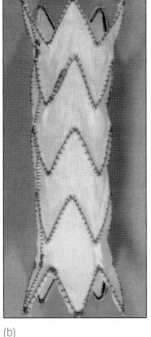

(a)   (b)

Figure 48.11

The Gore Thoracic Excluder™ (a) and Talent™ thoracic stent–graft (b).

Stent–grafts for repair of para-anastomotic aneurysms

One of the dreaded long-term complications of open repair of aortic and/or iliac aneurysmal or occlusive disease is the development of false or true para-anastomotic aneurysms (PAAAs). Studies indicate that 10–36% of aortoiliac replacements will result in PAA formation if followed for 15 years.[13] The risk of rupture of these lesions is real enough to warrant early treatment following their diagnosis. Open repair of PAAs carries a high morbidity and mortality rate due to the age and comorbidities of the patients as well as the hazard of reoperative aortic surgery.[14] Endovascular therapy for these lesions would be ideal given the poor outcomes associated with open repair. We have recently reported our experience with treatment of 35 PAAs of the aorta (abdominal and thoracic) and iliac arteries using stent–grafts.[15] Operative mortality was 0%, while initial success was 100%. There was one mortality at 30 days and a complication rate of 14.2%.

Devices used included homemade and commercially available aortouniiliac as well as bifurcated aortic prostheses. Some of the configurations of PAAs encountered in our patient population are seen in Figures 48.12–48.14. Tube grafts were used in several iliac and thoracic PAA cases. Figure 48.15 illustrates an iliac artery PAA which was successfully treated with a tube stent–graft. These results are a significant improvement over the high morbidity and mortality rates associated with open repair of PAAs. It seems reasonable to assert that endovascular therapy is the treatment of choice for PAAs of the aorta and iliac arteries. Since PAAs are highly variable in their location and number, the particular device suited to a particular lesion must be chosen based on these anatomic factors.

Endovascular therapy for arterial trauma

Direct injury to the arterial system may be iatrogenic or the result of blunt or penetrating injuries. Trauma to an artery can result in laceration, dissection, pseudoaneurysm formation, or traumatic arteriovenous fistula formation. The ability to treat major vascular injuries with a minimally invasive approach has obvious advantages.[16] Shorter operative times, less invasive techniques, and avoidance of placing exposed graft material in potentially contaminated fields are a few potential advantages. Patients with arterial trauma are frequently unstable or require attention to other injured systems and therefore pose a significant challenge. In addition, since trauma is not scheduled, the therapist must have enough devices available to treat injuries to arteries and veins of varying sizes.

Our early experience involved ePTFE grafts sutured to balloon-expandable stents, which were then mounted, on

Figure 48.12

Bilateral common liac artery PAAs and their treatment with a bifurcated aortoiliac stent–graft.

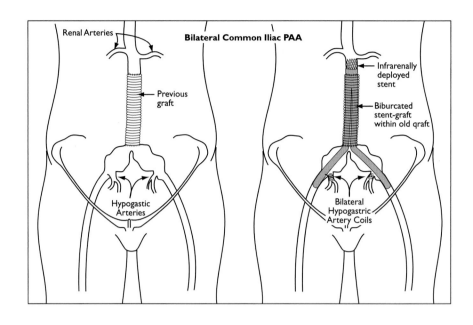

Figure 48.13

Proximal aortic and common iliac artery PAAs and their treatment with a bifurcated stent–graft.

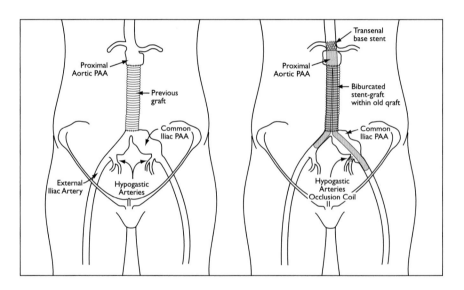

Figure 48.14

An iliac artery PAA at the arising at the distal anastomosis of a bifurcated aortoiliac graft. The lesion was treated with a tube stent–graft.

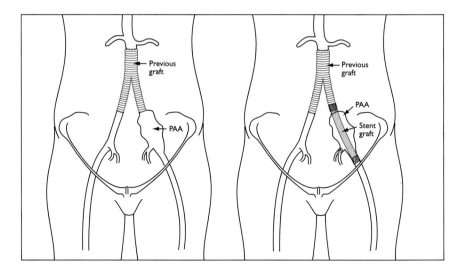

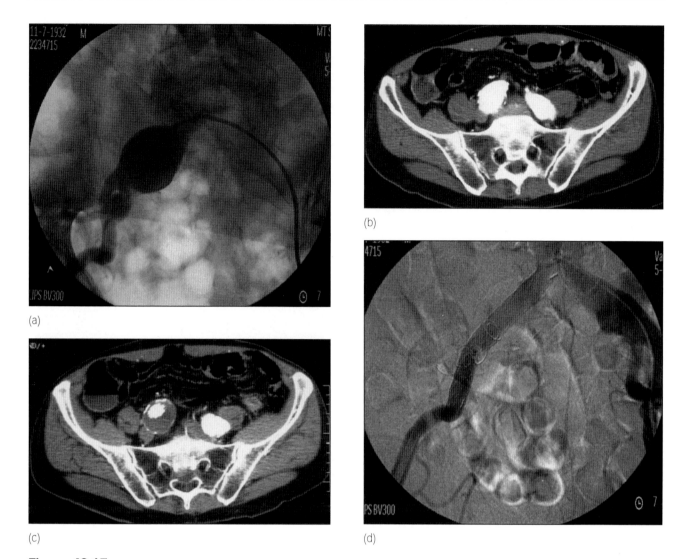

(a)

(b)

(c)

(d)

Figure 48.15

(a) and (b) angiogram and CT scan of a common iliac artery PAA. (c) and (d) CT scan and angiogram following successful exclusion of this PAA with a covered stent.

balloon catheters (Figure 48.16). The apparatus is then placed into a delivery sheath for placement via remote arteriotomy. (Figure 48.17). These devices can be made to various lengths and diameters, depending on the injured vessel.

The device can be used to obliterate a traumatic arteriovenous (AV) fistula, as shown in Figure 48.18. In the cases of AVFs and pseudoaneurysms, shorter devices are generally adequate. A pseudoaneurysm of the axillary artery caused by a gunshot wound is shown in Figure 48.19. This lesion was successfully treated by deploying a covered stent over the disrupted area of the artery (Figure 48.20). Schematic representations of the injury and endovascular treatment of an axillary artery pseudoaneurysm are shown in Figure 48.21.

It is now possible to use commercially available covered stents to treat injuries of the arterial tree. One of the devices currently available is the Wallgraft™ from Boston Scientific Medi-Tech Corporation (Natick, MA). This device features a self-expanding stent covered with thin polyester fabric (Figure 48.22). Such a system should prove to be useful in dealing with short segment arterial injuries in medium- to large-sized vessels. Injuries to the femoral, subclavian, iliac, axillary and, even, common carotid arteries may be effectively treated with this device. It is available in diameters from 5 to 12 mm and lengths of 20–70 mm. An example of a carotid artery pseudoaneurysm treated with a covered stent is shown in Figures 48.23–48.25.[17] Traumatic disruptions of the thoracic aorta have also been successfully treated with endovascular devices such as those seen in Figure 48.11.[18] With stent–grafts becoming available in many sizes and configurations, most arterial injuries will be approached initially with an attempt at endovascular therapy.

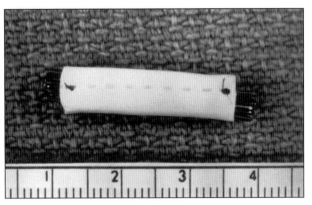

Figure 48.16
'Homemade' stent graft made from ePTFE graft sutured to stainless steel Palmaz stent.

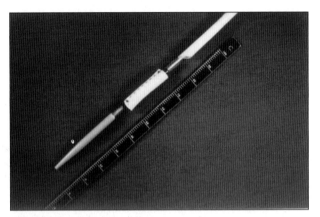

Figure 48.17
The device from Figure 46.19 is shown mounted on a balloon catheter, which will be back-loaded into the sheath shown.

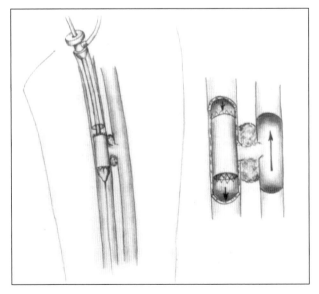

Figure 48.18
Diagram showing the exclusion of a femoral AV fistula with a covered stent.

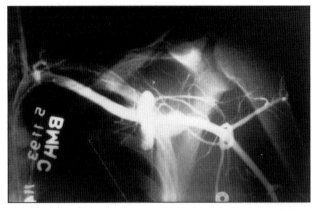

Figure 48.19
Axillary artery pseudoaneurysm caused by a gunshot wound.

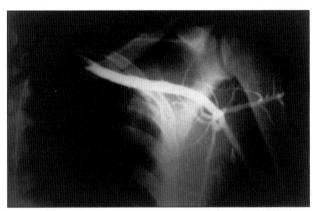

Figure 48.20
Successful exclusion of the pseudoaneurysm with a covered stent.

Covered stents in the treatment of arterial occlusive disease

Angioplasty and stenting of peripheral arterial occlusive lesions is gaining wider applicability as studies demonstrate improved results. The best results for this technology continue to be in cases of iliac artery occlusive disease. Shorter lesions tend to respond better to endovascular therapy. The use of covered stents allows an aggressive angioplasty to be performed while maintaining integrity of the arterial wall (Figure 48.26). It may also be helpful to reline the angioplastied arterial segment with a smooth prosthetic surface, although this concept is purely speculative. Stents coated with pharmacologic agents to prevent restenosis are being used in coronary arteries. These devices may be useful in peripheral arterial occlusive disease and are the subject of aggressive research.

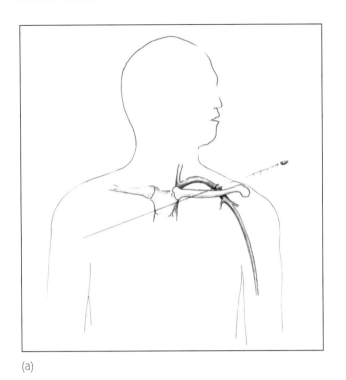

(a)

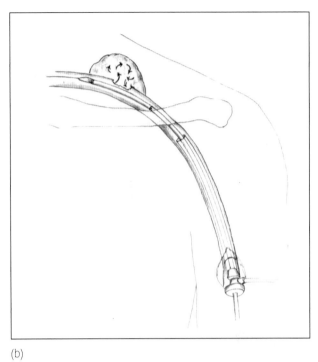

(b)

Figure 48.21
(a) An axillary artery pseudoaneurysm. (b) Endovascular device being introduced to exclude pseudoaneurysm.

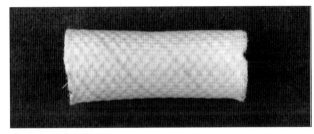

Figure 48.22
Wallgraft™ endoprosthesis, which may be used in the treatment of traumatic, occlusive, or aneurysmal lesions of medium- to large-sized arteries.

Summary

Since their introduction for the treatment of AAA in 1991, covered stents have become used with increasing frequency for a variety of pathologic arterial processes. These devices are especially suited to excluding lesions such as true or false aneurysms. The major benefits of endovascular therapy include, but are not limited to, less-invasive approach, shorter hospital stay, and faster recovery. Perhaps we will add improved overall outcomes to this list as long-term data become available. The results for para-anastomotic aneurysms seem to indicate that endovascular therapy should be the treatment of choice for these lesions. In addition, traumatic arterial injuries seem especially suited to endovascular repair with covered stents.

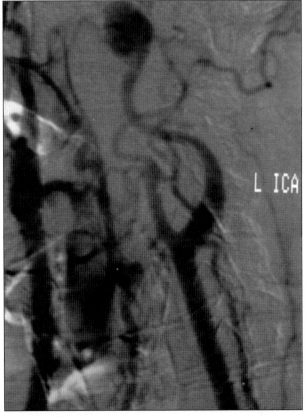

Figure 48.23
Angiogram of a carotid artery pseudoaneurysm.

Figure 48.24
Intraoperative image of the lesion shown in Figure 48.25.

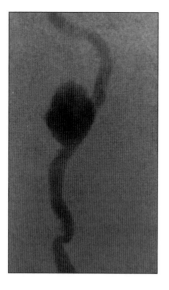

Figure 48.25
Completion angiogram, showing successful exclusion of carotid artery pseudoaneurysm.

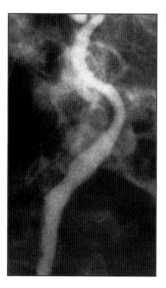

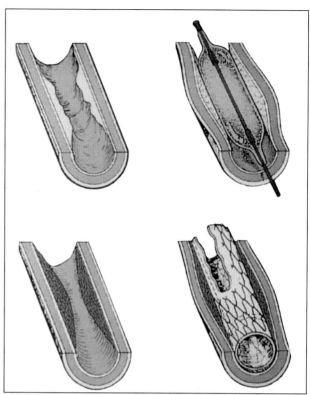

Figure 48.26
Balloon angioplasty of an atherosclerotic lesion. Angioplasty is followed by relining the arterial lumen with a covered stent.

The technology remains somewhat primitive and many lesions remain unsuitable for endovascular repair. As branch vessel technology and lower-profile devices become available, the scope of endovascular therapy will increase. At present, aggressive endovascular therapists can combine open and endovascular techniques to offer creative solutions to patients with complex arterial lesions. The role of covered stents in peripheral arterial occlusive disease has not yet been established. Data need to be collected to determine if covered or bioengineered stents will be of any use in the endoluminal treatment of lesions in the iliac or infrainguinal arterial tree.

References

1 Parodi JC, Palmaz JC, Barone HD. Transfemoral intraluminal graft implantation for abdominal aortic aneurysms. *Ann Vasc Surg* 1991; **5**: 491–9.

2 Moore WS. The EVT tube and bifurcated endograft systems: technical considerations and clinical summary. *J Endovasc Surg* 1997; **4**: 182–94.

3 Chuter TAM, Risberg B, Hopkinson BR et al. Clinical experience with a bifurcated endovascular graft for abdominal aortic aneurysm repair. *J Vasc Surg* 1996; 24: 655–66.

4 Makaroun MS. The Ancure endografting system: an update. *J Vasc Surg* 2001; **33**: S129–34.

5 Zarins CK, White RA, Schwarten D et al. for the investigators of the Medtronic AneuRx Multicenter Clinical Trial. AneuRx stent–graft vs open surgical repair of abdominal aortic aneurysms: multicenter prospective clinical trial. *J Vasc Surg* 1999; **29**: 292–308.

6 Zarins CK, White RA, Fogarty TJ. Aneurysm rupture after endovascular repair using the AneuRx stent–graft. *J Vasc Surg* 2000; **31**: 960–70.

7 Marin ML, Parsons RE, Hollier LH et al. Impact of transrenal aortic endograft placement on endovascular graft repair of abdominal aortic aneurysms *J Vasc Surg* 1998; **28**: 638–46.

8 Criado FJ, Wilson EP, Fairman RM et al. Update on the Talent aortic stent–graft: a preliminary report from the United States phase I and II trials. *J Vasc Surg* 2001; **33**: S146–9.

9   Greenberg RK, Lawrence-Brown M, Bhandari G et al. An update of the Zenith endovascular graft for abdominal aortic aneurysms: initial implantation and mid-term follow-up data. *J Vasc Surg* 2001; **33**: S157–64.

10 Matsumura JS, Katzen BT, Hollier LH, Dake MD. Update on the bifurcated EXCLUDER endoprosthesis: phase I results. *J Vasc Surg* 2001; **33**: S150–3.

11 Mitchell RS, Miller DC, Dake MD. Stent–graft repair of thoracic aortic aneurysms. *Semin Vasc Surg* 1997; **10**(4): 257–71.

12 Greenberg R, Resch T, Nyman U et al. Endovascular repair of descending thoracic aortic aneurysms: an early experience with intermediate-term follow-up. *J Vasc Surg* 2000; **31**: 147–56.

13 Edwards JM, Teeffey FA, Zierler RE, Kohler TR. Intra-abdominal para-anastomotic aneurysms after aortic bypass grafting. *J Vasc Surg* 1992; **15**: 344–53.

14 Allen RC, Schneider J, Longnecker L et al. Para-anastomotic aneurysms of the abdominal aorta. *J Vasc Surg* 1993; **18**: 424–32.

15 Morrissey NJ, Yano OJ, Soundarajan K et al. Endovascular repair of paraanastomotic aneurysms of the aorta and iliac arteries: preferred approach for a complex problem *J Vasc Surg* 2001; **34**: 503–12.

16 Marin ML, Veith FJ, Panetta TF. Transluminally placed endovascular stented-graft repair for arterial trauma. *J Vasc Surg* 1994; **20**: 466–73.

17 Reiter BP, Marin ML, Teodorescu VJ et al. Endoluminal repair of an internal carotid artery pseudoaneurysm. *J Vasc Intervent Radiol* 1998; **9**: 245–8.

18 Desphande A, Mossop P, Gurry J et al. Treatment of traumatic false aneurysm of the thoracic aorta with endoluminal grafts. *J Endovasc Surg* 1998; **5**: 120–5.

49

Interventions in aortoarteritis

KA Abraham and Sriram Rajagopal

Introduction

Non-specific aortoarteritis (Takayasu's arteritis) is a chronic inflammatory disease of unknown etiology primarily involving the aorta and its major branches.[1] Inflammation leads to stenosis or occlusion of the affected vessels and occasionally to dilation. Pulmonary artery involvement, coronary artery disease and valvular heart disease have also been described.[2] The disease is seen relatively more frequently in Asia, though cases have been reported worldwide. Clinical features are related to inflammation in the early stages and to the effects of stenotic or occlusive changes in the chronic stage with absent pulses, hypertension, congestive failure and ischemia in the territory of the involved vessels. Several diagnostic criteria have been proposed to identify this disease.[1,3–5] The disease has also been classified into subtypes based on the pattern of involvement.[3,5–9] Medical therapy consists of anti-inflammatory agents and immunosuppressants. There are a few reports of surgical treatment,[10–14] but catheter-based interventional treatment is increasingly being used with encouraging results.[15–38]

The pathology is strikingly different from atherosclerosis and influences both interventional and surgical treatment. The pathologic changes involve all three layers of the vessel wall. Histologically, the active phase is characterized by inflammation and granuloma formation, while the chronic phase shows extensive intimal and adventitial thickening with scarring of the media. The marked thickening of the adventitia and intima produce lesions which can be extremely resistant to balloon dilation. The perivascular and mural changes make surgery very difficult. The diffuse involvement of the vessels with the frequent occurrence of long lesions adds to the therapeutic challenge. Several prognostic factors have been identified which influence the natural history.[8,39–41] Revascularization, whether surgical or interventional, is preferably performed when the disease is not in an active phase (which is usually diagnosed by the presence of systemic signs and an erythrocyte sedimentation rate above 20 mm), as procedures done during the active stage have been associated with a poorer outcome.[13,42]

Technical aspects in general

Pre-procedural evaluation

This should include a complete clinical examination with a view to assess the extent of disease as well as indicate possible approaches for access. Disease activity, manifested by systemic signs and vessel tenderness as well as elevated erythrocyte sedimentation rate, should be ruled out. If activity is detected, the patient is treated with corticosteroids until activity is suppressed, deferring intervention, if possible, until this is achieved. Detailed non-invasive evaluation, particularly with duplex Doppler ultrasonography, and in selected cases computed tomography or magnetic resonance angiography, is useful before proceeding to angiography. Angiography remains the mainstay of investigation to document the extent and severity of disease and decide on the management approach. All patients are pretreated with aspirin (325 mg o.d.) and ticlopidine (250 mg twice-daily) for at least 48 h prior to the procedure.

Vascular access

The femoral artery is usually the preferred access site, as it permits the use of large introducers etc. (except in small children, where even this site may have limitations). In certain cases a brachial approach may be needed, particularly in subclavian artery lesions (in addition to a femoral approach), as the lesion may not be crossable from the femoral approach. If the brachial pulse is not palpable, an arteriotomy may be required. When both subclavians are blocked (as happens not infrequently) and if the aorta is also occluded, a trans-septal approach with a long kink-resistant sheath has been described for access to the central aorta and arch vessels.[38]

Crossing the lesion

Stenotic lesions can be crossed with appropriate steerable or hydrophilic wires. Hydrophilic wires (straight or angled) in conjunction with angled or straight catheters also permit crossing of most occlusions. Approaching an occlusion from both ends is sometimes required. Once a wire is through a lesion it can be snared using an appropriate snare and brought to a convenient access site. Subtotal occlusions, particularly in the carotids, may require use of a floppy-tip 0.014-inch coronary wire with an over-the-wire low-profile coronary balloon or a microcatheter, to cross the lesion. Once the balloon or catheter is across, it is used to exchange to a stiffer wire, preferably a 0.018-inch wire.

Angioplasty

The use of a long sheath (or a guiding catheter), where practicable, is helpful, not only for angiography during the procedure, but also for pressure measurements and during stent deployment. Whenever possible, a 0.035-inch extra-stiff wire should be placed across the lesion (exceptions obviously being the carotid or renal arteries). Use of balloons with the lowest profile and which are non-compliant with high burst pressures is advisable. The last two features are particularly important, as often quite high pressures have to be used. Aorto-ostial lesions are usually treated with balloon-expandable stents, particularly those with high radial force. Long lesions in the carotid or subclavian arteries can be treated with self-expanding stents.

Factors affecting procedure outcome and complications

Disease activity

Intervention is preferably avoided during the active phase.

Lesion length

Longer lesions appear to have a worse outcome and higher restenosis rate.[16,32]

High-pressure dilation

Though often required, this occasionally results in balloon rupture, which can be associated with damage to the vessel being treated.[42]

Balloon–artery diameter ratio

Conservative balloon sizing is advisable, as overdilation, particularly with high pressures, can be dangerous. Even with appropriate balloon sizing (i.e. not exceeding 1 : 1), fatal aortic rupture has been reported.[43]

Inadequate stent expansion

Despite use of high pressures, it may occasionally be impossible to expand a stent fully, leading to the angiographic appearance of a deformed stent, due to the vessel being extremely rigid. The use of rotational atherectomy to alter vessel compliance has been reported in this connection,[43] though burr size obviously restricts the use to small-diameter vessels. Inadequate stent expansion may increase restenosis risk.

Age of the patient

Children appear to have a higher restenosis rate than adults, at least for renal angioplasty.[44]

Lesions at specific sites
Descending thoracic aorta

Lesions at this site commonly present with hypertension and (particularly in children) congestive cardiac failure. The hypertension may be due to both a mechanical component and renal hypoperfusion, as the kidneys are perfused at relatively low pressure. The increased afterload contributes to the failure and may often result in significant systolic dysfunction of the left ventricle. Dramatic reversal of both congestive failure and ventricular dysfunction may be seen after successful angioplasty (Figures 49.1 and 49.2). Linear dissections are often seen after balloon dilation, but these often remodel favourably (Figure 49.3). Stents, either balloon-expandable or self-expanding, have been used to optimize angioplasty results.

Abdominal aorta

The stenosed segment may be suprarenal, infrarenal or extend across the renal arteries. If the lesion is close to the renal artery, placement of a wire in the renal artery is advisable to preserve access. Large series have been reported with more than 90% procedural success.[44] Complications have been relatively rare, and are usually long dissections which can be managed with stents. One case of extravasation with retroperitoneal leak has been reported.[44] Both hypertension and claudication are usually significantly improved.

Supraaortic arteries
Innominate and carotid arteries

Lesions in the arch vessels often involve multiple vessels. Not infrequently, the patient has only one vessel providing cerebral supply, and this may also be diseased (Figure 49.4). Lesions in the carotid are often long and diffuse, and can be technically very challenging. The use of coronary wires, long coronary or other low-profile balloons, and long self-expanding stents is required. The risk of embolization is extremely low. Care must be taken to ensure that the syndrome of cerebral hyperperfusion is avoided, as these patients often get adapted to cerebral perfusion at very low pressures when multiple vessels are affected (Figure 49.5).

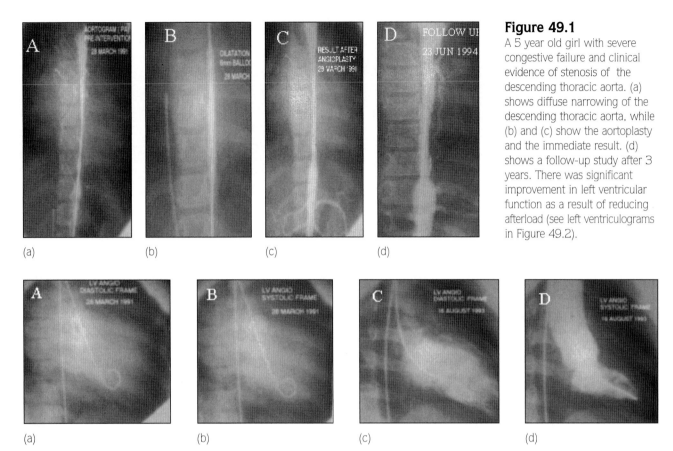

(a)   (b)   (c)   (d)

Figure 49.1
A 5 year old girl with severe congestive failure and clinical evidence of stenosis of the descending thoracic aorta. (a) shows diffuse narrowing of the descending thoracic aorta, while (b) and (c) show the aortoplasty and the immediate result. (d) shows a follow-up study after 3 years. There was significant improvement in left ventricular function as a result of reducing afterload (see left ventriculograms in Figure 49.2).

(a)   (b)   (c)   (d)

Figure 49.2
Left ventriculograms before (upper panel (a) and (b)) and at follow up (lower panel (c) and (d)) showing marked improvement in left ventricular function on follow up late after aortoplasty, with reduction of afterload. (Same patient as in Figure 49.1).

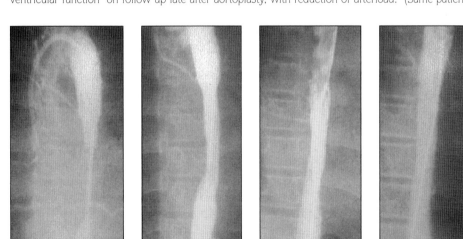

Figure 49.3
Serial aortograms of a patient who underwent dilatation of the descending thoracic aorta showing favourable remodelling of the aorta.

Figure 49.4
Angioplasty and stenting of tight stenosis of sole supra-aortic artery with aortoplasty in a young boy. Note total occlusion of innominate and left common carotid arteries with left vertebral artery providing sole supply to the brain.

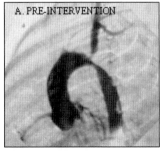
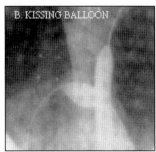
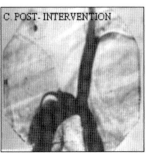

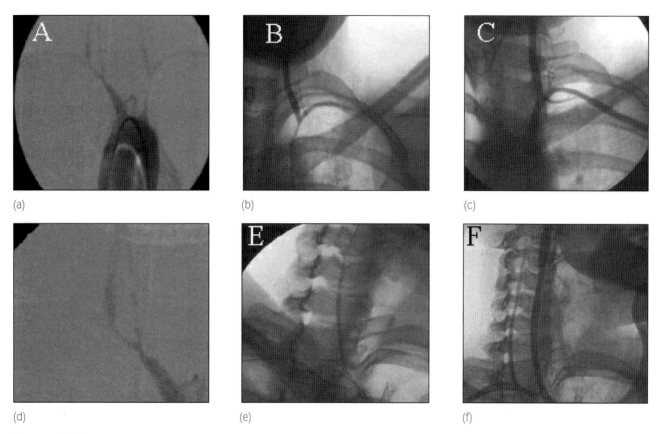

Figure 49.5
Young lady with marked narrowing of the distal innominate, right common carotid and right and left subclavian arteries and total occlusion of the left common carotid artery (a). The cerebral flow is mainly through the vertebral arteries. (b) and (c) show selective left subclavian angiograms before and after angioplasty and stenting of the left subclavian artery. (d) shows the 'string' like narrowing of the right common carotid artery as well as disease of the proximal right subclavian artery. (e) shows initial dilatation of the right common carotid artery with a long coronary balloon with a wire in the right subclavian artery, and (f) shows the final result after placement of a long self-expanding stent in the right common carotid artery with balloon angioplasty of the subclavian artery. The left subclavian artery was dilated first to improve flow through the left vertebral artery and the right common carotid artery was dilated the next day to avoid hyperperfusion syndrome.

Subclavian artery

Subclavian artery lesions are quite common and can be difficult to cross. A bidirectional approach (i.e. a combination of an antegrade and a retrograde approach) from both the aorta and the affected brachial artery is often required. Aorto-ostial lesions are usually treated with balloon-expandable stents, while distal lesions can be treated with self-expanding stents. Acute stent thrombosis and vessel rupture (requiring the use of a covered stent) have been described.[42]

Renal arteries

The overall success rate was 85% in a large series[44] and improved in the later part of the series with the use of a coaxial guiding catheter technique and the use of stents. Average balloon pressure required for angioplasty was 8.1

atmospheres (range 4–17 atmospheres). Major complications were rare. Restenosis after angioplasty was around 17% in patients restudied at 3–41 months. Eighteen patients underwent stent placement, and the procedure was technically successful in all. However, restenosis was reported in 36% of 11 patients, including 3 pediatric patients. All were successfully redilated.[44] Hypertension was reported to be cured in 40% and improved in 51%. Ostial lesions can occasionally prove very resistant, and incomplete stent expansion may occur despite high-pressure dilation (Figure 49.6).

Mesenteric arteries

Balloon angioplasty and stenting have occasionally been used to provide relief of abdominal angina.[36] The technical considerations are similar to those for other lesions described.

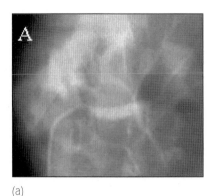
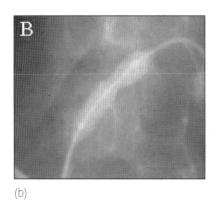
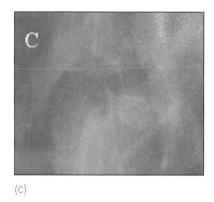

(a)   (b)   (c)

Figure 49.6
Resistant renal artery stenosis in a single functioning kidney in a nine year old boy. (a) shows tight ostial stenosis of the left renal artery. (b) shows the stent not fully expanding at the ostium despite use of a large balloon at high pressure (18 atm) and (c) shows a residual 'waist' on the stent.

Coronary arteries

Coronary ostial stenoses may present as myocardial ischemia or infarction. Successful stenting of unprotected left main coronary stenosis has been reported.[45]

Iliac vessels

Balloon angioplasty of iliac arteries with prolonged relief of claudication has been reported in a few cases.[44]

Conclusions

Percutaneous transluminal angioplasty, with stent implantation in selected situations, is a useful mode of treatment in aortoarteritis (Takayasu's disease) and appears to offer sustained improvement of patient status with an acceptably low complication rate. Future developments will include a better understanding of the pathophysiology of the disease and detection and management of disease activity, better hardware designed to meet the specific technical challenges posed by this disease, and more widespread application of interventional techniques.

References

1   Arend WP, Michel BA, Bloch DA et al. Criteria for the classification of Takayasu arteritis. The American College of Rheumatology. *Arthritis Rheum* 1990; **33**: 1129–34.

2   Kinare S, Gandhi M, Deshpande J. Non-specific aorto-arteritis (Takayasu's Disease) pathology and radiology. *Mumbai, Quest* 1998; 17–66.

3   Ishikawa K. Diagnostic approach and proposed criteria for the clinical diagnosis of Takayasu's arteriopathy. *J Am Coll Cardiol* 1988; **12**: 964.

4   Yoshitoshi Y, Masuyama Y, Koide K. Aortitis syndrome clinical features and characteristics in Japan. In: Eliakim, Neufeld, eds. *Cardiology 'Current Topics and Progress'.* Proceedings of the Fourth Asian Pacific Congress of Cardiology. Academic Press, 1968; 318.

5   Sen PK, Kinare SG, Kelkar MD, Parulkar GB. *Nonspecific Aortoartoritis. A Monography Based on a Study of 101 Cases.* Bombay, New Delhi: McGraw-Hill, 1973.

6   Ueno A, Awane Y, Wakabayachi A, Shimizu K. Successfully treated obliterative brachiocephalic arteritis (Takayasu) associated with elongated coarctation. *Jpn Heart J* 1967; **8**: 538.

7   Lupi-Herrera E, Sanchez-Torrez G, Marcushamer J et al. Takayasu's arteritis: clinical study of 107 cases. *Am Heart J* 1977; **93**: 94–103.

8   Ishikawa K. Natural history and classification of occlusive thrombo-aortopathy (Takayasu's Disease). *Circulation* 1978; **57**: 27.

9   Lie JT. The classification and diagnosis of vasculitis in large and medium sized vessels. *Pathol Ann* 1987; **22**(Part 1): 122.

10 Pokrovsky AV. Nonspecific aortoarteritis. In: Rutherford RB, ed. *Vascular Surgery*, 2nd edn. Philadelphia, Pa: WB Saunders, 1989: 217–37.

11 Neelakandhan KS, Muralidhar R, Unnikrishnan M, Ravimandalam K. Abdominal aortic aneurysm repair in a patient with bilateral autotransplanted kidneys. *Thorac Cardiovasc Surgeon* 1994; **42**(2): 128–30.

12 Weaver FA, Yellin AK, Campen DH et al. Surgical procedures in the management of Takayasu's arteritis. *J Vasc Surg* 1990; **12**: 429–37.

13 Pokrovsky AV, Sultanaliev JA, Spiridonov A. Surgical treatment of vasorenal hypertension in non-specific aortoarteritis (Takayasu's disease). *J Cardiovasc Surg* 1983; **24**: 111–18.

14 Tada Y, Sato O, Ohshima A et al. Surgical treatment of Takayasu's arteritis. *Heart Vessels* 1992; Suppl 7: 159–67.

15 Fava MP, Foradori GB, Garcia CB et al. Percutaneous transluminal angioplasty in patients with Takayasu arteritis: five year experience. *J Vasc Intervent Radiol* 1993; **4**: 649–52.

16 Joseph S, Mandalam KR, Rao VR et al. Percutaneous transluminal angioplasty of the subclavian artery in non specific aortoarteritis: results of long-term follow up. *J Vasc Intervent Radiol* 1994; **5**: 573–80.

17 Sharma S, Thatai D, Saxena A et al. Renovascular hypertension resulting from nonspecific aortoarteritis in children: midterm results of percutaneous transluminal renal angioplasty and predictors of restenosis. *Am J Roentgenol* 1996; **166**: 157–62.

18 Tyagi S, Verma PK, Gambhir DS et al. Early and long-term results of subclavian angioplasty in aortoarteritis (Takayasu disease): comparison with atherosclerosis. *Cardiovasc Intervent Radiol* 1998; **21**: 219–24.

19 Sawada S, Tanigawa N, Kobayashi M et al. Treatment of Takayasu's aortitis with self-expanding metallic stents (Gianturco stents) in two patients. *Cardiovasc Intervent Radiol* 1994; **17**: 102–5.

20 Bahl VK, Chandra S, Taneja K. Self-expanding Wallstent for management of severe abdominal coarctation due to non-specific aortoarteritis. *Indian Heart J* 1997; **49**: 189–91.

21 Rao AS, Ravimandalam K, Rao VRK et al. Takayasu arteritis: initial and long-term follow-up in 16 patients after percutaneous transluminal angioplasty of the descending thoracic and abdominal aorta. *Radiology* 1993; **189**: 173–9.

22 Martin EG, Diamond NG, Casarella WJ. Percutaneous transluminal angioplasty in non-atherosclerotic disease. *Radiology* 1980; **135**: 27–37.

23 Saddekni S, Sniderman KW, Hilton S, Sos TA. Percutaneous transluminal angioplasty for Takayasu's arteritis. *J Can Assoc Radiol* 1982; **33**: 205–7.

24 Yagura M, Sano J, Akioka H et al. Usefulness of percutaneous transluminal angioplasty for aortitis syndrome. *Arch Intern Med* 1984; **144**: 1465–8.

25 Khalilullah M, Tyagi S, Lochan R et al. Percutaneous transluminal balloon angioplasty of the aorta in patients with aortitis. *Circulation* 1987; **76**: 590–600.

26 Dong Z, Li S, Lu X. Percutaneous transluminal angioplasty for renovascular hypertension in arteritis: experience in China. *Radiology* 1987; **162**: 477–9.

27 Park JH, Han MC, Kim SH et al. Takayasu's arteritis: angiographic findings and results of angioplasty. *AJR* 1989; **153**: 1069–74.

28 Kumar S, Mandalam KR, Rao VR et al. Percutaneous transluminal angioplasty in non specific aortoarteritis (Takayasu's disease): experience of 16 cases. *Cardiovasc Intervent Radiol* 1989; **12**: 321–5.

29 Gu ZM, Lin JR, Li JM, Pan WM. Transluminal catheter angioplasty of abdominal aorta in Takayasu's arteritis. *Acta Radiol* 1988; **29**: 509–13.

30 Tyagi S, Kaul UA, Nair M et al. Balloon angioplasty for renovascular hypertension in Takayasu's arteritis. *Am Heart J* 1993; **125**: 1386–93.

31 Tyagi S, Jolly N, Khalilullah M. Multivessel angioplasty in Takayasu's arteritis. *Indian Heart J* 1993; **45**: 215–7.

32 Sharma S, Shrivastava S, Kothari SS et al. Influence of angiographic morphology on the acute and longer-term outcome of percutaneous transluminal angioplasty in patients with aortic stenosis due to nonspecific aortitis. *Cardiovasc Intervent Radiol* 1994; **17**: 147–51.

33 Tyagi S, Kaul UA, Satsangi DK, Arora R. Percutaneous transluminal angioplasty for renovascular hypertension in children: initial and long-term results. *Pediatrics* 1997; **99**: 44–9.

34 Sharma S, Gupta H, Saxena A et al. Results of renal angioplasty in nonspecific aortoarteritis (Takayasu disease). *J Vasc Intervent Radiol* 1998; **9**: 429–35.

35 Sharma S, Sharma S, Bahal VK, Rajani M. Stent treatment of obstructing dissection after percutaneous transluminal angioplasty of aortic stenosis caused by non specific aortitis. *Cardiovasc Intervent Radiol* 1997; **20**: 377–9.

36 Tyagi S, Verma PK, Kumar N, Arora R. Stent angioplasty for relief of chronic mesenteric ischemia in Takayasu arteritis. *Indian Heart J* 1997; **49**: 315–18.

37 Gu ZM, Gui L, Wang JH et al. Role of aorto-angioplasty in hypertension caused by Takayasu's arteritis. *Chinese Med J* 1991; **104**: 363–8.

38 Joseph G, Krishnaswami S, Barush DK et al. Transseptal approach to aortography and carotid artery stenting in pulseless disease. *Cathet Cardiovasc Diagn* 1997; **40**: 416–20.

39 Ishikawa K. Survival and morbidity after diagnosis of occlusive thromboaortopathy (Takayasu's disease). *Am J Cardiol* 1981; **47**: 1026.

40 Ishikawa K. Patterns of symptoms and prognosis in occlusive thromboaortopathy (Takayasu's disease). *Am Coll Cardiol* 1986; **8**:1041.

41 Subramanyam R, Joy J, Balakrishnan KG. Natural history of aortoarteritis (Takayasu's disease). *Circulation* 1989; **80**: 429–37.

42 Joseph G, Kumar S. Angioplasty and stenting for supra-aortic vessels and descending thoracic aorta in inflammatory disease (aortoarteritis). In: Henry M, Amor M, eds. *Tenth International Course Book of Peripheral Vascular Intervention*. Paris: Europa Edition, 1999.

43 Sharma S, Pinto RJ. Fatal aortic rupture following balloon angioplasty of aortic restenosis in aortoarteritis. *Catheter Cardiovasc Diagn* 1995; **36**: 132–3.

44 Tyagi S, Arora R. Angioplasty and stenting of abdominal aorta, renal and iliac arteries in primary inflammatory aortoarteritis. In: Henry M, Amor M, eds. *Tenth International Course Book of Peripheral Vascular Intervention*. Paris: Europa Edition, 1999.

45 Abraham KA, Rajagopal S. Balloon angioplasty and stenting of unprotected left main in aortoarteritis. In: Henry M, Amor M, eds. *Tenth International Course Book of Peripheral Vascular Intervention*. Paris: Europa Edition, 1999.

46 Yajima M, Numano E, Park YB, Sagar B. Comparative studies of patients with Takayasu arteritis in Japan, Korea and India. *Jpn Circ J* 1994; **58**: 9–14.

47 Neelakandhan K. Surgical considerations in aortoarteritis. In: Henry M, Amor M, eds. *Tenth International Course Book of Peripheral Vascular Intervention*. Paris: Europa Edition, 1999.

48 Karthik R, Abraham KA, Sriram R et al. Angioplasty and stenting of solitary supraaortic artery and aortoplasty by kissing balloon technique. *J Invas Cardiol* 1999; **11**(6): 375–8.

50

Limb salvage in critical limb ischemia

Emilio Calabrese

Introduction

Critical limb ischemia (CLI) occurs when blood flow to a limb is inadequate in order to maintain reasonable metabolic requirements of the tissues at rest.

Pain at rest, in the extremity involved, initially appears only when the limb is elevated and improves in the recumbent position. As the disease advances, rest pain persists in any position and becomes less responsive to conventional pain treatment.

Ischemic ulcerations are a more advanced stage of CLI and usually appear near bone prominences.

Gangrene results from complete tissue death and may be limited to the extremities of the toes or fingers, or it may involve a significant part of the limb.

Fontaine (Table 50.1) and Rutherford (Table 50.2) devised useful clinical classifications of the various stages of CLI. The low blood flow and the presence of certain metabolic diseases will reduce the host defenses against infectious agents. When bacteria attacks necrotic tissue, it is capable of rapidly extending the gangrenous area by producing thrombosis of the surrounding microcirculation and inducing further tissue destruction. Impairment of arterial perfusion is thus only a part of the cause of limb-threatening lesions. Diabetes, with its neuropathy and impaired resistance to infection, adds further

complication to the effects of arteriosclerosis and arterial occlusion.[1] Each year, 2.5% of all diabetics develops a foot ulcer. Three variables are independent predictors of this complication: absence of Achilles tendon reflexes, low transcutaneous pO_2 ($TcpO_2$ <30 mmHg), and an abnormal esthesiometry plantar test performed with a 5.07 monofilament. Absent vibratory sensation is not a significant risk factor.[1] Reopening obstructed vessels may not suffice to save a limb in many diabetic patients,[2] who will instead need further care: one will have to treat the lesions of the bone, joints, and soft tissue of the foot, along with providing strict control of the infection and the metabolic derangements.[3] The rare patients with true Buerger's disease will need complete abstension from smoking to maintain any hope of successful limb salvage. Trauma, both minor and major, and lack of appropriate hygiene, will further complicate the issue.[4]

Due to the complexity of the problem, which is not merely limited to addressing the issue of arterial occlusion, a whole field of medical care dedicated to limb salvage has been developed. Coordinating care efforts of orthopedists, diabetologists, internists, general and vascular surgeons, interventional radiologists, plastic surgeons, psychologists, microbiologists, nurses, and hospital administrators provides a better possibility of achieving results by devising a multifaceted approach to limb salvage.[5–10]

Table 50.1	Fontaine classification
Stage	Symptoms
I	Asymptomatic
II	Intermittent claudication
II-a	Pain-free, claudication walking >200m
II-b	Pain-free, claudication walking <200m
III	Rest pain/nocturnal pain
IV	Necrosis/gangrene

Arterial approach

Infrarenal aorta

Severe stenosis of the infrarenal aorta, producing a significant drop in distal blood flow, may be associated with CLI. Stenosis of the aorta can be dilated and a nitinol stent can be inserted to maintain patency. Either large net (Boston

Table 50.2 AHA/Rutherford classification

Grade	Category	Clinical description	Objective criteria
0	0	Asymptomatic – not hemodynamically significant	Normal treadmill/ stress test
I	1	Mild claudication	Completes treadmill exercise, ankle pressure after exercise <50 mmHg but >25 mmHg less than BP
	2	Moderate claudication	Between categories 1 and 3
	3	Severe claudication	Cannot complete treadmill exercise and ankle pressure after exercise <50 mmHg
II	4	Ischemic rest pain flat or barely pulsatile	Resting ankle pressure <40 mmHg, flat or barely pulsatile ankle or metatarsal Pulse Volume Recording; toe Pressure <30 mmHg
	5	Minor tissue loss: non-healing ulcer; focal gangrene with diffuse foot ischemia	Resting ankle pressure <60 mmHg, ankle metatarsal Pulse Volume Recording flat or barely pulsatile; toe Pressure <40 mmHg
III	6	Major tissue loss: extending above trans-metatarsal level, functional foot no longer salvageable	Resting ankle pressure <60 mmHg, ankle metatarsal Pulse Volume Recording flat or barely pulsatile; toe Pressure <40 mmHg

Scientific's Symphony®) or tight net (Cordis' SMART®) nitinol stents can be used: generally a 14-mm stent will be adequate and will be inserted through a 7F introducer. Inserting larger stents such as 16- or 18-mm Bard's Memotherm® will require a larger introducer and is seldom indicated. The stent should completely cover the stenotic area and, of course, should not encroach the ostium of the renal arteries. The stenosed aorta is then dilated with a 12-mm or 14-mm balloon. Palmaz-type, balloon expandable stents can also be successfully utilized in this position. Figure 50.1 shows a case of ischemia of the left allux associated with infrarenal aortic stenosis, which responded to percutaneous transluminal angioplasty (PTA) and stenting.

Iliac artery

Stenosis or occlusion of a common or external iliac artery is rarely associated with CLI, unless a second tandem lesion is present in the thigh or in the leg, or unless a diabetic patient has developed a foot infection. In the presence of sequential lesions, the iliac artery has to be treated first, while the distal femoral or infragenicular lesion may often not require treatment at this stage. Simultaneous iliac and femoral artery treatment, in critical ischemia, will increase the operative mortality. Balloon dilation, with or without stenting, will provide an effective increase in blood flow, but local additional debridement procedures on the ischemic lesions are also needed. When stenting is indicated, both self-expandable and balloon expandable stents can be used

in the common iliac, while only self-expandable stents should be used in the external iliac, because this vessel is sharply bent during flexion of the thigh. In experienced hands, endovascular procedures are usually successful on the iliac artery, and surgery is rarely needed. Long stenosis and complete short- and long-segment obstructions can be approached either in a transbrachial manner, or in a contralateral or omolateral one, through the femoral artery. When recanalization of a completely obstructed iliac artery fails, one could consider optimization of the contra-lateral artery to prepare for a cross-over bypass. Hybrid, combined interventional and surgical procedures are an acceptable approach. Percutaneous transluminal angioplasty should thus be the primary choice of treatment for iliac artery disease (Figure 50.2) and, only when endovascular recanalization is not successful should surgical bypass be considered as an option.[11]

Femoral bifurcation

Simultaneous occlusion or tight stenosis of the profunda and superficial femoral artery (SFA) are often associated with gangrene and they are most often seen in diabetic patients. Lesions in this area are usually approached by surgical endarterectomy because PTA, without stenting of the origin of the superficial femoral artery, is associated with prompt restenosis and occlusion. Recent studies which involve the insertion of highly flexible nitinol stents in the ostium of the superficial femoral artery, that extend up into the distal part of

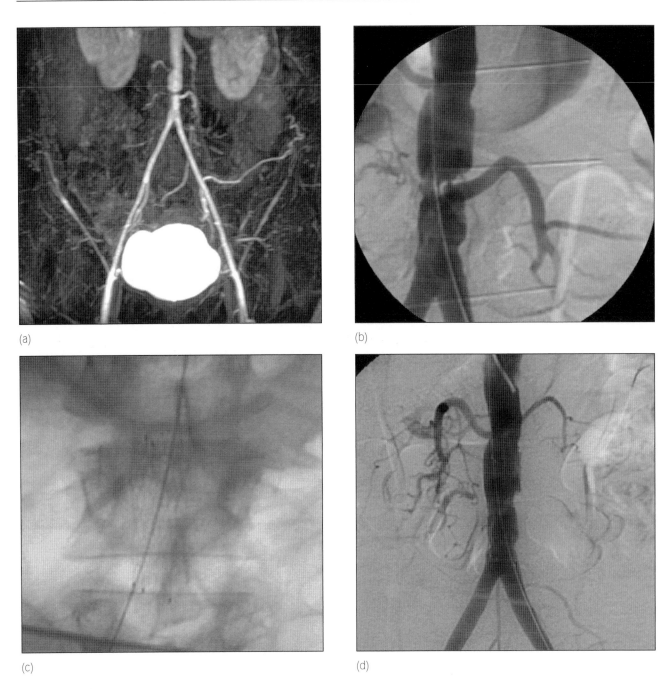

(a)

(b)

(c)

(d)

Figure 50.1
(a) A magnetic resonance angiogram (MRA) showing a short critical stenosis of the infrarenal aorta. (b) Angiogram confirming the stenosis and showing a large lumbar artery arising from the stenotic area. (c) Self-expandable Symphony 14/40 nitinol stent inserted in the aorta. (d) Percutaneous transluminal angioplasty (PTA) of the aorta completed. The lumbar artery has been sacrificed. Additional PTA and stenting of the right iliac artery has also been performed.

the common femoral artery, have been offering promising results (E. Calabrese pers. comm.). When a long segment of the superficial femoral artery is completely occluded, then a surgical bypass is, as of today, the best option, provided that a distal vessel suitable for anastomosis is present.

Some patients may be treated with profundaplasty alone, either surgical[12] or endovascular.[13] Simple profundaplasty, without stenting or patching, is generally deemed to encounter early failure and poor results. Ostial lesions may be treated by inserting a nitinol stent, extending from the

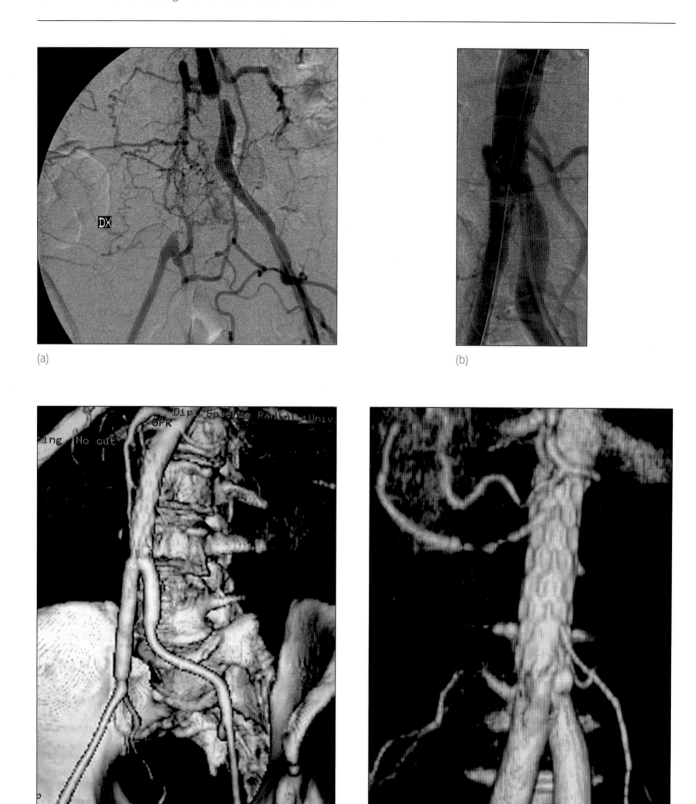

(a)

(b)

(c)

(d)

Figure 50.2

(a) Occlusion of the right iliac artery, severe stenosis of the left iliac ostium, tapering and stenosis of the distal aorta. (b) SMART® stents in both iliac arteries and Symphony® stent in the aorta. (c) Follow-up multislice computed tomography (CT) scan. (d) Detail of the aortic bifurcation with triple stenting.

common femoral artery to the profunda beyond the point of critical stenosis (Figure 50.3). Balloon-expandable stents should never be inserted in this position (Figure 50.4). When the procedure is performed, it is essential to check the patency and position of the stent while the thigh is completely flexed. Highly flexible nitinol stents (Abbott/JoMed Xpert® or SelfX® and Guidant Dynalink®) are preferred. There is a caveat concerning interventional procedures on the profunda femoris: past experience with surgical profundaplasty has shown that extensive gangrene will almost never heal with this procedure alone.[12] In such cases, one will only achieve a lowering of the level of amputation (from above to below the knee, usually). Profundaplasty is much more effective in Fontaine class III patients, where it will significantly improve rest pain, and in small ischemic ulcerations. Interventional profundaplasty for limb salvage may require 1 or 2 months to show its maximum effect, due to the slow development of an improved collateral circulation. Extreme attention to the control of ongoing infection should be given, during the first several weeks after the procedure, to allow time for collateral vessels to develop and improve distal perfusion.

Superficial femoral artery

Stenosis, either single or multiple, and short- or long-segment occlusions of the SFA, are associated with ulceration or gangrene solely in diabetic patients or in patients who have arteritis, recent trauma, or infection. Tandem arterial lesions, either proximal iliac or distal infragenicular, may also be responsible for the appearance of gangrene. A short, severe stenosis may enhance gangrene due to neuropathy and infection so much that it may induce rapidly extending tissue destruction. A simple PTA, or a stent-supported PTA, will improve the blood flow to the lesion and enhance the healing.[14–17] Local treatment is needed to control infection, to limit tissue loss, and to provide functional reconstruction of the foot. When SFA stenosis is present together with an iliac lesion, they should not be treated both at the same time: the iliac stenosis, especially if severe, retains priority. When an SFA occlusion is present, together with infragenicular disease, treatment should be initially limited to the SFA only, unless extensive gangrene is present, requiring a massive increase in blood flow.

When ostial lesions of the SFA are present, they are best treated either by surgery or by insertion of nitinol stents across the lesion. Preliminary data show that self-expanding nitinol stents delivered from the common femoral to the proximal part of the SFA, which cross and cover the ostium of the profunda, do not produce occlusion of the profunda, neither in the immediate term nor at 1-year follow-ups. Occasionally, double-crossed bifurcation stenting of the profunda and superficial femoral artery has been reported, but long-term follow-up is not yet available.

In long-segment occlusions of the SFA, a surgical bypass is currently the best option, when good runoff vessels are present. Percutaneous transluminal angioplasty is preferred

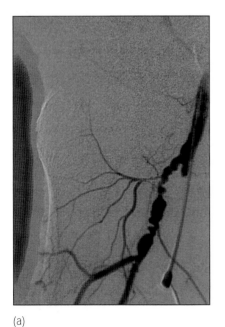

(a)

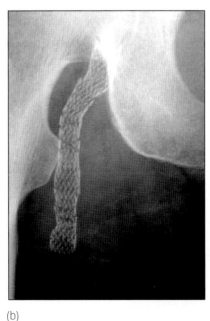

(b)

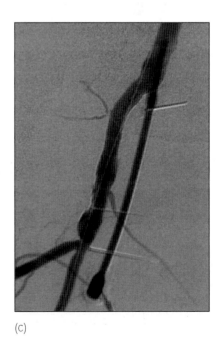

(c)

Figure 50.3

(a) Occlusion of the superficial femoral artery and stenosis of distal iliac and profunda. (b) Insertion of JoMed SELFX® nitinol stent.
(c) Percutaneous transluminal angioplasty and stenting are complete.

when there is severe limb infection or when there is no suitable point for distal anastomosis. Several studies with the use of sequential long-segment stenting have shown controversial results. Some of these series were marred by the use of balloon expandable stents, which are exposed to external compression and may easily deform and occlude. Picking up the deformation of a stent as a cause of stenosis or occlusion of a previously performed PTA requires multiple-angle angiograms, three-dimensional reconstruction angioplasty or intravascular ultrasound (IVUS). In a study done at the Cleveland Clinic by Gray et al. in 1997,[18] which showed poor results of long-segment femoral stenting, part of the failure could be attributed to the use of Palmaz stents in the exposed femoral position and to the fact that segmental pressure measurements, with high pressure cuffs applied over the stents, were used to assess patency. External compression and severe, temporary stent deformation by the inflating cuffs (Figure 50.5), could have influenced the long-term patency; it is in no doubt recommendable that these pressure cuffs never be used in assessing patency of a PTA in a limb. Nitinol stents seem to fare best in the thigh position, where balloon expandable stents are liable to external compression and occlusion. Sequential, multiple nitinol stents (Figure 50.6) may provide a viable option for limb salvage when severe infection or poor runoff increases the risk for a surgical bypass.[19] It seems that distal vessel runoff has less influence on the medium, and possibly, long-term patency of long-segment femoral artery stenting in limb salvage. Drug-eluting stents (Cordis Sirolimus® project) are under evaluation in this area and they are giving promising results showing an excellent medium-term patency rate with a follow-up now exceeding 18 months. The SIROLIMUS study has been showing an

excellent performance of the nitinol SMART® stent in the femoral artery in this well designed multicenter study.[48] With further improvement in the drug delivery system and in the design of the stents, one may expect that long segment stenting may compete with surgical bypass in selected cases. The drug involved influences the earlier stages of endothelial ingrowth, and initial studies suggest a reduction of in-stent restenosis. It is necessary to remember, though, that elution of the drug ceases within a few months from insertion.

Sirolimus®, Tacrolimus®, and even Thalidomide, with its limiting action on endothelial proliferation, may achieve a significant role in the future in preventing intra-stent stenosis.

When there are multiple points of stenosis, the combination of a surgical bypass with trans-bypass angioplasty and stenting of distal vessels, provides a significant increase in distal flow with adequate runoff to protect the patency of the surgical bypass, while avoiding the insertion of a large number of stents in the SFA.[20]

Popliteal artery

The retrogenicular segment of the popliteal artery is a very critical area where both PTA and stented PTA have often failed. A study of the behavior of the popliteal artery during knee movement has shown a better way to choose and position stents in this area (E. Calabrese pers. comm.). Balloon expandable stents are obviously excluded here, as they should also be avoided in any limb, in the thoracic outlet and in the distal external iliac artery, because they are liable to flexion, external compression, and deformation. Even

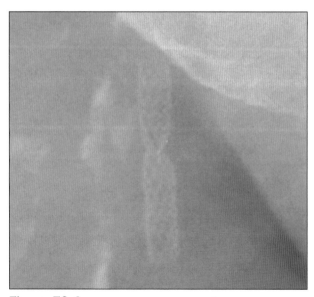

Figure 50.4
Balloon expandable stent deformed by flexion at the groin.

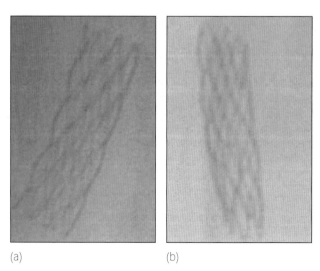

(a) (b)

Figure 50.5
(a) Thrombosed Palmaz® stent in the superficial femoral artery.
(b) A different angle shows the presence of pressure deformity of the stent.

self-expanding stents, to be delivered in the popliteal artery, need to be highly flexible. Boston Scientific's Symphony® and Bard's Memotherm® do not permit longitudinal flexion at all, and they are not appropriate for popliteal stenting. Cordis' SMART®, in its current version, has up to six interlacing links in its parallel rings structure. This partially limits the tangential flexibility of the stent and produces excessive rigidity of the stented artery and a tendency to a premature fracture of the struts undergoing repeated flexion. Several patients with retrogenicular implantation of Cordis' SMART® have maintained patency for well over 1 year, in spite of strut fractures and temporary deformation of the stent under flexion. It is in any case preferable to utilize more flexible stents in this position, until modifications of the SMART® structure along with its fatigue studies are available for popliteal stenting.

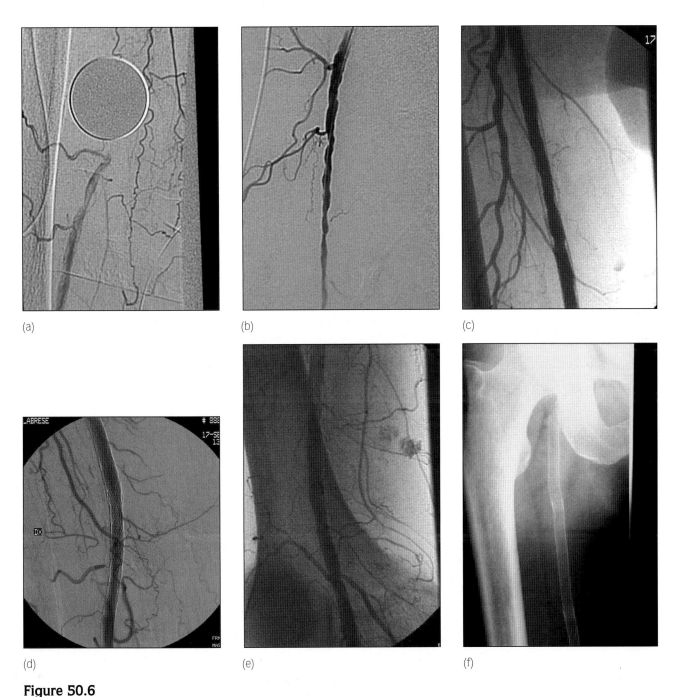

(a) (b) (c)

(d) (e) (f)

Figure 50.6

(a) Diffuse disease of the proximal superficial femoral artery. A previous femoropopliteal bypass had failed. (b) Complete occlusion of both the bypass and the distal superficial femoral artery. (c–e) Follow-up angiogram 27 months after stents insertion: (c) proximal femoral artery; (d) adductor canal; and, (e) distal femoropopliteal junction. (f) X-rays of the six stents.

JoMed's Selfx® has only three inter-ring links, which make this device extremely flexible and suitable for being positioned behind the knee and in the area of the profunda femoris. These stents may still fracture, due to the long-term fatigue that continuous knee flexion produces; however, they lend a better shape to the stented artery and they do not bend unduly under flexion, maintaining a patent lumen throughout the movement cycle of the knee joint. Correct positioning of the stents, both in the proximal and distal part of the popliteal artery, will determine early and late patency. When an isolated stent is put solely in the retrogenicular area, it may rapidly occlude, because although it looks perfect when seen on a straight knee angiography, the stent will produce arterial distortion during flexion of the knee, which causes damage to the intima and a rapidly progressing stenosis. Proximally, a popliteal stent should come up to reach the adductor canal. Distally, a popliteal stent should terminate either 2 or 3 cm above the take-off of the tibialis anterior or, better, it should enter the tibialis anterior itself or the tibioperoneal trunk for a significant length. A flexion dynamic angiography that, by reaching 90° angulations, shows eventual deformation of the arteries and kinking of the nitinol struts, will assess the correct positioning of the stent in each patient. Positioning of stents in the popliteal area is deemed to fail unless flexion angiography is done and ruled satisfactory (Figure 50.7).

Simple PTA of the popliteal artery may provide short-term patency, but a calcified vessel can suffer fragmentation of the dilated plaque during flexion with subsequent stenosis, embolism, and occlusion. Simple PTA may remain a viable option in discrete, brief stenosis with no significant calcifications, but it still needs a final control with a dynamic flexion angiography.

Infrapopliteal vessels

Patients with diabetes and in Fontaine class IV or Rutherford class 5 & 6, usually show multiple stenosis, occlusions of all the infragenicular vessels, or stenosis of the only remaining patent distal artery. The tibialis posterior often occludes first and the peroneal is usually the last one to go. Patent peroneal vessels often reinhabit the distal tibialis vessels at the ankle, thus providing the sole source of perfusion. Restoring patency of just one of the three infrapopliteal vessels will be sufficient, especially when one of the two tibialis arteries is being reopened. The two tibialis vessels reach the foot directly, taking part of the formation of the plantar arch circulation, so that they provide direct vascularization to the most distal lesions in a better way than the peroneal artery does. When all vessels are

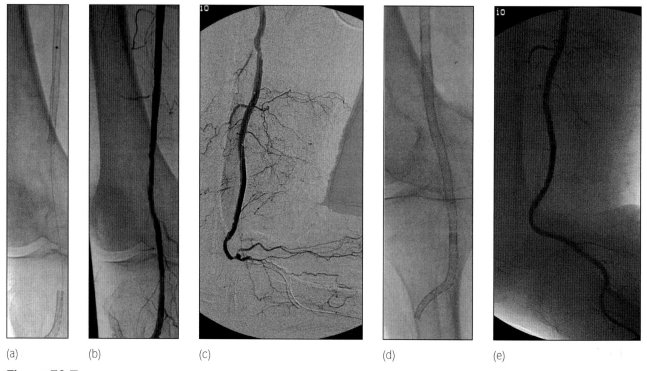

(a)   (b)   (c)   (d)   (e)

Figure 50.7
Demonstration of the need for a flexion angiogram when stenting behind the knee: (a) one stent above and one stent below the knee to treat two spot lesions; (b) perfect angiogram on a straight leg; (c) angiogram under flexion shows complete obstruction to flow; (d) insertion of two more stents to obtain sequential continuity; and, (e) final angiogram under flexion shows a satisfactory flow.

severely stenotic or occluded, restoring patency within the tibialis anterior or posterior should probably have priority. Simultaneous, multiple vessel infragenicular angioplasties could be dangerous, because a failure may completely wipe out any circulation to the distal part of the limb and may further compromise the chance for a surgical bypass.[21–23] Infrapopliteal PTA is a procedure widely performed in diabetic patients and its results are quite encouraging in terms of limb salvage. Even if the primary patency does not exceed 50% at 10 months, its limb salvage is comparable with the best surgical series. The recent addition of self-expanding small stents (Cordis' SMART®, SciMed'sRadius®, and JoMed's Petite® and the more advanced Abbott/JoMed Xpert® designed by Schaffner), inserted below the knee, has further improved the results in terms of patency and limb salvage with the Xpert® showing consistently better long-term patency rate thanks to its tighter net structure and flexible design (Figure 50.8). (E. Calabrese pers. comm.).

Diffuse obliteration of main vessels

In Buerger's disease (thromboangiitis obliterans) all main arteries in the limbs may be obliterated and only collateral flow, albeit well developed, may be present. While it is not feasible to recanalize long segments of occluded arteries in these patients, it is important to resolve all approachable proximal stenoses to increase the flow descending into the collaterals. If a severe stenosis of the proximal common iliac artery is present in a patient with all main vessels obliterated beyond the external iliac, this stenosis should be dilated and stented (Figure 50.9). This may provide an improvement in the distal flow beyond a subcritical level, and may help save the limb. Medical therapy and abstention from smoking is the current mainstay of treatment[24–26] and intensive stationary cycling may assist in developing a more effective collateral circulation. Iloprost®[27] helps in the treatment and unusual surgical procedures such as omentopexy[28] also seem to help. Immunomodulator drugs, such as Thalidomide, are currently under evaluation for the treatment of the disease.

Vessels not suitable for revascularization procedures

Deeming a patient non-operable rarely depends on the severity of the disease. More often, incomplete diagnostic studies, lack of appropriate equipment, limited knowledge and inexperience in the field of limb salvage, and fear of losing control when confronted with infected lesions might make a physician declare a limb not salvageable. This may lead to the excessive use of palliative measures with limited effectiveness (e.g. hyperbaric chambers, neural nerve stimulators) and to the amputation of many salvageable legs. Introducing a National Registry of Amputations and introducing a centralized, second opinion protocol before proceeding to major amputations will certainly increase the number of legs rescued.

Upper limb salvage

Ischemic problems in the upper limb, aside from embolic ones, are more common in nephropathic patients who have dialysis fistula. If a radial-artery-to-vein Cimino shunt has been performed in a patient with incomplete palmar arch or with diseased or absent ulnar artery, severe ischemia of the hand may ensue.

This is best treated by PTA of the ulnar artery if feasible, or by brachial-to-distal-radial-artery bypass with inverted saphenous vein graft.

A bypass may be needed in those patients who have undergone several shunting procedures because of the occlusion of previous arteriovenous (AV) fistulas, and who now suffer multiple occlusions in several sites of the arm and forearm. Occasionally, patients who have a latero–lateral or latero–terminal AV fistula may develop a steal syndrome. The blood will flow from the palmar arch back into the AV fistula, thus producing finger ischemia. Some of these patients benefit from distal ligation of the radial artery; others may require an additional procedure such as a distal bypass.[29,30]

Non-vascular approach
All vessels patent, gangrenous extremity

Patients may develop gangrene in spite of perfectly patent main vessels down to the ankle. Occlusion and stenosis at the pedal arterial arch may produce distal ischemia and techniques are under development to approach disease in this area (a case of palmar arch PTA is described elsewhere is this chapter). Emboli traveling to the digital arteries may produce distal ischemia of the toes. Distal embolic occlusion may be very difficult to treat with urokinase: adjunctive measures, such as vasodilators and sympathetic block, may assist in limiting the extension of gangrene. Intravenous heparin and surgical or endovascular control of the primary source of emboli, if identified, will further help reduce ischemic episodes. Severe prolonged vasospasm and prolonged exposure to freezing temperature may produce frostbite and gangrene. As a rule, the initial appearance of frostbite should not prompt to immediate amputation. By utilizing lukewarm thawing of the

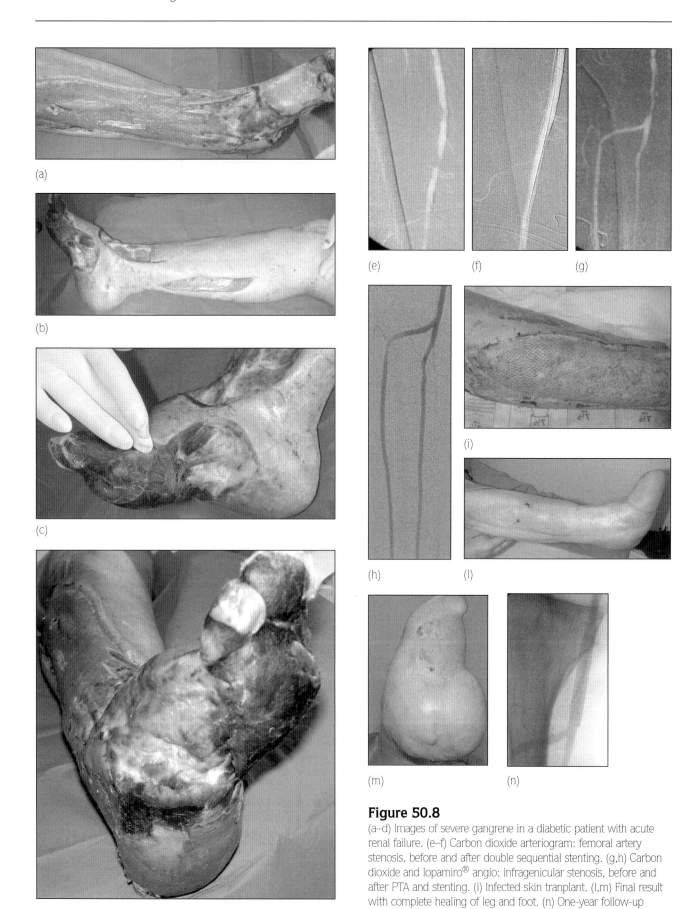

Figure 50.8

(a–d) Images of severe gangrene in a diabetic patient with acute renal failure. (e–f) Carbon dioxide arteriogram: femoral artery stenosis, before and after double sequential stenting. (g,h) Carbon dioxide and Iopamiro® angio: infragenicular stenosis, before and after PTA and stenting. (i) Infected skin tranplant. (l,m) Final result with complete healing of leg and foot. (n) One-year follow-up angio shows patency of the 6/40 Cordis SMART® stent.

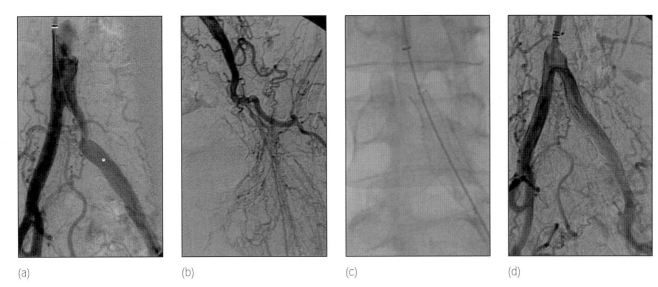

(a)   (b)   (c)   (d)

Figure 50.9
(a, b) Patient with severe thromboangiitis obliterans and no patent main vessel distal to the left external iliac artery. Stenosis of the proximal part of the left common iliac artery. (c, d) Percutaneous transluminal angioplasty and stenting (Cordis SMART®) of the left common iliac performed through a brachial access.

extremity and by patiently waiting for demarcation of the irreversible lesion, one may spare a significant amount of tissue and retain a functional foot or limb.

Chemical and iatrogenic damage to the arteries due to accidental injection of certain medications in an arterial line while the patient is in the intensive care unit may produce severe damage to the extremity: vasodilators and local care can sometimes provide limited help. Local anesthetic, when used to perform minor procedures on digits, may produce local gangrene if the vial contains small doses of epinephrine (adrenaline), a drug which is sometimes combined with the local anesthetic to prolong its action. Immediate injection of Regitine® (phentolamine) in the area infiltrated with epinephrine may partially limit the damage.

Extravasation of solutions containing high concentration of K^+, dopamine, norepinephrine (noradrenaline) or of several other drugs may also produce gangrene of tissues surrounding a vein. Regitine® will still help in dopa and epi lesions if administered within minutes. Using only central venous lines to infuse solutions with a K^+ concentration above 50 mmol/liter will best prevent K^+ lesions.

Bacterial infection

Anaerobes and Enterobacteriaceae, as well as certain aggressive streptococcal strains, may produce rapidly enlarging gangrenous areas: prompt Gram stain, cultural identification, and surgical debridement with irrigation and mechanical cleansing of lesions will assist the appropriate antibiotics in controlling the problem. Clostridia, streptococci, and certain Enterobacteriaceae should mostly be feared because of the rapidity with which they extend the damage, while Pseudomonas and staphylococci usually produce slowly expanding lesions. Local antibiotics have no use, while solutions such as povidone–iodine (an aqueous iodine solution) will be of greatest aid. Alkaline chlorine solutions may enhance Pseudomonas growth, while 0.5% acetic acid solutions applied locally will provide significant control of the growth of most Enterobacteriaceae, when associated with systemic antibiotics. To reach a wound, antibiotics need patent arteries to be able to travel to their target point, so that synchronization of debridement and PTA or surgical bypass is paramount. While drainage of abscesses should be done immediately upon seeing an infected patient, more extensive debridement should always be preceded first by approximate identification of the bacteria and its probable sensitivity to chosen antibiotics and then by revascularization. Providing too early a revascularization before identification of bacterial strains and initiation of proper antibiotic coverage may produce uncontrollable septicemia. Combinations of antibiotics covering streptococci, staphylococci and anaerobes and Enterobacteriaceae (metronidazole + amikacin + ampicillin) may be used during the first couple of days while awaiting culture results. Gram stain should always be used for guidance. Antiobiotic coverage requires intelligent interpretation of sensitivity tests: Serrata is sensitive to Beta-lactam in vitro, but asbolutely resistant in vivo.[31–33] Methicillin-resistant *staph.* may be sensitive to Imipenem in vitro, but will not respond to the drug in vivo; Rifampicin and Ciprofloxacin rapidly induce resistance when used alone against *Staph.* and Ciprofloxacin is not to be used alone in presence of *Streptococcus.*

Extensive gangrene

Extensive gangrene is best approached by immediate vascular evaluation and arteriogram, assessment of the infection, endovascular revascularization, and debridement.

No matter how severe the infection, all patients should be thoroughly studied. When joints are involved, all exposed cartilage should be completely excised and an arthrodesis with external fixators should be done to stabilize the extremity. Leaving even small fragments of exposed articular cartilage will strongly prevent wound healing and will promote persistent infection. A rotating, high-speed file will provide the best system to ablate the cartilage covering and to provide a smooth surface for arthrodesis. Insertion of screws for the external fixators should be planned in such a way as to completely avoid those areas where the only remaining patent vessel is running. The fixators are left in place for 6 months, initiating partial weight bearing when the wound has begun to heal.

Opportunistic Pseudomonas infection

Recurrent contamination of superficial extensive wounds with *Pseudomonas* is frequent, and antibiotics may not provide sufficient coverage. Alkaline solutions containing chlorine may sometimes enhance superficial contamination with Enterobacteriaceae. Povidone–iodine is generally ineffective, whereas continuous soaking with an 0.5% acetic acid solution will provide excellent control, because these bacteria do not thrive in an acidic environment.

Borderline renal failure

Patients with moderate elevation of creatinine may suffer most from interventional procedures, when nephrotoxic iodine contrast is utilized. Gadolinium may be a less nephrotoxic agent, but it is extremely expensive to use. Carbon dioxide arteriograms may be the best choice in most patients because they are inexpensive, simple to perform,

and harmless to the kidneys. Carbon dioxide may sometimes provide even better visualization of vessels than traditional iodinated contrast. To limit additional nephrotoxicity, antibiotics should be carefully selected and dosage should be adjusted according to creatinine clearance. Aminoglycosides and imipenem–cilastatin compounds require special attention in patients with renal failure.

Chronic terminal renal failure and dialysis

Nephropathic patients fare worst in limb salvage procedures and their wounds are often infected with methicillin-resistant staphylococci or with *Pseudomonas*, especially when diabetes complicates the picture.[34]

Vancomycin is a very helpful drug when *Staphylococcus* is present is these patients, because it cannot pass through the filters of most artificial kidneys and injections can be given once every 5 days, while checking serum levels of the drug. Carbon dioxide arteriograms reduce the problem of fluid overload seen with iodine contrast injections.

Pain

Ischemia produces severe suffering and many patients would accept a major amputation simply to free themselves from pain. They sleep in a chair to keep their legs down for some relief, but the resulting dependent edema compounds the problem. Successful revascularization procedures provide prompt pain relief, unless extensive tissue damage and infection perpetuate the problem. When repeated debridements and medications are needed, the implantation of an epidural catheter with a tunneled subcutaneous reservoir will reduce the discomfort during the healing phase. When revascularization procedures fail, then epidural Marcaine® (bupivacaine) will buy some time, while medical therapy and local care will attempt to save the limb. Addiction to pain medications is a common problem among patients with CLI and so is deprivation of sleep.

Spinal cord stimulators rarely succeed in helping patients with ischemic pain, although they may be of some assistance when causalgia is the problem.

Depression

Psychological assistance is often needed because depression is a common finding in patients who have suffered for a long time because of intense pain and deprivation of sleep. Some may even choose immediate amputation to relieve their suffering and to avoid dealing with long-term care and painful wound dressings. Motivating the family to provide support and giving professional psychological care to the patients will be of substantial help. Brain-dopamine modulator drugs, such as Prozac® (fluoxetine), will be of some help. A continuous effort should be made toward the patient to increase his self-esteem, his motivation to fight against the disease, and respect for the body itself. Without an appropriate and dedicated psychological support, an otherwise technically perfect limb salvage procedure may simply fail and make the patient choose the quickest road: toward amputation.[35,36]

Coronary disease

Heavy smoking, high cholesterol, and diabetes render ischemic heart disease strongly prevalent among patients with CLI. It is generally asymptomatic, because of the limited physical activity of these patients. Effort tests are unfeasible, so one must rely on dipyridamole technetium scans. Scans may fail to pinpoint a severe heart problem such as a simultaneous right coronary and left main trunk stenosis, a highly lethal disease. Dobutamine echocardiograms, in turn, may altogether miss a right coronary stenosis. A normal electrocardiogram at rest does not, of course, rule out coronary disease. Selective coronary arteriograms should be done in all cases when peripheral vascular disease is present in multiple sites and when dealing with patients with severe limb ischemia. Aggressive treatment of coronary lesions should be swiftly planned and carried out, because a myocardial infarction has a prohibitively high mortality when it occurs right after a revascularization procedure. In addition, a symptomatic patient may soon notice chest pain when their peripheral lesions improve, because they start walking and moving around more actively.

Extracranial carotid artery disease

B-mode Doppler ultrasound scans are very efficient in diagnosing carotid stenosis, and recently introduced endovascular stenting techniques have simplified its treatment in high-risk patients.

Cancer

Malignancies are somehow more prevalent in patients with limb ischemia, many of whom have a history of heavy cigarette smoking. Routine chest-X-rays are mandatory and can occasionally pick up an asymptomatic lung cancer still amenable to cure. Bladder cancer also seems to be more common in these patients, but further studies are needed to confirm these observations.

Survival issue

Patients with limb-threatening ischemia are plagued with a severely shortened life span due to coronary artery disease, cerebrovascular ischemia, and cancer. Most series show a 40% 5-year survival rate in this population. Achieving high limb salvage results in the few surviving patients is a technical feat, and a medical failure. Because it makes little sense to save a leg and see the patient die shortly thereafter, an aggressive follow-up program needs to be enacted.

Aside from these considerations, any patient who has a very short life span due to a concomitant terminal disease should not be deprived of the right to receive limb salvage procedures, even for the sole purpose of treating unbearable ischemic pain.

Limb loss

Failures in limb-saving procedures occur. It is the responsibility of the medical team to prepare the patient and the family for the amputation, to arrange for the psychological and logistical support, to perform the procedure itself, and to help plan a future without a limb.

Death

An operative mortality exceeding 5% can be expected in limb salvage procedures, when one deals with elderly sick patients with multiple organ failure and advanced cardiovascular disease.[43] Additional late mortality occurs most commonly during the first year; over 50% die within 5 years and few patients survive over 10 years. Attentive, post-procedure intensive care and careful follow-up should improve the survival.

Additional tools for treatment
Hyperbaric chamber

The use of hyperbaric oxygen (HO) in treating gangrene and infection is controversial, especially when non-clostridial species are concerned. Because HO is not the mainstay of treatment, appropriate antibiotics, surgical debridement, and revascularization should have top priority. Relying on the doubtful therapeutic effects of HO to save an infected or ischemic limb may lead to a loss of precious time, which could have been devoted to more effective procedures. In addition, other patients who are being treated in the same room as the septic patient are exposed to an unjustified contamination risk.

Hyperbaric oxygen will be of great help when treating diver's emboli, an air embolism due to accidental intra-arterial or an intravenous injection of air. It may be of some help when split-thickness skin transplants are applied to patients.[37] It could also speed up the growth of granulation tissue. Hyperbaric oxygen may sometimes be useful, but it is certainly not essential, in the treatment of ischemia or infected non-clostridial gangrene, and its cost can hardly be justified, except when dealing with gas embolism.[39–41]

Sympathectomy

Resection of sympathetic ganglia provides prompt and lasting relief when treating causalgia, but it rarely helps in ischemic pain. Results in limb salvage are marginal and even as a supportive measure to enhance patency in small-vessel bypass, surgical sympathectomy is better replaced by epidural anesthesia and infusion of dextran 40.[42]

Spinal cord stimulation

Since its introduction in the 1970s, spinal cord stimulation (SCS) has found its niche in the treatment of patients not suitable for arterial reconstruction. No prospective randomized study has shown clear evidence of the efficacy of SCS *alone* in limb salvage and in controlling ischemic pain. Its cost and its technical problems, associated with lead displacement and its marginal efficacy, severely restricts indications and use.[43,44]

Fasciotomy

Revascularization of severely ischemic limbs may produce swelling of the muscles within the tight compartments of the leg. The appearance of weakness in dorsiflexion of the toes and pain in the leg in spite of excellent blood flow and a warm foot should suggest the possibility of acute compartment syndrome. Measuring the pressure in the anterior compartment will provide a useful indication. Fasciotomy should be used liberally to decompress the muscles. Delaying a much-needed fasciotomy even for a few hours may produce irreversible damage to the limb.

Medical therapy

Prostaglandin,[27] heparin, urokinase,[45] antiplatelet drugs, and a careful assessment of the coagulation profile are essential tools in the management of CLI.

Home care

Prolonged hospital stays are expensive and they disrupt the life of the patients and their families. Home visits by nurses or regular wound dressings as outpatients in a podiatry day-care clinic reduce expenses and discomfort for the patient and the public health service. Training a cooperative and suitable family member to perform daily medications, along with supervised progress assessment, is of great help when patients reside in remote areas.

Betadine solutions used for long-term care should be diluted 1:10 to avoid damage to the granulation tissue. The 1:10 Betadine to sterile water solution should be discarded every other day and a fresh solution prepared. Use of VAC (vacuum assisted closure) employing a high negative pressure portable pump connected to a polyurethane sterile sponge, will markedly speed up the growth of granulation tissue, but will require well trained professionals. Advanced dressing techniques may also require extensive training, so it will often be better to keep the home wound treatment technique as simple as possible, and monitor through videophone or email photos the progress of the wound.

Internet

Sending electronic medical charts for on-line consultation to a specialized limb salvage center is a valid tool. Transmission of daily or weekly progress of a wound through JPEG scans (compressed electronic images) to the coordinating center helps in guiding the treatment and deciding when it is time for an in-hospital consultation and further surgery. Supervising long distance wound dressing procedures with a simple net-meeting live camera technique helps in training local professionals and family members when some basic computer knowledge is available *in loco*. Electronic cameras, possibly with a minimum 1,2 megapixels resolution, are relatively inexpensive and easy to use, if a computer connected to the Internet is available.

Even low-resolution photographs that can be transmitted through cellular phones or palm handheld computers may suffice in following up most of the wound progress.

Telephone support

The availability of a 24 hours a day call center that may answer common medical questions to patients who are undergoing home treatment for limb salvage is useful, especially in those cases when computer expertise is limited.

The call center should have well-trained personnel, possibly young physicians, nurses or senior medical students under close supervision, who undergo specific training for this purpose. Complete electronic medical records should be available to the operator, with photographs of the wound progress for comparison.

Solutions to simple questions such as clarification of techniques for wound dressing and assistance in the handling of simple complications will reduce the number of repeated hospital admissions and the overloading of day-care centers. The call center should also be alert in identifying suspect serious complications and directing the patient to the nearest medical center. Furthermore, the call center may assist local physicians in emergency rooms when they see these patients, by providing them with the clinical history and the details of the procedures they underwent, along with the protocols and reports on their progress, also suggesting further care.

To this purpose, a national center for limb salvage has been created and is being expanded in Italy; it provides training to physicians, support to patients, an Internet electronic consultation site **www.cnsdiabetes.org**, and a telephone assistance call center.

Preventive medicine

Diet, weight loss, control of diabetes, foot hygiene, avoidance of smoking, and proper physical activity will help reduce the incidence of CLI. Primary care physicians, educators, and the government itself could have a prominent part in the field of prevention.[3,4,46]

Procedures that may assist in preventing major amputations should be offered to all patients, regardless of age, provided they would be able to use their limbs for walking and self-sufficiency. Younger patients require efficient and esthetically pleasing extremities, while many elderly patients may be quite satisfied with the capability to move around their home without assistance. In rare instances, preserving a limb, which cannot be utilized for walking, may be justified, even if only out of respect toward the self-consciousness and dignity of the individual.

There are some morbidity, mortality and costs involved when limb salvage procedures are performed, but they are no match compared with the mortality, morbidity, and high social and personal costs involved in major amputations, not to mention to the degree of permanent invalidity implied in such procedures.[46,47]

References

1   McNeely MJ, Boyko EJ, Ahroni JH et al. The independent contributions of diabetic neuropathy and vasculopathy in foot ulceration: how great are the risks? *Diabetes Care* 1995; **18**: 216–9.

2   Millington JT, Norri TW. Effective treatment strategies for diabetic foot wounds. *J Fam Prac* 2000; **49**(11 suppl): S40–8.

3   Levin ME. Preventing amputation in the patient with diabetes. *Diabetes Care* 1995; **18**: 1383–94.

4   Litzelman DK, Slemenda CW, Langefeld CD et al. Reduction of lower extremity clinical abnormalities in patients with non-insulin-dependent diabetes mellitus. A randomized, controlled trial. *Ann Intern Med* 1993; **119**: 36–41.

5   Stiegler H, Standl E, Frank S, Mendler G. Failure of reducing lower extremity amputations in diabetic patients: results of two subsequent population-based surveys 1990 and 1995 in Germany. *Vasa* 1998: **27**: 10–14.

6   Panayiotopoulos YP, Tyrrell MR, Arnold FJ, Korzon-Burakowska A, Amiel SA, Taylor PR. Results and cost analysis of distal (crural/pedal) arteries revascularization for limb salvage in diabetic and non-diabetic patients. *Diabetic Med* 1997; **14**: 214–20.

7   Muller IS, de Grauw WJ, van Gerwen WH et al. Foot ulceration and lower limb amputation in type 2 diabetic patients in Dutch primary health care. *Diabetes Care* 2002; **25**: 570–4.

8   Inglese L, Graziani L, Tarricone R. Percutaneous treatment of peripheral obstructive arteriopathy: the reasons for a choice. *Ital Heart J* 2000; **1**(9 suppl): 1138–47.

9   Ragnarson, Tennvall G, Apelqvist J. Prevention of diabetes-related foot ulcers and amputations: a cost–utility analysis based on Markov model simulation. *Diabetologia* 2001; **44**: 2077–87.

10   Tennvall G, Apelqvist J, Eneroth M. Costs of deep foot infections in patients with diabetes mellitus. *Pharmacoeconomics* 2000; **18**: 225–38.

11   Calabrese E, Kjellmer B, Rotolo M. Complex vascular reconstructions: extraperitoneal and thoracoabdominal approach to the aorta. *Adv Vasc Path* 1989; **1**: 455–8.

12   Towne JB, Bernhard VM, Rollins DL, Baum PL. Profundaplasty in perspective: limitations on the long term management of limb ischemia. *Surgery* 1981; **90**: 1037–46.

13   Motarjeme A, Keifer JW, Zuska AJ. Percutaneous transluminal angioplasty of the deep femoral artery. *Radiology* 1980; **135**: 613–7.

14   Zdanowski Z, Albrechtsson U, Lundin A et al. Percutaneous transluminal angioplasty with or without stenting for femoropopliteal occlusions? A randomized controlled study. *Int Angiol* 1999; **18**: 251–5.

15   Cejna M, Thurnher S, Illiasch H et al. PTA versus Palmaz stent placement in femoropopliteal artery obstructions: a multicenter prospective randomized study. *J Vasc Intervent Radiol* 2001; **12**: 23–31.

16   Jahnke T, Voshage G et al. Endovascular placement of self-expanding nitinol coil stents for the treatment of the femoropopliteal obstructive disease. *J Vasc Interven Radiol* 2002; **13**: 257–66.

17   Grimm J, Muller-Hulsbeck S, Jahnke T, Hilbert C, Brossmann J, Heller M. Randomized study to compare PTA alone versus PTA with Palmaz stent placement for femoropopliteal lesions. *J Vasc Intervent Radiol* 2001; **12**: 35–42.

18   Gray BH, Sullivan TM, Childs MB, Young JR, Olin JW. High incidence of restenosis/reocclusion of stents in the percutanous treatement of long segment superfcial femoral artery disease after suboptimal angioplasty. *J Vasc Surg* 1997; **25**: 74–83.

19   Calabrese E:.Long segment PTA in limb salvage (in critical limb ischemia). EURO-PCR 2001: the Paris Course on Revascularization, Paris, May 2001.

20 Steckmeier B, Parzhuber A, Verrel F, Kellner W, Reininger C. Simultaneous vascular and endovascular surgery of complex vascular diseases. *Langenbeck's Archiv für Chirurgie – Supplement – Kongressband* 1998; **115**: 532–7.

21 Dorros G, Jaff MR, Dorros AM, Mathiak LM, He T. Tibioperoneal (outflow lesion) angioplasty can be used as primary treatment in 235 patients with critical limb ischemia – five-year follow-up. *Circulation* 2001; **104**: 2057–62.

22 Dorros G, Jaff MR, Murphy KJ, Mathiak L. The acute outcome of tibioperoneal vessel angioplasty in 417 cases with claudication and critical limb ischemia. *Cathet Cardiovasc Diag* 1998; **45**: 252–6.

23 Soder HK, Manninen HI, Jaakkola P et al. Prospective trial of infrapopliteal artery balloon angioplasty for critical limb ischemia: angiographic and clinical results. *JVIR* 2000; **11**:1021–31.

24 Shionoya S. Diagnostic criteria of Bueger's disease. *Int J Cardiol* 1998; **66**(suppl 1): S243–5; discussion S247.

25 Papa MZ, Rabi I, Adar R. A point scoring system for the clinical diagnosis of Bueger's disease. *Eur J Vasc Endovasc Surg* 1996; **11**:335–9.

26 Kobayashi M, Nakagawa A, Nishikimi N, Nimura Y. Immunohistochemical analysis of arterial wall cellular infiltration in Bueger's disease (endarteritis obliterans). *J Vasc Surg* 1999; **29**: 451–8.

27 Fiessinger JN, Schafer M. Trial of Iloprost versus aspirin treatment for critical limb ischaemia of thromboangiitis obliterans. The TAO Study. *Lancet* 1990; **335**: 555–7.

28 Talwar S, Choudhary SK. Omentopexy for limb salvage in Buerger's disease: indications, technique and results. *J Postgrad Med* 2001; **47**: 137–42.

29 Duncan H, Ferguson L, Faris I. Incidence of the radial steal syndrome in patients with Brescia fistula for hemodialysis: its clinical significance. *J Vasc Surg* 1996; **4**: 144–7.

30 Katz S, Kohl RD. The treatment of hand ischemia by arterial ligation and upper extremity bypass after angioaccess surgery. *J Am College Surg* 1996; **183**: 239–42.

31 Wheat LJ, Allen SD et al. Diabetic foot infections. Bacteriological analysis. *Arch Intern Med* 1986; **146**: 1935–40.

32 Wack C, Wolfle KD, Hauser H, Bohndorf K, Loeprecht H. Diabetic foot – uncontrollable infections despite successful revascularization. *Langenbeck's Archiv für Chirurgie – Suppl – Kongressband* 1997; **114**: 569–71.

33 Eckman MH, Greenfield S, Mackey WC et al. Foot infections in diabetic patients: decision and cost-effectiveness analyses. *JAMA* 1995; **273**: 712–20.

34 Attinger CE, Ducic I, Neville RF, Abbruzzese MR, Gomes M, Sidawy AN. The relative roles of aggressive wound care versus revascularization in salvage of the threatened lower extremity in the renal failure diabetic patient. *Plas Reconstr Surg* 2002; **109**: 1281–90.

35 Cavigelli A, Fischer R, Dietz V. Socio-economic outcome of paraplegia compared to lower limb amputation. *Spinal Cord* 2002; **40**: 174–7.

36 Refaat Y, Gunnoe J, Hornicek FJ, Mankin HJ. Comparison of quality of life after amputation or limb salvage. *Clin Orthopaed Rel Res* 2002; **397**: 298-305.

37 Tan CM, Im MJ, Myers RA, Hoopes JE. Effects of hyperbaric oxygen and hyperbaric air on the survival of island skin flaps. *Plas Reconstr Surg* 1984; **73**: 27–30.

38 Calabrese E, Rotolo M, Sottile A, Kjellmer B. Terapia intensiva in chirurgia vascolare. *Minerva Angiologica* 1990; **15**: 79–81.

39 Bakker DJ. Hyperbaric oxygen therapy and the diabetic foot. *Diabetes/Metabolism Res Rev* 2000; **16**(suppl 1): S55–8.

40 Faglia E, Rampoldi A, Morabito A et al. Change in major amputation rate in a center dedicated to diabetic foot care during the 1980s: prognostic determinants for major amputation. *J Diabetes & Its Complications* 1998; **12**: 96–102.

41 Wunderlich RP, Peters EJ, Lavery LA. Systemic hyperbaric oxygen therapy: lower-extremity wound healing and the diabetic foot. *Diabetes Care* 2000; **23**: 1551–5.

42 Rutherford RB, Jones DN, Bergentz SE et al. The efficacy of dextran-40 preventing early postoperative thrombosis following difficult lower extremity bypass. *J Vasc Surg* 1984; **1**: 765–73.

43 Swiigris JJ, Olin JW, Mekhail NA. Implantable spinal cord stimulator to treat the ischemic manifestations of thromboangiitis obliterans (Buerger's disease). *J Vasc Surg* 1999; **29**: 928–35.

44 Spincemaille GH, Klomp HM, Steyerberg EW et al. Technical data and complications of spinal cord stimulation: data from a randomized trial on critical limb ischemia. *Stereotac Funct Neurosurg* 2000; **74**: 63–72.

45 Patel ST, Haser PB, Bush HL Jr, Kent KC. Is thrombolysis of lower extremity acute arterial occlusion cost-effective? *J Surg Res* 1999; **83**:106–12.

46 Ollendorf DA, Kotsanos JG, Wishner WJ et al. Potential economic benefits of lower-extremity amputation prevention strategies in diabetes. *Diabetes Care* 1998; **21**: 1240–5.

47 Calabrese E. Salvataggio d'arto in gangrena. *Minerva Angiologica* 1990; **5**: 95–7.

48 Duda SH, Pusich B, Richter G et al. Sirolimus-eluting stents for the treatment of obstructive superficial femoral artery disease. Six-month results. *Circulation* 2002; 1505–9.

51

Embolization in peripheral territory

Claudio J Schönholz, Esteban Mendaro, Sergio Sierro and
Denisse Hurvitz

The continuous development and improvement of materials
and techniques in recent years has led to a wider spectrum of
methods for transcatheter occlusive therapy. Since the 1970s
the percutaneous treatment of multiple and varied
pathologies with detachable balloons, big particles and
rudimentary coils has been introduced.[1-3] Advances in agents
for embolization and in catheter and guide-wire technology
have increased the reach of the interventional radiologist in
treating a variety of pathologic conditions that were
traditionally treated by surgery. The proper use of
embolization techniques requires an understanding of the
vascular anatomy and pathology, the tools used to deliver
embolic agents, and the embolic agents themselves.

Embolic agents

An ideal embolic agent would be precisely sized,
nonclumping, highly radiopaque, nontoxic, nonallergenic, and
inexpensive.[4] It would allow easily controlled delivery
through conventional or microcatheter systems to a specific
vascular territory, and would provide reliable occlusion for
the desired length of time. It is the task of the interventional
radiologist to find the appropriate embolic agent to match the
clinical indication.

Methods for embolization can be categorized by the
duration of the effect and the type of agent. Resorbable
agents generally give temporary occlusion, although
permanent occlusion may result, especially when there is
poor collateral flow and necrosis occurs. Nonresorbable
agents usually give permanent occlusion. The types of agents
include liquids, particulates, mechanical devices, and
coagulants. Liquid and particulate agents tend to give distal
occlusion, whereas mechanical agents are generally larger
and tend to give proximal vessel occlusion.[4,5]

Commonly used embolization materials

These materials can be divided into the following groups;
details of some of these are given below.

- *Biodegradable particles:*
  Gelatin sponge (Gelfoam®)
  Microfibrillar collagen (Avitene®)
  Starch microspheres (Spherex®).
- *Permanent particles:*
  Polyvinyl alcohol sponge (Ivalon®, Contour®)
  Acrylic microspheres (Embospheres®).
- *Liquids:*
  Ethanol
  Iodized oil (Lipiodol®)
  Glue (*n*-butyl-cyanoacrylate – Histoacryl®)
  Ethibloc®
  Hypertonic glucose
- *Mechanical agents:*
  Metallic coils, Fibered coils, GDC
  Detachable balloons
  Covered stent–grafts
  Vascular occlusors

Biodegradable particles

Gelfoam®

Gelfoam is a gelatin sponge that causes vascular occlusion by
mechanical obstruction, induction of thrombosis, and
inflammation of the vessel wall. The gelatin dissolves and
permits recanalization of the artery within days to weeks.[6]
Since it does not cause permanent occlusion, Gelfoam is

useful in treating benign sources of bleeding such as trauma, or for temporary devascularization of masses immediately before resection to minimize blood loss. Gelfoam® powder is 40–60 μm and causes occlusion of vessels 100–200 μm in diameter. Gelfoam powder is good for preoperative embolization of tumors or organs.

Microfibrillar collagen

Avitene® is a preparation of collagen fibers.[7] The fibers are 5 μm in diameter by 70–100 μm in length, and they cause vascular occlusion at the 25–250 μm level. Avitene causes a granulomatous reaction. Recanalization of the vessels begins at about a week and continues over 1 to 2 months. Collagen is useful for tumor embolization, either preoperatively or palliatively, and has been used for chemoembolization in the liver. It can be used mixed with Gelfoam and Ivalon®.

Permanent particles

Polyvinyl alcohol (PVA – Ivalon®)

Polyvinyl alcohol (PVA) is an inert plastic sponge that is ground into coarsely shaped particles of graded dimensions from 100 to 1000 μm. It causes permanent mechanical occlusion of the vessel lumen with subsequent ingrowth of thrombus and fibrin. The irregular, cratered surface of the particles makes them prone to clump into aggregates, so that occlusion occurs at the level of vessels larger than the nominal size of the particles used. Like Gelfoam, PVA particles tend to float in contrast, so the syringe must be pointed upward during injection to avoid clumping at the back of the barrel. It is used in cases of distal devascularization, such as preoperative tumors or in cases of hemoptysis in bronchial embolization.

Microspheres (Embospheres®)

This permanent embolic agent has the advantage of a regular shape and precise targeted level occlusion due to its calibrated size. This agent is used as the other permanent particles, with similar indications.

Mechanical agents

Coils

These permanent occlusive agents are available in varying wire sizes, lengths, coil diameters, and shapes. The conventional steel coil embolus consists of a short length of guide wire with multiple polyester strands attached transversely along most of its length between the turns of the wire. These devices come prepackaged and stretched out in metal cartridges, eliminating the need for a special mandrel introducer and permitting their delivery through conventional 5F, 0.035- and 0.038-inch tapered catheters using conventional, floppy guide wires. They are used, for instance, in cases of pseudoaneurysms or arteriovenous fistulae (AVFs), leading to the occlusion of the afferent feeding channel. The 0.018 or 0.010-inch platinum Guglielmi detachable coils (GDC) coils are recommended for use with 0.018–0.010-inch inner lumen catheters, such as the Tracker® 18 or Excel® 014. These modern microcoils are used in the treatment of cerebral aneurysms. There are many reports of its use in peripheral territory also.[8,9]

Liquid agents

Unlike particles, which by virtue of their size are arrested at a precapillary level, liquid sclerosants can pass to the capillary level and through to the venous circulation.[10] This feature makes them desirable agents in the treatment of vascular malformations. Vascular occlusion occurs from a combination of thrombosis and destruction of the vessel endothelium, which is usually permanent. Liquid sclerosants (e.g. ethanol) are more challenging to use than particulates due to their deeper penetration into tissue, making their distribution harder to control and increasing the risk of nontarget embolization.

NBCA (n-isobutyl cyanocrylate)

It is a liquid, rapidly plastic adhesive agent that polymerizes immediately upon contact with any ionic surface (blood, endothelium), which makes necessary the use of a coaxial technique with microcatheters.[11] It is a permanent occlusive agent, not radiopaque, so it needs ethiodized oils or tantalum powder to be opacified.[12,13] Due to its precision delivery, NBCA is used for arteriovenous malformations (AVMs) in cerebral or peripheral territories. Great experience of the operator in the management of the agent and in endovascular microcatheter techniques is required to avoid complications, because of the rapid action and strong adhesive quality of the agent.

Ethanol

Ethanol is a very powerful sclerosing agent that causes parietal necrosis and thrombosis. It is used for organ ablation or tumor devascularization.[14] The distribution of the ethanol is difficult to control, and it is important to avoid reflux at the moment of embolization.

Transcatheter peripheral embolization: some clinical indications

Pelvis and extremities transcatheter embolization

Trauma

Before undertaking transcatheter therapy for arterial lesions, it is important to understand the surgical alternatives for treatment and their risks and benefits. Radiologic management is primarily limited to embolotherapy, the intentional occlusion of a vessel. The technique of embolization depends on the type and location of the vascular lesions. In trauma, a temporary occluding agent such as gelatin sponge is theoretically advantageous because many of these lesions will heal.[15,16] Alternatively, fibered coils and platinum microcoils, although permanent, offer the advantage of speed and precise positioning. The success rate for transcatheter embolization has been reported to be between 85 and 100%.

High-flow priapism

Priapism is caused by an imbalance in penile blood inflow and outflow. High-flow priapism presents an uncontrolled arterial inflow to the corpora cavernosa generally due to a post-traumatic arteriocavernosal fistula.[17–20] The endovascular treatment consists in superselective embolization of the feeding vessel of the AVF. Platinum microcoils, sometimes associated with Gelfoam, make this procedure feasible with good clinical outcome.[21–25] (Figure 51.1).

Uterine fibroid embolization

Uterine fibroid embolization is a promising procedure in the treatment of uterine leiomyomata with good clinical results.[26–30] This alternative treatment is a minimally invasive technique with low complication rates, very good clinical efficacy, and a significant reduction in fibroid size and, consequently, in symptoms.[31–39] The bilateral uterine artery embolization is performed with permanent particulated agents (PVA, 300–500μm).[32] In some cases, Gelfoam is also used. (Figure 51.2).

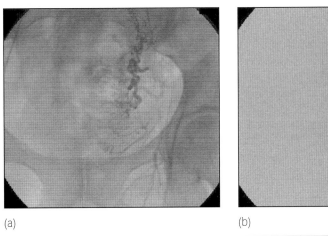

(a)

(b)

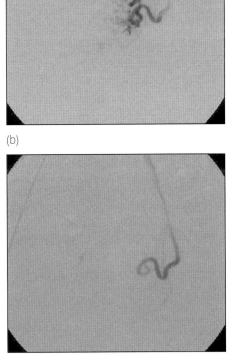

(c)

(d)

Figure 51.1

High flow priapism. (a) Selective internal pudendal angiogram. Traumatic fistula to cavernosal body. (b) Superselective catheterization with a 3F microcatheter. (c) Angiogram post-embolization: note a platinum microcoil occluding the feeding artery. (d) Selective internal pudendal angiogram: note the fistula occlusion.

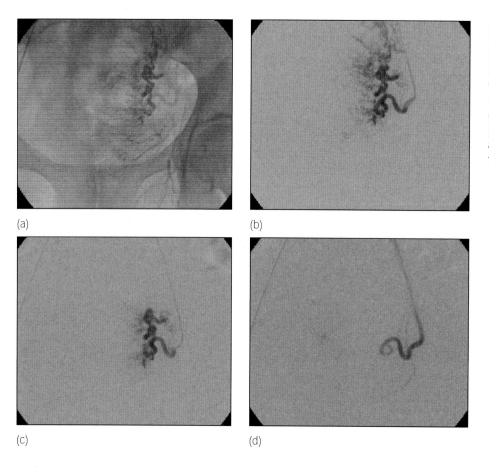

(a)

(b)

(c)

(d)

Figure 51.2
Uterine fibroid embolization. (a,b) Selective internal iliac angiogram demonstrates uterine fibroid vascularization. (c) Selective uterine artery angiogram. (d) Post-embolization with polyvinyl alcohol (PVA) angiogram demonstrates fibroid devascularization.

Bronchial embolization in the treatment of hemoptysis

Once the site of hemorrhage is known, attention can be confined to embolization of bronchial arteries and collaterals supplying that area.[40] Transcatheter embolization requires a stable catheter position. When a stable catheter position cannot be obtained with these catheters, coaxial catheterization can be performed. Distal embolization should be performed whenever possible. Special attention must be paid to detect the presence of a spinal artery for avoiding neurologic complications. The most commonly used embolic materials for bronchial artery embolization include Gelfoam and PVA particles.[41,42]

Gelfoam (gelatin sponge) is the most commonly used material. It is a readily available, slowly resorbable material that can be used as individual pledgets, torpedoes, or part of a slurry. Polyvinyl alcohol is the other commonly used particulate embolic material that is permanent in nature and available in several particle sizes. Particles in the 300–500-μm range and 500–700-μm range are compatible with coaxial systems and are used routinely.[43,44] Bronchial artery embolization has been shown to be a very effective technique for the immediate control of hemoptysis of inflammatory origin. In general, the long-term control rate of hemoptysis is approximately 70–94% (Figure 51.3).

Splenic embolization

Trauma

The goal of embolization in splenic trauma is to stop active bleeding while preserving as much splenic tissue as possible. This is achieved with the use of coils (stainless steel coils) as occlusive agents, embolizing the splenic artery or one of its branches.[45,46] They are relatively safe, fast, easy to use, and inexpensive, with good clinical and angiographic results. Gelfoam can also be used in association with coils, to assure the complete vessel occlusion.[47] (Figure 51.4).

Hypersplenism

The more conventional technique of splenic embolization i.e., particulate embolization of the spleen, is employed in hypersplenism.[48–50] The goal is permanent reduction of splenic substance. The technique is performed with particulated permanent agents such as PVA or microspheres.[51]

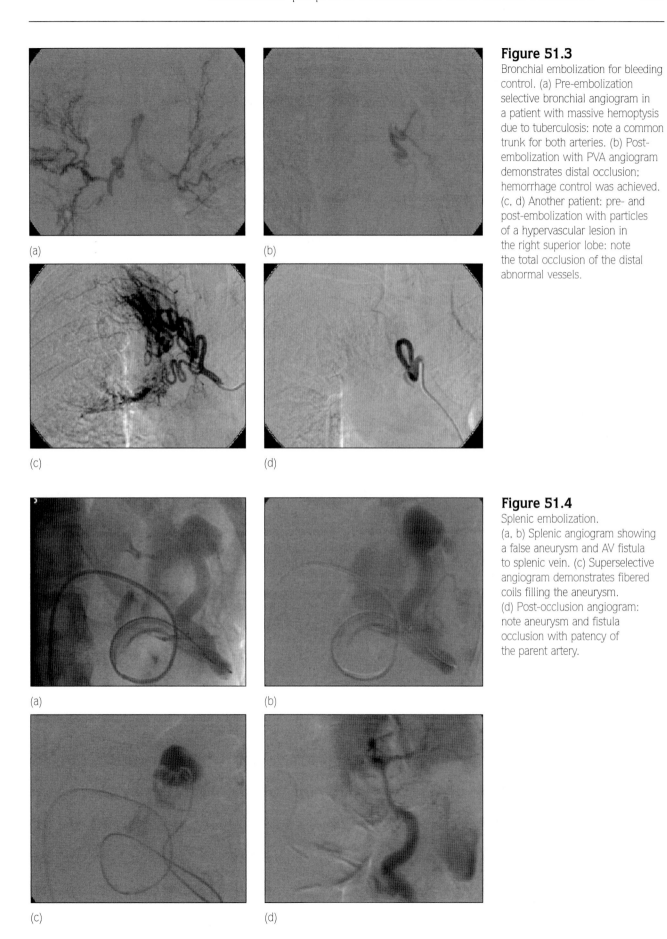

Figure 51.3
Bronchial embolization for bleeding control. (a) Pre-embolization selective bronchial angiogram in a patient with massive hemoptysis due to tuberculosis: note a common trunk for both arteries. (b) Post-embolization with PVA angiogram demonstrates distal occlusion; hemorrhage control was achieved. (c, d) Another patient: pre- and post-embolization with particles of a hypervascular lesion in the right superior lobe: note the total occlusion of the distal abnormal vessels.

(a)

(b)

(c)

(d)

Figure 51.4
Splenic embolization.
(a, b) Splenic angiogram showing a false aneurysm and AV fistula to splenic vein. (c) Superselective angiogram demonstrates fibered coils filling the aneurysm.
(d) Post-occlusion angiogram: note aneurysm and fistula occlusion with patency of the parent artery.

(a)

(b)

(c)

(d)

Hypervascular tumor embolization

Embolization of a variety of tumors has been performed, preoperatively or as an isolated therapy.[52,53] Embolization of tumors is done for preoperative vascular control and to palliate unresectable lesions. In general, the isolated use of mechanical agents to occlude proximal vessels has a limited role, especially if the organ is to remain in the patient, since collateral flow will quickly result in reperfusion. Even in organs with end arteries, such as the kidney, agents traveling to the distal, small-vessel level give a more definitive occlusion, which is achieved with particulate agents.[54,55] (Figure 51.5).

Hepatic malignancies: chemoembolization

Many pharmacological agents have been used for hepatic artery infusion.[56] The most frequently used drugs for chemoembolization are doxorubicin, cisplatin, and mitomycin.

A number of embolic agents have been used to treat liver tumors. The agents are broadly categorized into mechanical and particulate (further subdivided into permanent and temporary). Mechanical agents such as coils, differing little from proximal surgical ligation of a vessel, have little role in the primary management of liver tumors. In these cancer patients, the most experience has been accumulated with the embolic agents Gelfoam, PVA, and Lipiodol.[57]

Proponents of embolization alone advocate PVA particles because they provide permanent occlusion. Since the hepatic artery is to be intentionally embolized, confirmation of portal vein patency is essential. In the presence of portal vein thrombus, hepatic chemoembolization can be safely performed if collateral flow is adequate. Fever and abdominal pain ('postembolization syndrome') occur commonly after such procedures and can be effectively treated with nonsteroidal anti-inflammatory agents. (Figure 51.6).

Peripheral aneurysms, pseudoaneurysms and arteriovenous malformations

Aneurysms–Pseudoaneurysms

The major indications for treating aneurysms are to prevent hemorrhagic or thromboembolic complications. Less

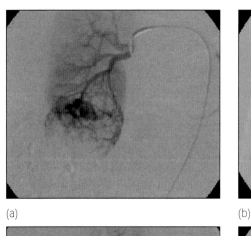
(a)

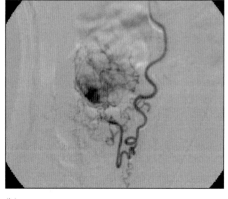
(b)

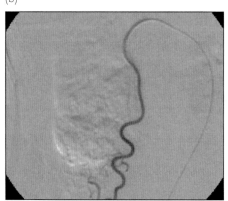
(c) (d)

Figure 51.5
Renal cell carcinoma embolization.
(a) Selective right renal angiogram demonstrates a well-marginated, small vascular mass in the inferior pole of the right kidney.
(b) Selective capsular artery angiogram shows that this artery is also involved in tumor vascularization.
(c, d) Post-embolization angiograms demonstrate tumor occlusion with patency of the main branches.

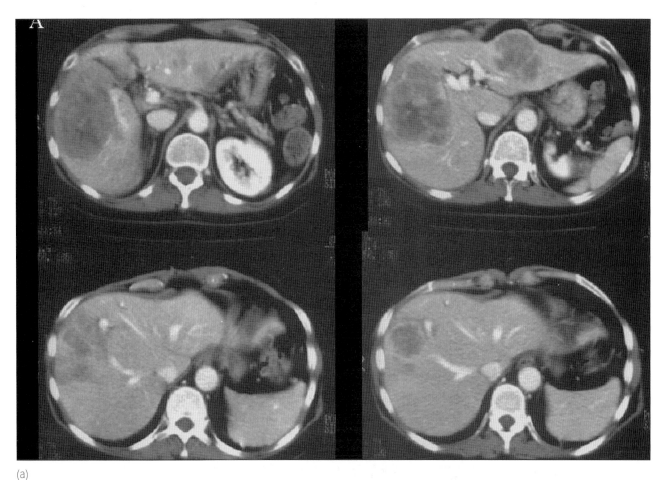

(a)

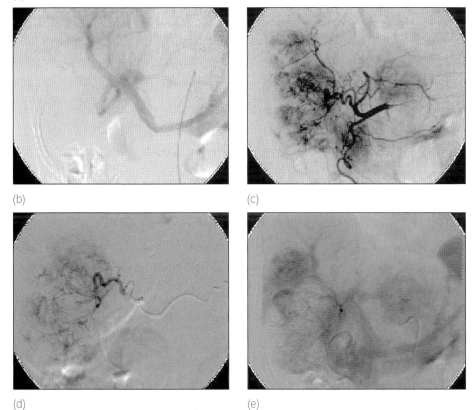

(b)

(c)

(d)

(e)

Figure 51.6

(a). Contrast-enhanced computed tomography (CT) scan of the liver demonstrates a large heterogeneous mass involving the right lobe of the liver confirmed as hepatocarcinoma: note another lesion involving the left lobe of the liver. (b) Selective superior mesenteric artery angiography: venous phase showing portal vein patency. (c) Selective common hepatic artery angiography demonstrating a large hypervascular mass corresponding to the lesions seen on the CT. (d) Selective injection of a branch of the right hepatic artery through the microcatheter, demonstrating hypervascular supply of the dominant lesion. (e) Post-chemoembolization with doxorubicin, polyvinyl alcohol (PVA) particles, and Lipiodol angiogram showing devascularization of the treated lesion (compare with c).

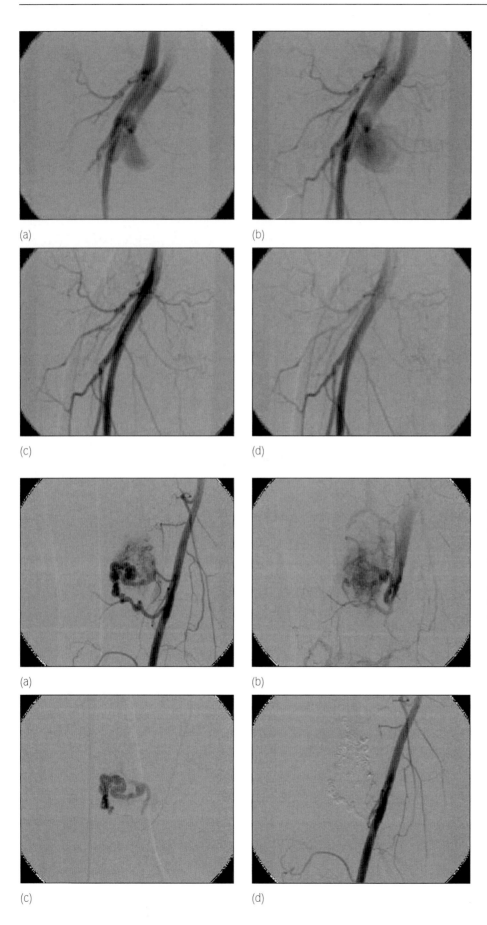

(a)

(b)

(c)

(d)

Figure 51.7
(a, b). Selective superficial femoral artery angiography showing a false aneurysm and arteriovenous fistula to the femoral vein in a patient with an iatrogenic groin hematoma. (c, d). Completion angiogram after implanting a covered stent–graft (Hemobahn, Gore). Note the total occlusion of the pseudoaneurysm and the associated fistula.

(a)

(b)

(c)

(d)

Figure 51.8
(a) Selective right superficial femoral artery with a congenital arteriovenous malformation (AVM) at the level of the thigh – arterial phase. (b) Venous phase. (c) Superselective injection with a 3 Fr catheter placed in one of the feeding arteries. (d) Post-embolization angiogram after the injection of 0.8 ml of Histoacryl. No filling of the AVM in noted.

frequently, they may create difficulties due to the mass effect on adjacent structures (of greater concern intracranially). Percutaneous occlusion is effective when the sac and origin of the aneurysm is securely closed.

For aneurysmatic lesions, mechanical agents can provide occlusion for all of these methods:

- placing a stent or endovascular graft, closing the orifice of an aneurysm, is an alternative method of occlusion while preserving the vessel. (Figure 51.7).
- fibered coils and microcoils are also a good indication for this kind of lesion, filling the aneurysm sac or occluding the afferent vessel.

Arteriovenous malformations

These lesions may cause complications due to hemorrhage, mass effect, high-output heart failure, or local ischemia due to vascular steal. They are best treated by eradicating the nidus, so the isolated occlusion of feeding vessels with mechanical devices frequently only results in at best temporary benefit as collateral vessels enlarge to supply the malformation. The smaller mechanical agents, such as 0.018 microcoils, have a role because they can be placed closer to the nidus. Liquid agents such as NBCA (Histoacryl®), which occlude the malformation nidus, have demonstrated excellent results with very low recurrence rates. Malformations that are simple AVFs or in which eradication of the nidus is not essential, such as pulmonary arteriovenous malformations, are well treated by mechanical embolization devices. In such cases, depending on the branching pattern, the length of the artery supplying the malformation, and the size of the artery, the decision is made to either embolize the feeding artery with coils or with detachable balloons for occlusion. (Figure 51.8)

References

1. Dawbain G, Lussenhop AJ, Spence WT. Artificial embolization of cerebral arteries: report of use in a case of arteriovenous malformation. *JAMA* 1960; **172**: 1153–5.
2. Tadavarthy SM, Moller JH, Amplatz K. Polyvinyl alcohol (Ivalon): a new embolic material. *AJR* 1975; **125**: 609–16.
3. Gianturco C, Anderson JH, Wallace S. Mechanical devices for arterial occlusion. *AJR* 1975; **124**: 428–35.
4. Castañeda-Zuñiga WR, Tadavarthy SM. *Interventional radiology.* Baltimore: Williams & Wilkins, 1992.
5. Greenfield AJ, Athanasoulis CA, Waltman AC. Transcatheter vessel occlusion: selection of methods and material. *Cardiovasc Intervent Radiol* 1980; **3**: 222–8.
6. Jander HP, Russinovich NAE. Transcatheter Gelfoam embolization in abdominal, retroperitoneal, and pelvic hemorrhage. *Radiology* 1980; **136**: 337–44.
7. Diamond NG, Casarella WJ, Bachman DM, Wolff M. Microfibrillar collagen hemostat: a new transcatheter embolization agent. *Radiology* 1979; **133**: 775–9.

8. Morse SS, Clark RA, Puffenbarger A. Platinum microcoils for therapeutic embolization: nonneuroradiologic applications. Technical note. *AJR* 1990; **155**: 401–3.
9. Tisnado J, Beachley MC, Cho SR. Peripheral embolization of a stainless steel coil. *AJR* 1979; **133**: 324–6.
10. Goldman ML, Philip PL, Sarrafizadeh MS. Bucrylate, a liquid tissue adhesive for transcatheter embolization. *Appl Radiol* 1984; **Nov/Dec**: 89–94.
11. Dotter CT, Goldman ML, Rosch J. Instant selective arterial occlusion with isobutyl-2–cyanoacrylate. *Radiology* 1975; **114**: 227–30.
12. Frenny PC, Bush WH, Kidd R. Transcatheter occlusive therapy of genitourinary abnormalities using isobutyl-2-cyanoacrylate. *AJR* 1979; **133**: 647–56.
13. Cromwell LD, Kerber CW. Modification of cyanoacrylate for therapeutic embolization: preliminary experience. *AJR* 1981; **137**: 781–5.
14. Ellman BA, Parkhill BJ, Curry TS et al. Ablation of renal tumors with absolute ethanol: a new technique. *Radiology* 1981; **141**: 619–26.
15. Matalon T, Athanasoulis CA, Margolies MN et al. Hemorrhage with pelvic fractures: efficacy of transcatheter embolization. *AJR* 1979; **133**: 859–67.
16. Ben-Menachem Y, Handel SF, Ray RD, Child TL III. Embolization procedures in trauma: a matter of urgency. *Semin Intervent Radiol* 1985; **2**: 107–17.
17. Gujral S, MacDonagh RP, Cavanagh PM. Bilateral super-selective arterial microcoil embolisation in delayed post-traumatic high flow priapism. *Postgrad Med J* 2001; **77**(905): 193–4.
18. Logarakis NF, Simons ME, Hassouna M. Selective arterial embolization for post-traumatic high flow priapism. *Can J Urol* 2000; **7**(3): 1051–4.
19. Colombo F, Lovaria A, Saccheri S et al. Arterial embolization in the treatment of post-traumatic priapism.
20. Callewaert P, Stockx L, Bogaert G, Baert L. Post-traumatic high-flow priapism in a 6-year-old boy: management by percutaneous placement of bilateral vascular coils. *Urology* 1998; **52**(1): 134–7.
21. Moscovici J, Barret E, Galinier P et al. Post-traumatic arterial priapism in the child: a study of four cases. *Eur J Pediatr Surg* 2000; **10**(1): 72–6.
22. Ji MX, He NS, Wang P, Chen G. Use of selective embolization of the bilateral cavernous arteries for posttraumatic arterial priapism. *J Urol* 1994; **151**(6): 1641–2.
23. Puppo P, Belgrano E, Germinale F et al. Angiographic treatment of high-flow priapism. *Eur Urol* 1985; **11**(6): 397–400.
24. Walker TG, Grant PW, Goldstein I et al. 'High-flow' priapism: treatment with superselective transcatheter embolization. *Radiology* 1990; **174**(3 Pt 2): 1053–4.
25. Webber RJ, Thirsk I, Moffat LE, Hussey J. Selective arterial embolization in the treatment of arterial priapism. *J R Coll Surg Edinb* 1998; **43**(1): 61.
26. Uterine artery embolization in a 10–week cervical pregnancy with coexisting fibroids. *Int J Gynaecol Obstet* 2001; **72**(3): 253–8.
27. Ravina JH. Fibroma: surgical myomectomy or embolization or GnRH analogs? Embolization of uterine fibroma: a new treatment. *Gynecol Obstet Fertil* 2001; **29**(1): 66–7.

28 Spies J, Niedzwiecki G, Goodwin S et al. Training standards for physicians performing uterine artery embolization for leiomyomata: consensus statement developed by the Task Force on Uterine Artery Embolization and the Standards Division of the Society of Cardiovascular & Interventional Radiology – August 2000. *J Vasc Interv Radiol* 2001; **12**(1): 19–21.

29 McLucas B, Adler L, Perrella R. Uterine fibroid embolization: nonsurgical treatment for symptomatic fibroids. *J Am Coll Surg* 2001; **192**(1): 95–105.

30 Pelage J, Le Dref O, Jacob D et al. Uterine artery embolization: anatomical and technical considerations, indications, results and complications. *J Radiol* 2000; **81**(12–Fmc): 1863–72.

31 Worthington-Kirsch RL, Fueredi GA, Goodwin SC, et al. Polyvinyl alcohol particle size for uterine artery embolization. *Radiology* 2001; **218**(2): 605–6.

32 Braude P, Reidy J, Nott V et al. Embolization of uterine leiomyomata: current concepts in management. *Hum Reprod Update* 2000; **6**(6): 603–8.

33 Golfieri R, Muzzi C, De Iaco P et al. The percutaneous treatment of uterine fibromas by means of transcatheter arterial embolization. *Radiol Med (Torino)* 2000; **100**(1–2):48–55.

34 Lund N, Justesen P, Elle B et al. Fibroids treated by uterine artery embolization. A review. *Acta Obstet Gynecol Scand* 2000; **79**(11): 905–10.

35 Dubel GJ, Ferland RJ, Murphy TP, Frishman G. The emerging role of uterine artery embolization in the management of symptomatic uterine fibroids. *Med Health R I.* 2000; **83**(10): 305–11.

36 Brunereau L, Herbreteau D, Gallas S et al. Uterine artery embolization in the primary treatment of uterine leiomyomas: technical features and prospective follow-up with clinical and sonographic examinations in 58 patients. *Am J Roentgenol* 2000; **175**(5): 1267–72.

37 McLucas B, Adler L, Perrella R. Uterine fibroid embolization: nonsurgical treatment for symptomatic fibroids. *J Am Coll Surg* 2001; **192**(1): 95–105.

38 Pelage J, Le Dref O, Jacob D et al. Uterine artery embolization: anatomical and technical considerations, indications, results and complications. *J Radiol* 2000; **81**(12–Fmc): 1863–72.

39 Reidy JF, Spies JB, Walker WJ. Polyvinyl alcohol particle size for uterine artery embolization. *Radiology* 2001; **218**(2): 605–6.

40 Remy J, Arnaud A, Fardou H et al. Treatment of hemoptysis by embolization of bronchial arteries. *Radiology* 1977; **122**: 33–7

41 Cohen AM, Doershuk CF, Stern RC. Bronchial artery embolization to control hemoptysis in cystic fibrosis. *Radiology* 1990; **175**: 401–5.

42 Vujic I, Pyle R, Parker E, Mithoefer J. Control of massive hemoptysis by embolization of intercostal arteries. *Radiology* 1980; **137**: 617–20.

43 Stoll JF, Bettman MA. Bronchial artery embolization to control hemoptysis: a review. *Cardiovasc Intervent Radiol* 1988; **11**: 263–9.

44 Wholey MH, Chamorro HA, Gopal R et al. Bronchial artery embolization for massive hemoptysis. *JAMA* 1976; **236**: 2501–4.

45 Fisher RG, Ben-Menachen Y. Embolization procedures in trauma: the abdomen – extraperitoneal. *Semin Intervent Radiol* 1985; **2**: 148–57.

46 Richman SD, Green WW, Kroll R, Casarella WJ. Superselective transcatheter embolization of traumatic renal hemorrhage. *AJR* 1977; **128**: 843–4.

47 Castañeda-Zuñiga WR, Hammerschmidt DE, Sanchez R, Amplatz K. Nonsurgical splenectomy. *AJR* 1977; **129**: 805–11.

48 Chuang VO, Reuter SR. Experimental diminution of splenic function by selective embolization of the esplenic artery. *Surg Gynecol Obstet* 1975; **140**: 715–20.

49 Alwmark A, Bengmark S, Gullstrand P et al. Evaluation of splenic embolization in patient with portal hypertension and hyperesplenism. *Ann Surg* 1982; **196**: 518–24.

50 Owman T, Lunderquist A, Alwmark A, Borjesson B. Embolization of the spleen for treatment of splenomegaly and hypersplenism in patients with portal hypertension. *Invest Radiol* 1979; **14**: 457–64.

51 Castañeda-Zuñiga WR, Hammerschmidt DE, Sanchez R, Amplatz K. Nonsurgical splenectomy. *AJR* 1977; **129**: 805–11.

52 Chuang VP. Superselective hepatic tumor embolization with tracker-18 catheter. *J Intervent Radiol* 1988; **3**: 69–71.

53 Coldwell DM. Hepatic arterial embolization utilizing a coaxial catheter system technical note. *Cardiovasc Intervent Radiol* 1990; **13**: 53–4.

54 Almgard LE, Fernstrom I, Haverling M. Treatment of renal adenocarcinoma by embolic occlusion of the renal circulation. *Br J Urol* 1973; **45**: 474–9.

55 Kaisary AV, Williams G, Riddle PR. The role of preoperative embolization in renal cell carcinoma. *J Urol* 1984; **131**: 641–6.

56 Chuang VP, Wallace S. Hepatic arterial redistribution for intra-arterial infusion of hepatic neoplasms. *Radiology* 1980; **135**: 295–9.

57 Shimizu T, Sako M. Hirota S. Intraarterial infusion therapy with polysaccharide solution as a carrier of anticancer agents. *Nippon Acta Radiol* 1988; **48**: 702.

52

Hemodialysis access intervention

Kamran Ahrar

In the United States alone, over 200 000 patients with end-stage renal disease are maintained on long-term dialysis.[1] The creation and maintenance of long-term vascular access are essential components of a multidisciplinary approach to the care of patients on hemodialysis. This chapter describes percutaneous interventions for maintenance of native arteriovenous fistulas (AVFs) and synthetic bridge grafts.

Native arteriovenous fistulas

The creation of an endogenous fistula by surgical anastomosis of an artery and vein represents a major advance in vascular access surgery. At this time, Brescia–Cimino (BC) type AVFs remain the preferred method of access for patients on long-term hemodialysis (Figure 52.1). The BC AVF is created by performing a side-to-side anastomosis of the radial artery and cephalic vein at the level of the wrist.[2] Dilatation and arterialization of the draining vein of the AVF is referred to as maturation, a process that takes 1–2 months. If the vein becomes large enough and provides sufficient flow for hemodialysis, the long-term patency should be excellent.[3,4] However, nonmaturation occurs in 11–27% of cases and appears to be even more common among patients who are elderly or who have diabetes.[5,6] Several other forearm AVFs offer similar to the excellent patency rate reported for BC AVFs.[4,7,8] However, a more proximal location of the AVF may predispose the patient to increased risk of arm swelling or distal ischemia (Figure 52.2).[9] Other complications of AVFs include low flow states (due to stenoses), thrombosis, prolonged bleeding, and pseudoaneurysm.[10]

Native AVFs offer distinct advantages over synthetic bridge grafts. The rate of revision for native AVFs (0.07 revision/access per year) is significantly lower than that for polytetrafluorethylene (PTFE) grafts (0.5 revision/access per

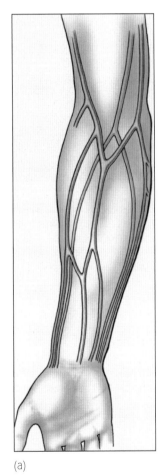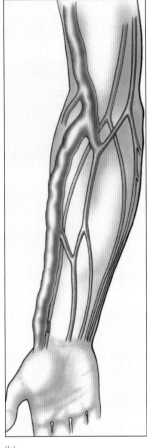

(a)   (b)

Figure 52.1
Creation and maturation of a Brescia–Cimino radiocephalic arteriovenous fistula. (a) Normal arterial and venous anatomy of the forearm. (b) Side-to-side anastomosis of the radial artery and cephalic vein at the level of the wrist. Also demonstrated is dilatation and arterialization of the cephalic vein. which provide easy access for needle placement.

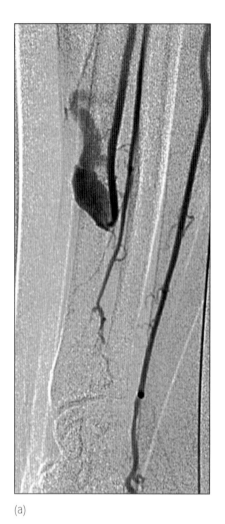
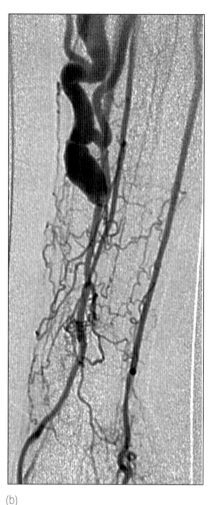
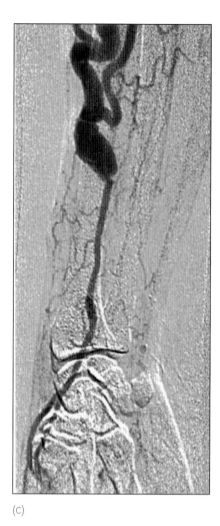

(a)　　　　　　　　　　　　　　　　(b)　　　　　　　　　　　　　　　　(c)

Figure 52.2
Creation of an arteriovenous fistula proximal to the wrist, causing hand ischemia. (a) Early phase of brachial arteriogram demonstrates preferential flow of blood from the radial artery into the cephalic vein. (b, c) Delayed images of the same arteriogram depicted in Part A demonstrate reversal of flow in the distal radial artery.

year). In addition, the infection rate for native AVFs is minimal, compared with 9% for PTFE grafts. Consequently, there are few published reports of percutaneous interventions for the salvage of AVFs.[11–17] The sections that follow describe the causes of poor function and failure of AVFs and outline approaches to reversing these problems.

Intervention in arteriovenous fistulas that fail to mature

AVFs typically mature within 1–2 months after their creation. However, maturation depends on two factors: adequate inflow and sufficient outflow venous resistance. If an AVF does not mature within 4 months, another type of access must be established.[18] Because the sites available for hemodialysis fistulas are limited, attempts to explore the etiology of nonmaturation and to treat the underlying cause are warranted. The adequacy of inflow is evaluated by arteriography. In cases of an upper extremity fistula, arteriography reveals the inflow extending from the aortic subclavian ostium to the anastomosis. Any flow-limiting stenoses may be treated by percutaneous transluminal angioplasty (PTA) in standard fashion. The venous limb may be the cause of nonmaturation of the fistula. Side branches in the draining vein provide alternative drainage. The alternative drainage decreases the resistance in the main outflow vein and may prevent adequate arterialization of the outflow vein. These side branches may be eliminated by suture ligation or coil embolization.[19,20]

Interventions in thrombosed or poorly functioning arteriovenous fistulas previously used for dialysis

Information gained during physical examination of dysfunctional fistulas is invaluable in directing percutaneous intervention. Lack of palpable thrill in the fistula suggests either inadequate inflow or access thrombosis. Thrombosed AVFs may be salvaged by pharmacologic thrombolysis, mechanical thrombectomy, or both. Although some investigators have reported mobilization of the thrombus to the central veins and pulmonary circulation,[11] it is important to remember that native arteriovenous fistulas may have a much larger clot burden in comparison to synthetic bridge grafts. The technical success rates for declotting of native AVFs (81–95%) are slightly lower than those for synthetic bridge grafts (89–100%). However, the lower success rates of AVFs are offset by their excellent patency rates. Primary 12-month patency rates of 50–64% and secondary 12-month patency rates of 81–100% have been reported.[11,13,16,17] In addition, the revision rate associated with native AVFs is lower than that associated with synthetic bridge grafts.[21]

Unlike synthetic bridge grafts, native AVFs may remain patent despite extremely low blood flow velocities. A hand-held Doppler may help detect slow flow and prevent an erroneous diagnosis of thrombosis. Patent AVFs are characterized by a palpable thrill over the anastomosis. A prominent pulse at the anastomosis upon physical examination suggests stenosis of the outflow vein. This suspicion is confirmed by the findings of elevated venous pressure and increased recirculation values during hemodialysis. A pull-back venography is performed to evaluate the venous outflow channel from the fistula to the right atrium. Central venous stenosis is commonly encountered in patients with a history of having a subclavian temporary dialysis catheter (Figure 52.3). Venous stenosis may also develop in the draining vein as a result of a high flow rate, high pressure, and turbulence (Figure 52.4). In such cases, angioplasty of the venous stenoses may be performed in the usual fashion. If angioplasty is not successful, vascular stents may be placed, but deployment of stents in the segment of the vein used for hemodialysis needle placement should be avoided. Decreased inflow is suggested by decreased thrill at the anastomosis or by a vein that lies flat in the subcutaneous tissues (Figure 52.5). A common site of stenosis is an area within 1 cm from the anastomosis. Such cases of stenosis may be treated with angioplasty through the fistula. Several 2- to 3-min inflations may be necessary to break the stenosis. More proximal stenoses may be encountered as a result of atherosclerosis and may be treated with angioplasty. Loss of access, or distal ischemia, or both may result from progression of atherosclerosis, from thrombosis of angioplasty site, or from a flow-limiting intimal tear.

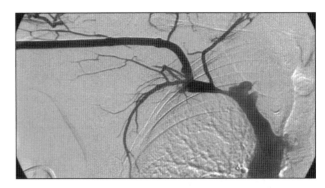

(a)

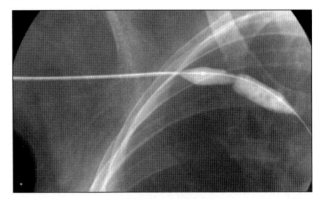

(b)

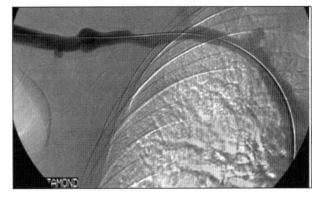

(c)

Figure 52.3
Catheter-induced, central venous stenosis causing pulsatile flow in the cephalic vein. (a) Fistulogram demonstrates high-grade stenosis of the medial subclavian vein. (b) Balloon angioplasty was performed through a basilic vein access. The waist in the angioplasty balloon demonstrates the resilient nature of these stenoses, requiring high-pressure balloon for effective angioplasty. (c) Venogram after angioplasty shows successful treatment of the stenotic lesion.

Complications

Major complications occur in fewer than 1% of reported cases of AVFs and may include severe rupture of a vein resulting in loss of access, sepsis-related death, myocardial

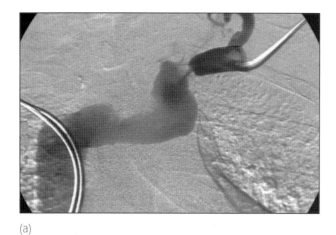

(a)

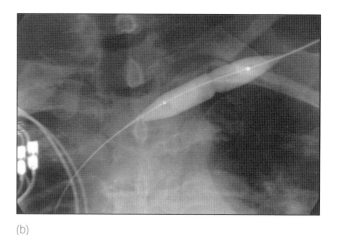

(b)

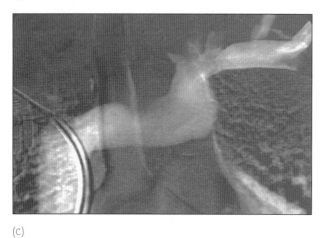

(c)

Figure 52.4

Cephalic vein stenosis causing high venous pressure in the fistula. (a) Pull-back venography through the radiocephalic fistula demonstrates stenosis of the central cephalic vein. (b) Angioplasty was performed through the fistula. (c) Fistulogram following angioplasty shows good result.

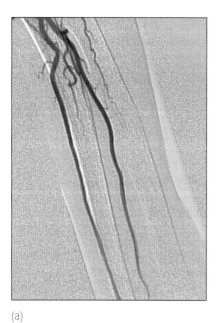

(a)

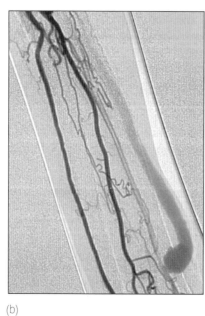

(b)

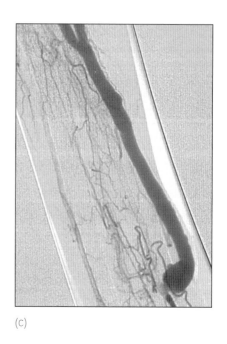

(c)

Figure 52.5

Lack of a palpable thrill due to inadequate arterial inflow. (a) Early phase of brachial arteriogram demonstrates the ulnar and interosseous arteries. There is no flow in the radial artery. (b, c) Delayed images of the same arteriogram shown in (a) demonstrate reversal of flow in the distal radial artery and confirm occlusion of the proximal radial artery.

infarction, pulmonary edema, intracranial hemorrhage complicating thrombolysis, or ischemia of the hand or distal runoff bed. Minor complications are more common and may include minor rupture of a vein (1.7–35%), thrombosis of the fistula during angioplasty (2–7%), bacteremia (3%), formation of a pseudoaneurysm (6%), and embolization of a thrombus from the fistula to the arterial circulation (6–24%).[11,20,22]

Synthetic bridge grafts

When an AVF cannot be created, the alternative is to create a synthetic bridge graft.[23] Most commonly, PTFE grafts are placed in straight or loop fashion in the forearm or upper arm.[24–27] There are multiple permutations for inflow and outflow sites. Loop grafts in the forearm are interposed between the brachial artery and the brachial vein. In the upper arm, a loop graft may be interposed between the high brachial artery or axillary artery and the high brachial vein. Synthetic bridge grafts are prone to complications, including stenosis, thrombosis, and pseudoaneurysms. The lifespan of synthetic grafts is shorter than that of AVFs.[3] If all the sites in the upper extremities have been exhausted, a loop graft between the superficial femoral artery and vein or the greater saphenous vein may be created.[28] Another alternative site for a graft is the anterior chest wall, where the arterial inflow may be directed from the axillary or subclavian vessels and the outflow may be directed into the ipsilateral or contralateral axillary or jugular vein.[29] Compared with grafts in the upper extremity, grafts in the lower extremity or in the chest wall may have higher rates of vascular steal syndrome and infection.

For synthetic PTFE grafts, the primary patency rate at 1 year is at least 70%.[26,30–32] The most common cause of graft failure is stenosis of the outflow vein, resulting in graft thrombosis.[32] Exposure of the draining vein to high-velocity, high-pressure, and turbulent blood flow promotes neointimal hyperplasia that in turn results in venous stenosis. Progression of venous stenosis markedly reduces the flow of blood in the graft, eventually leading to graft thrombosis.

Intervention in failing synthetic bridge grafts

Screening for impending failure of synthetic bridge grafts

Progressive neointimal hyperplasia, encountered at the venous anastomosis, is the most common cause of graft thrombosis. Furthermore, thrombotic events that cannot be resolved are the leading cause of access loss. Either percutaneous intervention with angioplasty or surgical

revision to correct stenosis dramatically reduces the rate of graft thrombosis and loss.[33–35] As venous stenoses progress, they increase the intra-access pressure while decreasing the rate of blood flow. Each institution should implement an organized monitoring program to identify failing grafts by regular assessment of several clinical and functional hemodialysis parameters. Clinical indicators of a failing graft include conversion of a thrill to a pulsatile flow, difficulty with needle placement, prolonged bleeding after needle withdrawal, or persistent swelling of the arm.[36–39] Useful measurements to monitor for stenosis in arteriovenous grafts include intra-access flow, static venous pressures, dynamic venous pressures, and recirculation.[33,38,40,41] Direct measurements of flow detect not only outflow lesions but also inflow and intragraft stenoses. It is anticipated that direct measurement of intra-access flow will eventually replace measurement of venous pressure and recirculation. Persistent abnormalities in any of these parameters should prompt referral for venography.

Treatment of failing synthetic bridge grafts

Venous stenoses causing more than a 50% decrease in lumen diameter that are associated with at least one abnormal clinical or physiological variable must be treated in order to prevent graft thrombosis.[42] Central venous stenoses are better treated with angioplasty than with surgical treatment, which requires thoracotomy.[43] Vascular stents may be deployed in elastic central venous stenoses or if a stenosis recurs within 3 months.[43] The vast majority of central venous stenoses are due to placement of temporary dialysis catheters in the subclavian veins. Angioplasty of these stenotic lesions usually requires large-diameter balloons (10–12 mm or larger) with high-burst pressure (> 17 mmHg). The choice of appropriate treatment of venous stenosis at or near the anastomosis is controversial.[44,45] Surgical revision using a jump graft may extend the access further up the arm to a more central location. On the other hand, angioplasty helps in conserving the available veins for future use (Figure 52.6). Also, with angioplasty, the graft is immediately available for hemodialysis, thus obviating the need for placement of a temporary hemodialysis catheter. Finally, redilation is an easy and safe procedure that is more acceptable to patients than are repeated surgical revisions. Most commonly, stenoses are solitary and are less than 6 cm long and thus lend themselves to successful angioplasty. A 6-month primary patency rate of 40–50% is expected for these lesions.[42] Longer stenoses and those lesions that have been dilated several times have less favorable patency rates than more focal lesions dilated for the first time. A lesion that requires more than two angioplasties within 3 months should be referred for surgical revision.[18]

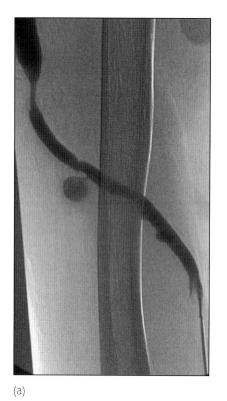
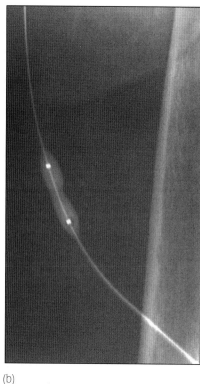
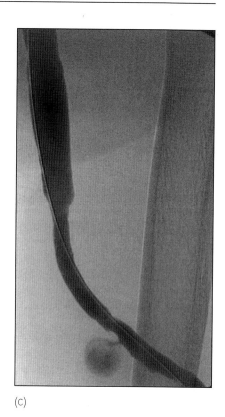

(a)
(b)
(c)

Figure 52.6
Stenosis at the venous anastomosis of a straight arteriovenous graft, causing pulsatile flow, prolonged bleeding, and enlarging pseudoaneurysm. (a) The fistulogram demonstrates significant stenosis at the venous anastomosis. A pseudoaneurysm is also identified. (b) Angioplasty was performed prior to graft thrombosis. (c) Fistulogram following balloon angioplasty demonstrates a good result. The pseudoaneurysm remained stable and did not require any other intervention.

In a few cases, stenosis at the arterial anastomosis may limit inflow and prevent successful hemodialysis.[46–48] The arterial anastomosis may be imaged through the graft. Manual compression or balloon occlusion of the graft with injection of contrast into the arterial limb of the graft provides reflux into the feeding artery, thus outlining the arterial anastomosis. Lesions at this location may be accessed through the graft and treated with PTA. Direct brachial artery puncture is an alternative for lesions that cannot be accessed through the graft.

Intervention in thrombosed synthetic bridge grafts

The traditional therapy for thrombosed arteriovenous grafts has been surgical thrombectomy with or without revision.[30,49,50] Over the past 15 years, percutaneous techniques have been investigated and have become widely utilized for hemodialysis access salvage.[51] Percutaneous procedures are particularly suitable for arteriovenous grafts because these grafts are easily accessible and contain only a small amount of fresh thrombus. In more than 85% of thrombosed arteriovenous grafts, stenosis of the venous outflow is the underlying cause of graft failure and can be treated using endovascular techniques. Percutaneous techniques also allow for evaluation of the rest of the graft, including the arterial anastomosis, the graft body, and the entire venous outflow (Figure 52.7). Percutaneous techniques also allow abnormalities involving any of these segments to be treated through the graft in a single session, and dialysis can be performed immediately after the procedure.

Pre-procedural patient assessment

Graft infection is an absolute contraindication for percutaneous declotting. Revascularization of an infected graft may lead to bacteremia and fatal sepsis.[52] Patients with graft infection should be treated with antibiotics followed by surgical removal of the graft. Before every diagnostic or therapeutic procedure, physical examination by the interventional radiologist is necessary to detect any signs of infection, including redness, tenderness, warmth, or swelling. These signs may be subtle, and the more ominous signs of infection, such as purulent discharge or skin breakdown over the graft, are rare.

Patients undergoing hemodialysis are chronically anemic. Additional blood loss may occur during an endovascular procedure, increasing the risk of an acute cardiac event.[53] Patients undergoing mechanical thrombectomy are at higher risk than are patients who undergo pharmacologic declotting. Thrombectomy devices can cause blood loss in two ways: (1) mechanical destruction of red cells and (2) aspiration of whole blood along with thrombus fragments. Patients with severe anemia may require blood transfusion before percutaneous declotting procedures.

Percutaneous graft declotting techniques

Early attempts at percutaneous declotting of arteriovenous grafts involved prolonged infusion of streptokinase through a needle or short catheter.[54] This technique restored graft patency in only 52% of the reported cases and was complicated by frequent bleeding and allergic reactions. Eventually, simple pharmacologic declotting procedures were replaced by pharmacomechanical thrombolysis with the use of forced periodic injections of thrombolytic agents (i.e., the pulse spray technique.[55] The prolonged and labor-intensive nature of pharmacomechanical thrombolysis has led to the development of other techniques, including mechanical thrombectomy.[53]

Four basic steps are common to any percutaneous intervention for salvage of thrombosed arteriovenous grafts (Figure 52.8).[53] First, a venogram is performed to evaluate the central and peripheral native veins. The second step involves removal of the thrombus from the graft. In the third step, all significant stenoses are treated with PTA, atherectomy, vascular stents, or a combination of these techniques. Finally, the organized clot at the arterial anastomosis (i.e., the arterial plug) is removed to restore flow into the graft. Although most physicians perform these steps in the order presented below, there are several variations of this scheme.

Venography. Access is gained via the arterial limb of the graft, with the puncture directed towards the venous outflow (Figure 52.8b). A catheter is placed in the outflow vein, and venography is performed to evaluate the central and peripheral veins. The most common finding in cases of thrombosed arteriovenous grafts is a focal stenosis at the venous anastomosis.[51] Occasionally, long-segment stenosis or multiple segmental stenoses or occlusions are identified in the native veins. Compared with shorter lesions, long-segment stenoses and occlusions may be better treated surgically; however, the true extent of the lesion may not be determined until after blood flow is reestablished (Figure 52.9). Even if the results of percutaneous intervention are not durable, successful declotting allows for the graft to function while a surgical revision is being planned.

Removal of the thrombus. Simple pharmacologic graft thrombolysis was soon replaced by pulse-spray pharmacomechanical thrombolysis (PSPMT). This technique involves forceful injection of a thrombolytic agent through infusion catheters, theoretically macerating the clot and exposing a larger surface area to the fibrinolytic agent.[55] For this purpose, the graft is accessed with two 5F (French) sheaths, one directed towards the arterial anastomosis and the other to the venous anastomosis. Two pulse-spray catheters are then placed in the graft in a crisscross fashion. A mixture of urokinase and heparin is infused by forceful periodic injection of small aliquots in each catheter. Urokinase is no longer available in the United States; other thrombolytic agents are utilized. Those interventionalists who use tissue plasminogen activator (tPA) do not mix heparin with tPA because it may cause a precipitate. In this case, heparin is administered intravenously. With pharmacomechanical thrombolysis, 75–94% of grafts are salvaged.[51] Primary patencies range from 25 to 34% at 6 months; secondary patencies may reach up to 80%.

The development of thrombectomy devices has increased the efficiency and speed of thrombus removal, thereby eliminating the need for thrombolytic agents and reducing the overall procedure time. Several mechanical thrombectomy devices are available for use in hemodialysis grafts.[53] Regardless of type, the thrombectomy device is introduced through a sheath placed adjacent to the arterial anastomosis and is advanced to the venous anastomosis (Figure 52.8c). The device is activated and is moved through the venous limb of the graft, either aspirating or macerating the thrombus. At this time, venous angioplasty procedures are performed to

Figure 52.7

Angiogram of a 2-year-old arteriovenous graft demonstrates stenosis at the arterial anastomosis, as well as intragraft stenoses, pseudoaneurysms, and stenosis at the venous anastomosis.

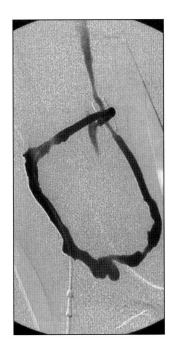

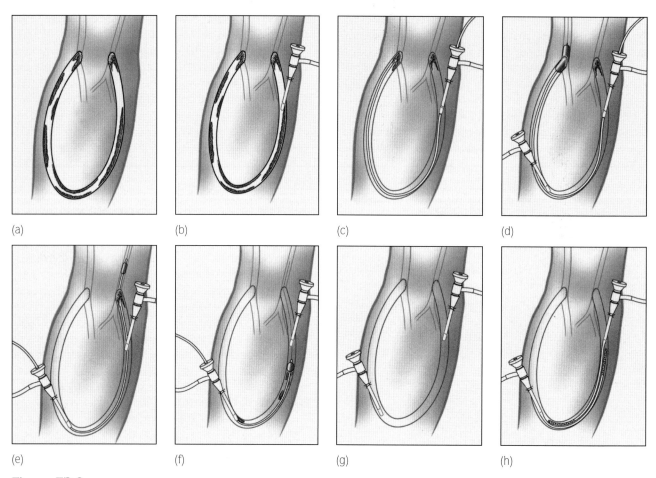

(a)   (b)   (c)   (d)

(e)   (f)   (g)   (h)

Figure 52.8

Interventions in thrombosed synthetic bridge grafts. (a) Thrombosed loop graft. Three different components are depicted: the arterial plug, intragraft thrombus, and stenosis at the venous anastomosis. (b) Access is obtained in the arterial limb of the graft near the arterial anastomosis. A vascular sheath is placed towards the venous outflow. (c) A mechanical thrombectomy device is used for maceration and/or removal of thrombus. Alternatively, the thrombus can be macerated and displaced into the venous outflow using a balloon catheter. (d) The venous anastomosis is treated with angioplasty. A second vascular sheath is placed in the venous limb of the graft. The thrombectomy device is advanced to the arterial anastomosis, and the residual thrombus is removed from the arterial limb. (e) An embolectomy balloon is advanced beyond the arterial anastomosis into the feeding artery. (f) The arterial plug is dislodged into the graft. Brisk flow displaces these fragments into the venous outflow. (g) After removal of the thrombus, a fistulogram is performed to evaluate the graft, the arterial supply, and the venous outflow tract. (h) Vascular sheaths can be replaced with crossing dialysis catheters for immediate dialysis. Alternatively, the vascular sheaths can be removed, and hemostasis may be achieved with manual compression or purse-string sutures.

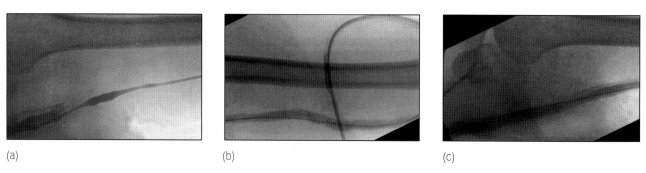

(a)   (b)   (c)

Figure 52.9

Apparent long-segment stenosis of the venous outflow due to inadequate flow and spasm. (a) Pull-back venography demonstrates an apparent long-segment stenosis of the venous outflow tract. (b) Fistulogram after declotting and focal angioplasty of the venous anastomosis demonstrates good flow through the graft and the venous anastomosis. (c) Venogram demonstrates good flow in the venous outflow tract without any interventions in this segment.

establish a patent venous outflow tract (Figure 52.8d). The device is then reintroduced into the graft through a second sheath placed closer to the venous anastomosis and is advanced to the arterial anastomosis without disturbing the arterial plug. The rest of the arterial limb is treated in the same fashion.

Venous angioplasty procedures. Most stenoses are encountered at or near the venous anastomosis.[51] These lesions are difficult to dilate and typically require a high-burst pressure balloon that is 10–20% larger than the draining vein (i.e., balloons 5–8 mm in diameter) (Figure 52.10a). If initial dilation is not successful, repeated prolonged (1- to 2-min) dilatations may be necessary to overcome the stenosis. Directional atherectomy may help weaken the stenotic segment.[56] Ultimately, a metallic stent may be placed to overcome the elastic recoil.[51]

Removal of the arterial plug. The arterial plug is composed of densely packed red blood cells and fibrin and is often adherent to the wall of the graft at the arterial anastomosis. Plug mobilization is the final and important step in declotting arteriovenous grafts.[12,57,58] An embolectomy balloon is advanced beyond the anastomosis into the feeding artery (Figure 52.8e). The balloon is partially inflated and is pulled back into the graft (Figure 52.8f). At times, three or four passes of the embolectomy balloon may be necessary to remove the adherent clot from the arterial anastomosis. Once the plug is pulled into the graft, brisk flow is re-established and displaces the plug to the pulmonary circulation. The arterial plug is small (0.3 ml) and allowing its embolization to the pulmonary circulation is thought to represent only a minimal risk. Alternatively, the plug may be mobilized into the graft and macerated using a mechanical thrombectomy device.[59]

In the lyse-and-wait technique, a variation of the approach presented above, most dissolution of the clot occurs outside the interventional suite.[60] A mixture of urokinase and heparin, or other thrombolytic agent, is injected slowly into the graft through a small angiocatheter placed near the arterial anastomosis. This approach allows for dissolution of the clot while the patient is in the waiting area. Approximately 30–60 min later, the patient is placed on the angiographic table, and the venous outflow is evaluated, the venous stenoses are treated, and the arterial plug is dislodged.

Regardless of the technique used for percutaneous declotting, a clinical success rate of 85% or better is expected.[51] The reported primary patency rates are 37–58% at 3 months and 18–39% at 6 months. The secondary patency rates are 62–80% at 6 months and 57–69% at 12 months. If the access thromboses more than two times within a 1-month period and a correctable lesion is identified, surgical revision must be considered.

Complications

Minor complications occur in 10% of cases of graft declotting and major complications in 1%.[57,58] Minor complications include small hematomas, limited perigraft bleeding, and contrast reactions. Serious complications include angioplasty rupture or dissection, symptomatic peripheral arterial emboli, or bleeding that requires transfusion. Asymptomatic arterial emboli may occur more frequently than is reported and may be treated percutaneously.[61] Symptomatic pulmonary emboli are rare.[62]

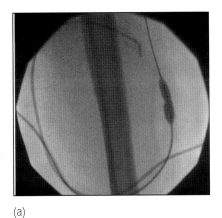
(a)

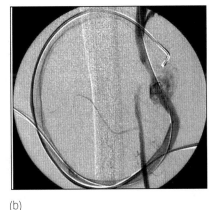
(b)

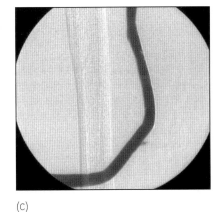
(c)

Figure 52.10
Rupture of the venous anastomosis after angioplasty. The graft was salvaged by placement of a vascular stent. (a) Angioplasty of the venous anastomosis requiring multiple dilatations of the lesion. (b) Fistulogram following angioplasty demonstrates active extravasation and expanding hematoma. (c) Fistulogram after placement of a Wallstent demonstrates no further extravasation.

References

1 USRDS 1996 Annual Data Report. The USRDS 1996 morbidity and mortality study. In: *Renal data system*. Bethesda, MD: National Institute of Diabetes and Digestive and Kidney Diseases, 1996: 46–67.

2 Brescia MJ, Cimino JE, Appel K, Hurwich BJ. Chronic hemodialysis using venipuncture and a surgically created arteriovenous fistula. *N Engl J Med* 1966; **275**: 1089–92.

3 Chazan JA, London MR, Pono LM. Long-term survival of vascular accesses in a large chronic hemodialysis population. *Nephron* 1995; **69**: 228–33.

4 Coburn MC, Carney WI Jr. Comparison of basilic vein and polytetrafluoroethylene for brachial arteriovenous fistula. *J Vasc Surg* 1994; **20**: 896–902; discussion 903–4.

5 Hakaim AG, Nalbandian M, Scott T. Superior maturation and patency of primary brachiocephalic and transposed basilic vein arteriovenous fistulae in patients with diabetes. *J Vasc Surg* 1998; **27**: 154–7.

6 Miller PE, Tolwani A, Luscy CP et al. Predictors of adequacy of arteriovenous fistulas in hemodialysis patients. *Kidney Int* 1999; **56**: 275–80.

7 Dagher FJ. The upper arm AV hemoaccess: long term follow-up. *J Cardiovasc Surg (Torino)* 1986; **27**: 447–9.

8 Matsuura JH, Rosenthal D, Clark M et al. Transposed basilic vein versus polytetrafluoroethylene for brachial-axillary arteriovenous fistulas. *Am J Surg* 1998; **176**: 219–21.

9 White G. Planning and assessment for vascular access surgery. In: Wilson S (ed.), *Vascular Access*. St. Louis, MO: Mosby-Year Book, 1996: 6–12.

10 Moray G, Karakayali H, Yildirim S et al. Fifteen years of experience in vascular access surgery. *Transplant Proc* 1998; **30**: 764–6.

11 Zaleski GX, Funaki B, Kenney S et al. Angioplasty and bolus urokinase infusion for the restoration of function in thrombosed Brescia–Cimino dialysis fistulas. *J Vasc Interv Radiol* 1999; **10**: 129–36.

12 Vorwerk D, Sohn M, Schurmann K et al. Hydrodynamic thrombectomy of hemodialysis fistulas: first clinical results. *J Vasc Interv Radiol* 1994; **5**: 813–21.

13 Vorwerk D, Schurmann K, Muller-Leisse C et al. Hydrodynamic thrombectomy of haemodialysis grafts and fistulae: results of 51 procedures. *Nephrol Dial Transplant* 1996; **11**: 1058–64.

14 Lay JP, Ashleigh RJ, Tranconi L et al. Result of angioplasty of Brescia–Cimino haemodialysis fistulae: medium-term follow-up. *Clin Radiol* 1998; **53**: 608–11.

15 Castellan L, Miotto D, Savastano S et al. The percutaneous translumina, angioplasty of Brescia–Cimono arteriovenous fistulae. An evaluation of the results. *Radiol Med (Torino)* 1994; **87**: 134–40.

16 Overbosch EH, Pattynama PM, Aarts HJ et al. Occluded hemodialysis shunts: Dutch multicenter experience with the hydrolyser catheter. *Radiology* 1996; **201**: 485–8.

17 Turmel-Rodrigues L, Sapoval M, Pengloan J et al. Manual thromboaspiration and dilation of thrombosed dialysis access: mid-term results of a simple concept. *J Vasc Interv Radiol* 1997; **8**: 813–24.

18 NFK-DOQI clinical practice guidelines for vascular access. National Kidney Foundation–Dialysis Outcome Quality Initiative. *Am J Kidney Dis* 1997; **30**: S137–240.

19 Aruny J. Maintaining native arteriovenous fistulas for dialysis access. *Tech Vasc Interv Radiol* 1999; **2**: 199–207.

20 Beathard GA, Settle SM, Shields MW. Salvage of the nonfunctioning arteriovenous fistula. *Am J Kidney Dis* 1999; **33**: 910–16.

21 Hodges TC, Fillinger MF, Zwolak RM et al. Longitudinal comparison of dialysis access methods: risk factors for failure. *J Vasc Surg* 1997; **26**: 1009–19.

22 Turmel-Rodrigues L, Pengloan J, Blanchier D et al. Insufficient dialysis shunts: improved long-term patency rates with close hemodynamic monitoring, repeated percutaneous balloon angioplasty, and stent placement. *Radiology* 1993; **187**: 273–8.

23 Rapaport A, Noon GP, McCollum CH. Polytetrafluoroethylene (PTFE) grafts for haemodialysis in chronic renal failure: assessment of durability and function at three years. *Aust N Z J Surg* 1981; **51**: 562–6.

24 Rittgers SE, Garcia-Valdez C, McCormick JT, Posner MP. Noninvasive blood flow measurement in expanded polytetrafluoroethylene grafts for hemodialysis access. *J Vasc Surg* 1986; **3**: 635–42.

25 Rizzuti RP, Hale JC, Burkart TE. Extended patency of expanded polytetrafluoroethylene grafts for vascular access using optimal configuration and revisions. *Surg Gynecol Obstet* 1988; **166**: 23–7.

26 Munda R, First MR, Alexander JW et al. Polytetrafluoroethylene graft survival in hemodialysis. *JAMA* 1983; **249**: 219–22.

27 Tellis V, Veith F. Vascular access. In: Haimovici H (ed.), *Vascular Surgery*. East Norwalk, CT: Appleton and Lange, 1989: 806–25.

28 Taylor SM, Eaves GL, Weatherford DA et al. Results and complications of arteriovenous access dialysis grafts in the lower extremity: a five year review. *Am Surg* 1996; **62**: 188–91.

29 McCann RL. Axillary grafts for difficult hemodialysis access. *J Vasc Surg* 1996; **24**: 457–61; discussion 461–2.

30 Palder SB, Kirkman RL, Whittemore AD et al. Vascular access for hemodialysis. Patency rates and results of revision. *Ann Surg* 1985; **202**: 235–9.

31 Raju S. PTFE grafts for hemodialysis access. Techniques for insertion and management of complications. *Ann Surg* 1987; **206**: 666–73.

32 Albers FJ. Causes of hemodialysis access failure. *Adv Ren Replace Ther* 1994; **1**: 107–18.

33 Schwab SJ, Raymond JR, Saeed M et al. Prevention of hemodialysis fistula thrombosis. Early detection of venous stenoses. *Kidney Int* 1989; **36**: 707–11.

34 Roberts AB, Kahn MB, Bradford S et al. Graft surveillance and angioplasty prolongs dialysis graft patency. *J Am Coll Surg* 1996; **183**: 486–92.

35 Besarab A, Sullivan KL, Ross RP, Moritz MJ. Utility of intra-access pressure monitoring in detecting and correcting venous outlet stenoses prior to thrombosis. *Kidney Int* 1995; **47**: 1364–73.

36 Beathard GA. The treatment of vascular access graft dysfunction: a nephrologist's view and experience. *Adv Ren Replace Ther* 1994; **1**: 131–47.

37   Beathard GA. Physical examination of AV grafts. *Semin Dial* 1992; **5**: 74.

38   Beathard GA. Thrombolysis versus surgery for the treatment of thrombosed dialysis access grafts. *J Am Soc Nephrol* 1995; **6**: 1619–24.

39   Trerotola SO, Scheel PJ, Powe NR et al. Screening for dialysis access graft malfunction: comparison of physical examination with US. *J Vasc Interv Radiol* 1996; **7**: 15–20.

40   Windus DW, Audrain J, Vanderson R et al. Optimization of high-efficiency hemodialysis by detection and correction of fistula dysfunction. *Kidney Int* 1990; **38**: 337–41.

41   Collins DM, Lambert MB, Middleton JP et al. Fistula dysfunction: effect on rapid hemodialysis. *Kidney Int* 1992; **41**: 1292–6.

42   Aruny JE, Lewis CA, Cardella JF et al. Quality improvement guidelines for percutaneous management of the thrombosed or dysfunctional dialysis access. Standards of Practice Committee of the Society of Cardiovascular & Interventional Radiology. *J Vasc Interv Radiol* 1999; **10**: 491–8.

43   Beathard GA. Percutaneous transvenous angioplasty in the treatment of vascular access stenosis. *Kidney Int* 1992; **42**: 1390–7.

44   Marston WA, Criado E, Jaques PF et al. Prospective randomized comparison of surgical versus endovascular management of thrombosed dialysis access grafts. *J Vasc Surg* 1997; **26**: 373–80; discussion 380–1.

45   Bitar G, Yang S, Badosa F. Balloon versus patch angioplasty as an adjuvant treatment to surgical thrombectomy of hemodialysis grafts. *Am J Surg* 1997; **174**: 140–2.

46   Saeed M, Newman GE, McCann RL et al. Stenoses in dialysis fistulas: treatment with percutaneous angioplasty. *Radiology* 1987; **164**: 693–7.

47   Roberts AC, Valji K, Bookstein JJ, Hye RJ. Pulse-spray pharmacomechanical thrombolysis for treatment of thrombosed dialysis access grafts. *Am J Surg* 1993; **166**: 221–5; discussion 225–6.

48   Valji K. Transcatheter treatment of thrombosed hemodialysis access grafts. *Am J Roentgenol* 1995; **164**: 823–9.

49   Etheredge EE, Haid SD, Maeser MN et al. Salvage operations for malfunctioning polytetrafluorethylene hemodialysis access grafts. *Surgery* 1983; **94**: 464–70.

50   Brotman DN, Fandos L, Faust GR et al. Hemodialysis graft salvage. *J Am Coll Surg* 1994; **178**: 431–4.

51   Gray RJ. Percutaneous intervention for permanent hemodialysis access: a review. *J Vasc Interv Radiol* 1997; **8**: 313–27.

52   Davis GB, Dowd CF, Bookstein JJ et al. Thrombosed dialysis grafts: efficacy of intrathrombic deposition of concentrated urokinase, clot maceration, and angioplasty. *Am J Roentgenol* 1987; **149**: 177–81.

53   Vesely T. Techniques for using mechanical thrombectomy devices to treat thombosed hemodialysis grafts. *Tech Vasc Interv Radiol* 1999; **2**: 208–16.

54   Zeit RM, Cope C. Failed hemodialysis shunts. One year of experience with aggressive treatment. *Radiology* 1985; **154**: 353–6.

55   Bookstein JJ, Fellmeth B, Roberts A et al. Pulsed-spray pharmacomechanical thrombolysis: preliminary clinical results. *Am J Roentgenol* 1989; **152**: 1097–100.

56   Gray RJ, Dolmatch BL, Buick MK. Directional atherectomy treatment for hemodialysis access: early results. *J Vasc Interv Radiol* 1992; **3**: 497–503.

57   Valji K, Bookstein JJ, Roberts AC et al. Pulse-spray pharmacomechanical thrombolysis of thrombosed hemodialysis access grafts: long-term experience and comparison of original and current techniques. *Am J Roentgenol* 1995; **164**: 1495–500; discussion 1501–3.

58   Trerotola SO, Lund GB, Scheel PJ et al. Thrombosed dialysis access grafts: percutaneous mechanical declotting without urokinase. *Radiology* 1994; **191**: 721–6.

59   Lazzaro CR, Trerotola SO, Shah H et al. Modified use of the arrow-trerotola percutaneous thrombolytic device for the treatment of thrombosed hemodialysis access grafts. *J Vasc Interv Radiol* 1999; **10**: 1025–31.

60   Cynamon J, Lakritz PS, Wahl SI et al. Hemodialysis graft declotting: description of the 'lyse and wait' technique. *J Vasc Interv Radiol* 1997; **8**: 825–9.

61   Trerotola SO, Johnson MS, Shah H, Namyslowski J. Backbleeding technique for treatment of arterial emboli resulting from dialysis graft thrombolysis. *J Vasc Interv Radiol* 1998; **9**: 141–3.

62   Kinney TB, Valji K, Rose SC et al. Pulmonary embolism from pulse-spray pharmacomechanical thrombolysis of clotted hemodialysis grafts: urokinase versus heparinized saline. *J Vasc Interv Radiol* 2000; **11**: 1143–52.

53

Superior and inferior vena cava interventional management

João Martins Pisco

Introduction

Superior vena cava (SVC) syndrome was first described by Hunter in 1757.[1] As a consequence of vena cava obstruction there is an increase of venous hypertension with congestion and edema, dilation of veins of the involved area and, in the late stages, development of the superior and inferior vena cava syndromes.

SVC syndrome has a dramatic clinical presentation. Patients with SVC syndrome present with swelling of the face, neck and arms, dilated tortuous collateral veins over the chest wall and periscapular region, respiratory distress, severe headache, alterations in the state of consciousness, cyanosis, cough, hoarseness, dysphasia and cognitive dysfunction due to cerebral venous hypertension, conjunctival edema and blurred vision. SVC syndrome may be the first sign of a bronchogenic or mediastinal tumor or it may appear during the course of the disease. Obstruction of the superior vena cava, in most cases, is caused by venous compression or by invasion by malignant tumors.

Bronchogenic carcinoma is the cause of the syndrome in 85% of cases, the small type being the most frequent. SVC syndrome occurs in about 3–15% of patients with brochogenic carcinoma and 3–8% of patients with lymphoma.

SVC syndrome has a benign cause in 15% of cases. The main benign causes are mediastinal fibrosis, radiation fibrosis, benign tumor, central venous catheters, thoracic aortic aneurysm and thrombosis secondary to invasive monitoring devices, such as cardiac pacemaker electrodes, and pulmonary artery and central venous monitoring catheters.

Bilateral subclavian vein thrombosis may result in thrombosis of the SVC. Thrombosis of the SVC does not usually occur with unilateral subclavian vein thrombosis due to the inflow from the contralateral vein. The different entities cause progressive reduction in bloodflow and secondary thrombosis.

The clinical presentation of inferior vena cava (IVC) syndrome depends on the degree and length of obstruction, the presence or absence of collaterals and the level of obstruction. Patients may be asymptomatic if there is enough collateral circulation. Usually, there is venous dilation and incapacitating swelling of the abdomen, lower limbs, pelvis, scrotum or labia, and legs.

There is renal vein thrombosis and infarction when the middle segment of the IVC is occluded. Obstruction of the hepatic segment of the IVC may result in Budd–Chiari syndrome, hepatomegaly and ascites. Patients with Budd–Chiari syndrome have abdominal distension, hepatomegaly, lower leg varicosity, varices of the abdominal wall and ascites.

The causes of IVC obstruction are malignant (retroperitoneal, caval, pelvic, kidney, adrenal and liver tumors) and benign (retroperitoneal fibrosis, radiation therapy, liver cirrhosis, webs, membranes and idiopathic).

Indications

Radiation therapy and chemotherapy, which comprise the conventional treatment for SVC syndrome caused by bronchogenic tumor usually take 3 weeks before improvement of the symptomatology, and the success rate is over 90%. The symptoms of SVC syndrome are quite distressing, and although life-expectancy is short, 3–10 months, because of immediate relief of symptoms and consequent improvement of the quality of life following stent placement, stenting may be the first-choice treatment, and should be followed by conventional therapy.

Following successful treatment, recurrences develop in 10–20% of patients due to tumor ingrowth, fibrosis, edema or thrombosis. Less than 50% respond a second time, and alternative treatment is required. Interventional management is important in patients whose disease is refractory to standard therapy, who develop benign post-radiation fibrosis, who respond too slowly to conventional treatment, who have recurrences or who have acute and severe symptoms.

Owing to recoil of the vein wall, to the thinner vein wall and to the thinner muscular layer of the vein wall, or owing to fibrosis or extrinsic compression and the firm nature of malignant tumors, large vein obstruction due to malignancy responds poorly to angioplasty. A stent is mandatory in order to keep the lumen open, to prevent elastic recoil, to obtain a good therapeutic result and to prevent occlusion. The SVC syndromes caused by central catheters and membranous obstructions of the IVC are exceptions and they respond well to angioplasty. Surgery is usually not effective and is associated with morbidity and mortality.

Percutaneous stent placement in the SVC was first reported by Charnsangavej et al in 1986. Since then, there have been several series in the literature. Initially, the first stents to be used were the Gianturco or Röch modified Gianturco. These stents have expansible force and are useful to reopen narrowed lumens and maintain patency following percutaneous transluminal angioplasty (PTA) of the occluded IVC. However, this stent is poorly adapted to curved vessels. On the other hand, because of large stent interstices, the Gianturco stent may be prone to tumor ingrowth.

For tortuous vessels, the Wallstent has been used. Wallstent and Palmaz stents that have tighter interstices have been used more and more in order to prevent tumor ingrowth. In cases of total encasement of the SVC by tumor or a firm obstruction, a Palmaz stent is indicated.[2] Dacron-covered stents may be used when treatment with an uncovered stent is suboptimal or when there is tumor ingrowth.[3]

Technical considerations

Patients should have CT before the endovascular treatment to evaluate the nature of the obstruction, the length of stenosis, the presence of thrombus and the extent of collateral circulation.[4]

Before stent placement, venography of the SVC should be performed for confirmation and evaluation of the length, severity and location of the obstruction and the thrombosis above the lesion. The most frequent approach for stent placement is the right common femoral vein (Figure 53.1). However, if there is difficulty in crossing the occlusion, the right or left internal jugular vein or peripheral veins of the arms may be used.

A catheter is placed in the SVC by the femoral approach. Attempts are made to cross the stenosis or occlusion with a guidewire. In difficult cases, a 0.035-inch hydrophilic, curved guidewire can be used. If this is impossible, a guidewire introduced by arm access is advanced across the stenosis and is

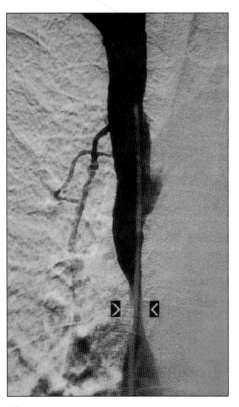
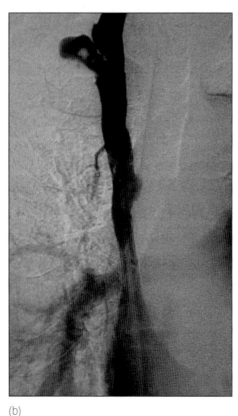

Figure 53.1
Superior vena cava flebography by femoral approach: (a) tight stenoses at distal end of SVC; (b) following stenting.

(a)   (b)

snared from the groin approach. If there is difficulty, the stenosis/occlusion is negotiated with a guidewire and catheter combination. Once the guidewire is placed through the occlusion, a pigtail catheter is positioned across the lesion and a venogram is obtained.

If it is impossible to cross the occlusion, in spite of all different attempts, and in obstructions complicated by thrombosis, thrombolysis is performed before stenting. Thrombolysis can be performed by thromboaspiration and/or by fibrinolysis. Thromboaspiration is performed through a 9F guiding catheter.

Local catheter-directed infusion of thrombolytic therapy leads to higher concentration of thrombolytic drug directly in the clot. As a result, there is faster dissolution of the thrombus, with reduced hemorrhagic complications. For fibrinolysis, an initial bolus of 250 000 IU/ of urokinase is given, followed by an infusion of 50 000 to 100 000 IU/h administered through a multi-sidehole catheter placed in the thrombus. Angioplasty combined with catheter-directed thrombolysis creates a channel through the thrombus, allowing an increased area to the fibrinolytic, with improvement of clot lysis. Later, the created channel allows the passage of the stent introducer.

During thrombolysis, heparin 24 000 IU is administered intravenously daily. Follow-up venography is performed daily, and thrombolysis is stopped when there is no residual thrombus, or most of the thrombus has been dissolved.

Partial thrombus is treated by stent deployment to wedge the thrombus against the vena cava wall without thrombolysis.

For stent placement, the patient receives 10 000 IU of heparin. Following stent placement, patients receive heparin for 2 days, 250 mg triclopidine for 4 weeks, and 100 mg aspirin for life. After the stent is in place, all lesions are dilated.

Before stent placement, the obstruction is crossed with a guidewire. Once the guidewire is placed across the vena cava stenosis/occlusion, there is a good possibility of a successful procedure. The lesion is dilated initially with a balloon catheter smaller than the diameter of the stent used. The purpose of that dilation is to evaluate the length of the stenosis, and the site of maximum stenosis where the central part of the stent should be placed, and to make easier the placement of the introductory sheath.

The diameter of the stent used should be 2–5 mm larger than the diameter of the normal vein below the stenosis and should be slightly longer than the length of the stenosis. When more than one stent is used, we start stenting from the cranial to caudal direction. For stent placement, an 8F to 10F, 80-cm sheath is introduced over the guidewire, through which the stent is placed.

High-grade stenosis may be impossible to cross with large catheters. Maintaining the guidewire under tension at both ends through dual venous access sites makes it possible for larger catheters to cross such lesions.[5]

Chest radiography can be done 48 h later to determine the position of the stent and the degree of expansion. Helical CT can also be performed 48 h later as baseline.

Results

Forty-five patients with SVC syndrome of malignant etiology were sent to us for stenting.

There were 9 females and 36 males, aged between 36 and 82 years, with a mean age of 59.3 years. Thirty-four of these patients had been treated before with radiotherapy or chemotherapy. Eighteen of them had failure and 16 recurrences of the syndrome. Only 11 had not had previous treatment. The flebography showed that there was occlusion of the SVC in 21 of the patients and tight stenosis in 24 of them.

There were 5 technical failures. In the remaining 40 patients, there were 3 thromboses at the time of stenting that were treated by fibrinolysis with urokinase. Fibrinolysis was performed in another 5 patients who had a complicated occlusion by thrombosis (Figure 53.2).

In the 40 patients in whom technical success was obtained, there was clinical success in all of them, with immediate relief that was complete in 28 and partial in 12.

On follow-up, stenting patency was considered if there was continued absence of symptoms and signs, as occurred in 18 patients between 2 and 13 months and in 14 up to their death. There was recurrence due to tumor ingrowth in 8 patients.

Discussion

In patients with SVC and IVC syndromes, the main purpose of stenting is immediate relief of the symptoms. Following successful stent placement, there is an increase of the vein lumen, and the metallic stent struts give enough mechanical support to the vein to maintain the venous lesions patent. As a consequence, there is re-establishment of normal blood-flow and immediate relief of the congestive symptoms.

In patients with SVC syndrome, the tension of the face and neck, headache, cyanosis, dyspnea, disturbances of consciousness and blurred vision improve almost immediately. The edema and pain of the face and neck regress on the following day and the edema and collateral circulation of the upper limbs, scapular region and the chest wall in 2 days.

Technical success is defined when an expanded stent is placed across the venous lesion and there is free flow of contrast through the stent. Establishment of a good antegrade flow is the best prophylactic against stent-related thrombosis.

The technical success rates for treatment of SVC obstruction of malignant etiology range from 81.3% to 100% for the Gianturco stent and from 86% to 100% for the Wallstent. The technical failures are due to the impossibility of introducing a guidewire through a chronic occlusion and consequent failure of deployment of the stent.[2] Among 45 patients with SVC syndrome of malignant etiology for stenting, we had 5 technical failures.

The two largest series of patients with benign obstruction of the SVC gave a technical success of 100%, with complete

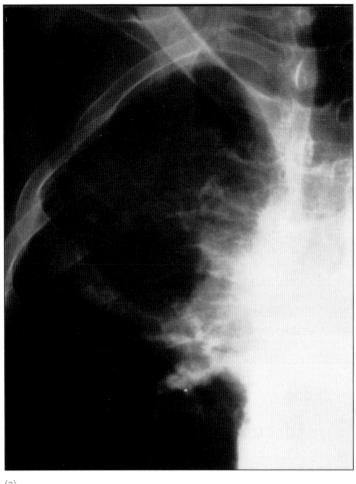

(a)

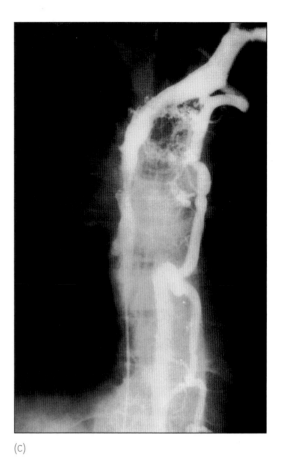

(c)

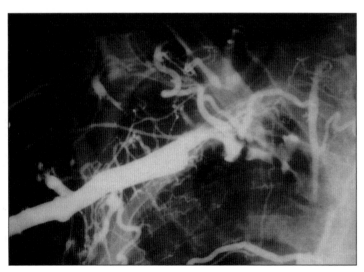

(b)

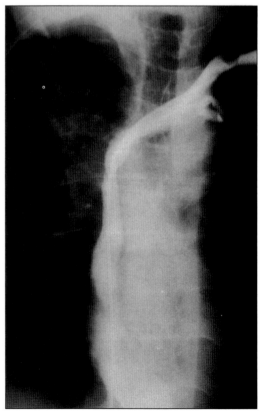

(d)

Figure 53.2

Superior vena cava flebography: (a) femoral approach – occlusion of SVC; (b) right arm approach – occlusion of SVC and subclavian vein, collateral circulation; (c) left arm approach – occlusion of SVC, drainage by azygous system; (d) femoral approach following fibrinolysis and stenting – venous drainage of upper body through SVC.

resolution of symptoms in all patients. There was only one recurrence due to shortening of a Wallstent, and this was treated with a second Wallstent. All the other stents remained patent during the follow-up period ranging from 1 to 36 months.[4,6]

Clinical success is considered when there is complete or partial resolution of edema, and tortuous collateral vein. Among 40 patients with SVC syndrome of malignant etiology in whom we placed stents, there was complete relief of symptoms in 28 patients and partial in 12.

As the treatment is palliative for most of the patients with malignant SVC syndrome, long-term follow-up does not apply to these patients, because short-term mortality is high. Therefore, the result of stenting is usually evaluated on the basis of success of the intervention at the time of the patient's death and not on long-term patency. Most of the patients become asymptomatic or less symptomatic after SVC stenting, and the stent is usually patent at the time of death. The patients are usually followed clinically during the first 48 h and then as outpatients.[7]

Patients with Budd–Chiari syndrome and IVC membranous obstruction are treated with interventional procedures. After puncture with a metallic needle such as the Brockenbrough needle or Colapinto needle, dilation is performed with a balloon catheter. For cases without satisfactory patency obtained by angioplasty and for the recurrences, stenting placement may be performed by placement of a Gianturco–Rösch stent.[3]

Angioplasty is the primary treatment for SVC syndrome of benign etiology, because the long-term patency rates of intravenous stents are as yet unknown, in spite of the early restenosis that may occur. However, stenting is performed if initial treatment including anticoagulation, thrombosis and angioplasty fails.

The recurrence rate of SVC syndrome following stenting ranges from 0% to 45% and is secondary to tumor ingrowth, radiation fibrosis or thrombosis of the stent.[8,9] The recurrences may be treated with thrombolysis, angioplasty or an additional stent placement.

Of 40 patients with SVC syndrome in whom we placed stents, there was recurrence due to tumor ingrowth in 8 patients. In the remainder, there was no recurrence between 2 and 11 months in 18 patients and up to their death in 14 patients.

The main complications reported are groin hematoma, early thrombosis, stent migration and pulmonary emboli; the overall complication rate is 3.2–7.8%.[7] We had three thromboses at the time of deployment of a Gianturco stent that were treated by fibrinolysis with urokinase.

References

1   Hunter W. History of aneurysm of the aorta with some remarks on aneurysm in general. *Med Observation Inquiries* 1757; **1**: 323.

2   Yim CN, Sane SS, Bjarnason H. Superior vena cava stenting. *Radiol Clin North Am* 2000; **38**: 409–24.

3   Xu K, He Fx, Zhang H et al. Budd–Chiari syndrome caused by obstruction of the hepatic inferior vena cava: immediate and 2–year treatment results of transluminal angioplasty and metallic stent placement. *Cardiovasc Intervent Radiol* 1996; **19**: 32–6.

4   Qanadli S, El Hajjam M, Mignon F et al. Subacute and chronic benign superior vena cava obstructions. Endovascular treatment with self-expanding metallic stents. *AJR* 1999; **173**: 159–64.

5   Takenchi Y, Arai Y, Kasahara T et al. Technical aspects of venous stenting in high-grade stenoses using a long guidewire between dual venous access sites. *Eur Radiol* 2000; **10**: 167–9.

6   Rosenblum J, Leef J, Massersmith R et al. Intravascular stents in the treatment of acute superior vena cava obstruction of benign etiology. *J Parenteral Enteral Nutrition* 1994; **18**: 362–6.

7   Nicholson AA, Ettles DF, Arnold A et al. Treatment of malignant superior vena cava obstruction: metal stent or radiation therapy. *JVIR* 1997; **8**: 781–8.

8   Cross C, Kramer J, Waignant J et al. Stent implantation in patients with superior vena cava syndrome. *AJR* 1997; **169**: 429–32.

9   Crowe M, Davies C, Caines P. Percutaneous management of superior vena cava occlusions. *Cardiovasc Intervent Radiol* 1995; **18**: 367–72.

54

Restenosis in peripheral intervention

Luc Bilodeau, Jean-François Tanguay and Martin Sirois

Advances in technology and technique refinements allow successful percutaneous transluminal approaches at enlarging abnormally narrowed vessel segments (either congenital or acquired) with re-establishment of end-organ distal functionality. This percutaneous transluminal angioplasty concept, where an intravascular balloon expansion creating a disruption of the target obstructive lesion and an overexpansion of the surrounding vascular structure, has proven so effective at reinstituting a functional vascular lumen that it now serves as the basis for interventional vascular therapy. However, restenosis or recurrence of a significant obstructive lesion after successful angioplasty remains the major limitation of vascular dilatation techniques. Fortunately, not every vascular site has the potential for a restenosis after intervention and better knowledge of the phenomenon has allowed either restenosis reduction or avoidance of prohibitively high restenotic vascular location for dilatation.

Restenosis can be defined as the recurrence of impaired lumen area after successful angioplasty. This phenomenon has been characterized classically by quantitative angiographic analysis, and most commonly, it is confirmed by a diameter stenosis of 50% or more at follow-up while a significant decrease in stenosis severity ($<50\%$ diameter stenosis) was obtained immediately after angioplasty, adjustments being made for inter- and intra-observer variability in individual laboratories.[1] This lumen impairment can also be characterized by numerous imaging modalities such as intravascular ultrasound, duplex sonography, angio-computed tomography (CT) scan and magnetic resonance imaging. Despite all these measurement techniques, restenosis is oftentimes diagnosed by recurrence of a patient's symptoms as a result of end-organ dysfunction, e.g. recurrent angina (coronary), recurrent claudication (lower limb), recurrent hypertension (renal artery). From these recurrent dysfunctions comes the need for reintervention or, more precisely, the need for target lesion revascularization (TLR) or target vessel revascularization

(TVR). Rates of TLR are classically lower than rates of TVR due to reintervention related to disease progression in the same vessel. Angiographically defined restenosis rates are also commonly higher than TVRs and TLRs due to some discrepancy between stenosis severity and patient symptoms. For instance, 4–16% of patients display angiographic evidence of restenosis after coronary angioplasty at a routine follow-up angiography without presenting angina.[2] Primary patency refers to a significant decrease in stenosis severity at follow-up after a single intervention whereas secondary patency corresponds to a result obtained after reintervention for a restenotic lesion.

Most restenosis occur within the first 6 months after intervention.[3,4] The underlying mechanism includes acute elastic recoil, local thrombotic and inflammatory reactions, intimal hyperplasia and negative arterial remodeling.[5] If a permanent stent is implanted during the angioplasty procedure, the instent restenosis is entirely explained by an intimal hyperplastic response partly influenced by a local thrombo-inflammatory process. The risk for restenosis is modulated by systemic factors, vessel and lesion morphology and, by mechanical damage caused by angioplasty. Diabetes through endothelial dysfunction, increased secretion of growth factors and enhanced platelet activity represent the most commonly associated systemic factors.[6–8] The other most powerful correlate of restenosis for a vascular segment is the occurrence of restenosis at another treated site on the same vessel type.[9] Lesion wise, plaque burden, obstruction length and vessel diameter[10,11] are all related to restenosis. In addition to vessel size, vessel type seems to play a major role in determining the risk for restenosis. Conductance vessels such as the aorta, carotids and iliac arteries are categorized as elastic arteries with their media composed mainly of fenestrated layers of elastin. Conversely, distributing vessels classified as muscular arteries such as the brachial, femoral and coronary arteries are characterized by a media composed mostly of smooth muscle cells, permitting active vessel diameter change in response to end-organ need. An aggressive restenotic process is much more common in muscular arteries, raising the hypothesis that vessels containing proportionally more smooth muscle might respond more vigorously to arterial injury.[12] In addition, elastic vessels stretch in response to balloon dilatation, but muscular arteries tear, resulting in more severe local injury. Finally, the more severe the injury caused by angioplasty, the more aggressive will be the hyperplastic response. This relationship has been well demonstrated in the porcine coronary model and it has been used to study anti-restenotic therapies.[13]

Restenosis after peripheral artery intervention represents a problem of different magnitude depending upon the target vessel type or location. Rates range from less than 5% in carotid arteries to as high as 80% in femoropopliteal locations. These extreme differences are explained by numerous factors, including muscular versus elastic type of arteries (as discussed previously), target vessel reference diameter, plaque burden and anatomical considerations. In other words, low restenosis rates will characterize an intervention in a large diameter elastic artery with moderate plaque burden where treatment was applied on the entire lesion length (healthy to healthy segments). Specifically, abdominal aorta stenoses are nearly restenosis-free after balloon angioplasty.[14,15] Carotid artery stenting is associated with 5–10% recurrent stenoses at 1 year[16,17] while subclavian artery stenoses show a 5–7% restenosis rate after balloon angioplasty with provisional stenting.[18,19] Renal artery balloon angioplasty without stenting is complicated by a prohibitively high recurrence rate if atherosclerosis is the underlying disease as opposed to fibromuscular dysplasia.[20,21] If properly covered with stents, restenosis rates reach 10–30% (ostial location).[22–24] Iliac procedures are associated with a 5-year patency rate of 72%.[25] The anti-restenotic effect of stenting in iliac arteries remains highly controversial.[26–31] Finally, the femoropopliteal muscular arteries represent the highest restenotic lesion location with recurrence rates as high as 84% after recanalization of vessel with poor distal run-off.[32] Long diffuse lesions and chronic total occlusion classically characterize femoropopliteal arterial disease. Multiple stent designs as well as covered stents have been suggested to improve long-term results but, so far, success has been limited.[32–35]

Histopathology of instent restenosis in patients with peripheral artery disease, as in coronary artery disease, demonstrates hypercellularity predominantly composed of smooth muscle cells. Directional atherectomy specimen in such instances reveals cellular proliferation and apoptosis exceeding that observed in native vessels. In a small series of 10 specimens, Kearney et al also showed that thrombus was present in 60% of cases with occasional inflammatory cells identified by CD-45 immunostaining.[36]

Overall, restenosis is considered to occur over four phases: phase I, elastic recoil within 24 hours; phase II, mural thrombus formation and organization within 2 weeks; phase III, neointimal proliferation and extracellular matrix synthesis within 3 months; and phase IV, inadequate compensatory enlargement of a vessel after angioplasty (inadequate vascular remodeling).[5,37] Elastic recoil and inadequate arterial remodeling may be reduced to an extent by coronary stenting. However, a permanent metallic prosthesis does not reduce neointimal proliferation, which is considered to be the primary mechanism of restenosis after stenting.[38]

Mural thrombus and restenosis

In an animal model of angioplasty, platelet deposition was noted to occur immediately after injury and was not detectable by 7 days; smooth muscle cell migration and proliferation in media have been noted as early as 36 hours after arterial injury and occur within 7 days.[39–41] Platelets were found to relate directly to intimal proliferation after arterial injury, and severe thrombocytopenia inhibited intimal thickening, an effect that correlated with the degree of thrombocytopenia.[42] Following arterial injury, platelets rapidly adhere to the site of injury by several adhesion receptors; thromboxane A_2 is generated; changes in GPIIb/IIIa complex occur which then bind to fibrinogen, subsequently leading to platelet aggregation and activation.[43] Activated platelets release among other factors, platelet-derived growth factor (PDGF), a potential smooth muscle cell (SMC) mitogen.[44]

PDGF is the most important growth factor released by activated platelets. The association between PDGF and vascular smooth muscle cell proliferation has been demonstrated in animal experiments,[45] in which the rise and augmented levels of PDGF-B following arterial injury correlated with neointimal cellular proliferation. Besides inducing proliferation, the primary effect of PDGF on vascular SMC could be the induction of migration, as PDGF is the strongest reported chemoattractant for vascular SMC.[46]

The expression of transforming growth factor-beta (TGF-β) Beta is reported to be increased in atherosclerotic vessels of rabbits following balloon injury;[47] and, direct transfer of TGFβ-1 gene into porcine arteries resulted in intimal hyperplasia and increased extracellular matrix production.[48] Serotonin and thromboxane A_2 are released by activated platelets and promote SMC proliferation, both alone, and synergistically when combined together.[49] P-selectin is a glycoprotein stored in α-granules of platelets, expressed upon activation of platelets. It is implicated in platelet–leukocyte interactions, and decreased neointimal formation has been demonstrated in P-selectin deficient mice.[50] Histamine released from activated platelets at the site of vascular injury is postulated to induce intimal hyperplasia via H1 receptors.[51] Interleukin-1 derived from platelets increases production of interleukin-6 and interleukin-8, which are important mediators of inflammation at the site of vascular injury.[52] Although platelet-activating factor induces proliferation in SMC cultures,[53] it has been demonstrated to have no influence on restenosis.[54]

Platelets, when activated, can enhance thrombin generation by five to sixfold.[55] Thrombin, a powerful mitogen, contributes to SMC proliferation by inducing platelet release of PDGF.[56] Thrombin may also exert a direct mitogenic stimulation on vascular SMC.[57] During organization of thrombus, thrombin becomes bound to extracellular matrix and remains in its active form,[58] being released gradually to exert a prolonged effect on SMC proliferation. These effects could be of significance as increased thrombin generation has been demonstrated following percutaneous transluminal coronary angiography (PTCA) in humans.[59]

Platelets, by their capacity to adhere to the sites of arterial injury, to form aggregates, and to secrete highly potent growth factors of which the most important is PDGF, appear to play an important role in neointimal proliferation and development of restenosis.

Intimal hyperplasia and restenosis

The aggressive dilation of vascular structures that accompanies angioplasty involves compression and fracture of atherosclerotic plaque and internal elastic lamina, and damage to the vascular endothelium. Whether accidental or deliberate, the damage to endothelial cells (ECs) and medial SMCs exposes the subendothelial connective tissue to blood borne elements. This exposure leads to a coordinated sequence of cellular events that includes: platelet adhesion, activation and aggregation, leukocyte adhesion and transmigration, monocyte/macrophage transmigration and transformation, and release of mitogenic and chemotactic growth factors.[60,61] These growth factors elicit a cascade of intracellular signaling pathways, and overexpression of genes critical to proliferation and migration of medial SMCs. As a consequence, intimal hyperplasia and restenosis occurs after coronary and peripheral vascular angioplasties (Fig. 54.1).

The intimal hyperplastic process following an angioplasty can be divided into four waves.[62,63] The first wave (0–3 days) is governed by proliferation of medial SMCs.[64,65] Although a number of mitogens including the acidic and basic fibroblast growth factors (aFGF, bFGF), insulin-like growth factors (IGFs), interleukin-1, thrombin and angiotensin II stimulate SMC proliferation in vitro,[64,65] it appears that bFGF released from dying medial SMCs is the predominant mitogenic factor for the first wave.[66] However, even though treatment with anti-bFGF antibodies can reduce medial SMC proliferation by more than 80%, it does not prevent intimal thickening.[67] The second wave (3–7 days) consists on the migration of medial

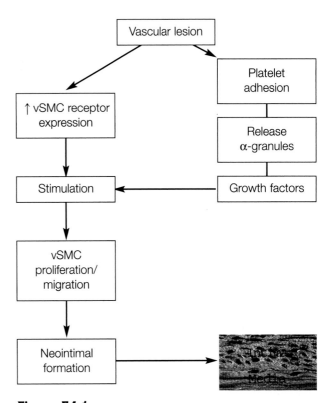

Figure 54.1
Benefits of drug eluting stents.

SMCs across the internal elastic lamina to the intima. If the medial SMC proliferation (first wave) is not a prerequisite for the induction of intimal thickening, it appears that the migration of medial SMCs is absolutely required for the development of intimal hyperplasia. Several molecules such as angiotensin II, bFGF, TGF-ß and the platelet-derived growth factor-BB (PDGF-BB) may act as SMC chemotactic factors during the second wave of cellular event.[68] Among these, the predominant mediator appears to be PDGF-BB.[69] Circulating platelets are the major source of PDGF release (all 3 isoforms – AA–AB–BB – are equally present in humans).[70,71] The PDGF receptor is a dimer of α and/or ß subunits, and exists as -$\alpha\alpha$, -αß, and -ßß isoforms. PDGF-AA binds to -$\alpha\alpha$ receptors, PDGF-AB binds to -$\alpha\alpha$ or -αß receptors, and PDGF-BB binds to -$\alpha\alpha$, -αß, and -ßß receptors with higher affinity for the -ßß receptor.[72]

In rats, administration of polyclonal antibodies to all forms of PDGF blocked the intimal hyperplasia mediated by a balloon catheter injury, even though the first wave of medial SMCs proliferation was not prevented.[73–75] Polyclonal antibodies specific for the PDGF-B chain block intimal hyperplasia, whereas antibodies specific for PDGF-A chain have no inhibitory effect.[76] Infusion of PDGF-BB causes a 10- to 20-fold increase in medial SMC migration but had little effect on intimal SMCs proliferation.[72] Banai et al showed in pigs that a selective PDGFR-ß tyrosine kinase blocker reduced neointimal formation in injured femoral arteries,[77] whereas in baboons, blockade of PDGFR-ß with specific antibodies inhibited intimal hyperplasia in the saphenous arteries after balloon angioplasty.[78] In addition, blockade of PDGFR-ß did not alter SMC proliferation in the injured wall suggesting that the decrease in intimal hyperplasia was due to the inhibition of medial SMC migration. These data support the conclusion that PDGF-BB regulates the movement of SMCs from the media into the intima and plays a critical role in intimal thickening. Involvement of the PDGF ligand-receptor interaction in vascular impairment is also supported by the presence of PDGF receptors and PDGF ligands in normal rat, pig, baboon and human arteries as well as in human atherosclerotic plaques and in injured rat and human arteries.[79–84] Another very interesting point playing in favor of regulating the PDGFR-ß activation is the fact that PDGFR-ß is specifically expressed in mesenchymal cells, such as SMCs and fibroblasts and that it is not expressed on ECs of large arteries (i.e. aorta, coronary, carotid).[85] Consequently, the inhibition of PDGFR-ß activity would not alter the ECs activity during the vascular healing process.

The third wave intimal hyperplastic response consists of the replication of SMCs within the intima. It is thought that half of the migrating SMCs will undergo three rounds of cell cycle proliferation in the intima, ultimately representing nearly 90% of the final cell count in the neointima. The other half of the migrating SMCs do not divide, and account for the remaining 10% of the intimal cell counts.[63] SMCs are observed within the neointima as soon as 3 days after the injury. Their number peaks within 2 weeks of injury and remains relatively constant for up to 1 year,[65] and no specific mitogenic factors have been identified.[65,73] The fourth wave implies an additional increase in intimal thickness mediated by the accumulation of extracellular matrix, connective tissue and increase of cell replication, which can be modulated by TGF-ß, bFGF and angiotensin II.[66,85–87]

Numerous pharmacological agents (calcium channel blockers, hypolipidemic agents, growth factors and their antagonists, antiplatelet agents, anti-inflammatory, inhibitors of cell cycle regulatory genes such as c-myb, c-myc, cdc2/cdk2, PCNA) and different anti-restenosis devices including brachytherapy, laser therapy, cryotherapy and others have been developed with the scope to prevent the intimal SMC proliferating phase. Most attempts have been unsuccessful. Among the most efficient approaches some either by their drastic and non-selective effects lead to necrosis and/or apoptosis of the exposed cells (SMCs and ECs), or block non-selectively the proliferation of SMCs and ECs.[88–107] In such cases, the vascular healing process as well as the recovery of vasoactive functions of the injured arteries may be altered and unachieved.

In native arteries, the ECs serve as a natural permeability barrier between blood borne elements and the media, produce molecules involved in vascular tone modulation (NO, PGI_2, PGE_2, PAF), and release SMC growth inhibitory factors which are important in the prevention of neointimal thickening.[106–110] Thus, the absence or limited re-endothe-

lialization of the arterial injury site may be a key element in the extent of the intimal hyperplasia, and in the vascular healing process. The migration of SMCs into the intima is likely to contribute to failure of re-endothelialization. This may be due to the fact that SMCs migrate into the intima before ECs. Since SMCs are releasing mediators that inhibit EC growth, absence of or incomplete re-endothelialization may result.[108,111] Postmortem studies in patients who died within a month after PTCA showed no evidence of re-endothelialization at the angioplasty site.[112]

Recent studies suggest that stimulating the re-endothelialization process of injured arteries reduces neointimal hyperplasia and promotes the injured arteries vasomotor function recovery. Reports showed that a single intra-arterial bolus injection of VEGF improved re-endothelialization at vascular injury sites, with a partial reduction of intimal thickening.[111,113,114] However, VEGF is also an inflammatory mediator,[109,115,116] and its delivery at high dosage as currently used in animal and clinical trials induces a secondary inflammatory reaction[109,117,118] which may antagonize its beneficial effect and even exacerbate neointimal formation.[119] Meurice et al showed in balloon injured rabbit iliac arteries that treatment with bFGF doubled the degree of re-endothelialization at 4 weeks post-injury. Although this bFGF-induced re-endothelialization was incomplete (60%), it was nevertheless sufficient to restore almost completely the acetylcholine-mediated relaxation.[120] However, since bFGF is a mitogenic factor for both ECs and SMCs, it did not prevent the intimal hyperplasia process.

Vascular remodeling and restenosis

Arterial remodeling is an important mechanism of restenosis,[37] particularly in non-stent interventions. The exact mechanisms involved in vascular remodeling remain elusive. Negative or constrictive remodeling can be mediated by the production and maturation of the extracellular matrix. Under the stimulation by TGF-ß, the myofibroblasts from the adventitia can produce an extracellular matrix rich in collagen that can transform itself by diverse integrin expression in a dense and fibrous scar with contraction.[121] A positive or adaptative vascular remodeling could be facilitated by the induction of matrix metalloproteinases (MMPs) to degrade the extracellular matrix and allow the artery to dilate and accommodate the neointima. Again the myofibroblasts from the adventitia may play an important role as they have been shown to express MMP-2, TIMP-1 and TIMP-2 (inhibitors of MMP) after balloon angioplasty.[122] A rapid and intense neovascularization has been described in the adventitia with thickening and negative remodeling in a porcine model.[123] Many experimental preparations in various animal model have suggested that remodeling was more important in restenosis than neo-intimal proliferation.[124] Intravascular ultrasound (IVUS) evaluation allowed the validation of the existence of negative remodeling in patients with restenosis.[125] These results were confirmed in postmortem histopathology analysis from coronary arteries several months after angioplasty.[126]

Restenosis prevention and treatment

Peripheral artery restenosis, as mentioned earlier, characterizes certain vessel types, sizes and locations. Muscular distributive vessels such as the superficial femoral arteries (SFA) represent the classical nidus for restenosis after angioplasty and as such, they have been considered optimal for investigation of innovative preventive measures or new treatment modalities. They also share some structural and pathological similarities with the extensively studied coronary arteries. As a consequence, some concepts applied in coronary angioplasty can, to a certain extent, show favorable results in SFAs. Among these, avoidance of intervention on a small caliber vessel with extensive plaque burden and, with existing collateralization offers a good example of lesion where in order to prevent complication angioplasty should be avoided. In addition, procedure wise, operators will aim at obtaining the largest lumen after procedure or the lowest residual stenosis (<30%), knowing the delicate balance between the severity of produced injury and the required acute gain in luminal area. Unfortunately, a debulking strategy via laser, cutting balloon, directional or rotational atherectomy in an attempt at increasing lumen gain while preventing vessel wall injury failed to demonstrate superiority over simple balloon angioplasty with or without stenting in the coronary vasculature.[127–130] Although mechanistically appealing, debulking in peripheral artery angioplasty to prevent restenosis has not been supported by randomized data. While stenting in coronary arteries has consistently showed an antirestenotic effect,[131–133] its efficacy in SFAs remains highly controversial.[134–137] Recently, local delivery of cytostatic agents such as sirolimus and paclitaxel using a stent platform and a polymer for carrier has proven extremely effective at reducing the instent hyperplastic response and the need for target lesion revascularization in coronary arteries.[138,139] Sirolimus is a macrocyclic lactone with immunosuppressive activity combining anti-inflammatory and antiproliferative effects through cell cycle arrest in G1 phase. A sirolimus-eluting nitinol self-expandable stent (SES) has been compared to a bare metal same design stent (BMS) for treatment of SFAs presenting stenosis greater than 70% in diameter and 7–20 cm in length. Thirty-six patients were enrolled in the 'Sirocco' trial. The primary endpoint was the instent mean percent diameter stenosis, as measured by quantitative angiography at

6 months (Fig 54.2). At follow-up, the instent mean percent diameter stenosis was 22.6% in the SES group versus 30.9% in the BMS group (p=0.294). However, the binary restenosis rate was 0% in the SES group and 23.5% in the BMS group.[140] No data exist yet regarding the use of paclitaxel eluting stents in peripheral arteries.

Three different non-stent based devices have also been proposed for restenosis prevention in peripheral arteries namely, brachytherapy, cryotherapy and photodynamic therapy. Radiation results in DNA breaks leading to cell death during cell division. The application of this antiproliferative technology has been extensively studied to treat instent restenosis in coronary arteries. The overwhelming efficacy of brachytherapy compared to simple balloon angioplasty in restenotic lesions has not been reproduced for de novo lesions. In peripheral interventions, brachytherapy was reported efficient both for restenosis prevention and treatment in SFAs, renal artery stenosis and arteriovenous dialysis shunts, in several small registries.[150–152] The most well documented randomized brachytherapy trial for prevention of restenosis in de novo SFA lesions is the Vienna-2 study.[144] One hundred and thirteen patients were enrolled in two groups, angioplasty alone (without stent) and angioplasty with brachytherapy using an iridium-192 source, a dose of

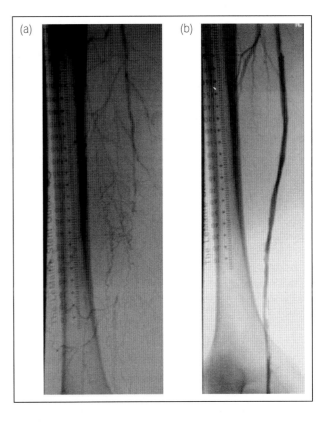

Figure 54.2

(a) Baseline occluded superficial femoral artery and (b) six months later control angiogram after two sirolimus-eluting nitinol self-expandable stents. (Courtesy of Dr Vincent Oliva, Notre-Dame Hospital, Montréal, Québec, Canada).

12 Gy at 3 mm (radial reference depth). At 6 months, binary angiographic restenosis was observed in 28.3% of the brachytherapy patients versus 53.7% in the control group. Two large randomized trials in their final phase, the Paris and the Vienna 05 studies, will address the issue of brachytherapy efficacy for de novo stented SFAs.

Cryotherapy, a technology derived from electrophysiology ablative equipment, has also been proposed to prevent restenosis. While applying subzero temperatures (refrigeration catheter using liquid nitrogen) to the target vessel wall intimal proliferation is inhibited by apoptosis induction to the target vessel wall, reduced smooth muscle cells proliferation and diminished vascular inflammatory response. A positive remodeling phenomenon has also been demonstrated.[145] Photodynamic therapy is based on administration of photosensitizer agents that localize selectively to the target tissue with subsequent activation by endovascular light. The photo-excited sensitizer generates highly reactive and cytotoxic singlet oxygen that induce irreversible cell damage and prevent neointimal proliferation. Small human registries have demonstrated the safety and feasibility of this technique.[146,147]

Finally, none of the systemic pharmacologic approaches already proposed for prevention of restenosis after coronary angioplasty have shown positive results in peripheral intervention.

Conclusion

Restenosis after peripheral arteries intervention remains a critical limitation of the technique. This late complication characterizes mainly distributive muscular arteries. Elastic recoil, mural thrombus formation, intimal hyperplasia and negative remodeling all contribute in different proportions to the recurrence of stenosis phenomenon. Proper lesion selection with optimal peri-procedural lumen enlargement and possibly stenting minimize the risk of restenosis. Adjunctive treatment for enhanced prevention of restenosis and treatment of instent restenosis will eventually be available. Most probably this treatment modality will be some local delivery of agents inhibiting platelet–leukocyte activation, smooth muscle cell migration, proliferation and secretion while maintaining vessel wall integrity and functionality.

References

1 Serruys PW, Foley DP, Kirkeeide RL, King SB. Restenosis revisited: Insights provided by quantitative coronary angiography (Editorial). *Am Heart J* 1993; **126**: 1243–67.

2 Miller JM, Obman EM, Moliterno DJ, Califf RM. Restenosis the clinical issues. In: Topol EJ (ed). Silent restenosis in clinical trials. *Textbook of Interventional Cardiology*. Philadelphia: WB Saunders, 2002.

3 Nobuyoshi M, Kimura T, Nosaka H et al. Serial angiographic follow-up of 229 patients. *J Am Cardiol* 1988; **12**: 616–23.

4 Serruys PW, Luitjen HE, Beatt KJ et al. Incidence of restenosis after successful coronary angioplasty: A time-related phenomenon. *Circulation* 1988; **77**: 361–71.

5 Dangas G, Fuster V. Management of restenosis after coronary intervention. *Am Heart J* 1996; **132**: 428–36.

6 Weintraub WS, Kosinski AS, Brown CL, King SB III. Can restenosis after coronary angioplasty be predicted from clinical variables? *J Am Coll Cardiol* 1993; **21**: 6–14.

7 Rensing BJ, Hermans WR, Dekers JW et al. Which angiographic variables best describes functional status 6 months after successful single vessel coronary balloon angioplasty? *J Am Coll Cardiol* 1993; **21**: 317–24.

8 Lambert M, Bonan R, Côté G et al. Multiple coronary angioplasty: A model to discriminate systemic and procedural factors related to restenosis. *J Am Coll Cardiol* 1988; **12**: 310–14.

9 Weintraub WS, Brown CL, Liberman HA et al. Effect of restenosis at one previously dilated coronary site on the probability of restenosis at another previously dilated coronary site. *Am J Cardiol* 1993; **72**: 1107–13.

10 Hirshfeld JWJ, Wchwartz JS, Jugo R et al. Restenosis after coronary angioplasty: A multivariate statistical model to relate lesion and procedure variables to restenosis. *J Am Coll Cardiol* 1991; **18**: 647–56.

11 Weintraub WS, Douglas JS, Ghazzal Z et al. Evaluation and prediction of clinical restenosis (Abstract). *Circulation* 1996; **94**: 1–90.

12 Schwartz RS. Animal model of human coronary restenosis. In: Topol EJ (ed). *Textbook of Interventional Cardiology*. Philadelphia: WB Saunders, 2002: 358–78.

13 Schwartz R, Huber K, Murphy J et al. Restenosis and the proportional neointimal response to coronary artery injury: Results in a porcine model. *J Am Coll Cardiol* 1992; **19**: 267–74.

14 Heeney D, Bookstein J, Daniels E et al. Transluminal angioplasty of the lower abdominal aorta. *Am J Radiol* 1986; **146**: 369–71.

15 Hallisey MJ, Meranze SG, Barker BC. Percutaneous transluminal angioplasty of the abdominal aorta. *J Vasc Interv Radiol* 1994; **5**: 679–87.

16 Yadav JS, Roubin GS, Iyer SS et al. Elective stenting of the extracranial carotid arteries. *Circulation* 1997; **95**: 376–81.

17 Henry M, Amor M, Masson I et al. Angioplasty and stenting of the extracranial carotid arteries. *J Endovasc Surg* 1998; **6**: 293–304.

18 McNamara TO, Greasler LE, Fisher JR et al. Initial and long-term results of treatment of brachiocephalic arterial stenosis and occlusions with balloon angioplasty, thrombolysis, stents. *J Invas Cardiol* 1997; **9**: 372–83.

19 Henry M, Amor M, Henry I et al. Percutaneous transluminal angioplasty of the subclavian arteries. *J Endovasc Surg* 1999; **6**: 33–41.

20 Schreiber JJ, Polh MA, Novack AC. The natural history of atherosclerotic and fibrous renal artery disease. *Urol Clin North Am* 1984; **11**: 383–92.

21 Weibull II, Berquist D, Jonsson I et al. Long-term results after percutaneous transluminal angioplasty of atherosclerotic renal artery stenosis: The importance of intensive follow-up. *Eur J Revasc Surg* 1991; **5**: 291–301.

22   Rees CR, Snead D. Results of United States multicenter trial of stents in renal arteries. *Abstract Cardiovasc Intervent Radiol* 1994; **17**(Suppl 2): S1–145.

23   Henry M, Amor M, Henry I et al. Stent placement in the renal artery: Three-year experience with Palmaz stent. *J Vasc Inter Radiol* 1996; **7**: 343–50.

24   Rees CR, Palmaz JC, Becker GJ et al. Palmaz stent in atherosclerotic stenosis involving the ostia of the renal arteries: Preliminary report of a multicenter study. *Radiology* 1991; **181**: 507–14.

25   Vogelzang RL. Long-term results of angioplasty. *J Vasc Interv Radiol* 1996; **7**(Suppl): 179.

26   Palmaz JC, Lagourd JC, Riviera JF et al. Stenting of the iliac arteries with the Palmaz stents. Experience from a multicenter trial. *Cardiovasc Intervent Radiol* 1992; **15**: 291–7.

27   Marin EC, Katzen BT, Benenati JF et al. Multi-center trial of the Wallstent in the iliac and femoral arteries. *J Vasc Interv Radiol* 1995; **6**: 843–9.

28   Henry M, Amor M, Ethevenot G et al. Palmaz stent placement in iliac and femoropopliteal arteries. Primary and secondary patency in 310 patients with two to four year follow-up. *Radiology* 1995; **197**: 167–74.

29   Richter GM, Roeren TM, Noelge G et al. Superior clinical results of iliac stent placement versus percutaneous transluminal angioplasty: Four year success rate of a randomized study (abstract). *Radiology* 1991; **181**: 161.

30   Tetteroo E, Van der Graaf Y, Bosch JL et al. Randomized comparison of primary stent placement versus angioplasty with selective stent placement in patients with iliac artery obstructive disease. In: Tetteroo E (ed). *The Dutch Iliac Stent Trial: Results from a Randomized Multicenter Study.* Utrecht, The Netherlands: FEBO Druk BV Enschede, 1997: 69–89.

31   Bosch JL, Hunink MGM. Meta-analysis of the results of percutaneous transluminal angioplasty and stent placement for aorto-iliac occlusive disease. *Radiology* 1997; **204**: 87–96.

32   Johnston KW. Femoral and popliteal arteries: Reanalysis of the results of balloon angioplasty. *Radiology* 1992; **183**: 767–71.

33   Chatelard P, Guibourt C. Long-term results with a Palmaz stent in the femoro-popliteal arteries. *J Cardiovasc Surg* 1996; **37**: 67–72.

34   Strecker EP, Boos IB, Gottmann D. Femoropopliteal artery stent placement: Evaluation of long-term results. *Radiology* 1997; **205**: 375–83.

35   Sapoval MR, Long AL, Raynaud AC et al. Femoro-popliteal stent placement: Long-term results. *Radiology* 1992; **184**: 833–9.

36   Kearney M, Pieczek A, Haley L et al. Histopathology of instent restenosis in patients with popliteal artery disease. *Circulation* 1997; **95**: 1998–2002.

37   Post MJ, Borst C, Kuntz RE. The relative importance of arterial remodeling compared with intimal hyperplasia in lumen narrowing after balloon angioplasty. *Circulation* 1994; **89**: 2816–21.

38   Currier JW, Faxon DP. Restenosis after percutaneous transluminal coronary angioplasty: Have we been aiming at the wrong target? *J Am Coll Cardiol* 1995; **25**: 516–20.

39   Markovitz JH, Roubin GS, Parks JM, Bittner V. Platelet activation and restenosis after coronary stenting: flow cytometric detection of wound-induced platelet activation. *Coronary Artery Disease* 1996; **7**: 657–65.

40   Clowes AW, Reidy MA, Clowes MM. Kinetics of cellular proliferation after arterial injury: smooth muscle cell growth in the absence of endothelium. *Lab Invest* 1983; **49**: 327–33.

41   Steele PM, Chesebro JH, Stanson AW et al. Balloon angioplasty: natural history of the pathophysiological response to injury in a pig model. *Circ Res* 1985; **57**: 105–12.

42   Moore S, Friedman RJ, Singhal DP et al. Inhibition of injury induced thromboatherosclerotic lesions by anti-platelet serum in rabbits. *Thromb Haemost* 1975; **35**: 70–81.

43   Fox JEB. *Platelet Biology and restenosis*. Restenosis Summit VIII, May 1996. The Cleveland Clinic Heart Center, p234.

44   Casscells W . Smooth muscle cell growth factors. *Prog Growth Factor Res* 1991; **3**: 177–206.

45   Uchida K, Sasahara M, Morigami N et al. Expression of platelet derived growth factor B-chain in neointimal smooth muscle cells of balloon injured rabbit femoral arteries. *Atherosclerosis* 1996; **124**: 9–23.

46   Bornfeldt KE, Raines EW, Nakano T et al. Insulin-like growth factor-1 and platelet derived growth factor-BB induce direct migration of human arterial smooth muscle cells via signalling pathways that are distinct from those of proliferation. *J Clin Invest* 1994; **93**: 1266–74.

47   Grant MB, Wargovich TJ, Bush DM et al. Expression of IGF-1, IGF-1 receptor and TGF-beta following balloon angioplasty in atherosclerotic and normal rabbit iliac arteries: an immunocytochemical study. *Regul Pept* 1999; **79**: 47–53.

48   Nabel EG, Shum L, Pompili VJ, et al. Direct transfer of transforming growth factor beta 1 gene into arteries stimulates fibrocellular hyperplasia. *Proc Natl Acad Sci* USA 1993; **90**: 10759–63.

49   Pakala R, Willerson JT, Benedict CR. Effect of serotonin, thromboxane A_2, and specific receptor antagonists on vascular smooth muscle cell proliferation. *Circulation* 1997; **96**: 2280–6.

50   Kumar A, Hoover JL, Simmons CA, et al. Remodeling and neointimal formation in the carotid artery of normal and P-selectin–deficient mice. *Circulation* 1997; **96**: 4333–42.

51   Miyazawa N, Watanabe S, Matsuda A et al. Role of histamine H1 and H2 receptor antagonists in the prevention of intimal thickening. *Eur J Pharmacol* 1998; **362**: 53–9.

52   Loppnow H, Bil R, Hirt S et al. Platelet-derived interleukin-1 induces cytokine production, but not proliferation of human vascular smooth muscle cells. *Blood* 1998; **91**: 134–41.

53   Stoll LL, Spector AA. Interaction of platelet-activating factor with endothelial and vascular smooth muscle cells in coculture. *J Cell Physiol* 1989; **139**: 253–61.

54   Herbert JM, Laplace MC, Mares AM, Dol F. Platelet-activating factor (PAF) is not an essential component of the cascade leading to smooth muscle cell proliferation following vascular injury. *J Lipid Mediat Cell Signal* 1995; **12**: 49–57.

55   Walsh PN, Schmaier AH. Platelet-coagulant protein interactions. In Colman RW, Hirsh J, Marder VJ, Salzman EW, (eds). *Hemostasis and Thrombosis: Basic Principles and Clinical Practice.* 3rd ed. 1994. Philadelphia: JB Lippincott Co, 629–51.

56   Maruyama I, Shigeta K. Regulation of the endothelial function by thrombomodulin and/or thrombin receptor. *Rinsho Ketsueki* 1994; **35**: 234–37.

57 McNamara CA, Sarembock IJ, Gimple LW et al. Thrombin stimulates proliferation of cultured rat aortic smooth muscle cell by a proteolytically activated receptor. *J Clin Invest* 1993; **91**: 94–8.

58 Wilner GD, Danitz MP, Mudd MS et al. Selective immobilization of alpha-thrombin by surface-bound fibrin. *J Lab Clin Med* 1981; **97**: 403–11.

59 Marmur JD, Merlini PA, Sharma SK et al. Thrombin generation in human coronary arteries after percutaneous transluminal balloon angioplasty. *J Am Coll Cardiol* 1994; **24**: 1484–91.

60 Ross R, Glomset JA. The pathogenesis of atherosclerosis. *N Engl J Med* 1976; **296**: 369–77.

61 Groves HM, Kinlough-Rathbone RL, Richardson M, Moore S, Mustard JF. Platelet interaction with damaged rabbit aorta. *Lab Invest* 1978; **40**: 194–9.

62 Popma JJ, Topol EJ. Factors influencing restenosis after coronary angioplasty. *Am J Med* 1990; **88**: 1N–16N.

63 Friedman RJ, Stemerman MB, Wenz B et al. The effect of thrombocytopenia on experimental atherosclerotic lesion formation in rabbits. Smooth muscle cell proliferation and re-endothelialization. *J Clin Invest* 1977; **60**: 1191–201.

64 Clowes AW, Schwartz SM. Significance of quiescent smooth muscle migration in the injured rat carotid artery. *Circ Res* 1985; **56**: 139–45.

65 Hanke H, Strohschneider T, Oberhoff M, Betz E, Karsch KR. Time course of smooth muscle cell proliferation in the intima and media of arteries following experimental angioplasty. *Circ Res* 1990; **67**: 651–9.

66 Schwartz SM, deBlois D, O'Brien ERM. The intima soil for the atherosclerosis and restenosis. *Circ Res* 1995; **77**: 445–65.

67 Lindner V, Reidy MA. Proliferation of smooth muscle cells after vascular injury is inhibited by an antibody against basic fibroblast growth factor. *Proc Natl Acad Sci USA*. 1991; **88**: 3739–43.

68 Olson NE, Chao S, Lindner V, Reidy MA. Intimal smooth muscle cell proliferation after balloon catheter injury: the role of basic fibroblast growth factor. *Am J Pathol* 1992; **140**: 1017–23.

69 Grotendorst GR, Seppa HEJ, Kleinman HK, Martin GR. Attachment of smooth muscle cells to collagen and their migration toward platelet-derived growth factor. *Proc Natl Acad Sci USA*. 1981; **78**: 3669–72.

70 Ihnatowycz IO, Winocour PD, Moore S. A platelet-derived factor chemotactic for rabbit smooth muscle cells in culture. *Artery* 1981; **9**: 316–17.

71 Jawien A, Bowen-Pope DF, Lindner V, Schwartz SM, Clowes AW. Platelet-derived growth factor promotes smooth muscle migration and intimal thickening in a rat model of balloon angioplasty. *J Clin Invest* 1992; **89**: 507–11.

72 Koyama N, Hart CE, Clowes AW. Different functions of the platelet-derived growth factor-α and -ß receptors for the migration and proliferation of cultured baboons smooth muscle cells. *Circ Res* 1994; **75**: 682–91.

73 Ferns GAA, Raines EW, Sprugel KH, Motani AS, Reidy MA, Ross R. Inhibition of neointimal smooth muscle accumulation after angioplasty by antibody to PDGF. *Science* 1991; **253**: 1129–32.

74 Clowes AW, Clowes MM, Reidy MA. Kinetics of cellular proliferation after arterial injury III. Endothelial and smooth muscle growth in chronically denuded vessels. *Lab Invest* 1986; **54**: 295–303.

75 Raines EW, Bowen-Pope DF, Ross R. Platelet-derived growth factor. In: MB Sporn, AB Roberts, (eds). *Peptide Growth Factors and their Receptors*. New York: Springer-Verlag, 1991, 173–262.

76 Rutherford C, Martin W, Salame M et al. Substantial inhibition of neo-intimal response to balloon injury in the rat carotid artery using a combination of antibodies to platelet-derived growth factor-BB and basic fibroblast growth factor. *Atherosclerosis* 1997; **130**: 45–51.

77 Banai S, Wolf Y, Golomg G et al. PDGF-receptor tyrosine kinase blocker AG1295 selectively attenuates smooth muscle cell growth in vitro and reduces neointimal formation after balloon angioplasty in swine. *Circulation* 1998; **97**: 1960–9.

78 Hart CE, Kraiss LW, Vergel S et al. PDGFß receptor blockade inhibits intimal hyperplasia in the baboon. *Circulation* 1999; **99**: 564–9.

79 Nabel EG, Yang Z, Liptay S et al. Recombinant platelet-derived growth factor B gene expression in porcine arteries induces intimal hyperplasia in vivo, *J Clin Invest* 1993; **91**: 1822–9.

80 Pompili VJ, Gordon D, San H et al. Expression and function of a recombinant PDGF gene in porcine arteries. *Arterioscler Thromb Vasc Biol* 1995; **15**: 2254–64.

81 Majesky MW, Reidy MA, Bowen-Pope DF et al. PDGF ligand and receptor gene expression during repair of arterial injury. *J Cell Biol* 1990; **111**: 2149–58.

82 Wilcox JN, Smith KM, Williams LT, Schwartz SM, Gordon D. Platelet-derived growth factor mRNA detection in human atherosclerotic plaques by in situ hybridization. *J Clin Invest* 1988; **82**: 1134–43.

83 Walker LN, Bowen-Pope DF, Ross R, Reidy MA. Production of platelet-derived growth factor-like molecules by cultured arterial smooth muscle cells accompanies proliferation after arterial injury. *Proc Natl Acad Sci USA*. 1986; **83**: 7311–15.

84 Tanizawa S, Ueda M, van der Loos CM, van der Wal AC, Becker AE. Expression of platelet derived growth factor B chain and ß receptor in human coronary arteries after percutaneous transluminal coronary angioplasty: an immunohistochemical study. *Heart* 1996; **75**: 549–56.

85 Clowes AW, Reidy MA, Clowes MM. Mechanism of stenosis after arterial injury. *Lab Invest* 1983; **49**: 208–15.

86 Daemen MJAP, Lombardi DM, Bosman FT, Schwartz SM. Angiotensin II induces smooth muscle cell proliferation in the normal and injured rat arterial wall. *Circ Res* 1991; **68**: 450–6.

87 Majesky MW, Lindner V, Twardzik DR, Schwartz SM, Reidy MA. Production of transforming growth factor β-1 during repair of arterial injury. *J Clin Invest* 1991; **88**: 904–10.

88 Popma JJ, Califf RM, Topol EJ. Clinical trials of restenosis after coronary angioplasty. *Circulation* 1991; **84**: 1426–36.

89 Lau KW, Sigwart U. Restenosis an accelerated arteriopathy: pathophysiology, preventive strategies and research horizons. In: Edelman ER (ed). *Molecular Interventions and Local Drug Delivery*. Cambridge: University Press, 1995, 1–28.

90 Simons M, Edelman ER, DeKeyser JL, Langer R, Rosenberg RD. Antisense c-myb oligonucleotides inhibit intimal arterial smooth muscle cell accumulation in vivo. *Nature* 1992; **359**: 67–70.

91 Morishita R, Gibbons GH, Ellison KE et al. Single intraluminal delivery of antisense cdc2 kinase and proliferating-cell nuclear antigen oligonucleotides results in chronic inhibition of neointimal hyperplasia. *Proc Natl Acad Sci USA* 1993; **90**: 8474–8.

92 Morishita R, Gibbons G, Ellison KE et al. Intimal hyperplasia after vascular injury is inhibited by antisense cdk2 kinase oligonucleotides. *J Clin Invest* 1994; **93**: 1458–64.

93 Abe J-I, Zhou W, Taguchi J-I et al. Suppression of neointimal smooth muscle cell accumulation in vivo by antisense cdc2 and cdk2 oligonucleotides in rat carotid artery. *Biochem Biophys Res Comm* 1994; **198**: 16–24.

94 Simons M, Edelman ER, Rosenberg RD. Antisense proliferating cell nuclear antigen oligonucleotides inhibit intimal hyperplasia in a rat carotid artery injury model. *J Clin Invest* 1994; **93**: 2351–6.

95 Bennett MR, Anglin S, McEwan JR et al. Inhibition of vascular smooth muscle cells proliferation in vitro and in vivo by c-myc antisense oligodeoxynucleotides. *J Clin Invest* 1994; **93**: 820–8.

96 Shi Y, Fard A, Galeo A et al. Transcatheter delivery of c-myc antisense oligomers reduces neointimal formation in a porcine model of coronary artery balloon injury. *Circulation* 1994; **90**: 944–951.

97 Edelman ER, Simons M, Sirois MG, Rosenberg RD. C-myc in vasculoproliferative disease. *Circ Res* 1995; **76**: 176–82.

98 Simons M, Rosenberg RD. Antisense nonmuscle myosin heavy chain and c-myb oligonucleotides suppress smooth muscle cell proliferation in vitro. *Circ Res* 1992; **70**: 835–43.

99 Ebbecke M, Unterberg C, Buchwald A, Stohr S, Wiegand V. Anti-proliferative effects of a c-myc antisense oligonucleotide on human arterial smooth muscle cells. *Basic Res Cardiol* 1992; **87**: 585–91.

100 Biro S, Fu YM, Yu ZX, Epstein SE. Inhibitory effects of antisense oligodeoxynucleotides targeting c-myc mRNA on smooth muscle cell proliferation and migration. *Proc Natl Acad Sci USA* 1993; **90**: 654–8.

101 Gunn J, Holt CM, Francis SE et al. The effect of oligonucleotides to c-myb upon vascular smooth muscle cell proliferation and neointima formation after porcine coronary angioplasty. *Circ Res* 1997; **80**: 520–31.

102 Waksman R, Robinson KA, Crocker IR et al. Endovascular low-dose irradiation inhibits neointima formation after coronary artery balloon injury in swine: a possible role for radiation therapy in restenosis prevention. *Circulation* 1995; **91**: 1533–9.

103 Waksman R, Robinson KA, Crocker IR et al. Intracoronary radiation before stent implantation inhibits neointima formation in stented porcine coronary arteries. *Circulation* 1995; **92**: 1383–6.

104 Carter AJ, Laird JR, Bailey LR et al. Effects of endovascular radiation from a b-particle-emitting stent in a porcine coronary restenosis model. *Circulation* 1996; **94**: 2364–8.

105 Meerkin D, Tardif J-C, Crocker IR et al. Effects of intracoronary ß-radiation therapy after coronary angioplasty: an intravascular ultrasound study. *Circulation* 1999; **99**: 1660–5.

106 Thorin E, Meerkin D, Bertrand OF et al. Influence of postangioplasty ß-irradiation on endothelial function in porcine coronary arteries. *Circulation* 2000; **101**: 1430–1.

107 Tanguay J-F, Goeffroy P, Sirois MG. Cryotherapy improves vascular remodeling after angioplasty. *Circulation* 1998; **98**: 1–674.

108 Casscells W. Migration of smooth muscle and endothelial cells: Critical events in restenosis. *Circulation* 1992; **86**: 723–9.

109 Clowes AW. Intimal hyperplasia and graft failure. *Cardiovasc Pathol* 1993; **2**: 179S–186S.

110 Asahara T, Chen D, Tsurumi Y et al. Accelerated restitution of endothelial integrity and endothelium-dependent function after phVEGF$_{165}$ gene transfer. *Circulation* 1996; **94**: 3291–302.

111 Casscells W. Growth factor therapies for vascular injury and ischemia. *Circulation* 1995; **91**: 2699–702.

112 Sirois MG, Edelman ER. VEGF effect on vascular permeability is mediated by synthesis of platelet-activating factor. *Am J Physiol* 1997; **272**: 2746–56.

113 Gravanis MB, Roubin GS. Histopathologic phenomena at the site of percutaneous transluminal coronary angioplasty: the problem of restenosis. *Hum Pathol* 1989; **20**: 477–85.

114 Asahara T, Bauters C, Pastore C et al. Local delivery of vascular endothelial growth factor accelerates reendothelialization and attenuates intimal hyperplasia in balloon-injured rat carotid artery. *Circulation* 1995; **91**: 2793–801.

115 Callow AD, Choi ET, Trachtenberg JD et al. Vascular permeability factor accelerates endothelial regrowth following balloon angioplasty. *Growth Factors* 1994; **10**: 223–8.

116 Burke PA, Lehmann-Bruinsma K, Powell JS. Vascular endothelial growth factor causes endothelial proliferation after vascular injury. *Biochem Biophys Res Commun* 1995; **207**: 348–54.

117 Senger DR, Galli SJ, Dvorak AM et al. Tumor cells secrete a vascular permeability factor that promotes accumulation of ascites fluid. *Science* 1983; **219**: 983–5.

118 Connolly DT, Heuvelman DM, Nelson R et al. Tumor vascular permeability factor stimulates endothelial cell growth and angiogenesis. *J Clin Invest* 1989; **84**: 1470–8.

119 Lindner V, Reidy MA. Expression of VEGF receptors in arteries after endothelial injury and lacks of increased endothelial regrowth in response to VEGF. *Arterioscler Thromb Vasc Biol* 1996; **16**: 1399–405.

120 Meurice T, Bauters C, Auffray J-J et al. Basic fibroblast growth factor restores endothelium-dependent responses after balloon injury of rabbits arteries. *Circulation* 1996; **93**: 18–22.

121 Geary RL, Nikkari ST, Wagner WD, Williams K, Adams MR, Dean RH. Wound healing: A paradigm for lumen narrowing after arterial reconstruction. *J Vasc Surg* 1998; **27**: 96–108.

122 Nakahara K, Okamoto E, Galis ZS, Scott NA, Wilcox JN. Adventitial expression of MMP-1, MMP-2, TIMP-1 and TIMP-2 during vascular remodeling after angioplasty of porcine coronary arteries. *Circulation* 1999; **100** (Suppl): I–700.

123 Pels K, Labinaz M, Hoffert C, O'Brien ER. Adventitial angiogenesis early after coronary angioplasty. Correlation with arterial remodeling. *Arterioscler Thromb Vasc Biol.* 1999; **19**: 229–38.

124 Schwartz RS, Topol EJ, Serruys PW, Sangiorgi G, Holmes DR. Artery size, neointima, and remodeling: Time for some standards. *J Am Coll Cardiol* 1998; **32**: 2087–94.

125 Mintz GS, Popma JJ, Pichard AD et al. Arterial remodeling after coronary angioplasty. *Circulation* 1996; **94**: 35–43.

126 Sangiorgi G, Taylor AJ, Farb A et al. Histopathology of percutaneous transluminal coronary angioplasty remodeling in human coronary arteries. *Am Heart J* 1999; **138**: 681–7.

127 Appelman YEA, Piek JJ, de Feyter PJ et al. Excimer laser coronary angioplasty versus balloon angioplasty used in long coronary lesions: The long-term results of the Amro trial. *J Am Coll Cardiol* 1995; **25**: 330.

128 Bonan R. Does cutting balloon angioplasty reduce restenosis in de novo lesions? Results of the global randomized trial. *TCT – Transcatheter Cariovascular Therapeutics* Washington, DC, USA, Sept 24–28, 2002.

129 Baim DS, Cutlip DE, Sharma SK et al. Final results of the balloon vs optimal atherectomy trial (Boat). *Circ* 1998; **97**: 322–31.

130 Reisman M, Buchbinder M, Sharma SK et al. A Multicenter Randomized Trial of Rotational Atherectomy vs PTCA: DART. *Circ* 1997; **96**(SupplA): 1–467.

131 Serruys PW, deJaegere P, Kiemeneis F et al. A comparison of balloon expandable stent implantation with balloon angioplasty in patients with coronary artery disease. *N Engl J Med* 1994; **331**: 489–95.

132 Fishman DL, Leon MB, Baim DS et al. A randomized comparison of coronary stent placement and balloon angioplasty in the treatment of coronary artery disease. *N Engl J Med* 1994; **331**: 496–501.

133 Serruys PW, Van Hout B, Bonnier H et al. Randomized comparison of implantation of heparin coated stents with balloon angioplasty in selected patients with coronary artery disease (Benestent-II). *Lancet* 1998; **352**: 673–81.

134 Cejna M, Thurnher SA, Illiasch H et al. PTA vs Palmaz stent placement in femoropopliteal artery obstructions: a multicenter prospective randomized study. *J Vasc Interven Radiol* 2001; **12**: 23–31.

135 Grimm J, Muller-Hulsbeck S, Jahnke T et al. Randomized study to compare PTA alone versus PTA with Palmaz stent placement for femoropopliteal lesions. *J Vasc Interv Radiol* 2001; **12**: 935–42

136 Muradin GS, Bosch JL, Stijen T et al. Balloon dilatation and stent implantation for treatment of femoropopliteal arterial disease: meta-analysis. *Radiology* 2001; **221**: 137–45.

137 Vroegindeweij D, Vos LD, Tielbeck AV et al. Balloon angioplasty combined with primary stenting versus balloon angioplasty alone in femoropopliteal obstructions: a comparative randomized study, *Cardiovasc Intervent Radiol* 1997; **20**: 420–5.

138 Morice MC. A randomized comparison of a sirolimus-eluting stent with a standard stent for coronary revascularization *N Engl J Med* 2002; **346**: 1773–80.

139 Grube E, Silber S, Hauptmann KE et al. Taxus I: Six and twelve month results from a randomized, double blind trial on a slow release paclitaxel eluting stent for deNovo coronary lesions. *Circulation* 2003; **107**: 559–64.

140 Duda SH, Pusich B, Richter G et al. Sirolimus-Eluting stents for the treatment of obstructive superficial femoral artery disease: six months results. *Circulation* 2002; **106**: 1505–9.

141 Böttcher HD, Schopohl B, Liermann D et al. Endovascular irradiation: a new method to avoid recurrent stenosis after stent implantation in peripheral arteries – technique and preliminary results. *Int J Radiat Oncol Biol Phys* 1994; **29**: 183–6

142 Waksman R, Laird JR, Jurkovitz CT et al. Intravascular radiation therapy after balloon angioplasty of narrowed femoropopliteal arteries to prevent restenosis: results of the PARIS feasibility clinical trial. *J Vasc Interv Radiol* 2001; **12**: 915–21.

143 Wolfram RM, Pokrajac B, Ahmadi R et al. Endovascular brachytherapy for prophylaxis against restenosis after long-segment femoropopliteal placement of stents: initial results. *Radiology* 2001; **200**: 724–9.

144 Minar E, Pokrajac B, Maca Th et al. Endovascular brachytherapy for prophylaxis of restenosis after femoropopliteal angioplasty: results of a prospective, randomized study. *Circulation* 2000; **102**: 2694–9.

145 Tanguay JF, Geoffroy P, Sirois M. Can single cryoapplication reduce restenosis after angioplasty? *Am J Cardiol* 1999; **84**(Suppl 6A): 61P.

146 Jenkins MP, Buonaccorsi GA, Raphael M et al. Clinical study of adjuvant photodynamic therapy to reduce restenosis following femoral angioplasty. *Br J Surg* 1999; **86**: 1258–63.

147 Rockson SG, Kramer P, Razavi M et al. Photoangioplasty for human peripheral atherosclerosis: results of a phase I trial of photodynamic therapy with motexafin lutetium (antrin). *Circulation* 2000; **102**: 2322–4.

55

Radioactive therapy

Ron Waksman

Introduction

As the manifestation of coronary atherosclerosis and peripheral artery disease is primarily evident in older patient populations, and with the generation of baby boomers nearing their 60s, the full impact of peripheral and coronary atherosclerosis in the USA is upon us. Vascular medicine is the fastest-growing field of medicine today. It is estimated that, in 1999, there were 270 000 peripheral endovascular procedures performed, and by the end of 2000 this rate is expected to increase to more than 550 000. Whereas coronary vascular procedures are increasing at a rate of 8% per year, there is greater growth in the frequency of peripheral procedures, estimated at 19% per year. Despite new advances such as stents, atherectomy devices, thrombectomy and endoluminal grafts, the restenosis rate after peripheral artery intervention continues to grow and compromise the overall success of these procedures.

Vascular brachytherapy is a promising technology with the potential to reduce restenosis rates. Clinical trials to evaluate the effectiveness and safety of this technology are still ongoing, with nearly 5000 patients enrolled in trials. Three-year follow-up of clinical and angiographic data collection on patients treated with intracoronary radiation for the prevention of restenosis has recently been released. These studies demonstrate different levels of efficacy and raise further questions regarding proper dosimetry, the incidence of edge effect, the late thrombosis phenomenon, and late restenosis. While the majority of vascular brachytherapy trials have focused on the use of radiation therapy for the prevention of coronary in-stent restenosis, more data are still needed to determine the effectiveness of beta and gamma sources, and the use of centering delivery systems.

Currently, the clinical experience with vascular brachytherapy for the peripheral system is limited, and planned trials are designed to evaluate the restenosis rates of several vascular sites with the use of endovascular radiation therapy following vascular intervention (i.e. balloon angioplasty, stent placement, atherectomy, or laser ablative techniques). Target sites for such preventive therapy have been identified as saphenous femoral artery lesions, renal artery stenosis, patients who are undergoing hemodialysis with the arteriovenous graft stenosis, a subclavian or brachiocephalic vein, and following transjugular intrahepatic portosystemic shunt (TIPS) procedures for patients with portal hypertension.

Mechanisms of restenosis

The use of percutaneous transluminal angioplasty (PTA) has considerably improved the revascularization rates of many patients. Unfortunately, the long-term efficacy of PTA is limited by its 6–12-month high rate of restenosis.[1] Restenosis following PTA occurs in response to the healing process associated with overinflation of the balloon during angioplasty and subsequent overstretching of the vessel. The main mechanisms of restenosis are acute recoil, intimal hyperplasia, and late vascular constriction (negative remodeling).[2–5]

In the peripheral system, restenosis following PTA is mainly seen in small and medium peripheral arteries, such as the saphenous femoral–popliteal arteries (SFA) and renal arteries. Although not as common, and found to have less of an effect on patency, lower rates of restenosis have also been reported in larger arteries, such as the aortoiliac and carotid arteries, following intervention.[6–12] Other sites affected by restenosis include bypass graft anastomosis, arteriovenous dialysis grafts (AVG) and following the placement of TIPS.[13] Factors which affect long-term vessel patency following PTA include the length of the lesion, the degree of the stenosis, the plaque burden, vessel size, and proximal and distal flow. For peripheral short focal lesions, short-term (6-month) patency rates as high as 75% have been reported. In contrast, more complex and longer areas of stenosis, those with poor distal run-off and those performed for limb salvage, may have a 6-month patency as low as 25%, and a 5-year patency of only 16%.[14]

Many attempts have been made to reduce restenosis by adding adjunct pharmacological therapy to PTA, or by the use of mechanical devices, including atherectomy, laser angioplasty, and intravascular stenting. It appears that instrumentation of these vessels by the balloon or the devices is responsible for inducing restenosis, as none of these alternative approaches significantly retard the neointimal hyperplasia or improve and preserve long-term vascular patency.[15–18] Indeed, the hyperplastic response post-revascularization remains an outstanding issue for all vascular interventional modalities.

Intraluminal delivery of radiation following vascular intervention is viewed as a viable solution to inhibit restenosis.[19–29] Exposing the vessels to low-dose radiation following angioplasty modifies wound healing by inhibiting the excessive neointima formation. Intravascular radiation in the peripheral system, however, requires special considerations when selecting the isotope and the delivery system to deliver the radiation to the target site.

Radiation physics and dosimetric considerations

Different isotopes on various platforms and systems have been developed for use in endovascular brachytherapy. The main platforms for radiation delivery are catheter-based systems and radioactive stents. Catheter-based systems contain a solid form such as line source wires, radioactive seeds or radioactive balloons, or non-solid sources such as radioactive gas and liquid-filled balloons.

As there are several different gamma and beta isotopes available, selecting the most appropriate one depends on the anatomy of the vessel, the properties of the treated lesion, and the proper identification of the target tissue that needs treatment. Anatomically important parameters which also need consideration include the diameter and the curvature of the vessel, the eccentricity of the plaque, the lesion length, the composition of the plaque, the amount of calcium, and the presence or absence of a stent in the treated segment. These factors influence which source to use, as different sources have varying properties which warrant using one over another.

Requirements for choosing the ideal radiation system for vascular brachytherapy should include dose distribution of a few millimeters from the source with a minimal dose gradient, low dose levels to surrounding tissues, and a dwell time less than 15 min. Other considerations for source selection include source energy, half-life for multiple applications, available activity, penetration, dose distribution, radiation exposure to the patient and the operator, shielding requirement, availability, and cost. An example of dose distribution of iridium-192 is presented in Figure 55.1.

In order to determine an accurate dosimetry, it is essential to identify the target tissue, the right dose, and the treatment margins. It has been argued that the adventitia is the target, but when considering the success of previous trials, it is difficult to deny the fact that the high dose exposure to the vessel wall and residual plaque may be essential to obtain efficacy.[30,31] The doses prescribed today in clinical studies are empirical; they are based on doses used in animal studies and the limited experience gained from treating other benign diseases. Since a wide range of doses demonstrated effectiveness in preclinical studies, a therapeutic window must exist that allows some flexibility in selecting the isotope for this application.

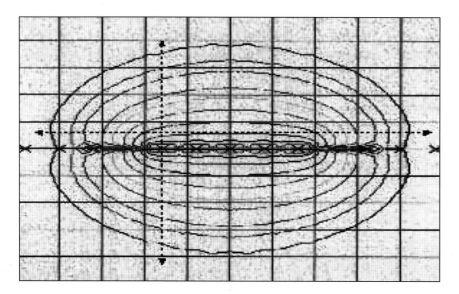

Figure 55.1

Example of dose distribution along an iridium-192 5–seed ribbon.

Understanding gamma radiation

Gamma rays are photons originating from the center of the nucleus and differ from X-rays, which originate from the orbital outside of the nucleus. Gamma rays have deep penetrating energies between 20 keV and 20 MeV which require an excess of shielding, as compared to beta and X-ray emitters. The only gamma ray isotope currently in use is iridium-192(^{192}Ir). There are isotopes that emit both gamma and X-rays, such as iodine-125(^{125}I) and palladium-103(^{103}Pd). These isotopes have lower energies, however, and require higher activity levels in order to deliver a prescribed dose in the acceptable dwell time (<15 min). Using these isotopes for vascular brachytherapy is difficult, as they are either not available in high activity levels or too expensive for this application. The dosimetry of ^{192}Ir is well understood and is associated with an acceptable dose gradient, as ^{192}Ir has less fall-off in dose than beta emitters. Iridium-192 is available in activities of up to 10 Ci, but because of high penetration, patients need to be transferred to the radiation oncology shielded room, as the average shielding of a catheterization laboratory will not be enough to handle more than 500 mCi source in activity. Focal stenosis in smaller-diameter arteries can be treated with lower activities of ^{192}Ir in the cath lab and will require an average of 20 min of dwell time for doses above 15 Gy when prescribed at 2-mm radial distance from the source.

Understanding beta radiation

Beta rays are high-energy electrons emitted by nuclei which contain too many or too few neutrons. These negatively charged particles have a wide variety of energies, including transition energies, particularly between parent and daughter cells, and a diverse range of half-lives from several minutes (^{62}Cu) up to 30 years (^{90}Sr/^{90}Y). Beta emitters are associated with a higher gradient to the near wall, as they lose their energy rapidly to surrounding tissue and their range is within 1 cm of tissue. Vascular brachytherapy using beta emitters appears promising, as safety levels are high when radiation exposure to non-targeted areas is low. In order to use beta emitters for the peripheral application, they must be in proximity with the vessel wall and should be used with as high an activity level as possible.

Radiation systems for the peripheral vascular system

Several radiation systems for peripheral endovascular brachytherapy have been suggested and are currently under development. These systems are as follows.

External radiation

External beam radiation is a viable option for the treatment of peripheral vessels. It allows a homogeneous dose distribution with the possibility of fractionation. To date, an attempt to treat SFA lesions and arteriovenous-dialysis grafts with external radiation has been reported without success in reducing the restenosis rate. The use of sterotactic techniques to localize the radiation to the target area may improve the results of this approach.

Radioactive stents

Radioactive stents are attractive devices since they require minimum shielding and are easy to use. The dosimetry of radioactive stents is even more complicated and depends on the geometry of the stent, which varies across stent designs. Current tested radioactive stents lack dose homogeneity across the entire length of the stent. This could affect the biological response to radiation, especially at the stent edges. The lack of even dose distribution may also result in an improper delivery to specific injured sites, causing additional growth. This problem, known as the edge effect, and identified as the major limitation of radioactive stents in coronary trials, may result from a stimulatory response from the vessel. Low-activity radioactive stents may be associated with an ineffective low dose rate. While radioactive stents with high activities may deliver toxic doses to the stented area that delay re-endothelialization, higher radiation doses might promote stent thrombosis and tissue necrosis to the area surrounding the stent. New studies are underway which will evaluate whether higher activities will minimize the edge effect phenomenon. Other approaches to improving the results with radioactive stents include changes to the geometry of the stent, and altering the isotope or the activity level at the stent's edges. A new approach with the use of radioactive Nitinol self-expanding stents utilizing gamma emitters is currently under investigation as a potential therapy for primary SFA lesions.

Catheter-based systems

Several catheter-based systems are available for the peripheral vascular system. However, the only system used in clinical trials is the MicroSelectron HDR (Nucletron-Odelft, Veenendaal, the Netherlands). The system uses a high-dose rate afterloader that consists of a computerized system which delivers a 3-mm stepping 10 Ci in activity of ^{192}Ir source into a centered closed-end lumen segmented balloon radiation catheter. There are many advantages to using a remote afterloading system for vascular brachytherapy. The remote

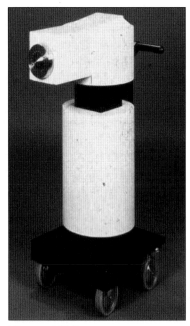

Figure 55.2
The MicroSelectron HDR afterloader
(Nucletron-Odelft, the Netherlands).

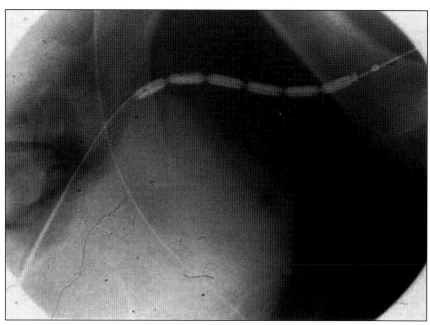

Figure 55.3
PARIS™ Centering Catheter (Guidant Corporation, Santa Clara, CA, USA).

afterloading system drives the radiation source quickly to the treatment site, avoiding radiation exposure to non-treated arteries. In addition, radiation exposure to the clinical personnel is eliminated by remotely programming the automatic advancement of the radiation source from a shielded safe to the treatment site. The radiation dose can be controlled and shaped by using the computerized afterloader device to accurately adjust the source position and treatment time. The afterloader continually monitors the radiation dose and automatically retracts the source into the shielded safe after treatment. Treatment time is automatically adapted for the radioactive decay of the source, and the afterloader can handle a very high-activity source (10 Ci), which results in shorter dwell times. The afterloader used in the MicroSelectron HDR system is shown in Figure 55.2.

The Peripheral Brachytherapy Centering Catheter (PARIS™ catheter) (Guidant, Santa Clara, CA, USA) is currently being used in the multicenter Peripheral Artery Radiation Investigational Study (PARIS). This catheter is a double-lumen catheter with multiple centering balloons near its distal tip. One lumen is for inflation of the centering balloon and the second lumen is for the guidewire and for the closed-end lumen sheath, which, once the catheter is in position, is introduced following removal of the guidewire. The inflated balloons engage the walls of the vessel and allow centering. The shaft diameter is a 7F closed end-lumen catheter (Figure 55.3), comes with balloons from 4 to 8 mm in diameter and 10–20 cm in length, and enables the catheter to be in the center of the lumen of large peripheral vessels during inflation. Other designs of catheter, such as the helical balloon,

will overcome the centering problem and provide flow and perfusion during centering.

Another catheter-based system which is available for use in the catheterization laboratory includes the use of a ^{192}Ir radioactive wire which is delivered manually or by hand into a closed-end lumen catheter. The activity of the source is limited to 500 mCi and the system is only practical to use for short lesions in small vessels (diameters <4.0 mm) that require a dwell time of 20 min. Similar to this gamma system, the eventual use of a catheter-based system using high-activity beta sources may also be an option for intermediate-sized vessels.

The angioplasty balloon is another platform which can be used to deliver radiation for the peripheral system. These balloons can be filled with either a liquid isotope such as ^{188}Re or ^{186}Re, or radioactive xenon-133 gas. The advantage of using these systems is the uniform dosimetry and proximity of the beta emitter to the vessel wall. Special care, however, is required when using the liquid-filled balloon to prevent spilling of the isotope outside of the balloon. The radioactive balloon catheter is particularly attractive for peripheral applications, since it is associated with apposition of a solid beta ^{32}P source attached to the inner balloon surface. With inflation of the balloon, the source is attached to the lumen surface. The system is limited to lesions <30 mm in length with one step, but can accommodate longer lesions with manual stepping. To date, there are no clinical data to support the use of this technology.

An alternative and attractive approach would be the use of low X-ray energy delivered intraluminally via a catheter. The emitter would be between 5 and 7 mm in length and 1.25–2.0 mm in diameter. It could be administered distally to the lesion and pulled back to cover the entire lesion length. If effective, it would alleviate the need for the use of radioisotopes in the catheterization laboratory. Miniaturizing the emitter is a technical challenge, and there are no preclinical data yet to support this theory.

Limitations to brachytherapy

Although clinical trials using vascular brachytherapy for both coronary and peripheral applications have demonstrated positive results in reducing restenosis rates, these trials have also identified two major serious complications related to the technology; late thrombosis and edge stenosis effects seen at the edges of radiation treatment segments. Late thrombosis is probably due to the delay in healing associated with radiation. It has been estimated that late thrombosis can be remedied through the prolonged administration of antiplatelet therapy following intervention.

Identified as a major limitation to radioactive stents and explained above, the edge effect phenomenon is not exclusive to stented lesions. The edge effect has also been known to occur with catheter-based systems utilizing both beta and gamma emitters, especially when the treated area is not covered with wide enough margins. The main explanation for the occurrence of the edge effect is a combination of low dose at the edges of the radiation source and an injury created by the device for intervention which is not covered by the radiation source. It is hypothesized that wider radiation margins of radiation treatment to the intervening segment may eliminate or significantly reduce the edge effect seen so far in all radiation trials.

Clinical trials

The first application of vascular brachytherapy for the prevention of restenosis was performed in the peripheral arteries and was initiated by Liermann and Schopohl (Frankfurt, Germany). Known as the Frankfurt Experience, the first pilot study of endovascular radiation was conducted in 30 patients with in-stent restenosis in their SFA.[32] The patients underwent atherectomy and PTA followed by endovascular radiation using the MicroSelectron HDR afterloader and a non-centering catheter. The gamma source ^{192}Ir was used to deliver a dose of 12 Gy, 3 mm into the vessel wall. The actual dose, however, varied from 8 to 28 Gy. No adverse effects from the radiation treatment were reported after up to 7 years follow-up. The 5-year patency rate of the target vessel was 82%, with only 3/28 (11%) stenosis within the treated segment reported. Late total occlusion developed in 2/28 patients (7%) after 16 and 37 months respectively.

The Emory experience

A subsequent pilot study was conducted at Emory University in 1994, which studied the effects of endovascular radiation in the SFAs of four patients following PTA and stenting. Of the four patients, one with a Palmaz stent needed subsequent surgery 1 year post-radiation therapy because of a crushed stent. The histology of the irradiated stent segment in this patient demonstrated minimal intimal hyperplasia surrounding the stent struts, thus indicating the inhibitory effect of radiation therapy in stented SFAs.

The Vienna experience

The effectiveness of the MicroSelectron HDR system was tested in a randomized placebo-controlled trial in Vienna using ^{192}Ir, a non-centering closed-end lumen catheter and a prescribed dose of 12 Gy in 100 patients following PTA to the SFA and the popliteal arteries. This study demonstrated a 50% reduction in the clinical restenosis rate in the irradiated group versus control.[33] The group from Vienna continued to investigate a series of patients with higher-dose 18 Gy and also a series of patients who were treated with primary stenting of the SFA followed by radiation therapy. The group receiving higher dosages experienced a late thrombosis rate of 10%. Prolonged antiplatelet therapy was initiated to further prevent this complication.

The PARIS trial

The PARIS Radiation Investigational Study is the first FDA-approved multicenter randomized double-blind control study involving 300 patients following PTA to SFA stenosis using a gamma radiation ^{192}Ir source. Utilizing the MicroSelectron HDR afterloader, the treatment dose is 14 Gy delivered via a centered segmented end-lumen balloon catheter. The primary objectives of this study are to determine angiographic evidence of patency and a reduction of >30% of the treated lesion's restenosis rate at 6 months. A secondary endpoint is to determine the clinical patency at 6 and 12 months by treadmill exercise and by the ankle–brachial index (ABI). The clinical endpoints are improvements in treadmill exercise time of >90 s, improvement of ABI of 0.10 compared to pre-PTA values, and an absence of repeat interventions to the treated vessel. This study was designed based on recently published recommendations and general principles of the evaluation of new interventional devices and technologies. The data from this study should ultimately determine whether endovascular radiation therapy has a role in prevention of restenosis in patients following PTA for SFA lesions.

In the feasibility phase of PARIS, 40 patients with claudication were enrolled. The mean lesion length was 9.9 ± 3.0 cm, with a mean reference vessel diameter of 5.4 ± 0.5 mm. Following successful PTA, a segmented balloon-centering catheter was positioned to cover the PTA site. The patients were transported to the radiation oncology suite and treated with radiation using a high-dose-rate MicroSelectron afterloader. The isotope used for this study was ^{192}Ir (maximum of 10 Ci in activity) and the prescribed dose was 14 Gy to 2 mm into the vessel wall. ABI and maximum walking time were evaluated with a repeat angiogram at 6 months. Radiation was delivered successfully in all but two patients (due to technical difficulties). There were no procedural, in-hospital, or 30–day complications in any of the treated patients. Maximum walking time on the treadmill was increased from 3.56 ± 2.7 min at baseline to 4.53 ± 2.7 min at 3 months ($p = 0.01$) and ABI was also improved from 0.7 ± 0.2 to 1.0 ± 0.2. Among the first 20 patients who returned for 5–month angiographic follow-up, there was only one patient who required revascularization of the treated site. There has been no evidence of arterial aneurysms or perforations. The 6–month angiographic follow-up was completed on 30 patients; 13.3% of them had evidence of clinical restenosis. The feasibility study of PARIS demonstrated that the delivery of high-dose-rate gamma radiation via a centering catheter is feasible and safe following PTA to SFA lesions. The randomization phase for this study is scheduled to be completed by the end of 2000, and results are expected in 2001.

Arterio-venous dialysis studies

A pilot study was initiated at Emory in 1994 to determine whether intravascular low-dose radiation retards neointimal hyperplasia in patients who had failed PTA at the distal venous anastomosis of AV dialysis grafts.[34]

Patients who failed prior PTAs to their AV graft and had <50% luminal stenosis were enrolled in the study and underwent balloon dilation at the narrowed segment. Following PTA, a sheath was placed across the lesion and a closed-end lumen 5F non-centered radiation delivery catheter was positioned at the angioplasty site. The catheter position was verified by radio-opaque marker bands on a dummy source wire that was placed into the catheter. The sheath and the catheter were fixed to the skin and the patients were transported to the radiation oncology suite. The patients were treated with a high-activity ^{192}Ir source delivered to the treatment site by a MicroSelectron HDR afterloader. The treatment dose was 14 Gy delivered to a depth of 2 mm into the arterial wall. After the radiation treatment, the sheath and the catheter were retrieved and the patients were sent home on the same day. Bimonthly clinical follow-up, including color-flow Doppler evaluation, was performed and the majority of the patients underwent angiographic follow-up at 6 months. Eleven patients with 18 lesions were treated. A 40% patency rate at 44 weeks was reported.

Although the procedure was successful in all patients, the long-term results of this study were similar to the practice reported so far by stand-alone PTA without radiation. In summary, this study demonstrated only the feasibility and safety of intravascular radiation therapy post-PTA using the MicroSelectron HDR afterloader for patients with AV dialysis graft stenosis.

This feasibility study had several limitations: the study population was small and heterogeneous; many patients had several PTA failures prior to the procedure; and there was heterogenicity with regard to the type of the treated grafted shunts. Several patients in this study had thrombotic events within 3 months following the procedure and underwent thrombectomy or lytic therapy. Although the prescribed dose was 14 Gy, the actual calculated dose given to the patients ranged between 7 and 90 Gy. This occurred because a centering catheter was not utilized in a large conduit. The effectiveness of intravascular radiation therapy in the AV dialysis grafts, however, is unclear. Utilizing a centered catheter to deliver radiation to large vessels will be essential to control the uniformity of the dose given to the vessel wall in such large conduits. Larger randomized studies are required to determine the value of this new technology for patients with AV dialysis graft failure.

A pilot study utilizing external radiation in a fractionated method for AV dialysis in 12 patients failed to keep any of these grafts within the first year. New studies on this application are currently underway using low-dose external radiation to reduce restenosis of vascular access for AV grafts of hemodialysis patients. Other studies using a centering device to deliver an accurate homogeneous dose of radiation following PTA are currently under design.

Recently, a new study was initiated at SCRIPPS, utilizing endovascular radiation therapy for the prevention of restenosis following transjugular intrahepatic portosystemic shunts (TIPS) for patients with portal hypertension. Overall, the restenosis rate due to intimal hyperplasia of TIPS at 6 months has been reported to be as high as 70%. Complete thrombosis as early as 2 weeks after the procedure has also been reported.[35] However, in the long term, brachytherapy may be the best means of preventing occlusion for these patients.

Other potential targets for vascular brachytherapy include renal arteries, and subclavian vein stenosis.

Conclusion

Despite new technologies and devices, restenosis remains the major limitation of intervention in the peripheral vascular system. The results from preliminary studies demonstrate that radiation has the potential to alter the rate of restenosis following intervention. With the further progression of these studies and their promising results, the use of vascular brachytherapy will dramatically change the practice of peripheral intervention, resulting in an improved long-term patency for our patients.

References

1   Tripuraneni P. Catheter-based radiotherapy for peripheral vascular restenosis. *Vasc Radiother Monitor* 1999; **1**(3): 70–7.

2   Haude M, Erbel R, Issa H, Meyer J. Quantitative analysis of elastic recoil after balloon angioplasty and after intracoronary implantation of balloon-expandable Palmaz–Schatz stents. *J Am Coll Cardiol* 1993; **21**: 2634.

3   Consigny PM, Bilder GE. Expression and release of smooth muscle cell mitogens in arterial wall after balloon angioplasty. *J Vasc Med Biol* 1993; **4**: 1–8.

4   Mintz GS, Popma JJ, Pichard AD et al. Arterial remodeling after coronary angioplasty. A serial intravascular ultrasound study. *Circulation* 1996; **94**: 35–43.

5   Isner JM. Vascular remodeling. Honey, I think I shrunk the artery. *Circulation* 1994; **89**: 2937–41.

6   Murray RR Jr, Hewews RC, White RI Jr et al. Long-segment femoro–popliteal stenoses: is angioplasty a boon or a bust? *Radiology* 1987; **162**: 473–6.

7   Johnston KW. Femoral and popliteal arteries: re-analyses of results of balloon angioplasty. *Radiology* 1992; **183**: 767–71.

8   Vroegindeweij D, Kemper FJ, Teilbeek AV et al. Recurrence of stenosis following balloon angioplasty and Simpson atherectomy of the femoropopliteal segment. A randomized comparative 1 year follow-up study using color flow duplex. *Eur J Vasc Surg* 1992; **6**: 164–71.

9   Rees CR, Palmaz JC, Becker GJ et al. Palmaz stent in atherosclerotic stenosis involving the ostia of the renal arteries: preliminary report of a multicenter study. *Radiology* 1991; **181**: 507–14.

10 Hunink MFM, Magruder CD, Meyerovitz MF et al. Risks and benefits fo femoropopliteal percutaneous balloon angioplasty. *J Vasc Surg* 1993; **17**: 183–94.

11 White GF, Liew SC, Waugh RC et al. Early outcome of intermediate follow-up of vascular stents in the femoral and popliteal arteries without long term anticoagulation. *J Vasc Surg* 1995; **21**: 279–81.

12 Kotb MM, Kadir S, Bennett JD, Beam CA. Aortoiliac angioplasty: is there a need for other types of percutaneous intervention? *JVIR* 1992; **3**: 67–71.

13 Dolmath BL, Gray RJ, Horton KM et al. Treatment of anastomotic bypass graft stenosis with directional atherectomy: short term and intermediate-term results. *J Vasc Int Radiol* 1995; **6**: 105–13.

14 Johnston KW. Femoral and popliteal arteries: reanalysis of results of angioplasty. *Radiology* 1987; **162**: 473–6.

15 Robinson KA. Arterial biologic response to ionizing radiation. In: Waksman R, Bonan R, eds. *Vascular Brachytherapy: State of the Art*. London: Remedica Publishing, 1999: 15–24.

16 Hillegass WB, Ohman EM, Califf RM. Restenosis: the clinical issues. In: Topol EJ, ed. *Textbook of Interventional Cardiology*, 2nd edn, Vol. 1. Philadelphia: WB Saunders, 1994: 415–35.

17 Pickering JG, Weir L, Jekanowski J et al. Proliferative activity in peripheral and coronary atherosclerotic plaques among patients undergoing percutaneous revascularization. *J Clin Invest* 1993; **91**: 1469–80.

18 Strandness DE, Barnes RW, Katzen B, Ring EJ. Indiscriminate use of laser angioplasty. *Radiology* 1989; **172**: 945–6.

19 Waksman R, Robinson KA, Crocker IR et al. Long term efficacy and safety of endovascular low dose irradiation in a swine model of restenosis after angioplasty. *Circulation* 1995; **91**: 1533–9.

20 Weidermann JG, Marboe C, Amols H et al. Intracoronary irradiation markedly reduces restenosis after balloon angioplasty in a porcine model. *J Am Coll Cardiol* 1994; **23**: 1491–8.

21 Weiderman JG, Marboe C, Amols H et al. Intracoronary irradiation markedly reduces neointimal proliferation after balloon angioplasty in swine: persistent benefit at 6-month follow-up. *J Am Coll Cardiol* 1995; **25**: 1456–61.

22 Mazur W, Ali MN, Dabhagi SF et al. High dose rate intracoronary radiation suppresses neointimal proliferation in the stented and balloon model of porcine restenosis. *Int J Radiat Oncol Biol Phys* 1996; **36**: 777–88.

23 Borok TL, Bray M, Sinclair I et al. Role of ionizing irradiation for keloids. *Int J Radiat Oncol Biol Phys* 1988; **15**: 865–70.

24 Van den Brenk HAS, Minty CCJ. Radiation in the management of keloids and hypertrophic scar. *Br J Surg* 1959/1960; **47**: 595–605.

25 Nickson JJ, Lawrence W, Rachwalsky I et al. Roentgen rays and wound healing: fractionated irradiation: experimental study. *Surgery* 1953; **34**: 859–62.

26 Insalsingh CHA. An experience in treating 501 patients with keloids. *Johns Hopkins Med J* 1974; **134**: 284–90.

27 Grillo HC, Potsaid MS. Studies in wound healing. *Ann Surg* 1961; **154**: 741.

28 MacLennon I, Keys HM, Evarts CM, Rubgin P. Usefulness of post-operative hip irradiation in the prevention of heterotrophic bone formation in a high risk group of patients. *Int J Radiat Oncol Biol Phys* 1984; **10**: 49–53.

29 Van den Brenk HAS. Results of prophylactic post-operative irradiation in 1300 cases of pterygium. *AJR* 1968; **103**: 723.

30 Mintz GS, Pichard AD, Kent KM et al. Endovascular stents reduce restenosis by eliminating geometric arterial remodeling: a serial intravascular ultrasound study. *J Am Coll Cardiol* 1995; **35A**: 701–5.

31 Waksman R, Rodriquez JC, Robinson KA et al. Effect of intravascular irradiation on cell proliferation, apoptosis and vascular remodeling after balloon overstretch injury of porcine coronary arteries. *Circulation* 1996; **96**: 1944–52.

32 Liermann DD, Bottcher HD, Kollath J et al. Prophylactic endovascular radiotherapy to prevent intimal hyperplasia after stent implantation in femoropopliteal arteries. *Cardiovasc Intervent Radiol* 1994; **17**: 12–16.

33 Minar E. SFA Brachytherapy: The Vienna Experience. *Cardiovascular Radiation Therapy III Syllabus* 1999: 431 (abstr).

34 Waksman R, Crocker IA, Kikeri D et al. Long term results of endovascular radiation therapy for prevention of restenosis in the peripheral vascular system. *Circulation* 1996; **94**(8) 1–300: 1745.

35 Raat H, Stockx L, Ranschaert E et al. Percutaneous hydrodynamic thrombectomy of acute thrombosis in transjugular intrahepatic portosystemic shunt (TIPS): a feasibility study in five patients. *Cardiovasc Intervent Radiol* 1997; **20**: 180–3.

56

Gene-based and angiogenesis therapy in cardiovascular diseases

Richard Baffour, Shmuel Fuchs and Ran Kornowski

What is gene therapy?

A gene (within each cell's DNA) is an inheritable (able to be passed on from one generation to the next generation) material found in every cell. Genes are necessary for each cell to 'know' how to grow and develop. In a way, genes may be thought of as 'cellular recipes'. Since organs are made up of many cells, it is necessary for the cells to grow and develop normally for the organ to function in a healthy manner.

Gene therapy involves the introduction of normal or modified genes into cells of a specific, predetermined organ. The purpose of this introduction is to correct or alter cellular functions such that the disorder will become corrected or be prevented. There has been much interest in using gene therapy to treat inheritable diseases, long-term health disorders, and cancer. Many clinical studies are underway worldwide in the treatment of inflammatory diseases, inheritable enzyme deficiency diseases, cancer, etc. Cardiovascular diseases have become a new aim for gene therapy research. Cardiovascular gene therapy is being evaluated for angiogenesis (the procedure of causing new blood vessel growth) in ischemic territories, the prevention of restenosis after angioplasty, and the treatment of atherosclerosis, hereditary forms of hypercholesterolemia, and congestive heart failure.

In vivo gene therapy (gene therapy performed within the cell of a living being either human or animal) usually relies on a vector to introduce the gene into the cell. Vectors are special biological complexes that are able to pass through the cellular membrane (outside barrier of each cell). A vector may be thought of as 'a vehicle with correct identification to cross a biological barrier' that permits the genetic material (DNA) to get inside the cell. Vectors currently in use include plasmids ('naked' DNA fragments) with or without liposome complexes, adeno-associated viruses, adenoviruses, and retroviruses. These viruses are replication deficient.

In adenoviral methods of delivery, the virus infects the cells bordering the point of injection. It does this with a very high degree of efficiency. The growth factor's DNA then travels from the cytoplasm of the cell to the nucleus, where it will be made into an active protein. The active protein is then secreted from the cell and travels throughout the heart to stimulate blood vessel growth where it is most needed and acts on nearby endothelial cells. With plasmids, a therapeutic gene ('naked' DNA) is injected into the target tissue and is taken up by the target cells. The newly introduced DNA segment can serve as a template for RNA to form new/deficient therapeutic proteins, although new DNA segments do not integrate into the native cellular DNA.

Table 56.1 specifies various vectors in investigational usage

Table 56.1 Characteristics of various vectors					
	Transfection efficacy	Host response	Target cells	DNA integration	DNA capacity
Plasmid DNA	Low	Against gene product	Cycling	No	Not limited
Retrovirus	Low	Against gene product	Cycling	Yes	Limited to viral size
Adenovirus	High	Against gene product and viral proteins	All	No	Limited by deletion size in virus
Adeno-associated virus	Unclear	Against gene product	Cycling> quiescent	Unclear	Limited to viral size
Oligonucleotide	High	Low	All	No	NA

NA, not applicable.

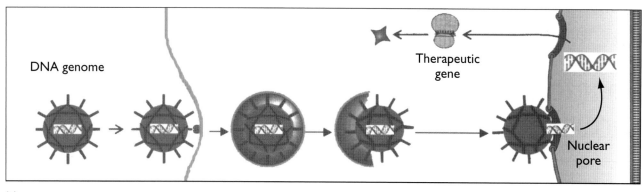

(a)

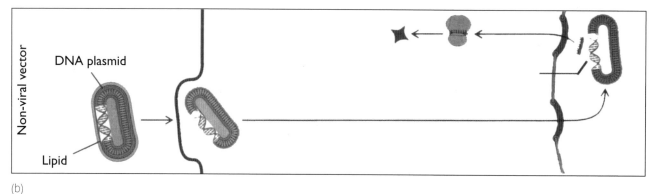

(b)

Figure 56.1

Representation of gene transfer using adenoviral vector or plasmid ('naked' DNA segment). (a) Adenoviral vector with the attached therapeutic gene infects cell through specific receptors. In the cytoplasm of the cell, the virus delivers the therapeutic gene to the nucleus through the nuclear pore where the gene is expressed. (b) Liposome delivers plasmid DNA through receptor-mediated endocytosis or fusion with cell membrane. Plasmid DNA is then released in the cytoplasm and transported to the nucleus, where the therapeutic gene is expressed.

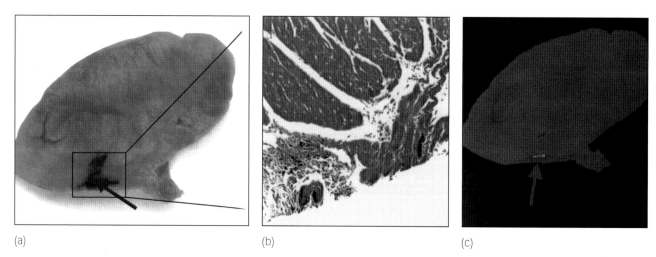

(a)   (b)   (c)

Figure 56.2

Gross (a) and microscopic (b) pathology of heart tissue (cross-section) injected with the adenovirus vector containing the ß-galactosidase reporter transgene and subsequently stained with X-gal solution. Note the areas of positive staining. Histopathology shows myocytes transfected by adenovirus-ß-galactosidase gene with typical nuclear as well as cytoplasmic staining (original magnification ×40).
(c) A representative injection site relative to fluorescent microsphere location shown under ultraviolet light. This shows successful gene delivery identified by co-injection of fluorescent beads and either ß-galactosidase marker or VEGF-121 isoform gene.

for gene therapy. Figure 56.1 shows schematics for gene therapy using adenoviral vector or plasmid (naked' DNA segment), and Figure 56.2 shows the pathology of heart tissue after gene transfer.

Angiogenic growth factors

Angiogenic growth factors are very powerful elements that cause blood vessels cells to grow. Endothelial cells are necessary to the structure of blood vessels. Growth factors or angiogenic genes have been demonstrated to show new blood vessel growth in animal studies and in the heart and leg of humans in phase I clinical trials.[1–21] There are several varieties of growth factors. Growth factors cause sprouting of new endothelial cells from existing blood vessels. These new blood vessels are then directed to grow towards the areas of maximal ischemia. The new blood vessels are then able to supply blood from a healthy area of the heart or peripheral limb into the unhealthy areas of the muscle. This identification of angiogenic growth factor 'prototypes', such as vascular endothelial growth factor (VEGF),[22–26] basic fibroblast growth factor (bFGF, or FGF2) and acidic FGF (aFGF, or FGF1), occurred in the late 1970s and early 1980s.[27–31] The practical application of these agents in cardiovascular ischemic syndromes had to await the development of technologies that allowed the angiogenic proteins to be produced in sufficient quantities, and subsequently the development of DNA technology and gene delivery techniques so that gene therapy studies became possible. Once these biotechnology breakthroughs were achieved, studies exploring the potential of various angiogenesis strategies to develop clinically relevant therapeutic approaches to both myocardial and leg ischemia have been conducted, so that over the past half-decade the field has moved forward with great momentum.

Using gene therapy constructs presents a potential advantage over 'simple' administration of angiogenic protein, since gene therapy can be considered a biological form of a sustained delivery system. A protein, injected once intramuscularly, would be unlikely to persist in the tissue long enough to exert an important biological effect. Once transfected, the target cell expresses gene product for days, weeks, or longer, depending on the specific tissue transfected and on the specific vector used.

Proof of the concept that gene therapy can improve collateral function in the heart was demonstrated by Giordano et al.[32] They found in a porcine model of myocardial ischemia (ameroid occlusion of the circumflex coronary artery) that a single-dose intracoronary administration of an adenoviral vector carrying the FGF5 transgene into the non-occluded coronary results in more than 90% 'first-pass' myocardial uptake, causing increased myocardial flow and function.

Hammond and colleagues have since demonstrated that FGF4 produces similar effects in restoring myocardial flow and function. Other investigators have also performed studies employing the rabbit hindlimb model of ischemia and have reported that injection into the femoral artery of the $VEGF_{165}$ transgene carried in a plasmid vector improves collateral flow.[33]

As stated above, a protein, injected once intramuscularly, would be unlikely to persist in the tissue long enough to exert an important biological effect. Although multiple injections of protein might well improve collateral flow,[34] such a strategy has practical limitations. Therefore, once it was demonstrated that an adenoviral vector carrying a reporter transgene efficiently expresses its gene product after intramyocardial injection,[35] this approach to gene delivery was explored as an approach for gene therapy.

Proof of the concept that intramyocardial injection could enhance collateral flow and improve impaired myocardial function was demonstrated in a porcine model of myocardial ischemia. This was achieved by the transepicardial injection of an adenoviral vector carrying the $VEGF_{121}$ transgene performed following thoracotomy.[36] The feasibility of catheter-based transendocardial delivery of angiogenic genes has recently been shown,[37,38] demonstrating that the direct injection of angiogenesis factors into the myocardium can be accomplished without the need for open chest thoracotomy.

Patient candidates for angiogenic gene therapy

Growth factors, given either as genes or peptides, have been demonstrated to induce new blood vessel growth in animal studies and in the heart and leg of humans in phase I clinical trials (testing safety and effectiveness).[32,33,35,36,37,39–45] By increasing the bloodflow with the growth of new blood vessels, they may cause the chest pain and other ischemic manifestations to decrease or even disappear. Research trials in cardiology include patients with severe anginal symptoms (symptoms of chest pain with very little exertion or at rest) who have been turned down for bypass surgery and angioplasty. Similarly, patients with advanced peripheral vascular disease who were poor candidates for conventional surgical revascularization and endovascular interventional therapy have undergone gene therapy research trials.[18,19] Almost all angiogenic gene therapy studies have involved attempts to enhance angiogenesis and collateral development in ischemic tissue beds. However, a recent report suggests that transfer of an angiogenic (VEGF) gene may also be effective in treating ischemic peripheral diabetic neuropathy in an experimental model of this disease.[46]

Routes of administration for gene delivery

Various delivery routes, including transcatheter, intraoperative intramyocardial injection, intrapericardial and catheter-based transendocardial, have been used to locally transfer angiogenic growth factors or genes in coronary studies.[35,37,38,47,48] Delivery routes used in peripheral vascular disease studies are transcatheter and direct injection into skeletal muscle.[18,19] Which of these approaches for both coronary and peripheral vascular disease are most safe and effective remains to be determined. Theoretically, it would seem that local gene delivery via direct intramuscular injection might be more effective than other routes, since genes can be targeted to specific ischemic areas of the myocardium or peripheral muscle.

Clinical experiences

Several clinical trials in both coronary and peripheral vascular disease studies have been reported (Table 56.2). In essence, nearly all of these studies were phase I trials, which demonstrated the safety and feasibility of growth factor or gene therapy. For example, in a preliminary study VEGF$_{165}$ protein was administered by the intracoronary route to establish the correct dose and infusion rates. In this study, three treatment

groups of patients, including a placebo-controlled group, were assessed at baseline and 60 days later. The assessments included exercise treadmill time, retinal photographs and angina class determination. However, a subsequent randomized double-blind phase II study (VIVA trial) using intracoronary followed by three intravenous doses of VEGF$_{165}$ protein showed no beneficial effect as assessed by treadmill exercise performance, the primary endpoint.[17] Indeed, there were similar performance improvements in treated and untreated patients. Similar disappointing results have been reported recently following intracoronary administration of basic FGF protein in a blinded randomized phase II trial.[49] Other investigators have reported enhanced angiogenesis and growth of collaterals after intramuscular injection of the plasmid encoding VEGF$_{165}$ in patients with critical limb ischemia.[18,19] However, these two studies had no controlled groups for comparison. In one of these studies, VEGF plasmid was transferred to the distal popliteal artery of a patient with an ischemic limb. At 4 and 12 weeks after gene transfer, follow-up assessments were performed. Angiography revealed collateral development, and intra-arterial Doppler bloodflow showed improvement.[18]

Ongoing clinical trials include two pioneering randomized controlled phase I studies using the electromagnetic catheter-based transendocardial injection technique (Biosense™ Johnson and Johnson, NJ, USA) of either VEGF-II plasmid or adenovirus containing the VEGF$_{121}$ transgene. These studies are designed to test the feasibility and safety aspects of such catheter-based approaches for transendocardial angiogenic gene delivery. The studies include appropriate 'control' patients who are blinded to the actual treatment. In addition, preliminary efficacy endpoints may reveal the potential efficacy of such pro-angiogenic intervention among patients by including subjective and objective efficacy measures of myocardial ischemia. In a recent study, similar to the discussed ongoing trials, Vale and colleagues used left ventricular (LV) electromechanical mapping (EMM) to assess infarcted, ischemic and normal myocardium before and after gene transfer.[50] They treated patients with chronic myocardial ischemia, not amenable to current therapeutic interventions, with direct myocardial injection of VEGF plasmid through a small incision in the left lateral chest. Sixty days after gene transfer, there was significant improvement in the areas of myocardial ischemia as assessed by LV EMM, suggesting increased perfusion of the ischemic myocardium as a result of gene therapy.[50]

The results of a phase II clinical trial of recombinant fibroblast growth factor-2 (FGF-2) protein in peripheral artery disease were recently presented.[51] The pre-specified efficacy analysis of change in peak walking time (PWT) at day 90 showed a positive trend in patients receiving a single bolus of FGF-2 compared to control patients or patients receiving a double bolus FGF-2 dose (34.1 vs 20.1 vs 14.1 increase vs baseline, $p=0.07$). Intra-coronary administration of Ad FGF-4 showed promising results in patients with coronary disease

Table 56.2   Clinical trials: gene therapy in coronary vascular disease (CVD) and peripheral vascular disease (PVD)

Reference	Treatment	Disease	Results
Rosengart et al (1999)[15]	VEGF	CVD	Collateral development + Myocardial function +
Losordo et al (1998)[16]	VEGF	CVD	Left ventricular ischemic zone − Collateral development +
Isner et al (1996)[18]	VEGF	PVD	Intra-arterial bloodflow + Angiogenesis + Development of spider angiomas
Baumgartner et al (1998)[19]	VEGF	PVD	Ankle–brachial index + Collateral development + Distal bloodflow + Development of transient lower limb edema
Isner et al (1998)[20]	VEGF	PVD	Non-healing ulcer healed Distal limb perfusion + Limb bloodflow + Collateral development + Development of transient ankle and calf edema +

+, stimulation; −, reduction.

who elected to undergo this mode of experimental treatment instead of coronary angioplasty or bypass surgery.[52] At 12 weeks following treatment, more patients receiving IC gene transfer had significant improvement in exercise treadmill time compared to placebo treated patients (45 vs 21.1).

Those recent trials have confirmed safety, feasibility and also suggested positive trends for either protein-based (peripheral artery disease) or gene-based (coronary disease) pro-angiogenesis interventions.

Potential hazards with gene therapy

It is conceivable that angiogenic agents that cause beneficial effects in chronic ischemic disease may cause unnecessary side-effects as well. For that reason, it is pertinent that the risk/benefit ratio should be taken into consideration before any therapeutic angiogenesis is instituted. Obviously, only a low risk ratio should be acceptable. Administration of angiogenic agents as treatment modality for chronic disease may be inappropriate in the presence of proliferative retinopathy, since these agents may enhance angiogenesis in this disease. Other areas of concern are undesired angiogenesis in normal tissues, and kidney damage. The angiogenic effects of growth factors appear to be restricted to injured or ischemic tissue, where there is upregulation of angiogenic receptor genes.[53,54] This may not necessarily apply to a normal organ, which has been exposed to high doses of angiogenic agents for an extended time.

Agents such as VEGF may cause increased vascular permeability that may lead to multiple organ edema.[53] Other potential undesired effects include growth of tumors and atherogenic plaque formation as demonstrated in some experimental studies.[56–60] It is reported that a patient with critical limb ischemia developed spider angiomas after phVEGF$_{165}$ gene transfer.[18] To our knowledge, there are no other clinical reports that suggest that angiogenic agents give rise to the growth of new tumor. Some angiogenic agents such as VEGF and bFGF proteins can cause hypotension following endovascular administration.[61–63] Similar responses are reported particularly in patients who receive rapid administration of high doses of bFGF.[14,21]

Prevention of atherosclerosis, restenosis and congestive heart failure

Atherosclerosis is a complex disease linked with multiple genes and risk factors such as family history, hypercholes-terolemia, hypertension, smoking, diabetes mellitus, and others. To date, it appears that only a few distinct causes of this disease are amenable to gene therapy. Animal and clinical studies have shown that gene replacement therapy can prevent genetic disorders, such as low-density lipoprotein (LDL) receptor deficiency, which cause premature athero-sclerosis.[64–66] In these studies, few patients with homozygous familial hypercholesterolemia were successfully treated with liver-directed LDL receptor gene transfer.

Another potential approach to prevent atherosclerosis is the use of genes which produce proteins that either impede this disease or stabilize susceptible lesions.[67] Gene therapy to prevent neointimal formation following coronary angioplasty and stenting may be a viable option to current therapeutic interventions, most of which have been unsuccessful in decreasing the numbers of restenoses.[68] Because there are several mechanisms involved in restenosis, such as smooth muscle cell proliferation, thrombosis, platelet activation and remodeling, transfer of multiple genes may be required to completely prevent restenosis.[68] Some studies have demonstrated decreased neointimal formation by transfer of different genes to the media of vessels after injury. For example, the transfer of human tissue inhibitor of the metalloproteinase 1 gene can prevent smooth muscle cell migration and neointimal formation in an in vitro human saphenous vein model.[69] Another theoretical approach may be the use of anti-restenotic gene-containing growth factor inhibitors that may decrease blood vessel supply to the neointima tissue.

Animal studies suggest that overexpression or downregulation of some myocardial genes may be an effective treatment for congestive heart failure, and this potentially may be applicable to similar disease in humans. Transfer of ß$_2$ adrenergic receptor genes has been shown to enhance heart function in transgenic mice with heart failure.[70] Similarly, transfer of a gene whose product inhibits the activity of ß-adrenergic receptor kinase, an enzyme that desensitizes and controls ß-adrenergic receptors, has been shown to prevent heart failure in a rabbit model of cardiomyopathy.[71]

Conclusions

Substantial knowledge has been acquired over recent years about the use of gene therapy as a treatment modality for cardiovascular diseases. However, much still needs to be learned before such treatment becomes successful in patients. In the past, efficient and safe deliveries of genes to the right targets were the major limitations of gene therapy. Better vectors and delivery systems have been developed over recent years with improved transfection efficiency and delivery to the target tissue, either the ischemic myocardium or peripheral limb. Preliminary clinical results are encouraging with regard to the feasibility and safety of gene therapy approaches applied to the cardiovascular system. Because of the complex nature of cardiovascular diseases, which involve multiple genes, the use of a single gene to treat a disease may not give the best possible result. Perhaps one should consider the idea of using multiple genes in combination, sequentially or in concert, to achieve a more effective intervention.

We should also be aware of serious complications and potential side-effects of gene therapy. Thus, cautiously controlled clinical trials must be completed to determine whether the risk/benefit ratio is sufficiently low such that the accompanying risks of gene therapy are overshadowed by the benefits achieved.

References

1 Banai S, Jaklitsch MT, Shou M et al. Angiogenic-induced enhancement of collateral blood flow to ischemic myocardium by vascular endothelial growth factor in dogs. *Circulation* 1994; **89**: 2183–9.

2 Takeshita S, Zheng LP, Brogi E et al. Therapeutic angiogenesis: a single intraarterial bolus of vascular endothelial growth factor augments revascularization in a rabbit ischemic hind limb model. *J Clin Invest* 1994; **93**: 662–70.

3 Pearlman JD, Hibberd MG, Chaung ML et al. Magnetic resonance mapping demonstrates benefits of VEGF-induced myocardial angiogenesis. *Nat Med* 1995; **1**: 1085–9.

4 Harada K, Friedman M, Lopez JJ et al. Vascular endothelial growth factor administration in chronic myocardial ischemia. *Am J Physiol* 1996; **270**: H1791–802.

5 Yanagisawa-Miwa A, Uchida Y, Nakamura F et al. Salvage of infarcted myocardium by angiogenic action of basic fibroblast growth factor. *Science* 1992; **257**: 1401–3.

6 Battler A, Scheinowitz M, Bor A et al. Intracoronary injection of basic fibroblast growth factor enhances angiogenesis in infarcted swine myocardium. *J Am Coll Cardiol* 1993; **22**: 2001–6.

7 Harada K, Grossman W, Friedman M et al. Basic fibroblast growth factor improves myocardial function in chronically ischemic porcine heart. *J Clin Invest* 1994; **94**: 623–30.

8 Uchida Y, Yanagisawa-Miwa A, Ikuta M et al. Angiogenic therapy of acute myocardial infarction (AMI) by intrapericardial injection of basic fibroblast growth factor (bFGF) and heparin sulfate (HS): an experimental study. *Circulation* 1994; **90**(suppl I): I–296 (abstr).

9 Unger EF, Banai S, Shou M et al. Basic fibroblast growth factor enhances myocardial collateral flow in a canine model. *Am J Physiol* 1994; **35**: H1588–95.

10 Lazarous DF, Scheinowitz M, Shou MN et al. Effects of chronic systemic administration of basic fibroblast growth factor on collateral development in the canine heart. *Circulation* 1995; **91**: 145–53.

11 Schumacher B, Pecher P, von Specht BU, Stegmann T. Induction of neoangiogenesis in ischemic myocardium by human growth factors: first clinical results of a new treatment of coronary heart disease. *Circulation* 1998; **97**: 645–50.

12 Sellke FW, Laham RJ, Edelman ER et al. Therapeutic angiogenesis with basic fibroblast growth factor: technique and early results. *Ann Thorac Surg* 1998; **65**: 1540–4.

13 Laham RJ, Sellke FW, Edelman ER et al. Local perivascular delivery of basic fibroblast growth factor in patients undergoing coronary bypass surgery: results of a phase I randomized, double-blind, placebo-controlled trial. *Circulation* 1999; **100**: 1865–71.

14 Unger EF, Goncalves L, Epstein SE et al. Effects of a single intracoronary injection of basic fibroblast growth factor in stable angina pectoris. *Am J Cardiol* 2000; **85**: 1414–19.

15 Rosengart TK, Lee LY, Patel SR et al. Angiogenesis gene therapy: phase I assessment of direct intramyocardial administration of an adenovirus vector expressing VEGF121 cDNA to individuals with clinically significant severe coronary artery disease. *Circulation* 1999; **100**: 468–74.

16 Losordo DW, Vale PR, Symes JF et al. Gene therapy for myocardial angiogenesis: initial clinical results with direct myocardial injection of phVEGF165 as sole therapy for myocardial ischemia. *Circulation* 1998; **98**: 2800–4.

17 Henry TD, Annex BH, Azrin MA et al. Double blind, placebo controlled trial of recombinant human vascular endothelial growth factor – the VIVA trial. *J Am Coll Cardiol* 1999; **33**(suppl A): 384A (abstr).

18 Isner JM, Pieczek A, Schainfeld R et al. Clinical evidence of angiogenesis after arterial gene transfer of phVEGF165 in patient with ischaemic limb. *Lancet* 1996; **348**: 370–4.

19 Baumgartner I, Pieczek A, Manor O et al. Constitutive expression of ph VEGF165 after intramuscular gene transfer promotes collateral vessel development in patients with critical limb ischemia. *Circulation* 1998; **97**: 1114–23.

20 Isner JM, Baumgartner I, Rauh G et al. Treatment of thromboangiitis obliterans (Buerger's disease) by intramuscular gene transfer of vascular endothelial growth factor: preliminary clinical results. *J Vasc Surg* 1998; **28**: 964–73.

21 Lazarous DF, Unger EF, Epstein SE et al. Basic fibroblast growth factor in patients with intermittent claudication: results of a phase I trial. *JACC* (in press).

22 Dvorak HF, Orenstein NS, Carvalho AC et al. Induction of a fibrin-gel investment: an early event in line 10 hepatocarcinoma growth medicated by tumor-secreted products. *J Immunol* 1979; **122**: 166–74.

23 Senger Dr, Galli SJ, Dvorak AM et al. Tumor cells secrete a vascular permeability factor that promotes accumulation of ascites fluid. *Science* 1983; **219**: 983–5.

24 Senger DR, Perruzzi CA, Feder J, Dvorak HF. A highly conserved vascular permeability factor secreted by a variety of human and rodent tumor cell lines. *Cancer Res* 1986; **46**: 5629–32.

25 Senger DR, Connolly D, Perruzzi CA et al. Purification of a vascular permeability factor (VPF) from tumor cell conditioned medium. *Fed Proc* 1987; **46**: 2102.

26 Connolly DT, Olander JV, Heuvelman D et al. Human vascular permeability factor. Isolation from U937 cells. *J Biol Chem* 1989; **264**: 20017–24.

27 Esch F, Baird A, Ling N et al. Primary structure of bovine pituitary basic fibroblast growth factor (FGF) and comparison with the amino-terminal sequence or bovine brain acidic FGF. *Proc Natl Acad Sci USA* 1985; **82**: 6507–11.

28 Gambarini AG, Armelin HA. Pituitary fibroblast growth factors. Partial purification and characterization. *Braz J Med Biol Res* 1981; **14**: 19–27.

29 Logan A, Berry M, Thomas GH et al. Identification and partial purification of fibroblast growth factor from the brains of developing rats and leucodystrophic mutant mice. *Neuroscience* 1985; **15**: 1239–46.

30 Baird A, Esch F, Gospodarowicz D, Guillemin R. Retina- and eye-derived endothelial cell growth factors: partial molecular characterization and identity with acidic and basic fibroblast growth factors. *Biochemistry* 1985; **24**: 7855–60.

31 Baird A, Esch F, Bohlen P et al. Isolation and partial characterization of an endothelial cell growth factor from the bovine kidney homology with basic fibroblast growth factor. *Regul Pept* 1985; **12**: 201–13.

32 Giordano FJ, Ping P, Mckirnan D et al. Intracoronary gene transfer of fibroblast growth factor-5 increases blood flow and contractile function in an ischemic region of the heart. *Nature Med* 1996; **2**: 534–9.

33 Witzenbichler B, Asahara T, Murohara T et al. Vascular endothelial growth factor-C (VEGF-C/VEGF-2) promotes angiogenesis in the setting of tissue ischemia. *Am J Pathol* 1998; **153**: 381–94.

34 Baffour R, Berman J, Garb JL et al. Enhanced angiogenesis and growth of collaterals by in vivo administration of recombinant basic fibroblast growth factor in a rabbit model of acute lower limb ischemia: dose–response effect of basic fibroblast growth factor. *J Vasc Surg* 1992; **16**: 181–91.

35 Guzman RJ, Lemarchand P, Crystal RG et al. Efficient gene transfer into myocardium by direct injection of adenovirus vectors. *Circ Res* 1993; **73**: 1202–7.

36 Mack CA, Patel SR, Schwartz EA et al. Biologic bypass with the use of adenovirus-mediated gene transfer of the complementary deoxyribonucleic acid for VEGF-12, improves myocardial perfusion and function in the ischemic porcine heart. *J Thorac Cardiovasc Surg* 1998: **115** 168–77.

37 Vale PR, Losordo DW, Tkebuchava T et al. Catheter-based myocardial gene transfer utilizing nonfluoroscopic electromechanical left ventricular mapping. *J Am Coll Cardiol* 1999; **34**: 246–54.

38 Kornowski R, Leon MB, Fuchs S et al. Electromagnetic guidance for catheter-based transendocardial injection: a platform for intramyocardial angiogenesis therapy. Results in normal and ischemic porcine models. *J Am Coll Cardiol* 2000; **35**: 1031–9.

39 Lazarous DF, Shou M, Stiber JA et al. Pharmacodynamics of basic fibroblast growth factor: route of administration determines myocardial and systemic distribution. *Cardiovasc Res* 1997; **36**: 78–85.

40 Lopez JJ, Laham RJ, Stamler A et al. VEGF administration in chronic myocardial ischemia in pigs. *Cardiovasc Res* 1998; **40**: 272–81.

41 Roth D, Maruoka Y, Rogers J et al. Development of coronary collateral circulation in left circumflex Ameriod-occluded swine myocardium. *Am J Physiol* 1987; **253**: (5 Pt 2): H 1279–88.

42 Hariawala MD, Horowitz JR, Esakof D et al. VEGF improves myocardial blood flow but produces EDRF-mediated hypotension in porcine hearts. *J Surg Res* 1996; **63**: 77–82.

43 Bauters C, Asahara T, Zheng LP et al. Site-specific therapeutic angiogenesis after systemic administration of vascular endothelial growth factor. *J Vasc Surg* 1995; **21**: 314–24.

44 Asahara T, Bauters C, Zheng LP et al. Synergistic effect of vascular endothelial growth factor and basic fibroblast growth factor on angiogenesis in vivo. *Circulation* 1995; **92**(suppl): II365–71.

45 Laham RJ, Rezaee M, Garcia L et al. Tissue and myocardial distribution of intracoronary, intravenous, intrapericardial, and intramyocardial ^{125}I-labeled basic fibroblast growth factor (bFGF) favor intramyocardial delivery. *JACC* 2000; **35**: 10A.

46 Schratzberger P, Schratzberger G, Silver M et al. Favorable effect of VEGF gene transfer on ischemic peripheral neuropathy. *Nature Med* 2000; **6**: 405–13.

47 Landau C, Jacobs AK, Haudenschild CC. Intrapericardial basic fibroblast growth factor induces myocardial angiogenesis in a rabbit model of chronic ischemia. *Am Heart J* 1995; **129**: 924–31.

48 Laham RJ, Hung D, Simons M. Therapeutic myocardial angiogenesis using percutaneous intrapericardial drug delivery. *Clin Cardiol* 1999; **22**(suppl 1): 16–9.

49 Chronos N et al.

50 Vale PR, Losordo DW, Milliken CE et al. Left ventricular electromechanical mapping to assess efficacy of ph VEGF$_{165}$ gene transfer for therapeutic angiogenesis in chronic myocardial ischemia. *Circulation* 2000; **102**: 965–74.

51 Lederman RJ. American College of Cardiology Meeting, April 2001.

52 Grines C et al. American College of Cardiology Meeting, April 2001.

53 Schaper W, Gorge G, Winkler B, Schaper J. The collateral circulation of the heart. *Prog Cardiovasc Dis* 1988; **31**: 57–77.

54 Lee PL, Johnson DE, Cousens LS et al. Purification and complementary DNA cloning of a receptor for basic fibroblast growth factor. *Science* 1989; **245**: 57–60.

55 Thurston G, Rudge JS, Ioffe E et al. Angiopoietin-1 protects the adult vasculature against plasma leakage. *Nature Med* 2000; **6**: 160–3.

56 Flugelman MY, Virmani R, Correa R et al. Smooth muscle cell abundance and fibroblast growth factors in coronary lesions of patients with nonfatal unstable angina. A clue to the mechanism of transformation from the stable to the unstable clinical state. *Circulation* 1993; **88**: 2493–500.

57 Schwarz ER, Speakman MT, Patterson M et al. Evaluation of the effects of intramyocardial injection of DNA expressing vascular endothelial growth factor (VEGF) in a myocardial infarction model in the rat – angiogenesis and angioma formation. *J Am Coll Cardiol* 2000; **35**: 1323–30.

58 Nabel EG, Yang ZY, Plautz G et al. Recombinant fibroblast growth factor-1 promotes intimal hyperplasia and angiogenesis in arteries in vivo. *Nature* 1993; **362**: 844–6.

59 Edelman ER, Nugent MA, Smith LT, Karnovsky MJ. Basic fibroblast growth factor enhances the coupling of intimal hyperplasia and proliferation of vasa vasorum in injured rat arteries. *J Clin Invest* 1992; **89**: 465–73.

60 Lazarous DF, Shou M, Scheinowitz M et al. Comparative effects of basic fibroblast growth factor and vascular endothelial growth factor on coronary collateral development and the arterial response to injury. *Circulation* 1996; **94**: 1074–82.

61 Horowitz JR, Rivard A, van der Zee R et al. Vascular endothelial growth factor/vascular permeability factor produces nitric oxide-dependent hypotension. Evidence for a maintenance role in quiescent adult endothelium. *Arterioscler Thromb Vasc Biol* 1997; **17**: 2793–800.

62 Ku DD, Zaleski JK, Liu S, Brock TA. Vascular endothelial growth factor induces EDRF-dependent relaxation in coronary arteries. *Am J Physiol* 1993; **265**: H586–92.

63 Wu HM, Yuan Y, McCarthy M, Granger HJ. Acidic and basic FGFs dilate arterioles of skeletal muscle through a NO-dependent mechanism. *Am J Physiol* 1996; **271**: H10897–93.

64 Kozarsky KF, McKinly DR, Austin LL et al. In vivo correction of low density lipoprotein receptor deficiency in the Watanabe heritable hyperlipidaemic rabbit with recombinant adenoviruses. *J Biol Chem* 1994; **29**: 13695–703.

65 Pakkanen T, Laitinen M, Hippelainen M et al. Enhanced plasma cholesterol lowering effect of retrovirus-mediated LDL receptor gene transfer to WHHL rabbit liver after improved surgical technique and stimulation of hepatocyte proliferation by combined partial liver resection and thymidine kinase–ganciclovir treatment. *Gen Ther* 1999; **6**: 34–41.

66 Grossman M, Rader DJ, Muller DW et al. A pilot study of ex vivo gene therapy for homozygous familial hypercholesterolaemia. *Nature Med* 1995; **1**: 1148–54.

67 Rader DJ. Gene therapy for atherosclerosis. *Int J Clin Lab Res* 1997; **27**: 37–43.

68 Kullo IJ, Simari RD, Schwartz RS. Vascular gene transfer from bench to bedside. *Arterioscler Thromb Vasc Viol* 1999; **19**: 196–207.

69 George SJ, Johnson JL, Angelini GD et al. Adenovirus-mediated gene transfer of human TIMP-1 gene inhibits smooth muscle cell migration and neointimal formation in human saphenous vein. *Hum Gene Ther* 1998; **9**: 867–77.

70 Shah AS, Lilly RE, Kypson AP et al. Intracoronary adenovirus-mediated delivery and overexpression of the beta (2)-adrenergic receptor in the heart: prospects for molecular ventricular assistance. *Circulation* 2000; **101**: 408–14.

71 White DC, Hata JA, Shah AS et al. Preservation of myocardial beta-adrenergic receptor signaling delays the development of heart failure after myocardial infarction. *Proc Natl Acad Sci USA* 2000; **97**: 5428–33.

57

Management of lipid disorders and other risk factors in patients with peripheral vascular disease

Deborah Levy and Thomas Pearson

Introduction

Atherosclerosis is a systemic disease. Peripheral vascular disease (PVD) is indicative of severe atherosclerosis in all vascular beds. The mortality associated with vascular disease results from coronary heart disease, as patients with PVD are three times more likely to die from cardiovascular causes.[1,2] This has led recent guidelines to consider PVD equivalent to coronary heart disease (CHD) because of equally great risk for subsequent myocardial infarction and CHD death.[3] The benefits of comprehensive risk factor reduction, including aggressive lipid management, have been demonstrated to reduce CHD mortality.[4] A risk factor reduction treatment plan for PVD will in turn reduce the risk of CHD.[5,6] Moreover, in several recent studies, subgroup analyses also revealed improvements in PVD outcomes, using similar risk factor modifications. Therefore, PVD patients should now be treated with the aggressiveness equal to those patients with established coronary disease. Indeed, efforts to identify asymptomatic PVD through screening with ankle–brachial blood pressure index (ABI) and other measures have as their rationale the identification of patients at high risk for CHD who would benefit from aggressive risk factor management.[7]

As with CHD, risk factor modification is part of optimal care of PVD patients.[8] This chapter reviews risk factor assessment and management of PVD patients. An approach to risk factor assessment for all PVD patients is described. This chapter lists comprehensive risk factor interventions recommended for PVD patients. The primary focus is management of lipid disorders, with attention to smoking, obesity, and exercise. A more comprehensive discussion of hypertension and diabetes can be found elsewhere in the book.

PVD as a coronary risk equivalent

Guidelines for risk factor modification including Prevention V[7] and ATP III[3] (Adult Treatment Panel III of the National Cholesterol Education Program), have established clinical PVD as a coronary heart disease *risk equivalent*. The following signs and symptoms are considered CHD risk equivalents:[3] femoral or carotid bruits on physical examination; symptomatic carotid disease, including transient ischemic attacks; symptoms of intermittent claudication; and/or decreased ABI < 0.9. Signs and symptoms of abdominal aortic aneurysm are also a CHD risk equivalent. Table 57.1 shows a comparison of annual risk and relative risk of death for PVD patients compared to persons without PVD. The absolute risk for death is consistently greater than 2% per year, the level of risk for myocardial infarction and CHD death defining a 'CHD risk equivalent.'

Comprehensive risk factor assessment in the patient with PVD

Clinical trials such as the Framingham Study have established that there is an epidemiological backing for cardiovascular risk factors. These risk factors include smoking, lipid disorders, diabetes, and hypertension, although smoking and diabetes are considered more closely correlated with peripheral vascular disease.

Initial risk factor screening will include establishing the patient's lifestyle traits (tobacco use, diet, physical activity), a full fasting lipid profile, a fasting glucose level, body mass index

Table 57.1 Annual risk and relative risk of death for persons with peripheral vascular disease (PVD) compared to persons without PVD. (Adapted with permission from Ref. 38)

Study	Ages	No. of subjects	Annual risk of death from all causes for PVD patients (percent per year)	Relative risk of death from all causes compared to patients without PVD (95% CI)[a]
Criqui et al.[31]	38–82	256 male 309 female	6.2 3.3	3.3 (1.9–6.0) 2.5 (1.2–5.3)
Vogt et al.[32]	≥65	1492 female	5.4	3.1 (1.7–5.5)
Leng et al.[33]	55–74	1592 (male and female)	3.8[b] 6.1[c]	1.6 (0.9–2.8)[b] 2.4 (1.6–3.7)[c]
Newman et al.[34]	≥65	5714 (male and female)	7.8	1.5 (1.2–1.9)
Newman et al.[35]	≥60	669 male 868 female	5.3 3.8	3.0 (2.8–5.3) 2.7 (1.6–4.6)
Kornitzer et al.[36]	40–55	2023 male	1.0	2.8 (1.4–5.5)

[a]CI = Confidence interval.
[b] = Patients with peripheral arterial disease with claudication.
[c] = Patients with peripheral arterial disease without symptoms.

Table 57.2 Risk factors for peripheral vascular disease (PVD) goals and assessment recommendations. (From Ref. 9)

Risk factor	Goal	Assessment techniques
Smoking	Complete cessation	Assess tobacco use, quantity and duration, including second-hand smoke at every visit
Blood pressure (BP) control	< 140/90 mm Hg or < 130/85 mm Hg (if heart failure or renal insufficiency) < 130/80 if diabetes	Measure BP at every visit. Consider ankle–brachial index (ABI) at baseline and at regular intervals
Lipid management – primary focus on low-density lipoprotein cholesterol (LDL-C)	LDL-C < 100 mg/dl	Check fasting lipid profile in all patients. Subsequent assessment based upon initial results
Lipid management – secondary focus on triglycerides (TG) and non-HDL cholesterol[a]	If TG ≥ 200, then non-HDL cholesterol should be < 130 mg/dl	Check fasting lipid profile in all patients. Subsequent assessment based upon initial results
Physical activity	Minimum goal: 30 min 3–4 days per week	Identify baseline level of activity, including frequency, type, and duration. Assess risk, preferably with exercise ECG, to guide activity prescription
Weight management	Body mass index (BMI) 21–25 kg/m^2	Measure weight and waist circumference, calculate BMI at every visit
Diabetes management	Normal fasting plasma glucose (<110 mg/dl) and near normal hemoglobin HbA$_{1c}$ (< 7)	Measure patient's blood glucose and nutritional intake. Measure HbA$_{1c}$ every 3 months if glucose > 110 mg/dl

[a]Non-HDL cholesterol = total cholesterol – high-density lipoprotein cholesterol (HDL-C).

(BMI) calculation, and blood pressure measurement. Goals for these risk factors are established (see Table 57.2).[9] Patients above the upper limits of normal require risk factor reduction. Thresholds and goals for risk factor modification in PVD are the same as those for CHD and equally aggressive treatment is required.

All smokers must be asked about their tobacco use at every visit and counseled on their smoking habits. Duration of use, as well as quantity should be recorded. Exposure to tobacco smoke in the work or home environment should also be determined. Some experts believe that the risk of PVD does not normalize after cessation of use. Addressing a patient's smoking status will enable smoking cessation recommendations tailored to that patient. Smoking cessation counseling is imperative to any comprehensive risk factor reduction plan, and will be discussed further in a subsequent section.

A screening brachial blood pressure, recorded separately from the ABI, will identify hypertensive patients. Antihypertensive therapy appropriate to the patient can be instituted, according to JNC-7 guidelines.[10]

A fasting lipid profile should include total cholesterol, high-density lipoprotein cholesterol (HDL-C), triglycerides, and calculated low-density lipoprotein cholesterol (LDL-C).[3] Goal lipid levels include total cholesterol < 200 mg/dl, LDL-C < 100 mg/dl, HDL-C > 40 mg/dl, and triglycerides < 150 mg/dl. Patients above these thresholds need to be evaluated for both dietary modifications and/or pharmacotherapy. Assessment should include the ruling out of secondary causes of lipid disorders such as hypothyroidism, obstructive liver disease, nephrotic syndrome, and uncontrolled diabetes.

A fasting serum glucose level above 126 mg/dl suggests diabetes. A second fasting serum glucose in this range constitutes a diagnosis of diabetes mellitus. Fasting glucose levels of 110–125 mg/dl indicate impaired glucose tolerance with the associated increased vascular risk.[11] Diabetic management will be addressed in another chapter of this book.

The level of physical activity or inactivity should be assessed initially. History should include type of exercise, duration of episodes of exercise, and the frequency with which these episodes occur. Patients may report a lower exercise tolerance, secondary to deconditioning or due to lower extremity pain.[7] Criqui noted that '... Less than half the patients with true [peripheral arterial disease] have possible or classic claudication ...'[12] Patients may also describe 'working through' claudication pain, or may be completely asymptomatic.[11] Recommendations regarding physical activity will follow, but generally include ≥ 30 min of moderate-intensity aerobic exercise at least 3 times weekly, preferably daily.

A baseline BMI and waist circumference measurement should be performed. A BMI between 18.5 and 24.9 incurs no additional vascular risk. A moderately increased vascular risk is associated with a BMI between 25.0 and 30. Very high risk patients have BMIs ≥25.0 and an increased waist circumference (at the level of the iliac crests; > 40 inches in men and > 35 inches in women) or between a BMI 30.0 and 39.9, with extremely high-risk status reserved for patients with BMIs greater than 40.0.[8]

A family history of CHD or PVD is a non-modifiable risk factor. A significant family history of premature cardiovascular disease exists in patients with known myocardial infarction or sudden death in a first-degree male relative who was younger than 55 or a female younger than 65.[7]

At the completion of the initial evaluation, those patients who remain at risk for PVD and its sequelae are those patients with positive risk factors; patients who smoke, have lipid disorders, are diabetic or have impaired glucose tolerance, have hypertension, are obese (BMI > 25.0) or have poor exercise capabilities or habits which warrant intensive risk factor modification. Complete risk factor evaluation enables the development of a comprehensive treatment plan, which is discussed in the next several sections.

Evidence for lipid modification to reduce morbidity and mortality in PVD patients

Numerous randomized control trials (RCTs) have recently been evaluated to assess the effects of lipid-lowering therapy in patients with lower limb atherosclerosis; they were reviewed by Leng et al.[2] in a recent meta-analysis. Table 57.3 identifies major trials of lipid-lowering pharmacotherapy in patients with peripheral vascular disease. Lipid lowering produced a marked reduction in mortality (odds ratio 0.21), but had little effect in non-fatal events. In 2 of 7 trials there was a significant overall reduction in disease progression by angiogram, although there were inconsistent changes in ABI and walking distance despite a general improvement in symptoms.

ABI improved 28.3% in the treatment group in the CORSI trial,[15] a significant improvement; however, some trials showed no improvement in ABI. Leng et al.[2] noted that of the trials that showed no change in ABI, a significant decrease in cholesterol was not achieved. Overall, the authors felt that lipid-lowering therapy may be useful in preventing deterioration of underlying disease and alleviating symptoms.

The KAPS study (Kuopio Atherosclerosis Prevention study) was an RCT focused on mostly male patients with a mean age of 57 with heterozygous familial hypercholesterolemia and known plaques in carotid and/or femoral arteries.[16] Patients in this study were treated with diet plus placebo or pravastatin (40 mg daily). One arm of the follow-up included serial high-resolution B-mode ultrasound measurements of intimal medial thickness (IMT) of carotid and femoral trees, over a 3-year period. Outcomes revealed a reduced rate of overall and annual progression of IMT of carotid arteries,

Table 57.3 Randomized controlled trials of lipid-lowering in peripheral vascular disease

| Trial | Demographics | | | Cardiovascular history | | | Outcomes measured | Results |
	Sex, M : F	Age	No	Coronary artery disease	Peripheral vascular disease			
St Thomas[37]	Both	<65	24	Hyper-lipidemia	Femoro-popliteal disease		Angiography	Total cholesterol lower in treatment group than control group
Lipid-lowering in limb atherosclerosis, Leng et al.[2] (a meta-analysis)	Both		698		Lower limb athero-sclerosis		Mortality, non-fatal events, direct tests of disease progression, indirect and direct measures of disease progression	Lipid-lowering treatment may be useful in prevention of underlying disease and alleviating symptoms
PQRST[18]		<71	303		Yes		To determine if probucol and diet, with cholestyramine will decrease or induce regression of femoral atherosclerosis in hypercholesterolemia	Regression not obtained by drug
POSCH[30]	Both	30–64	838	Carotid (survivors of single myocardial infarction)	Femoral		To ascertain whether the effective reduction of plasma total cholesterol and low-density lipoprotein cholesterol (LDL-C) levels and the increase of high-density lipoprotein cholesterol (HDL-C) induced by partial ileal bypass had a favorable impact on overall mortality and morbidity attributable to atherosclerotic coronary heart disease (ACHD)	At 5 years, statistical significance was obtained for differences in overall mortality and mortality from ACHD. There were no significant differences between the groups for cerebrovascular events, mortality from non-ACHD, and cancer
KAPS[16]	Men	44–65		Carotid	Femoral		A randomized, double-blind, trial to evaluate the effect of pravastatin on the arterial wall of carotid and femoral arteries as evaluated by B-mode ultrasound	Serum cholesterol was lowered in the pravastatin group, but not in the placebo group. There was differential progression in arterial deterioration between the pravastatin group and the control group, with that of the pravastatin group being lower and more constant. The control group showed increasing progression of arterial deterioration.

Table 57.3 (Continued)					
Trial	Demographics			Cardiovascular history	
	Sex, M : F	Age	No	Coronary artery disease	Peripheral vascular disease
CLAS[21]	Both	40–59	188	Coronary artery bypass graft in previous 3 months	PVD on angiogram

Outcomes measured	Results
Treatment intervention was colestipol, niacin, and diet vs placebo and diet. Mortality, non-fatal events, angiography, side effects	An overall regression of PVD (observed on repeat angiogram at 2 years) was attained in the colestipol (16%) versus placebo (4%) groups: no change was seen in 45% versus 37%, respectively; and a progression of PVD by angiogram was observed in 39% versus 59%, respectively. In contrast, the changes in lipid levels during the trial period were more significant: LDL–C levels (43% decrease on colestipol, 5% decrease on placebo); HDL levels (37% increase on colestipol, 5% decrease on placebo); HDL levels 37% increase on colestipol versus a 2% increase without the intervention; Triglycerides decreased 21% on colestipol versus 5% on placebo

although not of femoral arteries. Results indicated a significant improvement in the carotid plus femoral score in those who received lipid-lowering therapy instead of placebo.

The PQRST (Probucol Quantitative Swedish Regression Trial) examined dietary therapy in combination with pharmacotherapy in patients with and without symptoms of PVD.[17,18] Patients with diabetes or type III hyperlipidemias were excluded. Participants were randomized to either diet, diet plus cholestyramine (as relative placebo group), or cholestyramine plus probucol. Starting cholesterol levels of participants were approximately 350 mg/dl, reduced to approx 270 mg/dl over the 3-year trial duration. Probucol was ineffective when added to cholestyramine and diet in reducing indices of femoral artery atherosclerosis. Some critics suggest that the relative fall in HDL levels with probucol's addition to the therapy protocol, over diet plus cholestyramine, may have contributed to the lack of significant improvement in the treatment arm.[17,18]

In the Edinburgh Artery study, risk factors for PAD and CHD were compared in 1592 males and females aged 55–74.[19] Questionnaires were employed for regarding CHD risks: low HDL, high triglycerides and total cholesterol, diabetes, elevated systolic blood pressure, and smoking. A stronger association was discovered between smoking and PVD than any other risk factor, especially in the case of abdominal aortic aneurysms (AAA). Smoking was found to be the most significant risk factor for development of AAA. 'Claudicants' per questionnaire had a significantly increased risk of developing anginal symptoms. Furthermore, symptomatic patients with an ABI < 0.9 had similar incidence of cardiovascular events and death, compared with the symptomatic group.[5]

The 4S study, with later subgroup analyses, established that secondary prevention in patients with known CAD using an HMG-CoA (3-hydroxy-3-methylglutaryl coenzyme A) reductase inhibitor, simvastatin, was related to a statistically significant decrease in new or worsening IC symptoms from 3.6% to 2.3% in the simvastatin arm only, after 3 years.[20] The subpopulation in the 4S trial was expanded from diabetics to include all glucose-intolerant patients, as well. This subgroup showed a steady reduction of total and cardiovascular mortality with simvastatin.[20] The CLAS (Cholesterol Lowering Atherosclerosis Study) was an RCT that focused on 162 men, aged 40–59 years, who were status post-CABG (coronary artery bypass graft) and either non-smokers or ex-smokers for at least 6 months.[21] Participants were randomized to either diet plus placebo (n = 82) or colestipol and niacin (n = 80) for a period of 2 years. Outcomes included the progression of femoral atherosclerosis, assessed through angiographic segmental measurement and annual progression rate of computer-estimated atherosclerosis. The study established less progression of femoral segment atherosclerosis in the drug-treated arm of the study, by computer estimate and on segmental analysis. However, the difference from placebo was less than that seen in native and bypass coronary grafts.

Management of lipid disorders

The management of lipid disorders is an important component of a comprehensive risk factor reduction program. The short- and long-term benefits of lipid management in vascular disease have been well documented. Thresholds and goals have been set down by the NCEP – ATPIII,[3] and are outlined in Table 57.2. Goal lipid levels include total cholesterol < 200 mg/dl and LDL-C < 100 mg/dl. A secondary goal after attaining an LDL cholesterol level of < 100 mg/dl is, if the triglyceride level is > 200 mg/dl, a non-HDL-C of < 130 mg/dl. Triglyceride levels of > 150 mg/dl and HDL-C < 40 mg/dl might also be targets for therapy.

Thresholds for lipid lowering and goals of therapy

Once the full-fasting lipid profile has been completed, as part of PVD risk factor screening, tailored lipid-lowering pharmacotherapy can be initiated. Non-diabetic patients with LDL-C less than 100 mg/dl, HDL-C greater than 40 mg/dl, and triglycerides less than 150 mg/dl do not require lipid profile modification. All other patients should have this risk factor addressed.[3,4]

Patients with LDL-C levels greater than 100 mg/dl should be considered for lifestyle modification therapy, termed therapeutic lifestyle change (TLC).[3] Non-pharmacologic steps in risk factor reduction remain important. It may be appropriate to attempt a trial of dietary therapy in some patients with LDL-C levels between 100 and 130 mg/dl, with reassessment of lipid profiles after a trial period, though recent trials of statins suggested these patients do benefit from LDL-C reduction.[22]

Non-pharmacologic approaches to lipid lowering, including dietary modifications

The TLCs include modifications of diet, exercise, and body mass.

Daily recommendations of dietary therapy for elevated LDL-C are as follows:[3]

- ≤ 25–35% of total calories from fats
- < 200 mg/day of cholesterol
- ≤ 7% of total calories from saturated fats
- ≥ 50–60% of calories from carbohydrates
- approximately 15% of total calories from protein daily
- reduction in total calories to achieve desirable individual weight.

In addition to traditional dietary therapy, certain supplements may further lower serum lipid levels. These dietary additions include maintaining a high-fiber diet, adding viscous dietary fiber (10–25 g/day) and the use of stanols or sterol ester margarines (2 g/day).[22,23] A lowering of LDL cholesterol of 10–15% or more can be routinely achieved with the TLC approach.

A reduction in total calories plus an increase in exercise should allow the attainment of a desirable body weight. This is critically important for the management of the metabolic syndrome of high triglycerides and low HDL cholesterol levels.

Registered dieticians will benefit patients who find the above dietary recommendations difficult to implement on their own. Some registered dieticians work as part of organized lipid clinics or cardiovascular rehabilitation programs.

Lipid-lowering pharmacotherapy

If the TLC approach is unable to reach the goal of LDL-C < 100 mg/dl, pharmacotherapy agents can be considered. In general, if the LDL-C level is < 130 mg/dl at baseline, drug therapy can be initiated concurrently with the TLC approach.

Pharmacotherapy should address LDL-C levels first, with a goal LDL-C determined according to cardiovascular risk. A stepwise approach to pharmacotherapy is outlined in Figure 57.1. First-line therapy includes statins, bile acid sequestrants, or niacin. If the LDL-C goal has not been achieved after 6 weeks of well-tolerated therapy, the statin dose can be increased or a bile acid sequestrant or niacin can be initiated in combination therapy. Twelve weeks after initiating therapy, an LDL-C which remains elevated warrants referral to a lipid specialist. If the LDL-C goal is reached at any point, secondary goals of non-HDL cholesterol can be addressed if the triglyceride level is > 200 mg/dl. After achieving multiple lipid therapy goals, a fasting lipid profile should be re-checked every 4–6 months. Other laboratory tests should be monitored according to the pharmacologic agents being used to treat the dyslipidemia.

In the setting of an elevated LDL-C, if the triglycerides are less than 200 mg/dl, an HMG CoA reductase inhibitor, niacin, or a bile acid binding resin may be appropriate. If the triglycerides are between 200 and 400 mg/dl, an HMG CoA reductase inhibitor or niacin may appropriate. Finally, if the triglycerides are above 400 mg/dl, consider niacin, a fibrate, or an HMG CoA reductase inhibitor (Tables 57.4 and 57.5)

Close monitoring of the efficacy of lipid-lowering therapy is necessary to ensure that treatment goals are achieved. Studies in clinical settings suggest that the majority of patients are not optimally managed on their lipid-lowering therapies due to various factors, including patient non-compliance and lack of maximization of medical therapy. Hence, the benefits of lipid-lowering are often not attained.[24,25]

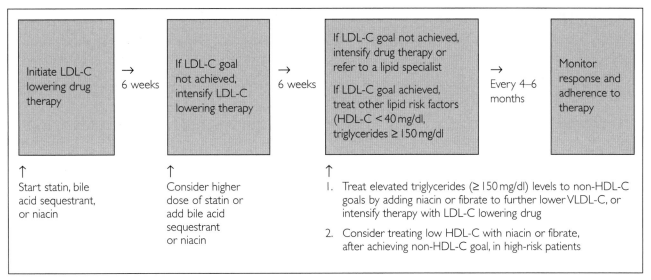

Figure 57.1
Procedure for implementing drug therapy to treat lipid abnormalities. (Adapted with permission from Ref. 3)

Table 57.4   Choices of lipid-lowering drugs for different lipid profile results

Lipid profiles			Lipid-lowering agents			
High LDL	Low HDL	High Triglycerides	Statins[a]	Niacin	Bile acid binders[b]	Fibrates
+	−	−	1	2	1	*
+	+	−	1	2	3	*
+	+	+	1	1	*	2
−	+	+	2	1	*	1
−	+	+	2	1	*	1
−	+	−	2	1	*	2

[a]Statins = HmG CoA reductase inhibitors.
[b]Bile acid binders = cholestyramine, colestipol.

Lipid profiles:
+ = pharmacotherapy indicated: low-density lipoprotein (LDL) > 100 mg/dl, high-density lipoprotein (HDL) < 35 mg/dl, triglycerides (Trigs) > 200 mg/dl
− = no pharmacotherapy indicated

Lipid-lowering agents:
1 = Agent of choice, best supporting evidence
2 = good indication, if #1 contraindicated or in combination therapy
3 = Indicated in some cases, or in combination therapy
* = no indication or contraindication

Comprehensive risk factor reduction

Lipid management is one component of a comprehensive risk factor reduction plan, which should also include smoking cessation, exercise, dietary modifications, and glycemic control in diabetics and those with impaired glucose tolerance. There are significant advantages to risk factor modification for PVD, in terms of reducing cardiovascular mortality and total mortality. Organized programs for cardiovascular rehabilitation, lipid management, and nutrition provide comprehensive diet, lifestyle, and exercise modification options in one setting.

Smoking cessation

A strong correlation exists between smoking and the development of PVD, more than any other single risk factor.[22] It is imperative that patients and their families be

Table 57.5 Lipid-lowering medication list. (Adapted from Ref. 26 with permission)

Medication	Standard dose	Lipid/lipoprotein effects	Initiation of treatment and contraindications	Side effects management and monitoring
HMG CoA reductase inhibitors				
Atorvastatin (Lipitor)	10–80 mg qd	LDL-C ↓ 18–55%	Start with 1 tablet of starting dose after p.m. meal, increase every 6 weeks	Abnormal LFTs – reduce dosage if > 2 times normal
Fluvastatin (Lescol, Lescol XT)	20–80 mg qhs	HDL-C ↑ 5–15%		Myopathy/myalgias – stop drug
Lovastatin (Mevacor, generic)	20–80 mg qhs	TG ↓ 7–30%	Do not use in patients with liver disease or concomitantly with cyclosporin, macrolide antibiotics, various antifungal agents, or P450 inhibitors. Concomitant use with fibrates or niacin increases risk of myopathy	Check fasting lipid profile, LFTs every 6 weeks until goal reached, then every 6 months
Pravastatin (Pravachol)	20, 40, 80 mg qhs			
Simvastatin (Zocor)	10, 20, 40, 80 mg qhs			
Niacin				
Niacin extended-release (Niaspan)	500 mg to 2 g qhs	LDL-C ↓ 5–25% HDL-C ↑ 15–35% TG ↓ 20–50%	Week 1–4: 500 mg qhs Week 5–8: 1000 mg qhs (2 × 500 mg) After week 8: titrate to patient response and tolerance, if necessary to maximum dose of 2 g qhs	Flushing – 1 aspirin 30 min prior to dose. Avoid taking with hot beverage, or on empty stomach. Nausea – take with meals
Niacin (generic, crystalline)	100 mg to 1 g qhs		Begin 100 mg tid and increase 100 mg tid/week to 500 mg tid. Check LFTs, glucose, and uric acid. If normal, proceed to 1 g tid, if necessary	Glucose intolerance – reduce dose. Gout – reduce dose. LFTs – reduced dose if > 2 times normal
Niacin dietary supplement (slow release)	250–500 mg qhs		Do not exceed 500 mg qhs	Check fasting lipid profile every 6 weeks until goal reached. Check glucose, AST, uric acid every 6 weeks until stable dose of drug, then every 6 months
			Do *not* use in patients with peptic ulcers, gout, liver disease, or diabetics with poor glycemic control. Relative contraindication: diabetes, hyperuricemia	
Combination therapy				
Niacin ER/lovastatin (Advicor)	500 mg/20 mg qhs to 2000 mg/40 mg qhs	LDL-C ↓ 30–55% HDL-C ↑ 20–35% TG ↓ 30–55%	For use when want to start Niaspan therapy in a patient already on lovastatin, and can switch to an equivalent dose of Advicor	See niacin and statin side effects management and monitoring
			Maintain at doses not to exceed 2000 mg/40 mg	
			See Niaspan and lovastatin contraindications	

Table 57.5 (Continued)

Medication	Standard dose	Lipid/lipoprotein effects	Initiation of treatment and contraindications	Side effects management and monitoring
Fibrates				
Fenofibrate (Tricor)	54–160 mg qd	LDL-C ↓ 5–20%	Do not use in patients with renal or hepatocellular diseases or with cholelithiasis	Nausea – Take with meals
Gemfibrozil (Lopid & generic	600 mg bid (generic or brand)	HDL-C ↑ 10–20%		Skin rash – stop drug
		TG ↓ 29–50%		Myositis – stop drug
				Fasting lipid profile every 6 weeks until goal reached
Bile acid sequestrants				
Cholestelam (Welchol)	3 tabs (625 mg) bid or 6 tabs (625 mg) qd	LDL-C ↓ 15–30% HDL-C ↑ 3–5%	Take with meals	Taste/texture – mix with pulpy juices or yogurt
				Bloating – reduce number of scoops per dose
Cholestyramine (Questran, Questran-lite)	2 scoops bid or tid of bulk form	TG or ↑	Begin with 1 scoop in a.m. 30 min before meal, increase to bid, then to 2 scoops bid	Heartburn – Let stand in liquid 10 min
				Constipation – fluids, fiber, stool softeners
Colestipol (Colestid)	4 colestipol tablets = 1 scoop or packet of powder			Drug interaction – take drugs 1 hour before or 4 hours after
			Do not use in patients with severe constipation, hypertriglyceridemia (TG > 400) or in type III hyperlipidemia	Fasting lipid profile every 6 weeks until goal reached
Ezetimibe				
Ezetimibe (Zetia)	10mg	LDL-C ↓ HDL-C ↑ 2% TG ↓ 12%	For use when single or double-agent therapy not sufficient to attain lipid goals, or if hepatotoxicity with other agents is a limiting factor. Often used in combination with a statin[39]	No specific tests needed, although often used with other agents. Check fasting lipid profile every 6 weeks until goal reached.

HDL-C = high-density lipoprotein cholesterol, LDL-C = low-density lipoprotein cholesterol, TG = triglycerides, qhs = at bedtime, qd = once daily, bid = twice daily, tid = three times daily, LTF = liver function tests (AST, ALT).

urged to stop smoking.[9,28] Patients can be provided with options for nicotine replacement, medical adjuncts to smoking cessation – including Wellbutrin (bupropion hydrochloride) – and referrals for counseling and formal smoking cessation programs. Physician smoking cessation counseling, even in 5–10 min sessions, has a major impact on the success rates of patients' smoking cessation attempts. A reliable method for counseling patients on smoking cessation is the ASK, ADVISE, ASSESS, ASSIST, and ARRANGE strategy.[28]

Exercise recommendations

Encourage all patients to develop a program including moderate intensity aerobic exercise, of at least 30 min duration, 3–4 times per week (preferably daily). Increased physical activity can be encouraged in activities of daily living, including walking at work and walking up stairs. In some patients, exercise will be accompanied by claudication pain. In this population, a supervised program will have further benefits in quantifying the improvements in duration and intensity regarding exercise tolerance. Long-term goals can be set based on with the patient's baseline exercise tolerance prior to the initiation of therapy.

In a review by Beard, after 6 months, significantly more favorable outcomes were observed in patients on an exercise than those who had undergone interventional procedures.[29]

[A] recent meta-analysis of 21 supervised exercise programs showed that training for at least 6 months, by walking to near maximum pain tolerance, significantly improved pain free and maximum walking distances … exercise was better [than percutaneous intraluminal angioplasty or surgery].[1]

Some sources feel that the maximum beneficial effect occurs with 5–6 hours of exercise per week.

In patients with suspected coronary disease, either an exercise test with electrocardiogram (ECG), exercise echocardiography, or exercise thallium scan is recommended prior to initiation of a rigorous exercise program. In patients limited by claudication, Persantine (dipyridamole) thallium scans or other provocative tests may be useful.

For patients with concomitant known coronary disease, and those with moderate to severe PVD, medically supervised exercise programs are recommended.[3] The exercise test can be used to prescribe levels of exercise.

Risk factor modification – initiation and compliance

Risk factor modification is part of the optimal care of all PVD patients. Although this is well recognized, the initiation of risk factor modification is often delayed until after acute interventions, when the patient returns to the outpatient setting. As with acute myocardial infarction, risk factor modification should be initiated when other treatment has begun. Many patients benefit from an organized setting in which full cardiovascular rehabilitation is addressed. Program types include cardiac rehabilitation programs, preventive cardiology clinics, and nurse care manager programs among others. Noncompliance presents a serious problem and the organized programs can be helpful.

Conclusions

Patients with PVD are at three times the risk of cardiovascular mortality than those without PVD.[1] There is a high prevalence of causal risk factors in this population, particularly those risk factors most closely associated with PVD such as smoking, lipid disorders, and diabetes. Patients diagnosed with PVD require a comprehensive risk factor assessment to provide guidelines for modification. Nutritional assessments are a component of risk factor modification, but many patients will still need lipid-lowering pharmacotherapy. There is ample evidence that lipid-lowering therapy decreases morbidity and mortality in PVD patients. Modification of lipid profiles is only one component of a comprehensive risk factor modification plan. Furthermore, risk factor modifying interventions should be initiated once the diagnosis of PVD is made. In cardiology, there is increasing evidence supporting lipid-lowering in the acute setting to decreases in the risk of plaque-ruptured thrombus. This can be extrapolated to PVD patients who need not wait weeks to months to benefit from lipid-lowering and other risk reduction therapy. PVD is common, and the most feared sequelae of PVD, namely myocardial infarction, sudden death, and stroke, are preventable by systemic risk factor modifications.

References

1 Beard JD. Chronic lower limb ischaemia. *BMJ* 2000; **320**: 854–7.

2 Leng GC, Price JF, Jepson RG. Lipid-lowering for lower limb atherosclerosis. *Cochrane Database of Systematic Reviews* [computer file]. (2):CD000123, 2000.

3 Expert Panel on Detection, Evaluation, and Treatment of High Blood Cholesterol in Adults. Executive Summary of the Third Report of the Executive Panel on Detection, Evaluation, and Treatment of High Blood Cholesterol (Adult Treatment Panel III). *JAMA* 2001; **285**: 2486–97.

4 AHA Guidelines for Primary Prevention of Cardiovascular Diseases and Stroke: 2002 Update: Consensus panel guide to comprehensive risk reduction for adult patients without coronary or other atherosclerotic vascular diseases. *Circulation* 2002; **106**: 388–91. The JNC 7 Report. *JAMA* 2003; **289**: 2560–72.

5 Campeau L, Hunninghake DB, Knatterud GL et al. Aggressive cholesterol lowering delays saphenous vein graft atherosclerosis in women, the elderly, and patients with associated risk factors. NHLBI post coronary artery bypass graft clinical trial. Post CABG Trial Investigators. *Circulation* 1999; **99**(25): 3241–7.

6 Hiatt WR. Drug therapy: medical treatment of peripheral arterial disease and claudication. *NEJM* 2001; **344**(21): 1608–21.

7 Greenland P, Abrams J, Aurigemma GP et al. Prevention Conference V: Beyond secondary prevention: Identifying the high-risk patient for primary prevention: noninvasive tests of atherosclerotic burden: Writing Group III. *Circulation (Online)* 2000; **101**(1): E16–22.

8 Fuster V, Pearson T (eds). 27th Bethesda conference: matching the intensity of risk factor management with the hazard for CAD events. *J Am Cardiol* 1996; **27**: 957–1047.

9 Smith SC, Blair SN, Bonow RO et al. AHA/ACC Guidelines for Preventing Heart Attack and Stroke in Patients with Atherosclerotic Cardiovascular Disease: 2002 Update. *Circulation* 2001; **104**: 1577–9.

10 The Seventh Report of the Joint National Committee on Prevention, Detection, Evaluation, and Treatment of High Blood Pressure. The JNC 7 Report. *JAMA* 2003; **289**: 2560–72.

11 Grundy SM, Benjamin IJ, Burke GJ et al. Diabetes and cardiovascular disease: A statement for health professionals for the American Heart Association. *Circulation* 1999; **100**: 1134–46.

12 Criqui MH. Peripheral arterial disease and subsequent cardiovascular mortality. A strong and consistent association. *Circulation* 1990; **82**(6): 2246–7.

13 Fowkes FGR, Housley E, Cawood EHH et al. Edinburgh Artery Study: Prevalence of asymptomatic and symptomatic peripheral arterial disease in the general population. *Int J Epidemiol* 1991; **20**: 384–92.

14 NHLBI Obesity Education Initiative Expert Panel. Clinical Guidelines on Education, Evaluation, and Treatment of Overweight and Obesity in Adults. *Obesity Res* 1998; 6(supplement): 515–2095.

15 Corsi C, Bocci L, Cipriani C et al. The effectiveness of glycosaminoglycans in peripheral vascular disease therapy: a clinical and experimental trial. *J Intern Med Res* 1985; **13**: 40–7.

16 Salonen R, Nyyssonen K, Porkkala E et al. Kuopio Atherosclerosis Prevention Study (KAPS). A population-based primary preventive trial of the effect of LDL lowering on atherosclerotic progression in carotid and femoral arteries. *Circulation* 1995; **92**(7): 1758–64.

17 Walldius G, Erikson U, Olsson AG et al. The effect of probucol on femoral atherosclerosis: the Probucol Quantitative Regression Swedish Trial (PQRST). *Am J Cardiol* 1994; **74**: 875–83.

18 Walldius G, Erikson U, Olsson AG et al. The effect of probucol on femoral atherosclerosis: A Probucol Quantitative Regression Swedish Trial (PQRST) Report. *Arterioscler Thromb Vasc Biol* 1995; **15**: 1049–56.

19 Duffield RGM, Lewis B, Miller NE et al. Treatment of hyperlipidaemia retards progression of symptomatic femoral atherosclerosis. *Lancet* 1983; **2**: 639–43.

20 Anonymous. Randomized trial of cholesterol lowering in 4444 patients with coronary heart disease: the Scandinavian Simvastatin Survival Study (4S). *Lancet* 1994; **344**: 1383–9.

21 Blankenhorn DH, Johnson RL, Nessim SA et al. The Cholesterol Lowering Atherosclerosis Study (CLAS): design, methods and baseline results. *Controlled Clinical Trials* 1987; **8**: 356–87.

22 Vuorio AF, Gylling H Turlola K et al. Stanol ester margarine alone and with simvastatin lowers serum cholesterol in families with familial hypercholesterolemia caused by the FH-North Karelia Mutation. *Aterio Thromb Vasc Biol* 2000; **20**: 500–6.

23 Law MR. Plant sterol and stanol margarines and health. *West J Med* 2000; **173**: 43–7.

24 Pearson TA, Laurora I, Chu H, Kafonek S. The Lipid Treatment Assessment Project (L-TAP): a multicenter survey to evaluate the percentages of dyslipidemic patients receiving lipid-lowering therapy and achieving low-density lipoprotein cholesterol goals. *Arch Inter Med* 2000; **160**: 459–67.

25 Pearson TA. Matching intensity of intervention with risk for coronary events: targets for LDL-C, HDL-C, and other risk factors. *Prevent Cardiol* 1999; **2**: 11–17.

26 Pearson TA. Bloch R et al. Strong preventive cardiology clinic lipid-lowering drug information sheet. *The Detection, Evaluation, & Management of High Blood Cholesterol in Adults: A Guide for Clinical Practice*. Guidelines for Cardiovascular risk reduction. *Primary Care* (special edition) 2000; **4**: 28.

27 Criqui MH. Peripheral arterial disease and subsequent cardiovascular mortality. A strong and consistent association. *Circulation* 1990; **82**(6): 2246–7.

28 Agency for Health Care Policy and Research. Treating Tobacco Use and Dependence. Public Health Services Report. US Department of Health and Human Services, June 2000.

29 Blankenhorn DH, Johnson RL, Nessim SA et al. The Cholesterol Lowering Atherosclerosis Study (CLAS): design, methods, and baseline results. *Control Clin Trials* 1987; **8**: 356–87.

30 Buchwald H, Boen JR, Nguyen PA et al. Plasma lipids and cardiovascular risk: a POSCH report. Program on the Surgical Control of the Hyperlipidemias. *Atherosclerosis* 2001; **154**(1): 221–7.

31 Criqui MH, Langer RD, Fronek A et al. Mortality over a period of 10 years in patients with peripheral arterial disease. *N Engl J Med* 1992; **326**: 381–6.

32 Vogt MT, Cauley JA, Newman AB et al. Decreased ankle/arm blood pressure index and mortality in elderly women. *JAMA* 1993; **270**: 465–9.

33 Leng GC, Lee AJ, Fowkes FG et al. Incidence, natural history and cardiovascular events in symptomatic and asymptomatic peripheral arterial disease in the general population. *Int J Epidemiol* 1996; **25**: 1172–81.

34 Newman AB, Shemanski L, Manolio TA et al. Ankle–arm index as a predictor of cardiovascular disease and mortality in the Cardiovascular Health Study. *Arterioscl Thromb Vasc Biol* 1999; **19**: 538–45.

35 Newman AB, Tyrrell KS, Kuller LH. Mortality over four years in SHEP participants with a low ankle–arm index. *J Am Geriatr Soc* 1997; **45**: 1472–8.

36 Kornitzer M, Dramaix M, Sobolski J et al. Ankle/arm pressure index in asymptomatic middle-aged males: an independent predictor of ten-year coronary heart disease mortality. *Angiology* 1995; **46**: 211–19.

37 Duffield RG, Lewis B, Miller NE et al. Treatment of hyperlipidaemia retards progression of symptomatic femoral atherosclerosis. A randomized controlled trial. *Lancet* 1983; **ii** 639–42.

38 Hiatt W. Drug therapy: Medical treatment of peripheral arterial disease and claudication. *NEJM* 2001; **344**(21): 1608–21.

39 Ballantyne CM, Houri J, Notarbartolo A, Ezetimibe Study Group. Effect of ezetimibe coadministered with atorvastatin in 628 patients with primary hypercholesterolemia: a prospective, randomized, double-blind trial. *Circulation* 2003; **107**: 2409–15.

58

Hemostasis and arterial 'closure' devices

William G Kussmaul III and Marc Cohen

Introduction

Hemostasis involves the interaction between three major components: circulating platelets, plasma coagulation proteins, and the vessel wall. The maintenance of blood fluidity under normal circumstances is dependent upon an intact and healthy endothelium. The response of all components to vascular injury – for example, the percutaneous arterial puncture used for percutaneous coronary and vascular interventions – is rapid and precise, working in a coordinated manner to stop bleeding and repair the vascular entry site. The relatively fragile platelet plug, initially formed in response to the vascular penetration, is anchored by the insoluble protein meshwork of fibrin, which stabilizes the thrombus and ultimately achieves stable hemostasis.[1]

Role of the endothelium in thrombosis

The only cellular surface within the body to which blood is normally exposed is the endothelial lining of the intimal surface of blood vessels. This endothelial lining possesses a remarkable resistance to thrombosis. In fact, the cascade of coagulation events is triggered only when blood comes into contact with any surface other than healthy endothelium. Dysfunctional endothelium, or non-endothelial surfaces such as components of damaged blood vessels, artificial surfaces, or extravascular tissues, can form the substrate for thrombosis. When the endothelial surface is damaged, circulating platelets adhere in a monolayer to the vessel wall. This platelet–vessel wall interaction, adhesion, is stimulated by the exposure of platelet-activating subendothelial components such as collagen. In addition, there is often loss of endothelial-derived thromboresistance provided by

prostacyclin and nitric oxide, which inhibit platelet activation, and promote vasodilatation. Adhesion of platelets is mediated primarily by the adhesive circulating macromolecule, von Willebrand's factor (vWF).[1]

Healthy vascular endothelium, therefore, plays a significant role in the maintenance of vascular homeostasis. Discoveries in the 1980s demonstrated that thrombin and aggregating platelets stimulate the release of endothelium-derived relaxing factor (nitric oxide), which dilates blood vessels, increases blood flow, inhibits platelet aggregation, and can thus help prevent the formation of occlusive thrombi.[2]

Role of procoagulant proteins in thrombosis

In vivo, coagulation is initiated by the exposure of tissue factor after endothelial damage. The exposure of tissue factor to circulating blood leads to the activation of factor X, which produces the prothrombinase complex. The prothrombinase complex, assembled on the surface of platelets, then catalyzes the conversion of prothrombin to thrombin. Thrombin, in turn, cleaves fibrinogen into fibrin. However, thrombin has another key role, as a direct and potent activator of platelets.[3]

Role of platelets in thrombosis

Activation and adhesion

Along with the coagulation and fibrinolytic systems, platelets participate in the maintenance and regulation of hemostasis. Platelets do not interact with normal endothelium, but readily adhere to damaged vascular tissue. When a vessel sustains a deep injury – for example, after rupture of an atherosclerotic plaque or vascular puncture – fibrillar collagen from the deeper vessel layers is exposed. This collagen, among other elements, activates the platelets and leads to the exposure of the surface platelet receptor, glycoprotein (GP) Ib, plus the subsequent binding to vWF. The platelets adhere to the subendothelium until a single layer of these cells has covered the damaged site. The platelet membrane receptor, GPIb, serves as the binding site for vWF at high shear rates and is essential for the initial contact of the platelets with the subendothelial surface. After platelets have adhered to the subendothelium, they spread over the surface of the injury. Once spread, the activated platelets recruit more platelets and form aggregates.

Platelet aggregation

When stimulated by exposure to damaged endothelium, platelets release the contents of their intracytoplasmic granules and produce thromboxane A_2 (TXA_2). The production and release of TXA_2 and adenosine diphosphate (ADP) leads to the recruitment of additional platelets and the formation of aggregates at the site of vessel wall damage. These platelet aggregates provide a surface for the localization and interaction of coagulation factors, enhancing the conversion of prothrombin to thrombin. Therefore, platelets and the coagulation system are intricately intertwined in the formation of a thrombus.[3,4] Recall that thrombin itself is a potent activator of platelet activation and aggregation.[5] Aggregation is mediated by the GPIIb/IIIa receptor.

The GPIIb/IIIa receptor is frequently referred to as the fibrinogen receptor. Agonist macromolecules convert platelets from a latent state to an activated state capable of binding soluble ligands. In the final process step, fibrinogen links adjacent platelets to one another and facilitates the process of aggregation. Specificity of the GPIIb/IIIa receptor is defined by two amino acid sequences in the fibrinogen molecule, which forms the 'molecular glue' for platelet aggregation. The arginine–glycine–aspartic acid sequence (RGD), is found in the extracellular adhesive macromolecules, fibrinonectin, vitronectin, vWF, and fibrinogen. The second sequence that binds fibrinogen to the GPIIb/IIIa receptor, lysine–glutamine–alanine–glycine–aspartic acid–valine, is present only on the fibrinogen macromolecule.[5]

Pharmacologic overview of the antithrombotic agents: impact on the coagulation cascade and platelet activation and aggregation

Before, during, and after percutaneous vascular interventions, all patients receive one or more drugs, usually several, that inhibit thrombosis. Therefore, each and every one of the antithrombotic agents used in vascular interventions can increase the likelihood of developing a bleeding or local vascular complication. The two complications that occur with some frequency (3–4%), which are exacerbated by antithrombotic therapy, are local hematoma, sometimes expanding into the retroperitoneal space, and/or arterial pseudoaneurysm.[6] Arteriovenous fistula may also be exacerbated by the use of antithrombotic therapy. However, the correlation between bleeding/local vascular complications and antithrombotic therapy is not a simple one. A major variable contributing to the risk of complications is the technique of the operator. It is very well established that 'too low' or 'too high', arterial punctures, away from the femoral head, will predispose the patient to bleeding complications irrespective of the antithrombotic therapy used during the vascular intervention. Furthermore, the risk of bleeding associated with a particular antithrombotic agent, such as the platelet receptor blocker abciximab, may be heavily confounded by the dose of intravenous heparin used. As demonstrated in the EPILOG trial, the risk of bleeding associated with abciximab and 'low dose' heparin was negligible compared with the significantly elevated risk of bleeding when heparin was used to achieve an activated clotting time (ACT) of > 300 s.[7]

Agents that inhibit the coagulation cascade

Heparin/low molecular-weight heparins

Molecules of heparin sulfate need to interact with circulating antithrombin III in order to provide an antithrombotic effect. Antithrombin III, synthesized in the liver, rapidly inhibits thrombin only in the presence of heparin.[8–10] The heparin/antithrombin III complex also inhibits activated factors IX, X, XI, XII, kallikrein, and plasmin. Clinical testing has established the value of intravenous unfractionated heparin in the prevention of periprocedural adverse thrombotic events occurring in the setting of PCIs. Based on a recent post-hoc analysis of six randomized trials, a target ACT > 350 s was identified as correlating with the fewest thrombotic events as well as the least risk of bleed.[11] The recent ESPRIT trial,[12] demonstrated that an ACT above 250 s, in the setting of a GPIIb/IIIa receptor blocker eptifibatide, was associated with a low rate of adverse events.

Low-molecular-weight heparins (LMWH) bind less avidly to plasma acute phase reactant proteins, have a higher bioavailability, and exert more durable and predictable therapeutic effects than unfractionated heparin. They are resistant to platelet factor IV and can inhibit factor Xa located on platelet surfaces. But not all LMWHs are the same. They differ in their molecular weights, and in their spectrum of anti-factor Xa:antithrombin activity. For example, dalteparin has a lower ratio of anti-factor Xa:antithrombin activity than enoxaparin.[13] LMWHs require less monitoring because they have a more predictable response, do not elevate the ACT very significantly, and carry a significantly lower risk of heparin-induced thrombocytopenia.[14]

The LMWHs have been evaluated for use in unstable coronary artery disease in several clinical trials. The FRISC (Fragmin During Instability in Coronary Artery Disease) study compared subcutaneous dalteparin with placebo,[15] and the FRIC (Fragmin in Unstable Coronary Artery Disease) study compared subcutaneously administered dalteparin with intravenous heparin.[16] Patients in all studies also received aspirin. Two large trials compared the LMWH enoxaparin versus unfractionated heparin; the ESSENCE (Efficacy and Safety of Subcutaneous Enoxaparin in Non Q-Wave Coronary Events) trial,[17] and the TIMI 11B study.[18] Both of these trials demonstrated superiority of enoxaparin to unfractionated heparin.[17–19] Based on these trials, the clinical application of the LMWHs in patients with acute coronary syndromes has increased dramatically. Since these drugs are long acting, with a sustained high level of anti-Xa activity, algorithms were developed for patients undergoing cardiac catheterization and PCI. Collet et al. treated patients coming to the catheterization laboratory within 8 hours of the last subcutaneous injection of LMWH, without administering any additional heparin, and observed no acute stent thrombosis and a bleeding rate of 1% heparin.[20] Recently, the NICE 3 registry was presented, also incorporating an 8-hour algorithm after subcutaneous injection of LMWH, and showed no significant increase in bleeding rate.[21]

Experience has accrued using LMWH enoxaparin as an intravenous bolus substituting for unfractionated heparin in the catheterization laboratory during PCI. Kereiakis et al.[22] showed that this substitution was not associated with any increase in bleeding even with the vascular sheaths being pulled after 4 hours.

Direct thrombin inhibitors

Thrombin plays a key role not only in coagulation but also in platelet aggregation. Some selective thrombin inhibitors of small molecular weight have been studied for their antiplatelet and antithrombotic activity and potential clinical use.[23]

Hirudin, a direct thrombin inhibitor isolated from the salivary glands of the medicinal leech, was compared with intravenous heparin in several studies, the GUSTO IIb (The Global Use of Strategies to Open Occluded Coronary Arteries) trial,[24] and the OASIS-2.[25] Neither of these studies resulted in widespread use of these agents in current clinical practice. However, both hirudin[26] and argatroban have been shown to be very useful in patients suffering from heparin-induced thrombocytopenia who are undergoing percutaneous vascular procedures.

Bivalirudin, a direct thrombin inhibitor, was used instead of heparin in order to assess the risk of ischemic or hemorrhagic complications in patients undergoing coronary angioplasty. The study concluded that bivalirudin was at least as effective as unfractionated heparin in preventing ischemic complications in patients who underwent angioplasty for unstable coronary syndromes, and was associated with a lower risk of bleeding and with significantly fewer bleeding complications.[27] Bivalirudin is now being evaluated, head to head, versus intravenous glycoprotein IIb/IIIa receptor blockers in low-risk PCI patients in the REPLACE trial.

Fibrinolytic agents

Whereas thrombolytic therapy has demonstrated benefits for patients with acute myocardial infarction, thrombolytic therapy is not recommended for patients without ST-segment elevation. Urokinase and tissue plasminogen activator (tPA) have been used to recanalize totally occluded venous bypass grafts in both the coronary circulation and in the peripheral circulation. These infusions are usually administered via indwelling catheters, which results in a higher than average risk of bleeding.

Agents that inhibit the action of platelets

Platelet deactivating agents

The orally active platelet inhibitor aspirin blocks the production of thromboxane by acetylating the enzyme cyclooxygenase. The action of aspirin on platelet cyclooxygenase is permanent (lasting the life of the platelet from 7 to 10 days), since platelets do not synthesize proteins. Therefore, repeated doses of aspirin produce a cumulative effect on platelet function. Barnathan et al.[28] was the first to show that preprocedural aspirin significantly reduced periprocedural ischemic events. Subsequently, another orally active platelet deactivating agent, ticlopidine, which blocks the effects of ADP as an agonist precipitating platelet aggregation, was found to have a synergistic benefit, when given along with aspirin in patients undergoing PCI with intravascular stents. However, an unacceptable side-effect profile, including a 1% incidence of severe neutropenia ($<0.45 \times 10^9$ cells/liter),[5,6] prompted interventional cardiologists to adopt clopidogrel. Clopidogrel was found to be as effective as ticlopidine in preventing stent thrombosis, but with fewer major side effects in the recently published CLASSICS trial.[29] Neither of these agents, which prevent platelet activation, is associated with a significant increase in the bleeding rate during percutaneous interventions above 1–2%.[5,6]

Intravenous platelet GPIIb/IIIa receptor blockers

Once platelets adhere at sites of mechanical vascular injury, they undergo activation and express functional GPIIb/IIIa receptors that bind to circulating adhesive ligand proteins, primarily fibrinogen. The fibrinogen molecule bridges between platelets, resulting in 'platelet aggregation.' The blockade of GPIIb/IIIa receptors, upon which platelet recruitment is dependent, became a viable therapeutic strategy for several logical reasons.[5,30]

Several important clinical trials have been conducted to evaluate the role of the GPIIb/IIIa inhibitors in the prevention of thrombotic complications expected after the 'controlled arterial injury' induced by vascular balloon angioplasty and stenting.[7,30–36]

Abciximab, a chimeric monoclonal antibody to the platelet IIb/IIIa receptor, has been shown to be effective in the prevention of platelet-mediated arterial thrombosis during PCI.[7,32,33] The EPIC trial established abciximab (ReoPro®) as the first GPIIb/IIIa receptor blocker to be beneficial in a large-scale trial.[32] The most important finding of the EPIC trial was the 35% reduction ($p = 0.008$) at 30 days in the frequency of the composite clinical end point (12.8% placebo vs 8.3% abciximab bolus and 12–hour infusion). This end point included death, nonfatal myocardial infarction, repeat revascularization – e.g. percutaneous transluminal coronary angioplasty (PTCA) or coronary artery bypass graft (CABG) and procedural failure requiring stent or intra-aortic balloon pump placement. However, the frequency of major bleeding complications in the bolus plus infusion group was double that of the placebo group (14% vs 7%; $p = 0.001$).[3] This prompted the EPILOG Trial.[7] This trial included 1500 patients and was designed to assess long-term outcome of treatment with abciximab with a lower dose of heparin during PTCA. The interim analysis of 2792 patients revealed a 56% reduction in the composite end point at 30 days (death, myocardial infarction, or urgent revascularization) in the abciximab plus low-dose heparin compared with placebo plus standard dose heparin (5.2% vs 11.7%; $p = 0.001$).

More importantly, this efficacy benefit was seen without any increase in the rate of major bleeding.[7] However, there remains a higher rate of thrombocytopenia with abciximab compared with placebo (5.6% vs 1.3%).[7,32,33]

Small molecule inhibitors of the platelet GPIIb/IIIa receptor, such as tirofiban and eptifibatide, with short half-lives (1.5–2.0 hours), and high affinity and specificity for the GPIIb/IIIa receptor, have also been evaluated in the setting of coronary intervention.[12,34–37] Eptifibatide, a synthetic cyclic heptapeptide, has been evaluated in the very large PURSUIT trial,[34] and in the catheterization laboratory-based ESPRIT[12] and IMPACT II trials.[35] In neither the ESPRIT[12] nor IMPACT II trials,[35] was there a significant excess in bleeding complications. Patients receiving eptifibatide in the earlier PURSUIT trial experienced a higher rate of major bleeding compared with those patients in the placebo group (10.6% vs 9.1%) and they also required more blood transfusions (11.6% vs 9.2%).[34]

Tirofiban, a non-peptide tyrosine derivative was evaluated in the catheterization laboratory-based RESTORE trial,[36] and in the PRISM-PLUS trials.[37] In the PRISM-PLUS trials 90% of patients underwent angiography and about 50% had coronary revascularization. In both of these trials, the rates of major bleeding were similar in all treatment groups.[36,37]

Antithrombotic therapy, with both oral and intravenous agents, has successfully reduced the rate of periprocedural thrombo-occlusive events in both high- and low-risk patients undergoing percutaneous vascular procedures. Identification of the optimal dose of unfractionated heparin, when used as an adjunct to the GPIIb/IIIa inhibitors, has allowed us to enjoy the benefits of these agents while minimizing the risk of vascular complications and bleeding.

Vascular closure devices

In 1995 VasoSeal (Datascope, Montvale, NJ, USA) became the first commercially available arterial hemostasis device. There are now four FDA-approved devices in use in the United States. Available devices have been reviewed extensively.[38]

The need for hemostasis devices arose from the observation that manual hemostasis can be uncomfortable, prolonged, and personnel-intensive. Bedrest for 4 to 8 hours afterwards inhibits early discharge from the hospital, a particular concern in the era of same-day/outpatient vascular procedures. Complications cause additional expense and discomfort.

Hemostasis devices have addressed some of these concerns, but not all. The most consistent result reported in the literature has been a dramatically decreased time to ambulation. Complication rates have not been reduced in most reports. The cost of the devices is a concern to many administrators.

VasoSeal

VasoSeal, the first available device,[39] consists of a collagen sponge weighing approximately 90 g. After insertion of a guide wire, the procedure sheath is removed and the tissues are dilated from the skin to the arterial wall, leaving a plastic sheath in place into which the collagen plug is delivered. Firm occlusive pressure is required on the femoral artery above the access site during and for at least 5 min after device deployment.

The results of three randomized clinical trials are available.[40–42] Femoral compression time was reduced compared with standard manual compression. Complications including bleeding and hematoma formation occurred at approximately the same incidence as with manual compression. Occasional episodes of arterial occlusion have been described, due to inadvertent intra-arterial delivery of collagen.[42,43]

Angio-Seal

Angio-Seal (St. Jude Medical, St Paul, MN, USA) is also a collagen device but is quite different from VasoSeal. Over a guide wire, the procedure sheath is removed and replaced with a delivery sheath advanced until the tip is just inside the artery. A 2 mm × 10 mm 'anchor' is extended through the sheath, then the sheath is pulled back as a collagen plug is snugged down on the outside of the artery, simultaneously pulling the reabsorbable anchor flat against the inside surface of the vessel. A suture connects the two components.

Initial case series[44,45] showed > 90% success of deployment with hemostasis within 5 min in most cases. Two randomized trials[46,47] have shown earlier time to hemostasis, ambulation and hospital discharge in comparison to manual hemostasis. Complication rates were modestly reduced in these studies, although the potential for infection[48,49] and arterial occlusion[50,51] exists.

Perclose

The only device involving a needle and suture technique, 'The Closer' (Abbott Laboratories, Abbott Park, IL, USA) and its predecessors ProStar and TechStar are inserted over a wire after removal of the procedure sheath. In the most recent device, an intra-arterial platform or 'foot' is extended, into which two needles are advanced capturing sutures stored within the shaft of the device. Removal of the needles forms a suture loop closing the arteriotomy site. The suture ends are tied off and clipped.

Initial experience with Perclose[52] showed a > 90% success rate. Three subsequent randomized trials have been reported. Compared with manual compression,[53,54] the device showed a high degree of success with equivalent complication rates and earlier time to ambulation. Patients receiving suture-mediated arterial closure experienced earlier ambulation than patients treated using a mechanical clamp technique,[55] but again the complication rate was not reduced. Arterial injury due to an entrapped device has been reported.[55]

Duett

The only device deployed through the existing procedure sheath, Duett (Vascular Solutions, Minneapolis, MN, USA) includes a central guide wire incorporating a balloon. Once extended beyond the sheath and inflated, the sheath is withdrawn as the balloon is pulled up against the interior of the arteriotomy site. A slurry of collagen and thrombin is then injected through the sheath onto the exterior of the arteriotomy site, after which the balloon is deflated and withdrawn. Light manual pressure is applied for 5 mins.

No randomized trials of Duett are available. Case series[56–61] have shown high success rates and few complications. Arterial occlusion has been reported.[57]

Cost issues

Hemostasis devices can cost upwards of US$200 per unit. Such a cost, multiplied by the number of cases to which the devices might be applied, causes concern and requires analysis in terms of cost-effectiveness. Factors in favor of the device could include a potential for less intensive personnel involvement during the shortened hemostasis process, earlier patient ambulation and discharge, and increased patient satisfaction.[59,60] Some of these factors are difficult to quantify in terms of dollars saved. Complications seem to occur with all devices at about the same rate as with manual hemostasis, so they cannot be used in the expectation of reducing such costs.

Comparison and contrast

The four available arteriotomy closure devices differ in many ways. Similarities include adding a degree of complexity and time to the vascular procedure, though with considerable time savings outside the laboratory in terms of the potential for earlier ambulation and discharge. All the devices require instruction and practice. A learning curve can be anticipated.[61]

Before deployment of any device, an iliac angiogram is recommended, as deployment below the femoral bifurcation may be dangerous. When atherosclerosis is present in the common femoral artery, devices with an intra-arterial component or step should not be used. In this setting, VasoSeal may be preferred.

None of the devices clearly reduces complication rates. Two observational comparisons[62,63] have been published. In one study, Perclose and VasoSeal were found equal in safety, although possibly less effective than a pneumatic balloon compression device in patients receiving a platelet IIB/IIIA receptor antagonist.[62] The other report [63] indicated a higher complication rate with Angio-Seal than with Perclose, in turn higher than VasoSeal. There are no prospective randomized comparisons between devices, so no objective evaluation of safety and effectiveness is possible.

Ease of use is a subjective matter. Deployment of VasoSeal requires two people, while all the other devices can be deployed by one operator. Angio-Seal may be the least complex in terms of the number of required steps. None of the devices are free from the risk of infection, and therefore most operators hesitate to employ them outside the sterile catheterization laboratory environment.

Only limited data are available concerning use of these devices in peripheral vascular procedures.[64] Applicability in this setting may be limited by the frequent presence of atherosclerotic femoral artery disease. Device-assisted hemostasis has excellent potential to facilitate same-day discharge after renal vascular interventions.

The use of platelet IIB/IIIA receptor inhibitors has become routine in coronary interventions and may prove useful in peripheral vascular interventions as well. These drugs clearly increase the potential for access site bleeding. Very limited data are available on the use of hemostasis devices in patients who have received these drugs.[62,65]

In summary, arterial sealing devices can be very useful, especially in terms of achieving earlier patient ambulation and discharge. If same-day discharge is not planned, they may still be useful in diminishing the time required to obtain arterial hemostasis, although cost remains an issue. Complication rates are not clearly lessened by their use. There are no randomized comparative data on which to base any conclusion concerning superiority of any device over others.

References

1   Schafer AI. Pathophysiology of thrombosis. In: Loscalzo J et al. (eds), *Vascular medicine: a textbook of vascular biology and disease*. Boston: Little Brown & Co, 1992: 307–33.

2   Rubanyi GM. Endothelium-derived vasoactive factors in health and disease. In: Rubanyi GM (ed.), *Cardiovascular significance of endothelium-derived vasoactive factors*. Mount Kisco, NY: Futura Publishing Co, 1991: xi–xix.

3   Stein B, Fuster V. Pharmacology of anticoagulants and platelet inhibitor drugs. In: Schlant RC, Alexander RW (eds), *Hurst's the heart*, Vol I, 8th edn. New York: McGraw-Hill, 1994: 1309–26.

4   Fuster V, Jang I. Role of platelet-inhibitor agents in coronary disease. In: Topol EJ (ed.), *Textbook of interventional cardiology*, Vol I, 2nd edn. Philadelphia: WB Saunders, 1994: 3–22.

5   Becker RC. Antiplatelet therapy. *Science & Medicine* 1996; **July/August**: 12–21.

6   Smith SC, Jr, Dove JT, Jacobs AK et al. ACC/AHA guidelines for percutaneous coronary intervention: a report of the American College of Cardiology/American Heart Association Task Force on Practice Guidelines (Committee to Revise the 1993 Guidelines for Percutaneous Transluminal Coronary Angioplasty). *J Am Coll Cardiol* 2001; **37**: 2239i–lxvi

7   The EPILOG Investigators. Platelet glycoprotein IIb/IIIa receptor blockade and low-dose heparin during percutaneous coronary revascularization. *N Engl J Med* 1997; **336**: 1689–96.

8   Olson St, Björk I. Regulation of thrombin by antithrombin and heparin cofactor II. In: Berliner, LJ (ed.), *Thrombin: structure and function*. New York: Plenum Press, 1992: 159–217.

9   Rosenberg RD. The heparin-antithrombin system: a natural anticoagulant mechanism. In: Colman RW, Hirsh J, Marder VJ, Salzman EW (eds), *Hemostasis and thrombosis: basic principles and clinical practice*, 2nd edn. Philadelphia: JB Lippincott, 1987: 1373–92.

10   Hirsh J. Heparin. *N Engl J Med* 1991; **324**: 1565–74.

11   Chew DP, Bhatt DL, Lincoff AM, et al. Defining the optimal activated clotting time during percutaneous coronary intervention: aggregate results from 6 randomized controlled trials. *Circulation* 2001; **103**: 961–6.

12   The ESPRIT investigators. Novel dosing regimen of eptifibatide in planned coronary stent implantation (ESPRIT): a randomised, placebo-controlled trial. *Lancet* 2000; **356**: 2037–44.

13   Hirsh J, Warkentin TE, Raschke R et al. Heparin and low-molecular-weight heparin: mechanisms of action, pharmacokinetics, dosing considerations, monitoring, efficacy and safety. *Chest* 1998; **114**(Suppl): 489510S.

14   Warkentin TE, Levine MN, Hirsh J et al. Heparin-induced thrombocytopenia in patients treated with low-molecular-weight heparins or UFH. *N Engl J Med* 1995; **332**: 1330–5.

15   Instability in Coronary Artery Disease (FRISC) Study Group. Low molecular weight heparin during instability in coronary artery disease. *Lancet* 1996; **347**: 561–8.

16   Klein W, Buchwald A, Hillis SE et al. Comparison of low-molecular-weight heparin with unfractionated heparin acutely and with placebo for 6 weeks in the management of unstable coronary artery disease. Fragmin in Unstable Coronary Artery Disease Study (FRIC). *Circulation* 1997; **96**: 61–8.

17   Cohen M, Demers C, Gurfinkel EP et al. A comparison of low-molecular weight heparin with unfractionated heparin for unstable coronary artery disease. Efficacy and safety of subcutaneous enoxaparin non-Q-wave coronary events study group. *N Engl J Med* 1997; **337**: 447–52.

18   Antman EM, McCabe CH, Gurfinkel EP et al. Enoxaparin prevents death and cardiac ischemic events in unstable angina/non-Q-wave myocardial infarction. Results of the thrombolysis in myocardial infarction (TIMI) 11B trial. *Circulation* 1999; **100**: 1593–601.

19   Antman EM, Cohen M, Radley D et al. for the TIMI 11 B (Thrombolysis in Myocardial Infarction) and ESSENCE (Efficacy and Safety of Subcutaneous Enoxaparin in non-Q-wave Coronary Events) Investigators. Assessment of the treatment effect of enoxaparin for unstable angina/non-Q wave myocardial infarction: TIMI 11 B–ESSENCE Meta-analysis. *Circulation* 1999; **100**: 1602–8.

20 Collet JPh, Montalescot G, Lison L et al. Percutaneous coronary intervention after subcutaneous enoxaparin pretreatment in patients with unstable angina pectoris. *Circulation* 2001; **103**: 658–63.

21 Ferguson J, Antman E, Bates E et al. the NICE 3 investigators. The use of enoxaparin and IIb/IIIa antagonists in acute coronary syndromes, including PCI: final results of the NICE 3 study. *J Am Coll Cardiol* 2001; **37**(Suppl A): 365A.

22 Kereiakes DJ, Grines C, Fry E et al. for the NICE 1 and NICE 4 investigators. Enoxaparin and abciximab adjunctive pharmacotherapy during percutaneous coronary intervention. *J Invas Cardiol* 2001; **13**: 272–8.

23 Markwardt F. Development of hirudin as an antithrombotic agent. *Semin Thromb Hemost* 1989; **15**: 269–82.

24 The GUSTO IIb investigators. A comparison of recombinant hirudin with heparin for the treatment of acute coronary syndromes. *N Engl J Med* 1996; **335**: 775–82.

25 Effects of recombinant hirudin (lepirudin) compared with heparin on death, myocardial infarction, refractory angina, and revascularization procedures in patients with acute myocardial ischemia without ST-segment elevation: a randomized trial. OASIS-2 investigators. *Lancet* 1999; **353**: 429–38.

26 Greinacher A, Janssens U, Berg G et al. for the Heparin-Associated Thrombocytopenia study (HAT) investigators. Lepirudin (recombinant hirudin) for parenteral anticoagulation in patients with heparin-induced thrombocytopenia. *Circulation* 1999; **100**: 587–93.

27 Bittl JA, Strony J, Brinker JA et al. Treatment with bivalirudin (Hirulog) as compared with heparin during coronary angioplasty for unstable or postinfarction angina. *N Engl J Med* 1995; **333**: 764–9.

28 Barnathan

29 CLASSICS.

30 Lefkovits J, Plow EF, Topol EJ. Platelet glycoprotein IIb/IIIa receptors in cardiovascular medicine. *N Engl J Med* 1995; **332**: 1553–9.

31 Tcheng JE. Glycoprotein IIb/IIIa receptor inhibitors: putting the EPIC, IMPACT II, RESTORE, and EPILOG trials into perspective. *Am J Cardiol* 1996; **78**: 35–40.

32 EPIC investigators. Use of monoclonal antibody directed against the platelet glycoprotein IIb/IIIa receptor in high-risk coronary angioplasty. *N Engl J Med* 1994; 330: 956–61.

33 The CAPTURE investigators. Randomized placebo-controlled trial of abciximab before and during coronary intervention in refractory unstable angina: the CAPTURE study. *Lancet* 1997; **349**: 1429–35.

34 The PURSUIT trial investigators. Inhibition of platelet glycoprotein IIb/IIIa with eptifibatide in patients with acute coronary syndromes. *N Engl J Med* 1998; **339**: 436–43.

35 The IMPACT-II investigators. Randomized placebo-controlled trial of effect of eptifibatide on complications of percutaneous coronary intervention: IMPACT-II. *Lancet* 1997; **349**: 1422–8.

36 The RESTORE investigators. Effects of platelet glycoprotein IIb/IIIa blockade with tirofiban on adverse cardiac events in patients with unstable angina or acute myocardial infarction undergoing coronary angioplasty. *Circulation* 1997; **96**: 1445–53.

37 PRISM-PLUS investigators. Inhibition of the platelet glycoprotein IIb/IIIa receptor with tirofiban in unstable angina and non Q-wave myocardial infarction. *N Engl J Med* 1998; **338**: 1488–97.

38 Sanborn TA, Kussmaul WG, Hinohara T. Percutaneous vascular hemostasis devices for arterial sealing after interventional procedures. In: Topol EJ (ed.), *Textbook of interventional cardiology*, 3rd edn. Philadelphia: WB Saunders, 1999: 693–700.

39 Ernst S, Tjonjoegin M, Scharder R et al. Immediate sealing of arterial puncture sites after cardiac catheterization and coronary angioplasty using a bio-degradable collagen plug: results of an international registry. *J Am Coll Cardiol* 1993; **21**: 851–5.

40 Schrader R, Steinbacher S, Burger W et al. Collagen application for sealing of arterial puncture sites in comparison to pressure dressing: a randomized trial. *Cathet Cardiovasc Diagn* 1992; **27**: 298–302.

41 Sanborn TA, Gibbs HH, Brinker JA et al. A multicenter randomized trial comparing a percutaneous collagen hemostasis device with conventional manual compression after diagnostic angiography and angioplasty. *J Am Coll Cardiol* 1993; **22**: 1273–9.

42 Camenzind E, Grossholz M, Urban P et al. Collagen application versus manual compression: a prospective randomized trial for arterial puncture site closure after coronary angioplasty. *J Am Coll Cardiol* 1994; **24**: 655–62.

43 Carere RG, Webb JG, Miyagishima R et al. Groin complications associated with collagen plug closure of femoral arterial puncture sites in anticoagulated patients. *Cathet Cardiovasc Diagn* 1998; **43**: 124–9.

44 de Swart H, Dijkman L, Hofstra L et al. A new hemostatic puncture closure device for the immediate sealing of arterial puncture sites. *Am J Cardiol* 1993; **72**: 445–9.

45 Aker UT, Kensey KR, Heuser RR et al. Immediate arterial hemostasis after cardiac catheterization: initial experience with a new puncture closure device. *Cathet Cardiovasc Diagn* 1994; **31**: 228–32.

46 Kussmaul WG, Buchbinder M, Whitlow PL et al. Rapid arterial hemostasis and decreased access site complications after cardiac catheterization and angioplasty: results of a randomized trial of a novel hemostatic device. *J Am Coll Cardiol* 1995; **25**: 1685–92.

47 Ward SR, Casale P, Raymond R et al. Efficacy and safety of a hemostatic puncture closure device with early ambulation after coronary angiography. Angio-Seal investigators. *Am J Cardiol* 1998; **81**: 569–72.

48. Cooper C, Miller A. Infectious complications related to the use of the Angio-Seal hemostatic puncture closure device. *Catheter Cardiovasc Interv* 1999; **48**: 301–3.

49 Eggebrecht H, Haude M, Baumgart D, Erbel R. Infectious complications related to the use of the Angio-Seal hemostatic puncture closure device. *Catheter Cardiovasc Interv* 2000; **49**: 352–3.

50 Eidt JF, Habibipour S, Saucedo JF et al. Surgical complications from hemostatic puncture closure devices. *Am J Surg* 1999; **178**: 511–6.

51 Goyen M, Manz S, Kroger K et al. Interventional therapy of vascular complications caused by the hemostatic puncture closure device Angio-Seal. *Catheter Cardiovasc Interv* 2000; **49**: 142–7.

52 Carere RG, Webb JG, Ahmed T, Dodek AA. Initial experience using Prostar: a new device for percutaneous suture-mediated closure of arterial puncture sites. *Cathet Cardiovasc Diagn*. 1996; **37**: 367–72.

53   Gerckens U, Cattelaens N, Lampe E-G, Grube E. Management of arterial puncture site after catheterization procedures: evaluating a suture-mediated closure device. *Am J Cardiol* 1999; **83**: 1658–63.

54   Baim DS, Knopf WD, Hinohara T et al. Suture-mediated closure of the femoral access site after cardiac catheterization: results of the STAND I and STAND II trials. *Am J Cardiol* 2000; **85**: 864–9.

55   Carere RG, Webb JG, Buller CEH et al. Suture closure of femoral arterial puncture sites after coronary angioplasty followed by same-day discharge. *Am Heart J* 2000; **139**: 52–8.

56   Silber S, Gershony G, Schon B et al. A novel vascular sealing device for closure of percutaneous arterial access sites. *Am J Cardiol* 1999; **83**: 1248–52.

57   Silber S, Tofte AJ, Kjellevand TO et al. Final report of the European multi-center registry using the Duett vascular sealing device. *Herz* 1999; **24**: 620–3.

58   Mooney MR, Ellis SG, Gershony G et al. Immediate sealing of arterial puncture sites after cardiac catheterization and coronary interventions: initial US feasibility trial using the Duett vascular closure device. *Cathet Cardiovasc Interv* 2000; **50**: 96–102.

59   Slaughter PM, Chetty R, Flintoft VF et al. A single center randomized trial assessing use of a vascular hemostasis device vs. conventional manual compression following PTCA: what are the potential resource savings? *Cathet Cardiovasc Diagn*. 1995; **34**: 210–14.

60   Brown CL, Freschi LA, Blincoe WA et al. A prospective, randomized trial and cost-effectiveness study of the VasoSeal collagen plug vs. manual arterial pressure in patients undergoing cardiac catheterization [abstract]. *Circulation* 1997; **96**: I-618.

61   Warren BS, Warren SG, Miller SD. Predictors of complications and learning curve using the Angio-Seal closure device following interventional and diagnostic catheterization. *Catheter Cardiovasc Interv* 1999; **48**: 162–6.

62   Chamberlin JR, Lardi AB, McKeever LS et al. Use of vascular sealing devices (VasoSeal and Perclose) versus assisted manual compression (Femostop) in transcatheter coronary interventions requiring abciximab (ReoPro). *Catheter Cardiovasc Interv* 1999; **47**: 143–7.

63   Shrake KL. Comparison of major complication rates associated with four methods of arterial closure. *Am J Cardiol* 2000; **85**: 1024–5.

64   Duda SH, Wiskirchen J, Erb M et al. Suture-mediated percutaneous closure of antegrade femoral arterial access sites in patients who have received full anticoagulation therapy. *Radiology* 1999; **210**: 47–52.

65   Lunney L, Karim K, Little T. Vasoseal hemostasis following coronary interventions with abciximab. *Cathet Cardiovasc Diagn* 1998; **44**: 405–6.

59

Our experience of endovascular treatment of some congenital heart defects

BG Alekyan, VP Podzolkov, VA Garibyan, MG Pursanov, EY Danilov, KE Cardenas, VF Kharpunov, TN Sarkisova and AV Ter-Akopyan

By the year 2003, we had performed endovascular procedures in more than 3800 patients with different congenital heart defects in the Bakoulev Scientific Center for Cardiovascular Surgery.

Balloon valvuloplasty in patients with congenital pulmonary artery and aortic valvular stenosis

Materials and methods

Transluminal balloon valvuloplasty was performed in 1208 patients. Seven hundred and twenty patients had an isolated pulmonary artery valvular stenosis, 203 congenital aortic valvular stenosis, and 186 cyanotic congenital heart defects.

Results

After the intervention, the systolic pressure gradient between the right ventricle (RV) and pulmonary artery (PA) fell on average from 120.9 ± 34.1 to 26.8 ± 14.5 mmHg. In the patients with congenital aortic valvular stenosis (Figure 59.1), the procedure led to a decrease in the systolic pressure gradient between the left ventricle (LV) and aorta from 106.8 ± 38.6 to 36.5 ± 20.7 mmHg. The patients with the cyanotic congenital heart defects showed an increase in blood oxygen saturation from (SaO_2) 65.1 ± 3.0 to 82.5 ± 2.8, and systolic pressure in the PA increased from 10.2 ± 4.5 to 18.6 ± 4.9 mmHg; in the patients with hypoplastic PA an increase in the size of the PA was noted.

Long-term follow-up (6 months to 15 years) studies were carried out in 390 (54.1%) patients with PA valvular stenosis, 128 (61.2%) patients with congenital aortic valvular stenosis, and 102 (54.8%) patients with cyanotic congenital heart defects. Good and satisfactory results of valvuloplasty of isolated PA stenosis were seen in 88.4% of the cases. In the

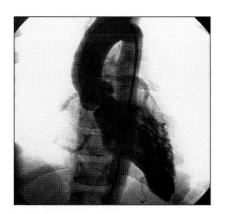 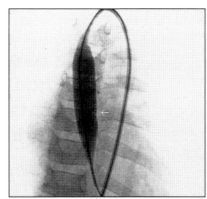 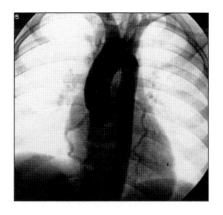

Figure 59.1
Transluminal balloon valvuloplasty of congenital aortic valvular stenosis.

patients with congenital aortic valvular stenosis, the good and satisfactory results were seen in 75.0% of all the cases, and in balloon valvuloplasty of PA valvular stenosis, in 68.6% of the patients.

Conclusions

Balloon valvuloplasty is an effective method of treatment of isolated PA valvular stenosis, congenital aortic valvular stenosis and PA valvular stenosis concomitant with cyanotic congenital heart defects.

Transluminal balloon angioplasty in the treatment of obstructive pathology of pulmonary arteries

Materials and methods

We have gained experience of transluminal balloon angioplasty of 177 obstructed segments of the PAs in 170 patients with congenital heart defects. The age of the patients varied from 6 months to 34 years. The patients were distributed into four groups. Group 1 comprised patients with isolated peripheral PA stenoses (14 segments in 8 patients) and PA narrowings after radical correction procedures (28 segments in 21 patients) and PA narrowings concomitant with isolated PA valvular stenosis (12 segments in 8 patients). Group 2 comprised patients who had undergone RV outflow tract reconstruction without VSD closure with PA stenoses (46 segments in 34 patients). Group 3 comprised patients with cyanotic heart defects (110 segments in 78 patients). Twenty-four of them had undergone balloon valvuloplasty of the PA only, 34 balloon valvuloplasty of the PA with balloon valvuloplasty of PA valvular stenosis, and 20 of them balloon valvuloplasty of the PA with balloon valvuloplasty of stenosed systemic–pulmonary anastomosis. The fourth group comprised patients who had undergone bi-directional cavapulmonary anastomosis and the Fontain procedure (22 segments in 20 patients).

Results

Balloon angioplasty in the first group was 60.9%, in the second group 73.9%, in the third group 64.5% and in the fourth group 86.4%.

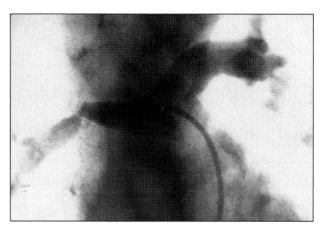
(a)

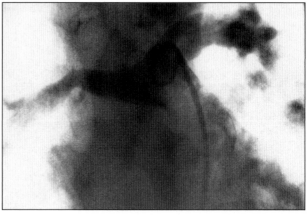
(b)

Figure 59.2
Transluminal balloon angioplasty of right pulmonary artery stenosis.

Conclusions

Thus, the efficacy of the balloon angioplasty was 71.4% on average (Figure 59.2). Thirty-six patients underwent PA stenting due to ineffectiveness of the angioplasty.

Use of stents in stenotic pulmonary arteries in patients with congenital heart defects

Materials and methods

Forty-eight stents were used to treat 44 stenosed segments of the pulmonary arteries in 36 patients. The patients' age varied from 3.5 to 27 years (mean 13.6 ± 6.2 years).

Results

After stenting the diameter of the stenosis increased on average from 5.5 ± 2.1 mm to 11.5 ± 2.1 mm ($p < 0.0005$), and the systolic pressure gradient fell on average from 51.1 ± 32.7 to 17.4 ± 17.9 mmHg ($p < 0.0005$). The ratio of systolic pressures in the RV and the aorta (RV/Ao) decreased from 0.79 ± 0.07 to 0.48 ± 0.06 ($p < 0.0033$). An immediate good effect of stenting was seen after dilation in 21 (95.5%) out of 22 segments of stenosed PA (Figure 59.3).

Serious complications were not seen. Three technical mistakes were noted: in one case the undeployed stent migrated into the lower lobe branch of the PA; in one case the stent was erroneously implanted into the trunk of the PA; and in one case the stent's position within the stenosis was suboptimal. Optimal position of the stents was obtained in 42 (88.5%) of 48 cases.

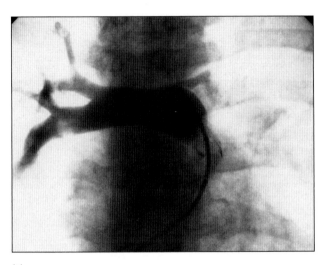

(a)

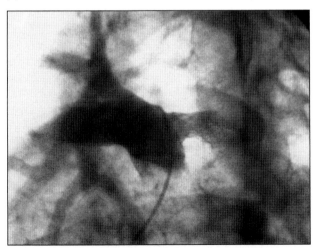

(b)

Figure 59.3
Stenting of stenosed left pulmonary artery.

Long-term follow-up studies were carried out in 24 (66.7%) patients in whom 32 stents had been implanted 6–38 months (mean 15 ± 11.6 months) after the procedure. In all of the cases, repeated catheterization and angiography were performed. All the stents were patent; no cases of migration were seen. Only in one case (4.1%) was a stent restenosed due to neointimal hyperplasia.

Conclusions

Stenting is an effective, but technically rather complicated, procedure. The rate of immediate success was 95.5%, with 4.1% of late restenoses.

Balloon angioplasty and stenting for aortic coarctation and recoarctation

Materials and methods

We have performed 184 transluminal balloon angioplasties (TLBAs) in 173 patients with coarctation (CoA) (122 patients) or recoarctation (ReCoA) (51 patients). In 13 cases aortic stenting was performed.

Results

Immediately after TLBA in patients with membranous CoA, the systolic pressure gradient between the ascending and descending aorta decreased from 41.0 ± 16.3 to 7.3 ± 6.7 mmHg; for patients with hypoplastic type of CoA from 40.1 ± 20.3 to 9.7 ± 8.2 mmHg, and in patients with ReCoA from 43.2 ± 24.2 to 9.5 ± 6.4 mmHg (Figure 59.4). Follow-up results of TLBA were studied 6 months to 15 years after the procedure in 105 patients (48.2%). In 40 patients with membranous-type CoA, the systolic pressure gradient was 9.8 ± 5.1 mmHg, in 35 patients with the hypoplastic type of CoA 17.5 ± 11.7 mmHg, and in 30 patients with ReCoA 9.6 ± 6.3 mmHg. Good and satisfactory results were seen in 98 (93.3%) patients with CoA and ReCoA. In 7 patients (6.7%), the systolic pressure gradient returned to the initial value, in 5 of them, repeated TLBA was carried out. Repeated TLBA was ineffective in two patients who had Palmaz stents (Cordis) implanted. In 13 patients after aortic stenting, mean SPG decreased from 50 ± 15 to 5 ± 3 mmHg (Figure 59.5). Aorto-aortic bypass grafting was performed in only 1 case.

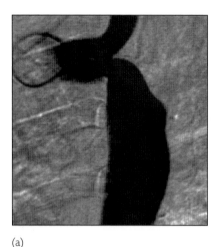
(a)

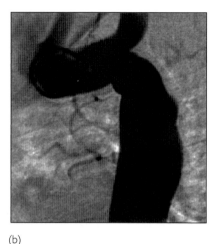
(b)

Figure 59.4
Transluminal balloon angioplasty of aortic recoarctation.

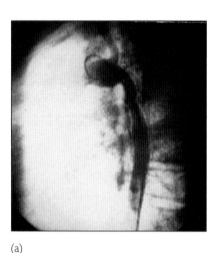
(a)

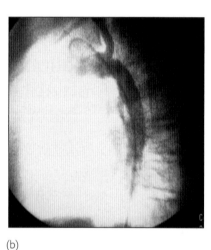
(b)

Figure 59.5
Stenting of aortic coarctation

Conclusions

Balloon angioplasty provided good and satisfactory long-term results in 92% of patients. The stenting of hypoplastic CoA and ReCoA provided excellent immediate and long-term results.

Transluminal balloon angioplasty of stenosed systemic–pulmonary and cavapulmonary anastomoses

Materials and methods

We have performed balloon angioplasty of the stenosed Blalock–Taussig anastomosis in 80 patients, Gore-tex anastomosis in 4 patients and bi-directional cavapulmonary anastomosis in 6 patients. All of the patients had severe cyanosis, dyspnea, rapid fatigue and decrease of physical capacities. We divided the anastomostic obstructions into three types: discrete obstructions, obstructions in extent and thrombosis. The vast majority of the patients fell into the first group.

We used balloons of the same diameter as the part of the vessel proximal to the stenosis in the cases of angioplasty of the stenosed Blalock–Taussig anastomosis, and the same as the prosthesis diameter in angioplasty of the Gore-tex anastomosis.

Results

After the balloon dilation of the narrowed anastomoses, the blood oxygen saturation increased from 62.4 ± 1.4 to 81.2 ± 1.2 on average, and systolic pressure in the PA increased from 16.4 ± 0.9 to 23.2 ± 1.8 mmHg. The angiometry showed more than a 1.5-fold increase of the stenosis diameter and more than a two-fold increase of the cross-sectional area in the zone of the stenosis.

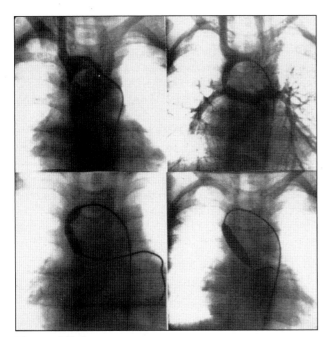

Figure 59.6
Recanalization and angioplasty of the Blalock–Taussig anastomosis.

Balloon angioplasty results were assessed as good in 63 (70.0%) patients (Figure 59.6), satisfactory in 24 patients (26.7%) and non-satisfactory in 3 patients (3.3%). We have achieved the best results in patients with discrete narrowings and thrombosed anastomoses. We also implanted the Corynphian stent (Cordis, J&J).

During and after the procedures, 3 (3.3%) patients had serious complications: pulmonary edema in 2 patients and pre-edematous state in one patient due to anastomosis hyperfunction.

Conclusions

Balloon angioplasty of the narrowed anastomoses may serve as an effective method of treatment and be a good alternative to the surgical procedure of repeated placement of systemic–pulmonary anastomoses.

Interventional procedures in the treatment of neonates with congenital heart defects

Materials and methods

We have performed more than 770 interventional procedures in patients from 16 hours to 12 months old. The patients with Rashkind and Park procedures (n = 570) were excluded from the study. Sixty (7.5%) patients were below 30 days of age. All patients were critically ill.

Results

In four cases, after an ineffective Rashkind procedure the restrictive atrial septal defect was dilated with balloons sized 6–12 mm. As a result, SaO_2 in those patients increased from $34.6 \pm 4.2\%$ to $60.2 \pm 3.9\%$. In 16 patients with critical valvular stenosis of the pulmonary artery (VSPA), transluminal balloon valvuloplasty (TLBV) was carried out. As a result, the systolic pressure gradient between the PA and the RV decreased from 112.6 ± 24.0 to 25.1 ± 14.8 mmHg, and SaO_2 increased from $74.0 \pm 8.4\%$ to $89.1 \pm 6.5\%$. Balloon valvuloplasty of VSPA was performed with good effect in four patients with tetralogy of Fallot, whose state was very critical, with SaO_2 below 40%. In 12 patients with critical valvular aortic stenosis (VAS), TLBV was carried out. As a result, the systolic pressure gradient between the LV and the aorta decreased from 89.2 ± 24.6 to 20.7 ± 12.8 mmHg, and left ventricular ejection fraction increased from 28.8 ± 10.3 to $39.4 \pm 9.2\%$. In two patients with type II pulmonary artery atresia patent ductus arteriosus was dilated. SaO_2 increased from 40% to 88%. Two patients (8.0%) died: the deaths were caused by balloon lesion of the left atrial wall during atrial septal defect (ASD) dilation and bilateral pneumonia after successful TLBV of valvular aortic stenosis.

Conclusions

Endovascular interventions are effective for the treatment of some congenital heart defects in critically ill infants during the first months of life (Figure 59.7).

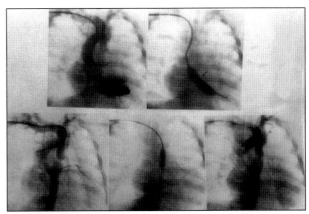

Figure 59.7
Simultaneous transluminal balloon valvuloplasty of aortic valvular stenosis and transluminal balloon angioplasty of aortic coarctation.

Interventional procedures for complex treatment of patients with pulmonary artery atresia

Patients with congenital or iatrogenous atresia of the pulmonary artery (PAA) are in the high-risk group for the radical or hemodynamic corrective procedures. Depending on the anatomy and hemodynamics of the defect, multistage methods of surgical treatment, including endovascular procedures, are being elaborated.

Materials and methods

At different stages of the treatment for PAA, we have performed 74 different interventional procedures in 65 patients. In 18 patients, after the reconstruction of the right ventricular outflow tract, TLBA of the 21 segments of the PA was performed for PA stenoses or hypoplasia (Figure 59.8).

In 6 patients, TLBA of the stenosed PA was performed using the approach through the systemic–pulmonary anastomosis. TLBA of the restricted Blalock–Taussig anastomosis was carried out in 11 patients, and in 2 of them simultaneous TLBA of the anastomosis and the PA was performed. In 2 patients, we performed TLBA of the stenosed aortopulmonary collaterals, with stenting in one case. In 2 cases, we performed dilation of closing PDA. In 19 cases, we have carried out embolization of the large aortopulmonary collaterals with Gianturco coils; 36 collaterals were closed completely with 80 coils (Figure 59.9). In 7 patients from this group, we have also performed dilation of the stenosed PA, with stent implantation in two cases.

Conclusion

In some cases, interventional surgical procedures are effective for the treatment of patients with PAA. They allow improvement of the anatomy and the hemodynamics of the pulmonary circulation, and preparation of this group of patients for radical or hemodynamic correction of the defect under favorable circumstances.

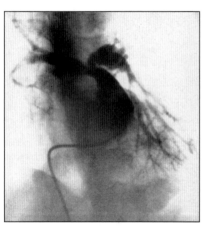

(a)

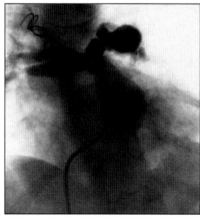

(b)

Figure 59.8
Transluminal balloon angioplasty of right and left pulmonary artery stenoses after reconstruction of the right ventricular outflow tract.

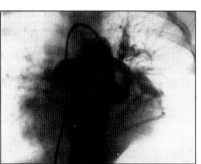

(a)

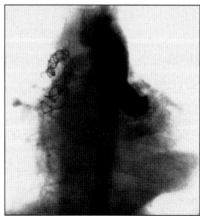

(b)

Figure 59.9
Embolization of the large aortopulmonary collaterals.

Use of occluders for the treatment of arteriovenous and venoarterial blood shunting

Purpose of the investigation

The aim was to demonstrate the possibilities of occluders in the treatment of 61 patients with following congenital heart defects: ASD, VSD aortopulmonary septal defect (APSD), patent ductus arteriosus (PDA), and communication between right PA and left atrium (LA).

Materials and methods

Five types of occluders have been used: Amplatzer Septal Occluder (ASO, AGA-Med, USA), Amplatzer Duct Occluder (ADO, AGA-Med), Buttoned atrial device (BAD, Sideris, Greece), Buttoned ventricular device (BVD, Sideris, Greece), and Patch Occluder (PO, Sideris, Greece).

The ASO was used in 53 cases, 39 with VSD, and 1 with APSD recanalization, and the ADO in 11 cases (PDA). The BAD was used in 7 patients: 2 with ASD, 2 with VSD and 4 with PDA. The PO was used in 2 cases of ASD, and the BVD was used for the closure of right PA–LA communication. The size of ASD closed varied from 8 to 34 mm, and PDA from 5 to 12 mm; APSD diameter was 4 mm,

Results

ASDs were successfully closed with the ASO in 37 patients (Figure 59.10); in 2 cases the defect could not be closed due to miscalculating of their sizes. The ASO was also successfully used for APSD closure, and the ADO for PDA closure. The BAD, BVD and PO were successfully implanted in all the cases. Immediately after the procedure, residual shunting was seen in 3 patients: 2 with ASD after BAD and PO implantation and 1 with right PA–LA communication (despite the shunting, SaO_2 increased from 68% to 92%). Follow-up results were studied in 11 patients with ASD and 2 patients with PDA 8.2 ± 2.4 months after the procedure. Only 1 patient had residual blood shunting after PO implantation.

Conclusions

The use of special occluders is an effective procedure with definite indications.

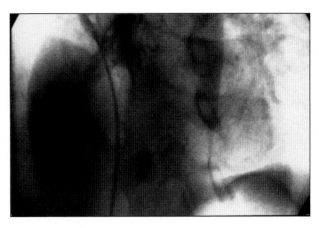
(a)

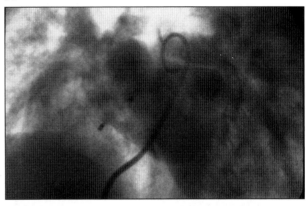
(b)

Figure 59.10
Successful closure of Amplatzer Septal Occluder with the atrial septal defect.

Endovascular surgery in the treatment of patients after radical and hemodynamic surgical procedures due to cyanotic congenital heart defects

Materials and methods

Forty-six patients underwent different endovascular procedures (70 procedures) over various periods (from 1 day to 5 years) after surgical procedures for radical or hemodynamic correction of congenital heart defects.

We performed 16 different endovascular procedures in 12 patients after the Fontain procedure. The heart failure class 2 comprised 3 patients, and the class 3 9 patients. Placement of fenestration in the atrial septum or intraatrial tunnel was performed in 5 patients (Figure 59.11). One patient, after the Fontain procedure (Kreizer modification), has undergone balloon

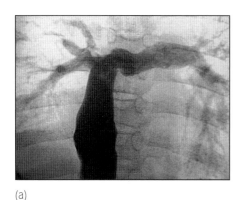

(a)

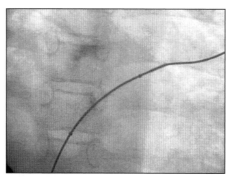

(b)

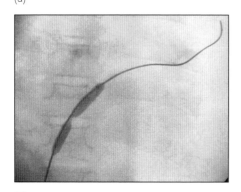

(c)

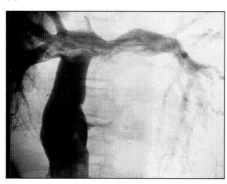

(d)

Figure 59.11
Placement of fenestration in intraatrial tunnel in a patient after the Fontain procedure in a modification of a total cavapulmonary anastomosis.

valvuloplasty of PA valvular stenosis. In addition, we performed the embolization of a residual communication between the RV and PA with a Gianturco coil in a patient after the procedure of placement of total cavapulmonary anastomoses and five balloon angioplasties of stenoses of peripheral branches of the PA, one of which, in the case of a rigid narrowing of the vessel, led to stenting. One patient with total cavapulmonary anastomoses underwent balloon angioplasty and stenting of the stenosed intraatrial tunnel. After the procedures were performed, heart failure class 1 was noted in eight patients, class 2 in three patients and class 3 in one patient.

Ten patients (12 procedures) after radical operations using conduits have undergone balloon dilation of stenosed conduits between the RV and PA (10 procedures) and balloon dilation of stenosed pulmonary arteries (2 procedures). Seven of the patients had heart failure class 2 and three class 3 NYHA. After the procedures, 8 patients fell into class 1 and 2 into class 2 NYHA. Twenty-four patients with peripheral PA stenoses have undergone balloon dilations of the stenotic segments (42 procedures) and 10 stents were implanted in 9 patients; before the procedures, 8 patients were in class 2 NYHA and 15 in class 3; after the procedures, 15 patients fell into class 1 and 9 into class 2.

Results

The procedures performed in the patients after the Fontain procedure provided relief of CHF symptoms, and in the

patients with stenosed conduits they decreased the right ventricular pressure and prolonged the lifetime of the conduits. The elimination of the peripheral stenoses led to the improvement of the PA anatomy and hemodynamics in the pulmonary circulation.

Conclusions

Endovascular procedures can be successfully used to treat postsurgical complications and eliminate obstructions.

Balloon dilation and stenting of brachiocephalic arteries in patients with supravalvular aortic stenosis

Materials and methods

We have performed 15 endovascular procedures in 13 patients with congenital pathology of brachiocephalic arteries. In 11 patients, supravalvular aortic stenosis was associated with congenital pathology of the left common carotid artery, and in 2 patients there were pathologies of the left common carotid artery and of the brachiocephalic trunk.

Results

As the first stage in preventing cerebral hypoxia during surgical correction of supravalvular aortic stenosis with cardiopulmonary bypass, the patients were submitted to balloon angioplasty of the affected brachiocephalic arteries (11 patients) and stenting (2 patients), which allowed us to perform surgical correction of supravalvular aortic stenosis without significant risk. After balloon angioplasty, the mean area of the stenosis increased from $10.8 \pm 0.4 mm^2$ to $19.7 \pm 0.7 mm^2$. The first stage of treatment in one patient with congenital supravalvular aortic stenosis associated with congenital stenosis of the left common carotid artery and brachiocephalic trunk consisted of balloon angioplasty of the left common carotid artery and brachiocephalic trunk stenosis. It allowed us to perform surgical correction of supravalvular aortic stenosis as the second stage. However, there was a need for implantation of the 'Smart' stent (Cordis) 3.5 years later due to restenotic lesion of the brachiocephalic trunk.

Angiographic and hemodynamic results after endovascular procedures were good (Figure 59.12). No complications were encountered.

Conclusions

Endovascular methods of treatment of stenoses of proximal segments of the aortic arch branches can be a method of choice in the complex treatment of patients with congenital supravalvular aortic stenoses.

Our experience of 350 transcatheter closures of patent ductus arteriosus

Materials and methods

Three hundred and fifty patients with PDA underwent attempted transcatheter closure. Patients were from 5 months to 74 years old. Native and recanalized PDA closure was performed using Gianturco coils (COOK) in 331 patients, 'DuctOccluder' (PFM) in 4 patients, Amplatzer Duct Occluder (AGA Med. Corp.) in 11 patients and the Buttoned device Sideris in 4 patients (in one case the combination of coil and button device was used). Duct diameter varied from 1.1 to 12.0 mm. Gianturco coils and 'DuctOccluder' have been used for duct diameters less than 4.0 mm. The coil diameter was twice the duct diameter. In 6 cases with duct diameters of 4.5–6.0 mm, we implanted two coils simultaneously using two delivery catheters. In 15 patients with concomitant congenital heart diseases (aortic stenosis, coarctation of the aorta, pulmonary artery valvular stenosis (PAVS), PAVS and peripheral stenosis), we performed one-step endovascular procedures such as balloon angioplasties and valvuloplasties and PDA embolization.

Results

Complete occlusion of the duct was achieved in 319 patients (94.4%) (Figure 59.13). In 4 cases we could not implant coils because of ductal kinking, incompatibility of the DuctOccluder

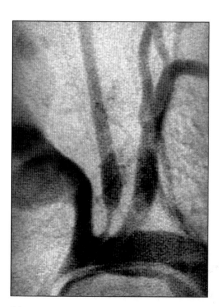 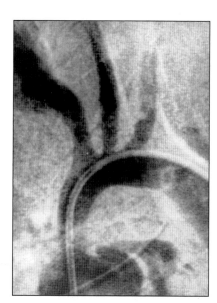

Figure 59.12
Transluminal balloon angioplasty of left common carotid artery.

(a) (b)

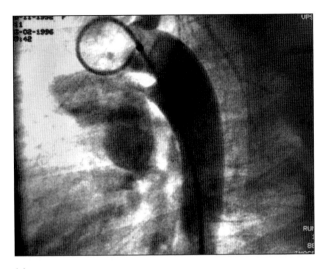

(a)

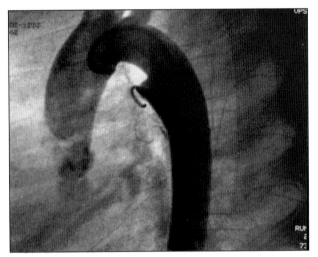

(b)

Figure 59.13
Transatheter patent ductus arteriosus closure using Gianturco coils.

and duct forms and PDA diameter greater than 6 mm. Coil migration to the PA occurred in 9 cases; all the coils were removed with a basket device. Complete closure was achieved in all the patients using the Amplatzer DuctOccluder and Buttoned device without complications. Long-term results (from 6 months to 6 years) were obtained in 230 patients. In 225 cases, we noted complete PDA occlusion; in 5 patients with incomplete duct closure, we performed repeated embolization, with coil implantation in 2 cases and the Buttoned device in 1 case.

Conclusion

Transcatheter closure of the PDA is an effective and non-traumatic method.

Transluminal coil embolization of the congenital coronary fistulae
Materials and methods

To 2003, 18 patients underwent attempted transluminal embolization of the coronary fistulae with Gianturco coils. Patients' age varied from 11 months to 44 years (mean 7.2 ± 2.7 years) and weight from 9 to 74 kg (mean 28 ± 3.1 kg). Localization and fistula diameter were determined after selective right and left coronary angiography. Four patients had the fistulae between the right coronary artery and RV, one between the posterior ventricular branch of the right coronary artery and RV, three between the right coronary artery and RA, two between the branch of the right

Figure 59.14
Transatheter closure of the coronary fistula between LAD and right ventricle.

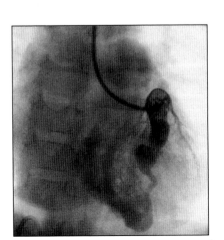

(a)

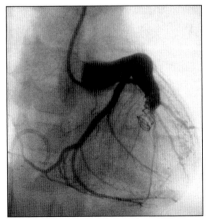

(b)

coronary artery and the trunk of the PA, four between the LAD and the RV, two between the Cx and the RV, and two between the Cx and the RA. Occlusive coil diameter was approximately twice the fistula diameter, and the number of the implanted coils was determined by the fistula size: from 2 to 20 coils were implanted in every patient.

Results

Complete coronary fistula occlusion was achieved in all of the nine cases (Figure 59.14). The following complications were noted: coil migration to the pulmonary artery in two patients (all the migrated coils were removed using a basket device), femoral artery thrombosis in two patients, and a wire-related perforation of the fistula in one case which led to immediate hemopericardium with complete fistula thrombosis.

Long-term results were obtained in 17 patients in 6 months to 16 years. All the patients led a regular life and had no complaints. A selective coronary angiography was carried out in 4 patients. Radionuclide test of myocardium was performed in 7 patients under loading conditions. The complete occlusion of the fistula was confirmed in all the cases.

Conclusion

Transluminal embolization of coronary fistulae is a safe and effective method.

References

1   Alekyan BG, Petrosyan YuS, Ilyin VN et al. Right subscapular artery approach for balloon valvuloplasty of congenital aortic valve stenosis in infants. *Cardiol Young* **3**(suppl 1): 75.

2   Alekyan BG, Petrosyan YuS, Coulson JC et al. Right subscapular artery for balloon valvuloplasty of critical aortic stenosis in infants. *Am J Cardiol* 1995; **76**: 1049–52.

3   Alekyan BG, Podzolkov VP, Pursanov MG et al. Transluminal balloon valvuloplasty of a stenosed systemic–pulmonary Blalock–Taussig anastomosis in congenital heart defects of 'blue' type *Grudnaya I serdechno-sosudistaya chirurgia* 1991; **11**: 10–14.

4   Alekyan BG, Podzolkov VP, Pursanov MG, Riumina EN. Stenting in a treatment of pulmonary artery pathology in patients with congenital heart defects. *Ann Chirurg* 1999; **6**: 91–100.

5   Alekyan BG, Pursanov MG. Stenting of pulmonary arteries in patients with congenital heart defects. *Ann Chirurg* 1998; 29–33.

6   Alekyan BG, Pursanov MG, Vedernikova LA et al. The first case of successful closure of aortopulmonary septum defect using 'Amplatzer Septal Occluder'. *Grudnaya I serdechno-sosudistaya chirurgia* 1998; **5**: 71–4.

7   Alekyan BG, Spiridonov AA, Harpunov VF et al. Transluminal balloon angioplasty and stenting in the treatment of aortic coarctation and re-coarctation. *Grudnaya I serdechno-sosudistaya chirurgia* 1996; **3**: 117–21.

8   Alekyan BG, Petrosyan YuS, Garibyan VA et al. Endovascular surgery in the treatment of congenital heart defects. *Ann Chirurg* 1996; **3**: 54–63.

9   Bockeria LA, Alekyan BG, Masura J et al. The first experience of transcatheter closure of atrial septal defect with 'Amplatzer Septal Occluder'. *Grudnaya I serdechno-sosudistaya chirurgia* 1998; **5**: 4.

10 Bockeria LA, Alekyan BG. Podzolkov VP. *Endovascular and Mini-Invasive Surgery of Heart and Vessels in Children*. Moscow, 1999.

60

Complications of peripheral interventions

Philip A Morales and Richard R Heuser

Since the first introduction of catheters in the vascular system for diagnostic or therapeutic purposes, the risk of adverse events (complications) occurring has existed. Fortunately, complications from diagnostic peripheral angiography or interventions are relatively uncommon and may be decreasing in frequency, in part due to advances in technology. As the role of percutaneous peripheral interventions increases, it is essential for those performing interventions to have a thorough understanding of the risks associated with the procedure, including the incidence and causes of complications. They should also understand the steps that should be taken to minimize the consequences when a complication occurs. These complications include the risks of the diagnostic study, in addition to the increased risks of the therapeutic modalities employed (i.e. thrombolysis, angioplasty, and stent placement).

The rate of complications varies, depending on how complications are defined and whether proper surveillance methods are employed to capture them.[1-4] Other factors influencing the complication rate are operator experience and never-ending technological improvements, which can either have a positive or negative impact on complications. For the individual patient, the risk of a complication occurring varies, depending on age, gender, vascular anatomy (renal artery, popliteal artery), clinical situation (intermittent claudication, critical limb ischemia), and the type of procedure (angioplasty, stenting).

One large review that continues to be referenced through the years is that of Becker et al.[1] They reviewed complications of 4662 published interventional procedures, which included peripheral and renal interventions. The total rate of complications observed was less then 10.1%, with the breakdown being 5.6% for major complications and less than 4.6% for minor complications. Major complications accounted for roughly half of the total complications; minor complications at the entry site (hematoma, pseudoaneurysm)

accounted for 3.7%. Surgery or other treatment was required in 2.5% of cases; limb or kidney loss was observed in 0.2%; and another 0.2% died. Of course, these complication rates were observed during the pre-stent era.

Another large review published more recently may reflect some of the same information from Becker's review.[5] Whereas the total numbers of procedures reviewed were in 3784 patients, the rates of complications were similar to the above: complications observed at the puncture site (bleeding, pseudoaneurysm, arteriovenous fistula) were 4.0%; complications observed at angioplasty site (thrombus, arterial rupture) were 3.5%. Dissection or embolization was observed in 2.7%, renal failure in 0.2%, and fatal myocardial infarction in 0.2%, and fatal cerebrovascular accident in 0.6%. Surgical repair was required in 2.0%, limb loss was observed in 0.2%, and mortality was 0.2%.

In one prospective series, a similar complication rate of 10.5% was noted, with 2.0% requiring operative repair.[2] Again, major complications constituted roughly half of the total complications. The most common complications in this series were thromboembolic vessel occlusions and puncture site injuries such as a hematoma or pseudoaneurysm. Less common were complications that occurred at the angioplasty site itself, including thrombosis, dissection, perforation, and occlusion.

Gardiner et al.[3] reviewed the complications of 453 angioplasties performed. The highest angioplasty complication rate occurred in the group with disease in the popliteal and distal vessels (19%). The lowest complication rate was observed in the group with iliofemoral disease (5%). Therefore, complications are also dependent on the location of the angioplasty. Complex lesions associated with long procedure times and multiple catheter manipulations and exchanges probably predispose to higher complication rates. Patient factors such as obesity can increase puncture site complications.

Complications can be classified as major (resulting in unplanned increase in the level of care, prolonged hospitalization, permanent adverse sequelae or death) or as minor with no long-term sequelae. They are also classified according to their specific site (puncture site, angioplasty site).

Puncture site

Adequate vascular access is essential in all diagnostic and interventional procedures. Consequently, it is not surprising that vascular complications at the puncture site are among the most common problems encountered. Potential complications include vessel thrombosis, bleeding, hematoma, pseudoaneurysm, or an arteriovenous fistula. If the bleeding is ongoing, then a poor puncture technique (i.e. arterial puncture above the inguinal ligament or posterior wall puncture), vessel laceration, excessive anticoagulation, or poor arteriotomy closure technique (i.e. manual compression, suture-mediated closure device) may be responsible.[6]

Comparison of complication rates between studies is difficult due to different complication definitions, different eras in which studies were performed, and different surveillance methods for capturing these complications. Pentecost et al.[5] reported the incidence of puncture site complications to be 4.0%, with bleeding/hematoma at 3.4%, pseudoaneurysm at 0.5%, and arteriovenous fistulae at 0.1%.

Vascular access

Familiarity and experience with the femoral artery makes it the most common site for vascular access. Reported vascular complications from the femoral artery site include significant blood loss, laceration of the femoral artery, retroperitoneal hematoma, pseudoaneurysm, arteriovenous fistula, arterial thrombosis, ischemia, femoral neuropathy, and infection. Overall complication rates have been reported from as low as less than 1% to greater than 10%.[1,6]

Other vascular access sites include the radial, brachial, and popliteal artery via retrograde approach. The retrograde radial and brachial approaches are useful for direct access to the subclavian arteries and less so for access to the arterial system below the aorta (i.e. iliac, femoral arteries). The retrograde popliteal artery approach is useful to gain direct access to the ipsilateral femoral artery. Antegrade femoral artery access is more technically challenging and less often used. This approach is very useful to gain direct access to the ipsilateral femoral and popliteal arteries. Complications from these access sites are similar to those from the retrograde femoral artery access site.[6,7]

Risk factors for the development of local vascular complications include female gender, increased body weight, uncontrolled high blood pressure, a large heparin dose, prolonged heparin use after intervention, use of a IIb/IIIa platelet inhibitor, older age, severity of peripheral vascular disease, low platelet count, and a need for a repeat intervention.

Bleeding/hematoma

Uncontrolled bleeding from the arterial puncture is the most common problem or complication encountered after the catheterization procedure.[6] Free bleeding may suggest a lacerated artery that may not respond by the placement of a larger French-size sheath. A hematoma, which is a collection of blood within the soft tissues, can form if this is not easily corrected. Usually, an uncomplicated hematoma will resolve within 1–2 weeks, as the blood is reabsorbed from the soft tissues. Rarely, a hematoma of significant size can compress the femoral nerve, causing a neuropathy.

A retroperitoneal bleed usually occurs with a femoral artery puncture (anterior or posterior wall) above the inguinal ligament. Although not clearly evident from the surface, a retroperitoneal bleed should be considered when there is unexplained hypotension, ipsilateral flank pain, and/or femoral neuropathy[8] that may not occur until a few hours after the procedure. A computed tomography (CT) scan or ultrasound will help confirm the diagnosis. These conditions can usually be treated by blood transfusion only, with a small percentage needing urgent vascular surgery.[8]

Pseudoaneurysm

Pseudoaneurysm occurs infrequently. Risk factors for the development of pseudoaneurysm have been reported to be the following: age greater than 70 years, female gender, multiple procedures during the index hospitalization, low platelet count, and hypertension.[9,10] One study reported that the puncture of the superficial femoral artery is an important but avoidable risk factor in the development of pseudoaneurysm.[9]

The need for active treatment depends on the size of the pseudoaneurysm, whether it has increased in size, and the need for continued anticoagulation. Very small pseudoaneurysms (< 1–2 cm in diameter) can be observed and they often close spontaneously (presumably by thrombosis). Somewhat larger pseudoaneurysms (2–3 cm in diameter) usually can be closed by ultrasound-guided compression, where the compression is aimed at the neck of the pseudoaneurysm. Large (> 3 cm) pseudoaneurysms are unlikely to spontaneously close; if ultrasound-guided compression fails in these cases, surgical correction is indicated because of the possibility of subsequent rupture with significant bleeding.[8] Success rates with ultrasound-guided compression are high in patients not receiving anticoagulation; they are lower but still reasonable in patients on anticoagulants.[11,12] Recently, the use of ultrasound-guided thrombin injection has been proved to be as efficacious as ultrasound-guided compression and is now considered the therapy of choice for femoral artery pseudoaneurysms.[13,14]

Arteriovenous fistula

Another local puncture site complication is the development of an arteriovenous fistula. Fistulas are not evident immediately and may take days to develop: they are recognized usually on routine follow-up by a to-and-fro continuous bruit over the puncture site.[15] The formation of an arteriovenous fistula usually occurs when entering either the superficial or profunda femoral artery and a venous branch, ultimately producing the fistulous connection.[16] Most arteriovenous fistulae after interventions are small and are not hemodynamically significant (Figure 60.1). Some will close spontaneously, whereas others remain unchanged for long periods. However, if these fistulae enlarge, then untoward long-term effects can occur, including accelerated atherosclerosis, an increase in arteriovenous shunting, and distal swelling and tenderness.

Symptomatic arteriovenous fistulae should undergo repair, but long-term observations have demonstrated that small asymptomatic fistulae usually remain stable and do not require surgical intervention. Recently, the use of a stent–graft on the arterial side of the fistula has been shown to be successful in a small cohort.[17]

Distal vessel complications

Distal embolization is an infrequent complication, occurring with a frequency up to 2.7%. Risk factors include a relatively large catheter or sheath size and severe peripheral vascular disease. Operator-induced access arterial dissection (Figure 60.2) or thrombus development also may be responsible. Symptoms and signs are typically those found for inadequate blood flow, including pain, pallor of the leg, cyanosis and coolness of the lower extremities, and lack of pulses.

Early corrective therapy is important in avoiding any increased morbidity or mortality associated with any delays. The first approach should be percutaneously with obtaining emergency vascular access through the contralateral vessel and performing angiography of the occluded side. Based on the arteriographic findings, local lytic therapy or angioplasty can be considered. If this fails, the second approach should be surgical. Systemic anticoagulation with heparin is advised. However, most operator-induced arterial dissections occur during retrograde advancement of the catheter or guide wire and the antegrade blood flow will usually 'tack down' the dissection or flap, requiring no further treatment.

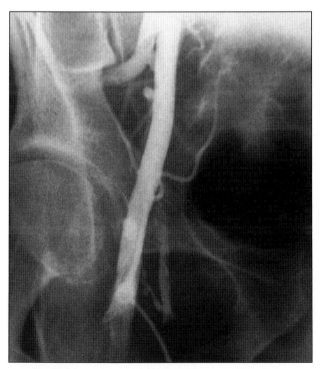

Figure 60.1
Angiographic appearance of an arteriovenous fistula with simultaneous filling of the right superficial femoral artery (left) and vein (right).

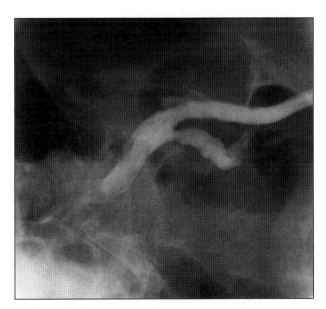

Figure 60.2
Angiographic appearance of a non-flow limiting arterial wall dissection of the left iliac artery caused by a guide wire.

Miscellaneous complications

A groin infection is a relatively rare complication that has been reported at a frequency of no higher than 0.2%.[6] A higher incidence should alert the laboratory to review the procedures for maintaining sterility. Risk factors may include performing a second procedure soon after the first at the same site with a hematoma present, or prolonged (> 24 hours) sheath placement at the access site. Another uncommon complication of an intervention is neuropathy. This may occur due to a large inguinal hematoma compressing the femoral nerve, a branch from a retroperitoneal bleed compressing the lumbar plexus, or from inadvertent injury to the femoral nerve during access. In most cases, recovery appears to occur slowly over time.

Femoral arteriotomy closure devices

Recently, femoral arteriotomy closure devices have been introduced in the catheterization laboratory.[18,19] They have evolved from the need to improve the closure of the arteriotomy created during the procedure and to decrease complications associated with manual or device compression.

Other benefits include the patient's overall comfort and ability to ambulate earlier. With several closure devices currently available, they are classified as fibrin/collagen-mediated devices (Angio-Seal™, Duett™)[20,21,23] or suture-mediated (Perclose™, Prostar-Plus™).[22] As with all new devices, there is a steep learning curve with the proper and safe use of them. The early use of these devices brought on reports from the surgical literature on complications that were considered different[24,25] and more devastating[26,27] than the usual complications experienced from manual compression (Figure 60.3). Dangas et al.[28] concluded that the early experience of arteriotomy closure devices did bring a comparatively higher rate of complications compared with manual compression. Although there was a higher rate of hematoma formation (9.3% vs 5.1%, $p < 0.001$) and incidence of bleeding (5.2% vs 2.5%, $p < 0.001$) with the closure devices, the rates of pseudoaneurysm and arteriovenous were similar between the two groups. On the contrary, Fram, et al.[1,29] reported a large series of patients with complication rates no different from those reported in the literature. Still other studies have shown that the use of closure devices can be safe,[19,22] even in patients with peripheral vascular disease,[30] and shorten the time to ambulation.

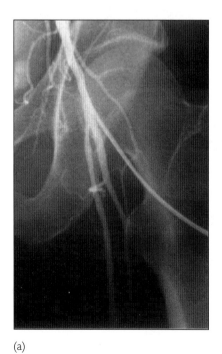

(a)

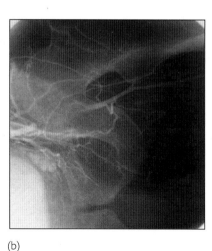

(b)

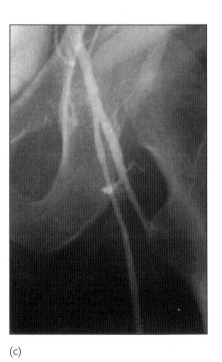

(c)

Figure 60.3
Femoral arterial thrombosis following deployment of a Duett™ closure device. (a) Patent right common femoral artery prior to deployment of the Duett™ device. (b) Acute arterial thrombosis in the right common femoral artery. (c) Recanalization of the right common femoral artery after thrombectomy therapy with the Angiojet™ system.

Angioplasty site

A second group of complications are related directly to the angioplasty site as well as distal to this site. These complications included acute vessel thrombosis, vessel dissection (Figure 60.4), perforation (Figure 60.5), and distal embolization. Bulky angioplasty equipment, high-profile compliant balloons, and lack of operator experience were part of the early years of peripheral intervention and the main reasons for complications to occur. With the miniaturization of the balloon catheter and its supporting equipment and the development of low-profile non-compliant balloons, these complications have decreased in frequency. Furthermore, the frequency of these complications has been greatly affected by the introduction of vascular stents. In the pre-stent era, most of these complications carried a substantial risk of mortality

and usually emergency surgery was the only option. Now, the true incidence of these complications (i.e. dissections), albeit smaller, may be under-reported. For example, a dissection at the site of angioplasty would be easily treated by the placement of a vascular stent with no significant adverse events, and would not be reported. Now with the recent introduction of covered stents, perforations and/or dissections can be treated percutaneously without the need for emergency surgery.[31]

Abrupt closure/thrombosis

In the era prior to stenting, balloon angioplasty carried the risk of abrupt closure or acute thrombosis of between 2 and

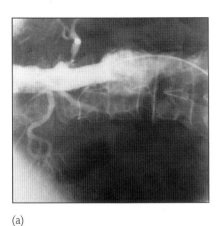
(a)

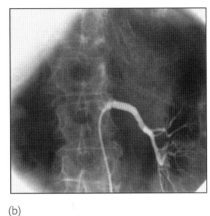
(b)

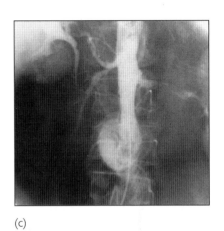
(c)

Figure 60.4
Renal artery dissection during angioplasty and stent placement. (a) Severe ostial stenosis of the left renal artery. (b) Angiogram following stent placement in the left renal artery. (c) Angiogram revealing dissection at the left renal artery.

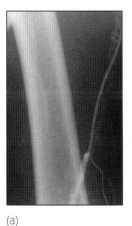
(a)

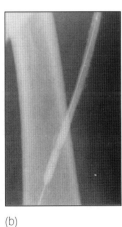
(b)

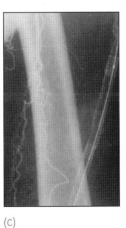
(c)

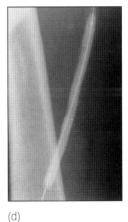
(d)

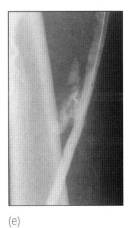
(e)

Figure 60.5
Superficial femoral artery perforation during angioplasty. (a) Total occlusion of the left superficial femoral artery. (b) Balloon angioplasty of the left superficial femoral artery. (c) Serial stent placements to a long segment of the left superficial femoral artery. (d) Post-stent balloon angioplasty. (e) Angiogram revealing perforation after post-stent balloon angioplasty.

4%.[1-3,5] Multivessel disease and complex lesions were predictors of acute occlusion during or after the procedure. Angiographic characteristics associated with abrupt closure with balloon angioplasty in early studies included long lesions, dissection, use of oversized balloons relative to the reference segment, residual stenosis of greater than 50%, intraluminal thrombus, and multivessel disease.

Abrupt closure mostly occurs shortly after balloon dilatation while the patient is still on the table, but a significant percentage may occur within the next 12 hours. It is rare for the adverse event to occur after 24 hours. Abrupt closure after balloon angioplasty is most commonly caused by dissection and is less likely to result from pure thrombosis, but it is frequently a combination of dissection and thrombus. Clinical features associated with an increased risk of abrupt closure include diabetes mellitus, inadequate antiplatelet therapy, female gender, and extreme age.

Stenting has essentially decreased abrupt closure at the end of the procedure to less than 1%. In most studies, it appears to be more effective than prolonged balloon inflation times. The superb angiographic results, ease of placement and a very low incidence of abrupt closure have urged most interventionalists to utilize stents in this situation.

Use of preprocedural aspirin has been shown to reduce abrupt closure during intervention. The dose of heparin intraprocedurally and the level of activated clotting time is unclear, but a level of greater than 300 s in the absence of a IIb/IIIa inhibitor has been suggested. With a IIb/IIIa inhibitor, a level of 250 s has been recommended, based on data showing less bleeding without an increase in recurrent ischemic events.

Acute/subacute stent thrombosis

Stent implantation has significantly transformed the therapy for peripheral vascular disease, with most of all interventions utilizing stents. With the introduction of stents, however, came the complication of acute and subacute stent thrombosis,[32] which initially had an unacceptably high rate of occurrence. A dramatic reduction in the rate of acute/subacute thrombosis has been related to improvements in deployment technique (i.e. high-pressure balloons) and post-stent placement antiplatelet therapy. For several years, different anticoagulation protocols were established and thoroughly investigated to determine their impact on decreasing the risk of subacute stent thrombosis.[33-6]. Recently, the combination of aspirin and clopidogrel has been shown to significantly reduce the incidence of subacute stent thrombosis.[35] Clopidogrel has replaced ticlopidine as the drug to prevent stent thrombosis in many centers because it has a simple dosing regimen and a safer hematological profile.[36] The vast majority of these post-stent antiplatelet/anticoagulation studies are with the use of coronary stents and not with peripheral stents. Given that the vascular biological response to stent placements may be somewhat similar in the coronary circulation compared to that in the peripheral circulation, many interventionalists will use the same if not similar antiplatelet regiment for post-stent placement therapy.

Systemic

Contrast-induced complications

Adverse effects of contrast media can be divided in two categories: anaphylactoid and toxic. Anaphylactoid reactions include urticaria, angioedema, bronchospasm, and cardiovascular collapse. Toxic effects include nausea, a hot flushing sensation, vascular congestion, metallic taste, arrhythmias – particularly bradycardia and asystole. The use of newer low-osmolar nonionic contrast media has decreased the incidence of adverse effects, especially arrhythmias.[6]

Contrast-induced nephropathy is generally defined as a greater than 0.5 mg/dl increase in serum creatinine within 48 hours of contrast exposure. The serum creatinine usually peaks within 4 to 5 days and in most cases returns to normal or near normal in 1–3 weeks. The incidence of contrast-induced nephropathy varies widely to as high as 70% in various populations undergoing catheterization.[37,38] The significant variation reflects the differences in the definition of nephropathy and the risk factors of the population undergoing the procedure.

The risk factors for developing contrast-induced nephropathy include pre-existing renal disease (serum creatinine > 1.5 mg/dl), diabetes mellitus, diabetic nephropathy, multiple myeloma, congestive heart failure, volume of contrast administered, and repeat dye exposure within 24 hours. Patients with pre-existing renal disease and diabetes seem to have the highest risk in developing contrast-induced nephropathy.

Until recently, the only effective strategy in preventing contrast-induced nephropathy was the use of aggressive hydration. Solomon et al.[39] revealed that saline infusion alone was superior to either mannitol or forced diuresis with furosemide in preventing contrast-induced nephropathy. Other trials using dopamine, aminophylline, or atrial natriuretic peptide have not shown any consistent benefit.[40,41] The use of fenoldopam mesylate, a selective dopamine A1 receptor agonist, and N-acetylcysteine (i.e. Mucomyst) are showing promise in the prevention of contrast-induced nephropathy:[38] they are currently the subjects of ongoing investigations into new renal protective agents. Other practical measures in preventing contrast-induced nephropathy are avoiding post procedural volume depletion, minimizing contrast volume use, and avoiding repeat contrast exposure within 48–72 hours.

Summary

Understanding the risks of peripheral interventions is essential for those performing invasive procedures. Given the variety of complex procedures now being performed, it is more difficult than ever to assess the various risks of these newer techniques. Minimizing vascular complications requires expertise with catheter insertion and manipulation, with balloon and stent sizing, and with anticoagulation regimens. New devices and techniques are rapidly being developed and are employed with enthusiasm. A careful evaluation of the potential complications associated with any new device is essential before it is accepted as an effective tool. When an adverse event does occur, the case should be reviewed to determine whether the event could have been avoided. A careful critical review of an interventionalist's own technique will only help to improve interventional outcomes and lower the risk of complications.

References

1   Becker GJ, Katzen BT, Dake MD. Noncoronary angioplasty. *Radiology* 1989; **170**: 921–40.

2   Matsi PJ, Manninen HI. Complications of lower-limb percutaneous transluminal angioplasty: a prospective analysis of 410 procedures on 295 consecutive patients. *Cardiovasc Intervent Radiol* 1999; **21**: 361–6.

3   Gardiner GA, Meyerovitz MF, Stokes KR et al. Complications of transluminal angioplasty. *Radiology* 1986; **159**: 201–8.

4   Leoni CJ, Potter JE, Rosen MP et al. Classifying complications of interventional procedures: a survey of practicing radiologists. *J Vasc Interv Radiol* 2001; **12**: 55–9.

5   Pentecost MJ, Criqui MH, Dorros G et al. Guidelines for peripheral percutaneous transluminal angioplasty of the abdominal aorta and lower extremity vessels. *Circulation* 1994; **89**: 511–31.

6   Baim DS, Grossman W. Complications of cardiac catheterization. In: *Cardiac catherization, angiography, and intervention*, 5th edn. Baltimore: Williams & Williams, 1996: 17–38.

7   Jenkins SJ. Vascular Access. In: Heuser RR (ed.). *Peripheral vascular stenting for cardiologists*. London: Martin Dunitz, 1999: 17–26.

8   Kent KC, Moscucci M, Mansour KA et al. Retroperitoneal hematoma after cardiac catherization: prevalence, risk factors, and optimal management. *J Vasc Surg* 1994; **20**: 905–10.

9   Moscucci M, Mansour KA, Kent KC et al. Peripheral vascular complications of directional coronary atherectomy and stenting: predictors, management, and outcome. *Am J Cardiol* 1994; **74**: 448–53.

10 Kent KC, McArdle CR, Kennedy B et al. A prospective study of the clinical outcome of femoral pseudoaneurysms and arteriovenous fistulas induced by arterial puncture. *J Vasc Surg* 1993; **17**: 125–31.

11 Moote DJ, Hilborn MD, Harris KA et al. Postarteriographic femoral pseudoaneurysms: treatment with ultrasound-guided compression. *Ann Vasc Surg* 1994; **8**: 325–31.

12 Cox GS, Young JR, Gray BR et al. Ultrasound-guided compression repair of postcatheterization pseudoaneurysms: results of treatment in one hundred cases. *J Vasc Surg* 1994; **19**: 683–6.

13 Calton WC, Franklin DP, Elmore JR et al. Ultrasound-guided thrombin injection is a safe and durable treatment for femoral pseudoaneurysms. *Vasc Surg* 2001; **35**: 379–83.

14 Reeder SB, Widlus DM, Lazinger M. Low-dose thrombin injection to treat iatrogenic femoral artery pseudoaneurysms. *Am J Roentgenol* 2001; **177**: 595–8.

15 Kent KC, McArdle CR, Kennedy B et al. Accuracy of clinical examination in the evaluation of femoral false aneurysm and arteriovenous fistula. *Cardiovasc Surg* 1993; **1**: 504–7.

16 Kim D, Orron DE, Skillman JJ et al. Role of superficial femoral artery puncture in the development of pseudoaneurysm and arteriovenous fistula complicating percutaneous transfemoral cardiac catheterization. *Cathet Cardiovasc Diagn* 1992; **25**: 91–7.

17 Meyer BT, Tautenhahn J, Halloul Z et al. Percutaneous treatment of rare iatrogenic arteriovenous fistulas of the lower limbs. *Int Surg* 1998; **83**: 198–201.

18 Aker UT, Kensey KR, Heuser RR et al. Immediate arterial hemostasis after cardiac catheterization: initial experience with a new puncture closure device. *Cathet Cardiovasc Diagn* 1994; **3**: 228–32.

19 Silber S, Gershony G et al. A novel vascular sealing device for closure of percutaneous arterial access sites. *Am J Cardiol* 1999; **83**: 1248–52.

20 Kussmaul WG, Buchbinder M, Whitlow PL et al. Femoral artery hemostasis using an implantable device (Angio-Seal) after coronary angioplasty. *Cathet Cardiovasc Diagn* 1996; **37**: 362–5.

21 Eggebrecht H, Haude M, von Birgelen C et al. Early clinical experience with the 6 French Angio-Seal device: immediate closure of femoral puncture sites after diagnostic and interventional coronary procedures. *Cathet Cardiovasc Interv* 2001; **53**: 437–42.

22 Baim DS, Knopf WD, Hinohara T et al. Suture-mediated closure of the femoral access site after cardiac catherization: results of the suture to ambulate and discharge (STAND I and STAND II) trails. *Am J Cardiol* 2000; **85**: 864–9.

23 Mooney MR, Ellis SG, Gershony G et al. Immediate sealing of arterial puncture sites after cardiac catheterization and coronary interventions: initial U.S. feasibility trial using the Duett vascular closure device. *Cathet Cardiovasc Interv* 2000; **50**: 96–102.

24 Pipkin W, Brophy C, Nesbit R. Early experience with infectious complications of percutaneous femoral artery closure devices. *J Vasc Surg* 2000; **32**: 205–8.

25 Nehler MR, Lawrence WA, Whitehill TA et al. Iatrogenic vascular injuries from percutaneous vascular suturing devices. *J Vasc Surg* 2001; **33**: 943–7.

26 Sprouse LR, Botta DM, Hamilton IN. The management of peripheral vascular complications associated with the use of percutaneous suture-mediated closure devices. *J Vasc Surg* 2001; **33**: 688–93.

27 Eidt JF, Habibipour S, Saucedo JF et al. Surgical complications from hemostatic puncture closure devices. *Am J Surg* 1999; **178**: 511–16.

28 Dangas G, Mehran R, Kokolis S et al. Vascular complications after percutaneous coronary interventions following hemostasis with manual compression versus arteriotomy closure devices. *J Am Coll Cardiol* 2001; **38**: 638–41.

29 Fram DB, Giri S, Jamil G et al. Suture closure of the femoral arteriotomy following invasive cardiac procedures: a detailed analysis of efficacy, complications, and the impact of early ambulation in 1200 consecutive, unselected cases. *Cathet Cardiovasc Interv* 2001; **53**: 163–73.

30 Balzer JO, Scheinert D, Diebold T et al. Postinterventional transcutaneous suture of femoral artery access sites in patients with peripheral arterial occlusive disease: a study of 930 patients. *Cathet Cardiovasc Interv* 2001; **53**: 174–81.

31 Scheinert D, Ludwig J, Steinkamp HJ et al. Treatment of catheter-induced iliac artery injuries with self-expanding endografts. *J Endovasc Ther* 2000; **7**: 213–20.

32 Sigwart U, Puel J, Mirkovitch V et al. Intravascular stents to prevent occlusion and restenosis after transluminal angioplasty. *N Engl J Med* 1987; **316**: 701–6.

33 Schatz RA, Baim DS, Leon M et al. Clinical experience with the Palmaz–Schatz coronary stent implantation with balloon angioplasty in patients with coronary artery disease. *N Engl J Med* 1994; **331**: 489–95.

34 Colombo A, Hall P, Nakamura S et al. Intracoronary stenting without anticoagulation accomplished with intravascular ultrasound guidance. *Circulation* 1995; **91**: 1676–88.

35 Berger PB, Bell MR, Rihal CS et al. Clopidogrel versus ticlopidine after intracoronary stent placement. *J Am Coll Cardiol* 1999; **34**: 1891–4.

36 Berger PB. Results of the Ticlid or Plavix Post-Stents (TOPPS) trial: do they justify the switch from ticlopidine to clopidogrel after coronary stent placement? *Curr Control Trials Cardiovasc Med* 2000; **1**: 83–7.

37 Porter GA. Contrast-associated nephropathy. *Am J Cardiol* 1989; **64**: 22E–26E.

38 Lepor NE. Radiocontrast nephropathy: the dye is not cast. *Rev Cardiovasc Med* 2000; **1**: 43–54.

39 Solomon R, Werner C, Mann D et al. Effects of saline, mannitol, and furosemide to prevent acute decreases in renal function induced by radiocontrast agents. *N Engl J Med* 1994; **331**: 1416–20.

40 Gare M, Haviv YS, Ben-Yehuda A et al. The renal effect of low-dose dopamine in high-risk patients undergoing coronary angiography. *J Am Coll Cardiol* 1999; **34**: 1682–8.

41 Abizaid AS, Clark CE, Mintz GS et al. Effects of dopamine and aminophylline on contrast-induced acute renal failure after coronary angioplasty in patients with preexisting renal insuffiency. *Am J Cardiol* 1999; **83**: 260–3.

61

Billing suggestions for peripheral vascular services

Roseanne R Wholey

Billing third-party carriers for the professional component of peripheral vascular services is a very complex responsibility that requires a detailed knowledge of anatomy as well as a comprehensive understanding of how to use the physicians' current procedural terminology (CPT) codes. CPT is the coding method developed by the Health Care Finance Administration (HCFA) for billing physician services to Medicare. Payment for CPT codes is based on a resource based relative value scale (RBRVS) for physician services performed, regardless of specialty.

Component coding and documentation

When submitting claims to third-party carriers for peripheral services, there are two components to consider:

- the surgical component, which includes both arteriotomy and percutaneous procedures: primarily the 30000 series CPT codes
- the supervision and interpretation (S&I) imaging component: the 70000 series CPT codes.

Many surgical services have a corresponding S&I code that can always be billed as a component of the surgical service. But there is not always a one-to-one correlation between a surgical code and an S&I code. Also, the procedures can vary significantly based on the puncture site(s), final position of the catheter(s), involvement of multiple vascular families, various transcatheter therapies, and the numerous imaging services that can be involved. Therefore, one approach does not apply to all situations.

From a documentation perspective, all services should be clearly spelled out. The coder (physician or someone specifically assigned by the practice) should know the puncture site, final position of the catheter within each vascular family, and all surgical and imaging services performed. The important thing to remember when submitting documentation to the third-party carriers is *that if it was not dictated, it was not done*.

Modifiers

Modifiers can assist the carriers in making proper payment determinations. A few important modifiers to consider when billing peripheral services are now considered.

–51 multiple surgical

Because there are frequently several surgical CPT codes billed on a claim form for a peripheral procedure, a –51 modifier helps the carrier to recognize the separately reimbursable multiple surgical services. These surgical services are subject to reductions in reimbursement by Medicare. The highest paid surgical service is reimbursed at 100% of the Medicare allowable. This service does not require a multiple surgical modifier. The subsequent surgical services require the addition of the –51 multiple surgical modifier and the next four services are paid at 50% of the Medicare allowable. If there are more than five surgical services, an operative report must be submitted documenting the services for a review by Medicare before an additional reimbursement can be considered. It is helpful to list the surgical codes in order of decreasing total relative value.

–59 distinct separate procedural service

This modifier can be used to indicate that a procedure was distinct or independent from other services performed on the same day. For example, if during a peripheral procedure a different vascular system is catheterized and the same catheter placement code is used more than once, i.e. bilateral renals, then a –59 modifier can be used to help the carrier recognize that the second catheter placement code is not a duplicate (see Example 3). This modifier can go before or after a –51 modifier.

–26 professional component

Peripheral vascular services are often performed in a hospital setting and the physician is billing for the S&I of the imaging studies while the hospital will bill for the *technical component*, i.e. operating budgets, supplies, overhead for utilities, capital equipment, short stay/patient stays. The technical component will also vary, dependent on inpatient vs outpatient procedures.

The physician bill for the 70000 series imaging codes should be submitted with a –26 professional component modifier, assuming the physician/group does not own the equipment which is being used. If the physician/group owns the equipment, then this modifier would not be used.

The imaging codes do not incur payment reductions and all 70000 series codes should be reimbursed at 100% of the Medicare allowable.

Three-sheet billing system

The following three-sheet billing system helps to identify the separately billable CPT procedure codes for peripheral vascular services.

Selective and non-selective vascular catheterizations

The first spreadsheet (Tables 61.1a and 61.1b) identifies the catheter placement codes for selective arterial and venous catheter placements in various vascular families as well as non-selective catheter placement codes. Each selective catheter placement within different vascular families should be coded separately to the highest level placement within each vascular family.

Dependent upon where it is positioned, selective catheterization can take on first-, second-, or third-order catheter placement. Let's look at an example. Needle puncture done from the ipsilateral side into the right femoral artery; the catheter is then manipulated through the superficial femoral artery (SFA) followed by popliteal and then eventually to anterior tibial:

- catheter initially placed in primary vessel, SFA (first order)
- catheter then manipulated through secondary vessel, popliteal (second order)
- catheter then finally positioned at the anterior tibial, which is a tertiary vessel (third order).

The highest level placement would be third order in the anterior tibial.

Non-selective catheterizations do not have first-, second-, or third-order catheter placement codes

Supervision and interpretation

The second sheet (Tables 61.2a and 61.2b) lists the various preprocedure imaging codes for arteriography and venography, respectively.

Transcatheter therapy

The third sheet (Table 61.3) identifies the various transcatheter therapies and the corresponding supervision and interpretation codes. (The 'open' or arteriotomy codes are used instead of the percutaneous codes when a cutdown is performed.)

The sheets (tables) can be utilized as a check sheet system for identifying the services performed. Also, a column can be added for the physician fee schedule. This column can be completed with a current fee schedule allowance, such as the Federal Register RVUs, the Medicare fee schedule, or any other fee schedule of choice for easy reference. Then that sheet can be the master charge sheet for that year. Based on the services performed, the number of sheets used may vary.

Case examples
Example 1: abdominal aortogram with runoff

If from a femoral puncture site the catheter is placed into the aorta and an abdominal aortogram with runoff is performed, only two sheets would be used. The non-selective catheter code 36000 on the first sheet (see Table 61.1b) would be checked and the aortogram with runoff code 75630 on the second sheet (see Table 61.2a) would be checked off.

Table 61.1a Procedural codes for selective vascular catheterizations

Selective vascular catheterizations	Procedural codes			
	1st order	2nd order	3rd order	Each additional order
Arterial vascular catheterizations (puncture-site dependent)				
Brachiocephalic (Right carotid/subclavian)	36215	36216	36217	36218
Left carotid	36215	36216	36217	36218
Left subclavian	36215	36216	36217	36218
Other vascular family (above diaphragm)	36215	36216	36217	36218
Celiac	36245	36246	36247	36248
SMA	36245	36246	36247	36248
IMA	36245	36246	36247	36248
Right renal	36245	36246	36247	36248
Left renal	36245	36246	36247	36248
Iliac ipsilateral internal	36245	36246	36247	36248
Common iliac contralateral	36245	36246	36247	36248
Common femoral ipsilateral	36140			
Antegrade femoral	36245	36246	36248	36248
Other vascular family (below diaphragm)	36245	36246	36248	36248
Right heart or pulmonary trunk only	36013			
Left pulmonary		36014	36015	36015
Right pulmonary		36014	36015	36015
Venous vascular catheterizations (puncture-site dependent)				
Right renal	36011	36012	36012	36012
Left renal	36011	36012	36012	36012
Jugular	36011	36012	36012	36012
Left adrenal		36012	36012	36012
Right adrenal	36011	36012	36012	36012
Epidural	36011	36012	36012	36012
Selective organ blood sampling				36500
Other venous vascular family	36011	36012	36012	36012

Table 61.1b Procedural codes for non-selective vascular catheterizations

Non-selective vascular catheterizations	(No catheter placement order) Procedural code
Aorta, catheter (femoral or axillary approach)	36200
Carotid or vertebral artery	36100
Retrograde brachial artery	36120
Extremity artery needle or intracatheter, unilateral	36140
Extremity artery needle or intracatheter, bilateral	36140 × 2
Aorta, translumbar	36160
Arteriovenous dialysis shunt	36145
Extremity vein needle or intracatheter, unilateral	36000
Extremity vein needle or intracatheter, bilateral	36000 × 2
Superior or inferior vena cava catheter	36010
Injection for contrast venography	36005

Table 61.2a   Supervision and interpretation (S&I) codes for arteriography

Arteriography	Code
Thoracic aortogram without serialography	75600
Thoracic aortogram	75605
Abdominal aortogram	75625
Abdominal aortogram with runoff	75630
Cervicocerebral (arch)	75650
Brachial, retrograde	75658
Carotid external, unilateral	75660
Carotid external, bilateral	75662
Carotid cerebral, unilateral	75665
Carotid cerebral, bilateral	75671
Carotid cervical, unilateral	75676
Carotid cervical, bilateral	75680
Vertebral, intracranial only	75685
Vertebral, intracranial and unilateral cervical	75685
Vertebral, intracranial and bilateral cervical	75685 × 2
Vertebral, cervical, unilateral	75685
Vertebral, cervical, bilateral	75685 × 2
Spinal selective each vessel	75705 ×
Extremity, unilateral	75710
Extremity, bilateral	75716
Renal, unilateral (with or without flush)	75722
Renal, bilateral (with or without flush)	75724
Visceral (with or without flush) each vessel	75726 ×
Adrenal, unilateral	75731
Adrenal, bilateral	75733
Pelvic each vessel	75736 ×
Pulmonary, unilateral	75741
Pulmonary, bilateral	75743
Pulmonary non-selective	75746
Arteriovenous dialysis shunt	75790
Each additional vessel after basic	75774 ×
Angio through existing catheter	75898

Table 61.2b   Supervision and interpretation (S&I) codes for venography

Venography	Codes
Extremity, unilateral	75820
Extremity, bilateral	75822
Inferior vena cava	75825
Superior vena cava	75827
Renal, unilateral	75831
Renal, bilateral	75833
Adrenal, unilateral	75840
Adrenal, bilateral	75842
Sinus or jugular	75860
Superior sagittal sinus	75870
Epidural	75872
Orbital	75880
Hepatic with hemodynamic evaluation	75889
Hepatic without hemodynamic evaluation	75891
Venous samplings (e.g. renins)	75893 ×

Table 61.1a) would be checked. Code 75710 would be checked on the second sheet (see Table 61.2a) for the unilateral extremity angiogram. On the third sheet (see Table 61.3), code 35474 PTA femoral artery and the corresponding S&I code 75962 would be checked off.

Suggested codes:
Surgical
35474   PTA femoral artery
36245-51   First-order catheter placement
Imaging
75710-26   Angiogram unilateral extremity
75962-26   PTA S&I

Suggested codes:
Surgical
36200   Catheter to aorta
Imaging
75630-26   Aortogram with runoff

Example 2: unilateral extremity angiogram, PTA of SFA

The coding would get more complicated if, from a right femoral puncture site, a catheter was placed into the right SFA and a unilateral extremity angiogram was performed prior to a percutaneous transluminal angioplasty (PTA) of the SFA. In this case, all three coding sheets are necessary. The first-order catheter placement code 36245 on the first sheet (see

Example 3: Bilateral renal angiograms and PTA of renals

Another example would be if from a right femoral puncture site a catheter is placed selectively into both right and left renal arteries for bilateral renal angiograms. Both renal arteries are subsequently angioplastied. In this case, two selective arterial catheter placement codes, 36245 and another 36245, on the first sheet (see Table 61.1a) would be selected for the catheter placement into both renal arteries. On the second sheet (see Table 61.2a) the bilateral renal angiogram code 75724 would be checked off. On the third sheet (see Table 61.3) two renal angioplasty codes, 35471 and 35471, would be indicated in addition to the two corresponding S&I codes of 75966 for the first vessel and 75968 for the S&I for the second vessel.

Table 61.3 Procedural codes and supervision and interpretation codes for transcatheter therapy, (S&I) atherectomy and ultrasound

Therapy	Arteriotomy procedural codes	Percutaneous procedural codes	S&I codes
Transcatheter therapy			
Infusion for thrombolysis		37201	75896
Infusion for non-thrombolytic		37202	75896
Embolization, non-neuro		37204	75894
Embolization, intracranial or spinal		61624	75894
Embolization, extracranial		61626	75894
Exchange previously placed arterial catheter during thrombolysis		37209	75900
Percutaneous transcatheter retrieval foreign body		37203	75961
PTA tibioperoneal artery and branches	35459	35470	75962
PTA renal or visceral artery	35450	35471	75966
PTA aorta	35452	35472	75966
PTA iliac artery	35454	35473	75962
PTA femoral – popliteal arteries	35456	35474	75962
PTA brachiocephalic arteries	35458	35475	75962
PTA venous	35460	35476	75978
PTA each additional peripheral vessel			75964
PTA each additional visceral vessel			75968
Cannula declotting with balloon catheter		36861	75894
Percutaneous placement of IVC filter		37620	75940
Angiography through existing catheter			75898
Intravascular stent	37207	37205	75960
Stent each additional	37208	37206	75960
Atherectomy			
Renal	35480	35490	75994
Visceral	35480	35490	75995
Aortic	35481	35491	75995
Iliac	35482	35492	75992
Femoral/popliteal	35483	35493	75992
Brachiocephalic	35484	35494	75992
Tibioperoneal trunk/branches	35485	35495	75992
Each additional visceral artery			75996
Each additional peripheral artery			75993
Ultrasound			
Intravascular ultrasound initial vessel		37250	75945
Intravascular ultrasound each additional vessel		37251	75946

IVC – inferior vena cava; PTA = percutaneous transluminal angioplasty.

Suggested codes:

Surgical

35471	PTA renal artery
35471-51-59	PTA renal artery
36245-51	First-order catheter placement
36245-51-59	First-order catheter placement

Imaging

75724-26	Angiogram bilateral renal arteries
75966-26	PTA S&I
75968-26	PTA S&I each additional vessel

Example 4: Unilateral extremity angiogram, SFA PTA, stent of SFA, PTA peroneal

Finally, from a left femoral puncture site the catheter is placed into the right iliac artery for a unilateral extremity angiogram. The catheter is then placed into the right SFA and the vessel is angioplastied with suboptimal results. A stent is subsequently deployed. The catheter is then placed more distally into the peroneal artery and this vessel is angioplastied.

Suggested codes:

Surgical

35470	PTA tibioperoneal trunk
35474-51	PTA femoral artery
37205-51	Stent
36247-51	Third-order catheter placement

Imaging

75710-26	Angiogram unilateral extremity
75960-26	Stent S&I
75962-26	PTA S&I
75964-26	PTA S&I each additional vessel

Reimbursement

It is important to remember that there is no guarantee that all services will be paid by the various payor plans. Individuals working for the third-party carriers may even misinterpret the regulations. Payment on services may initially be denied, requiring an appeal with additional documentation attached. It is helpful to diagram multiple services and highlight the procedures on the operative report. The diagnosis must also justify the services rendered and the ICD-9 diagnosis codes must be recorded to the highest level of specificity. It is a good idea to try to get policy guidelines from the carriers for these procedures if possible.

Index

AAA *see* abdominal aortic aneurysm
abciximab 329, 336, 351, 516
abdominal aortic aneurysm (AAA) 43–5, 65, 71, 194, 195, 234, 385–91, 413
abdominal aortic angiogram 8, 11, 12
abdominal aortic occlusion 363, 426
abdominal aortogram 10
ABI *see* ankle-brachial index
abrupt closure 537–8
abscesses 441
access sites 245
ACEIs *see* angiotensin-converting enzyme inhibitors
acidemia 164
ACT *see* activated clotting time
actinomycin 177, 178
activated clotting time (ACT) 164, 194
activated protein C 396
acute lower limb ischemia (ALLI) 163
acute stent thrombosis 538
addiction 442
adenovirus 493
ALLI *see* acute lower limb ischemia
altepase 165, 171
amaurosis 348
aminoglycosides 442
amputation 2, 163, 443
anastomosis 406
Ancure 414
anemia 463
anesthesia 394
AneuRx 414
aneurysm neck 73–4, 387
aneurysmal sac 398
aneurysms 182, 258, 302–3, 371
angina 475
Angio-Seal 517

angiogenic growth factors 495
angiographic patency 216
angiography 95, 164, 324
angiography suites 52
angioplasty 21, 22, 27, 35, 201, 204, 286, 310, 319, 426, 471, 537
angioscopy 108
angiotensin-converting enzyme inhibitors (ACEIs) 278
ankle-brachial index (ABI) 2, 15, 153, 191, 405
antecubital fossa 87–8
antegrade femoral catheterization 79–80
antegrade percutaneous popliteal approach 95–6
antibiotics 441
anticoagulation 306
antiplatelet therapy 15, 328, 329, 394, 396, 444
antithrombin III 396
antithrombotic agents 514–16
aorta 30
aortic aneurysms 30, 393–8
aortic arch 5
aortic coarctation 523–4
aortitis 372
aortoarteritis 150, 425–9
aortobifemoral bypass 201, 363
aortoiliac artery angioplasty 191–8
aortoiliac balloon angioplasty 192
aortoiliac occlusive disease 63–4, 191, 244
aortopulmonary septal defect (APSD) 527
apparent heart failure 300
APSD *see* aortopulmonary septal defect
archiving 55
arterial access techniques 79–85
arterial duplex ultrasonography 15
arterial embolization 323
arterial lesions 449
arterial occlusive disease 108, 420

arterial remodeling 478–9

arterial spasm 90

arterial traumas 258, 417–18

arteriosclerotic lesions 273

arteriovenous dialysis grafts (AVG) 485, 490

arteriovenous fistulas (AVFs) *see also* native arteriovenous fistulas 239, 258, 419, 439, 535

arteriovenous malformations (AVMs) 448, 454, 455

arteritis 309

aspirin 130, 192, 246, 326, 515

assisted primary patency 216

atherectomy 126

AtheroCath directional atherectomy catheter 135–6

atheroembolism 279, 289, 290

atheromatous ablation 138

atheromatous aneurysms 376

atherosclerosis 1, 293, 309, 324, 406, 476, 497, 501

atherosclerotic aneurysms 371

atherosclerotic plaque 328

attachment site 72–3

autogenous vein 62

AVFs *see* arteriovenous fistulas

AVG *see* arteriovenous dialysis grafts

AVMs *see* arteriovenous malformations

axillofemoral bypass 64

bacteremia 462

bacterial infection 441–2

balloon angioplasty 101–6, 181, 243, 323, 333, 523–4

balloon catheters 101–2, 488

balloon dilatation catheters 39–40

balloon expandable stents 41, 248

balloon valvuloplasty 521–2

basilar arteries 323

baskets 188

Behçet's syndrome 372

beta radiation 487

betadine 444

billing 541–6

biodegradable particles 447–8

bivalirudin 515

bleeding 534

BMI *see* body mass index

body mass index (BMI) 503

brachial access 245, 311, 408

brachial arteries 30
    access 83

brachiocephalic arteries 363, 528–9

brachiocephalic guide catheters 355

brachytherapy 259, 478, 479, 485, 489

bradycardia 334

brainstem 324

Brescia-Cimino type AVFs 457

bronchial embolization 450, 451

Budd-Chiari syndrome 473

Buerger's disease 431, 439

buttock claudication 231, 234, 398

bypass conduits 62

bypass stenosis 255–7, 485

CABG *see* coronary artery bypass grafting

calcium channel blockers 478

cancer 443

captopril renal scintigraphy 278, 302

carbon dioxide 295, 394

carbon dioxide angiography 10, 15, 398, 442

cardiac catheterization suites 52

carotid angioplasty and stenting (CAS) 334–8, 341–52, 355–61, 476

carotid arteries
    lesions 427
    pseudoaneurysm 419
    ultrasound 19, 27–9

carotid bifurcation 5, 19

carotid bruits 1

carotid embolization 316

carotid endarterectomy (CE) 21, 337, 341

carotid injections 6, 7

carotid plaques 20–1

carotid stenosis
    Doppler criteria 20
    surgical treatment 66–8

carotid stenting 21, 27, 333

CAS *see* carotid angioplasty and stenting

catheter-directed thrombolytic therapy (CDTT) 163, 171–4, 270

catheters 185–6, 244, 487–8

cavapulmonary anastomoses 524–5

CB *see* cutting balloon

CCA *see* common carotid artery

CCRAO *see* complete chronic renal artery occlusion

CDTT *see* catheter-directed thrombolytic therapy

CE *see* carotid endarterectomy

celiac angioplasty 305–7

cerebral embolization 350

cerebral ischemia 316

cerebral protection devices 312, 341, 345

cerebrovascular accidents 341

certification 57–9

CFA *see* common femoral artery

CHD *see* coronary heart disease

chemotherapy 469

children 426
cholesterol atheroembolism 279, 290
cholesterol emboli 394
chronic obstructive pulmonary disease (COPD) 371
chronic total occlusions (CTO) 153–60, 213
chylothorax 316
cilostazol 16, 244
claudication 243, 475
    buttock 231, 234
    intermittent 1, 2, 3, 16, 244
CLI see critical limb ischemia
clopidogrel 16, 130, 194, 326, 538
coils 448
collagen 448
common carotid artery (CCA) 342
common femoral artery (CFA) 393
complete chronic renal artery occlusion (CCRAO) 294
complications 259, 533–9
component coding 541
composite grafts 62
compression syndrome 309
computed tomography (CT) 153, 191, 202, 278, 294, 310, 324, 371, 475
congenital aneurysms 372
congenital coronary fistulae 530–1
congenital heart defects 521–31
congestive heart failure 281, 299, 497
contralateral access 245
contrast arteriography 15
contrast media 289, 538
contrast-induced nephropathy 538
Cook Zenith device 415
COPD see chronic obstructive pulmonary disease
Cordis-Quantum stent-graft 416
Corinthian stent 313
coronary arteries 429
coronary artery bypass grafting (CABG) 364
coronary heart disease (CHD) 244, 443, 476, 501
Corvita endoluminal graft 248, 402
coumadin 171
covered stents 248–9, 254–5, 259, 413, 420
CPT see current procedural terminology
cranial nerve palsies 341
critical limb ischemia (CLI) 431–45
crossover bypasses 63, 226
cryotherapy 478, 480
CTO see chronic total occlusions
current procedural terminology (CPT) codes 541
curved catheter 185
cutting balloon (CB) angioplasty 149–52
cyanotic congenital heart defects 527–8

DCA see directional coronary atherectomy
debris migration 349
debulking 123, 219–20, 479
debulking devices 45–6
deep vein thrombosis (DVT) 167, 171
delivery routes 496
depression 442–3
descending thoracic aortic aneurysms 45, 371–82, 426
device navigation 71–2
diabetes mellitus 2, 177, 313, 328, 431, 475, 497
diabetic neuropathy 495
diagnostic catheters 37–8
dialysis 442
diet 445, 506
difficult groin 82
digital subtraction angiography (DSA) 306, 341
dilatation 101
direct stenting 249
directional atherectomy 46, 116, 138
directional coronary atherectomy (DCA) 119
dissecting aneurysms 371, 533
distal arteries 129–33
distal embolism 300, 396, 405, 409, 439, 535
dizziness 327
dobutamine echocardiograms 443
Doppler imaging 19–23, 95
dosimetry 486
drug-eluting stents 177–80, 436
DSA see digital subtraction angiography
Duett 517
duplex sonography 15, 475
DVT see deep vein thrombosis
dyslipidemia 313
dystrophic aneurysms 372

ECA see external carotid artery
ECs see endothelial cells
edema 442, 473
EDV see end diastolic velocity
elastic recoil 328
electrocardiograms 443
electromechanical mapping (EMM) 496
ELGs see endoluminal stent-grafts
emboli protection devices (EPDs) 355
embolic agents 447–8
embolisms 116, 206, 209, 396–7, 447–55
EMM see electromechanical mapping
enarterectomy thrombosis 316
end diastolic velocity (EDV) 20
endarterectomy 21
endograft migration 390

endografts 42
endoleaks 231, 234, 388–9, 393, 395–6, 397–8
endoluminal grafts 43–5, 408
endoluminal stent-grafts (ELGs) 373, 374, 408
endometritis 233
endoprostheses 204–5, 209, 347, 414–22
endothelial cells (ECs) 477, 478
endothelium 513
endovascular equipment 35–48
endovascular intervention suite 51–6
endovascular therapy 1–3, 243
EPDs see emboli protection devices
epinephrine 441
erectile dysfunction 231
ethanol 448
excimer laser angioplasty 46, 221–3, 227
exercise 16, 509
external carotid artery (ECA) 342
external radiation 487
extracranial carotid artery disease 443
extracranial vertebral artery 323–9

facilities 59
false aneurysms 372
fasciotomy 444
fasting serum glucose 503
femoral access 79–82, 93, 108, 310–11, 375, 425,
    470
femoral aneurysms 406
femoral arteries
    balloon angioplasty 101–2
    closure devices 536
    thrombosis 369
femoral artery disease 177
femoral bifuraction 108, 432–3
femoropopliteal aneurysms 246
femoropopliteal artery occlusions 220–8, 243–59
femoropopliteal bypass 62
femoropopliteal lesions 244, 476
femoropopliteal PTA 246
femoropopliteal stenoses 245
femoropopliteal stenting 246
fever 393, 397, 405
fibreoptic guide wires 159
fibrinogen 164
fibrinolysis 203, 208–9, 244, 318, 515
fibroids 231
fibromuscular dysplasia 293, 301–2, 309, 316, 476
filters 312, 351
'flash' pulmonary edema (FPE) 293, 300
fluoroscopy equipment 53

foot hygiene 445
foot ulcerations 15
forceps 187, 189
foreign body retrieval 185–8
FPE see 'flash' pulmonary edema
Frontrunner TM CTO catheter 156
frostbite 439
functional neuroangiography 4–13

gadolinium 11, 294, 442
gamma radiation 487
gangrene 61, 196, 431, 439, 442
Gelfoam 447–8
gene therapy 180, 493–8
giant cell aortitis 372
Gianturco coils 236
glycoprotein IIb/IIIa inhibitors 336, 516
Gore Excluder endoprosthesis 415
graft failure 269
graft infection 462
growth factors 478
guide catheters 38–9
guide wire control system 157
guide wires 36–7, 219

hematomas 90–1, 259, 300, 533, 534
Hemobahn endoprosthesis 248
hemodialysis access 457–65
hemodynamic assessment 20
hemolysis 115
hemoptysis 450
hemorrhage 397
hemostasis 94, 513–18
heparin 96, 171, 394, 396, 444, 514–15
hepatocarcinoma 453
high-flow priapism 449
high-speed rotation 54
hirudin 515
histamine 476
histology 153
HMG-CoA 505
HO see hyperbaric oxygen
home care 444
Horner's syndrome 316
Horton's disease 372
hydration 538
hyperbaric oxygen (HO) 443–4
hypercholesterolemia 1, 371, 443, 497
hyperhomocysteinemia 2
hyperkalemia 164
hyperlipoproteinemia 220

hypersplenism 450
hypertension 1, 220, 299, 313, 475, 497
hypervascular tumor embolization 452
hypogastric artery 231–41
hypolipidemic agents 478
hypotension 334, 394

iliac aneurysms 239, 403, 406–7
iliac angioplasty 231
iliac artery 15, 31–2, 74, 196–7, 234, 235, 429, 432
iliac occlusions 201–11, 213–20, 227–8
iliofemoropopliteal aneurysms 406
illoprost 439
IMA see inferior mesenteric artery
imaging techniques 53–4
impotency 231
in-stent restenosis 177
infection 185, 398, 406
infectious aneurysms 372
inferior limb ischemia 363
inferior mesenteric artery (IMA) 12, 389
inferior vena cava (IVC) syndrome 469–73
inflammatory aneurysms 372
infragenicular PTA 263–7
infrainguinal occlusive disease 17, 61–3
infrapopliteal bypass 62–3
infrapopliteal vessels 3, 438–9
infrarenal aorta 431–2
inominate arteries 309, 350, 427
intermittent claudication 1, 2, 3, 16, 244
Internet 444
intestinal ischemia 396
intimal hyperplasia 273, 477–8
intracardiac thrombi 163
intravascular ultrasound (IVUS) 25–34, 104, 108, 137, 375, 403, 475
intravenous urography 278
introducer sheaths 35–6, 94
ipsilateral access 245
ischemia 244
ischemic sciatic neuropathy 398
ischemic ulcerations 196, 431
isotopes 486
IVC see inferior vena cava
IVUS see intravascular ultrasound

Jostent coronary stent graft 249

kidney rupture 301
kinking 408
kissing technique 203, 209, 312, 316

laparoscopic clipping 389
laser recanalization 204, 215, 222
lasers 116, 155, 219, 221–2, 478
LDL see low-density lipoprotein
lesions 201, 344–5, 533
limb salvage 167, 264, 431–45
lipid disorders 501–10
liquid agents 448
LMWH see low-molecular-weight heparin
loop snares 186–7, 189
lovastatin 1
low-density lipoprotein (LDL) receptor deficiency 497
low-molecular-weight heparin (LMWH) 515
lower extremity angiogram 9, 10
lower extremity bypass failure 269–74
lower limb arterial disease 22–3, 243
lower limb ischemia 272
lysis therapy 213

magnetic resonance angiography (MRA) 28, 29, 153, 278, 310, 324
magnetic resonance arteriography 15
magnetic resonance imaging (MRI) 202, 294, 310, 324, 475
malperfusion syndrome 377
Marfan syndrome 406
matrix metalloproteinases (MMP) 397, 478
maximum intensity projection (MIP) protocol 294
MDV see median density value
mechanical agents 448
mechanical recanalization 202–3
mechanical thrombectomy 45, 203, 209, 244, 396, 463
median density value (MDV) 343
Medtronic AVE stents 248
medullar ischemia 373
Megalink stents 248
MEPs see motor-evoked potentials
Mercaine 442
mesenteric angioplasty 305–7
mesenteric arteries 429
metalloproteinase-3 397
metalloproteinase-9 397
MI see myocardial infarction
microemboli 20
microfibrillar collagen 448
microspheres 448
MIP see maximum intensity projection
MMP see matrix metalloproteinases
modifiers 541–2
MollRing Cutter R 156
motor-evoked potentials (MEPs) 373

MPR *see* multiplanar reformatting
MRA *see* magnetic resonance angiography
MRI *see* magnetic resonance imaging
multiplanar reformatting (MPR) 294
multiple stents 267
multivascular atherosclerosis 363–9
mural thrombus 476–7
myocardial infarction (MI) 344, 356, 501

native arteriovenous fistulas 457–61
NBCA (n-isobutyl cyanocrylate) 448
neck dilatation 387
neck lymph fistula 316
neonates 525
nephrosclerosis 289
nephrotoxicity 289
neurofibromatosis 309
Nicolaides' method 343
nitinol 195, 248
nitinol stents 253–4
nitric oxide 513
non-covered stents 408
non-invasive testing 2

occluders 527
OCR *see* optical coherence reflectometry
omentopexy 439
optical coherence reflectometry (OCR) 156
optimal atherectomy 123–4
Orthner's disease 305
ostial lesions 286, 296, 328, 433
outpatient balloon angioplasty 105

P-selecting 476
PAA *see* pulmonary artery atresia
PAAAs *see* para-anastomotic aneurysms
paclitaxel 177, 178–9, 479
PAD *see* peripheral arterial disease
pain 442
pain-free walking distances (PFWD) 16
Palmaz stents 248, 251, 413, 470
para-anastomotic aneurysms (PAAAs) 417
parallax 54
paraplegia 379
Parodi endograft 385–6
patch angioplasty 166
patent ductus arteriosus (PDA) 527, 529–30
patient selection 244, 341–2
PAVS *see* pulmonary artery valvular stenosis
PDA *see* patent ductus arteriosus
PDGF *see* platelet-derived growth factor

PE *see* pulmonary edema
peak systolic velocity (PSV) 20
pedal pulse 1
pelvic angiogram 9
penile anatomy 231
pentoxifylline 16
Perclose 517
PercuSurge Guardwire 285–91, 312, 325, 341–52
percutaneous carotid intervention 334
percutaneous closure devices 47, 84–5
percutaneous declotting 463
percutaneous intentional extraluminal (subintimal)
    recanalization (PIER) 155
percutaneous intervention 153, 179
percutaneous peripheral atherectomy 107–16, 135–46
percutaneous transluminal angioplasty (PTA)
    aortoarteritis 429
    AVF nonmaturation 458
    balloon angioplasty 39, 101
    clinical trials 356
    extracranial vertebral artery 323–9
    femoropopliteal arteries 244
    iliac arteries 196, 201, 213, 432
    intravascular ultrasound 26
    lower extremities 271–2
    mesenteric ischemia 305
    multivascular atherosclerosis 364
    restenosis 485
    Rotablator 119, 138
    stent retrieval 188
    subclavian arteries 309–19
    superficial femoral artery 436
    superior vena cava 470
    thrombolysis 166
percutaneous transluminal coronary angiography (PTCA)
    477
percutaneous transluminal renal angioplasty (PTRA) 293,
    296–300
peripheral aneurysms 401–9, 452
peripheral arterial disease (PAD)
    clinical evaluation 15–17
    history 1
    non-interventional therapy 15–17
peripheral arteries
    balloon angioplasty 102–3
    restenosis 476
    stenosis 150
peripheral lesions 154
peripheral occlusive vascular disease (POVD) 101
peripheral vascular disease (PVD) 501–10
permanent particles 448

PFWD *see* pain-free walking distances
photoablation 219
phrenic nerve palsy 316
PIER *see* percutaneous intentional extraluminal (subintimal) recanalization
plaque morphology 20
plasma renin activity 278
plasminogen activators 163, 173
platelet-derived growth factor (PDGF) 476
platelets 476, 513–14
pleural effusions 316
plug mobilization 465
pneumothorax 316
polytetrafluoroethylene (PTFE)-covered stents 181–3, 243
polyvinyl alcohol (PVA) 448
popliteal access 95–9, 245
popliteal arteries 11, 32–3, 84, 406, 436–7
post-thrombotic syndrome (PTS) 171
post-traumatic aneurysms 372
postembolization syndrome 452
POVD *see* peripheral occlusive vascular disease
pravastatin 1
priapism 449
primary patency 216
primary stenting 249
privileges 58–9
procoagulent proteins 513
profundaplasty 433, 434
progressive neointimal hyperplasia 461
prospective observational studies 359–60
prostaglandin 444
prosthetic grafts 62
proteinuria 290
proximal brachial artery 88
Prozac 443
pseudoaneurysms 182, 259, 369, 402, 452, 533, 534
Pseudomonas infection 442
PSPMT *see* pulse-spray pharmacomechanical thrombolysis
PSV *see* peak systolic velocity
PTA *see* percutaneous transluminal angioplasty
PTCA *see* percutaneous transluminal coronary angiography
PTFE *see* polytetrafluoroethylene
PTRA *see* percutaneous transluminal renal angioplasty
PTS *see* post-thrombotic syndrome
pudendal arteriography 231
pulmonary angiogram 13
pulmonary artery atresia (PAA) 526
pulmonary artery valvular stenosis (PAVS) 529

pulmonary edema (PE) 294
pulmonary emboli 465
pulse-spray pharmacomechanical thrombolysis (PSPMT) 463
puncture needles 80–1
puncture site complications 259, 534
PVA *see* polyvinyl alcohol
PVD *see* peripheral vascular disease

qualifications 57
quantitative angiography 325

radial approach 94
radiation 309, 316, 479
radiation safety 55–6
radiation therapy 46–7, 469, 485–90
radioactive stents 487
randomized clinical trial (RCT) 355, 503
rapamycin 177, 178
RAS *see* renal artery stenosis
RAVEL 179
RCA *see* right coronary artery
RCT *see* randomized clinical trial
recanalization 214–15, 226–7
record management 55
rectosigmoidoscopy 396
Redha-Cut atherectomy catheter 143–5
Regitine 441
renal aneurysm 293
renal angioplasty 13, 285–91, 293–303, 366, 476
renal arteries
    lesions 428–9
    stents 41
    ultrasound 23, 30
renal arteriography 278
renal artery stenosis (RAS) 277–82, 285, 293–5
renal atheroembolism 290
renal biopsy 290
renal failure 394, 442
renal insufficiency 278
renovascular hypertension 277, 279–81
reoperation 270
reperfusion syndrome 164
restenosis 22, 46, 119, 149, 179, 217, 258, 259, 335, 405–6, 409, 475–80
reteplase 165, 166, 171
retrograde femoral approach 96
retrograde femoral catheterization 79–80
retrograde popliteal artery puncture 84–5
revascularization 243
rheolytic thrombectomy 270, 273–4

right coronary artery (RCA) stenosis 368
risk factors 2, 244, 497
road mapping 54, 223
Rotablator 107, 108, 138
Rotarex 119–27
rotational atherectomy 46, 107–16
rotational thrombectomy 119–26

SA see subclavian arteries
Safe-Cross TM TO RF Guidewire System 156
saphenous vein grafts 182, 243
screening tests 278
SCS see spinal cord stimulation
secondary patency 216
segmental infarction 301
self-expanding stents 41, 192–3, 248, 479
serotonin 476
SFA see superficial femoral artery
Shneddon's syndrome 305
sigmoid colon ischemia 396
simvasting 505
SIRIUS 179
SIROCCO 179
sirolimus 479
Smart Needle 95
SMC see smooth muscle cell
smoking 2, 220, 313, 431, 443, 445, 497, 503, 505, 507
smooth muscle cell (SMC) mitogen 476
spinal cord stimulation (SCS) 444
spinal liquid drainage 379
splenic embolization 450, 451
spot stenting 266
stable aneurysms 379
stent retrieval 188–9
stent-grafts 414–22
stenting 538
stenting indications 257–8, 305–6
stenting technique 286
stents 21, 27, 40–2, 177, 181, 195, 196, 247–9, 270, 272–3, 306, 360, 522–3
Strecker stent 248
streptokinase 165, 463
stroke 66, 344, 356, 363
subacute stent thrombosis 538
subclavian arteries (SA) 30, 309–19, 428
subclavian steal syndrome 309
subclavian thrombosis 314
subintimal angioplasty 129–33, 265
subintimal dissection 82
superficial femoral artery (SFA) disease 15, 32–3, 80, 129–33, 220, 224, 243, 435–6, 454, 479

superior mesenteric angiogram 11, 12
superior vena cava (SVC) syndrome 469–73
supraaortic arteries 427–9
suprainguinal puncture 82
suprarenal aortic aneurysm 74–7
surgical intervention 61–8, 153
surgical referrals 71–8
surgical revascularization 17
surpravalvular aortic stenosis 528–9
sutures 85
SVC see superior vena cava
sympathectomy 444
synthetic bridge grafts 461–5
systemic vasculitis 305

TAAs see thoracic aortic aneurysms
Takayasu syndrome 309, 316, 372, 425
Talent stent-graft 415
tantalum stent 306
target lesion revascularization (TLR) 475
target vessel revascularization (TVR) 475
TAXUS 179
TDM see transcranial Doppler monitoring
TEC see transluminal extraction-endarterectomy catheter
TEE see transesophageal echocardiography
telephone support 444–5
temporary stenting 189
TGF-β see transforming growth factor-beta
thalidomide 439
therapeutic lifestyle change (TLC) 506
thoracic aortic aneurysms (TAAs) 74–7, 417
thoracic aortogram 8
three-sheet billing system 542
thrombin 477, 515
thromboangiitis obliterans 431, 439
thromboaspiration 244
thromboendarterectomy 363
thrombolysis 163–8, 171, 270–1, 471
thrombosis 90, 115, 185, 258, 393, 396, 398, 513
thromboxane A_2 476, 514
thrombectomy 121, 126
TIA see transient ischemic attack
tibial arteries 33, 438
tibial artery angioplasty 263
ticlopidine 16, 326, 515
TIPS see transjugular intrahepatic portosystemic shunt
tirofiban 516
tissue plasminogen activator (tPA) 463
TLC see therapeutic lifestyle change
TLR see target lesion revascularization
tobacco 2

toe pressure (TP) 2
tortuosity 72
TP *see* toe pressure
tPA *see* tissue plasminogen activator
Trac-Wright catheter 143
training 57–9
transaxillary approaches 90–1
transbrachial approaches 87–9
transcatheter peripheral embolization 449–55
transcranial Doppler monitoring (TDM) 350
transesophageal echocardiography (TEE) 375
transforming growth factor-beta (TGF-ß) 476
transient ischemic attack (TIA) 66, 67, 163, 300, 323,
    344
transjugular intrahepatic portosystemic shunt (TIPS) 485,
    490
transluminal balloon angioplasty 522
transluminal coil embolization 530–1
transluminal extraction-endarterectomy catheter (TEC)
    119, 141–2
transluminal PTA 265
transradial approach 93–4
trauma 449, 450
trolley car technique 394
tubular necrosis 294
tumor growth 473
TVR *see* target vessel revascularization

UK *see* urokinase
ulnar artery 439
ultrasound 19, 191, 245, 325
    intravascular 25–34
unstable angina 281

upper limb salvage 439
urokinase (UK) 165, 167, 171, 396, 397, 444, 463
uterine artery embolization 232–3, 449
uterine leiomyomas 232

VA *see* vertebral artery
vancomycin 442
Vanguard endograft 385, 387
vascular access 534
vascular closure devices 516–18
vascular endothelial growth factor (VEGF) 495
vascular occlusion devices 47
vascular perforation 185
vascular snares 48
vasodilators 115
VasoSeal 517
VBI *see* vertebrobasilar insufficiency
vectors 493
VEGF *see* vascular endothelial growth factor
venography 463
venous stenoses 150–1, 461
vertebral angioplasty 324–5
vertebral artery (VA) 309, 312, 323
vertebral injections 8
vertebrobasilar insufficiency (VBI) 313, 323
von Willebrand's factor (vWF) 513
vWF *see* von Willebrand's factor

walking 244
Wallgraft 249, 402, 419
Wallstent 248, 470
warfarin 328
weight loss 445